Essentials of Orthopedic Surgery

Essentials of Orthopedic Surgery

Editor: Kristian Gilmore

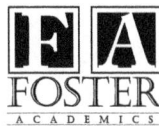

FA
FOSTER
ACADEMICS

www.fosteracademics.com

www.fosteracademics.com

FA
FOSTER
ACADEMICS

Cataloging-in-Publication Data

Essentials of orthopedic surgery / edited by Kristian Gilmore.
   p. cm.
Includes bibliographical references and index.
ISBN 978-1-63242-763-2
1. Orthopedic surgery. 2. Orthopedics. 3. Surgery, Operative. I. Gilmore, Kristian.
RD731 .E77 2019
617.3--dc23

Foster Academics,
118-35 Queens Blvd., Suite 400,
Forest Hills, NY 11375, USA

ISBN 978-1-63242-763-2 (Hardback)

Contents

Preface

This book has been a concerted effort by a group of academicians, researchers and scientists, who have contributed their research works for the realization of the book. This book has materialized in the wake of emerging advancements and innovations in this field. Therefore, the need of the hour was to compile all the required researches and disseminate the knowledge to a broad spectrum of people comprising of students, researchers and specialists of the field.

The surgical field of medicine concerned with the conditions associated with the musculoskeletal system is known as orthopedic surgery. The human musculoskeletal system consists of the bones of the skeleton, joints, ligaments, cartilage, tendons, muscles, etc. It gives humans the ability to move as it is a system which provides form, movement, support and stability to the body. Foot and ankle surgery is a sub-field of orthopedic surgery. It deals with the diagnosis, prevention and treatment of disorders related to the foot and ankle. Ankle arthroscopy, laser surgery and amputation are some of the common surgical methods to treat foot and ankle disorders. This book attempts to understand the multiple branches that fall under the discipline of orthopedic surgery and how such concepts have practical applications. It includes some of the vital pieces of work being conducted across the world, on various topics related to orthopedic surgery. Doctors and students actively engaged in this field will find this book full of crucial and unexplored concepts.

At the end of the preface, I would like to thank the authors for their brilliant chapters and the publisher for guiding us all-through the making of the book till its final stage. Also, I would like to thank my family for providing the support and encouragement throughout my academic career and research projects.

Editor

Early initiation of a strength training based rehabilitation after lumbar spine fusion improves core muscle strength

Dejan Kernc[1][*] [iD], Vojko Strojnik[1] and Rok Vengust[2]

Abstract

Background: To analyze the safety and effects of early initiation of rehabilitation including objective measurement outcomes after lumbar spine fusion based on principles of strength training.

Methods: The study recruited 27 patients, aged 45 to 70 years, who had undergone lumbar spine fusion. The method of concealed random allocation without blocking was used to form two groups. The strength training group started rehabilitation 3 weeks after surgery. Patients exercised twice weekly over 9 weeks focusing on muscle activation of lumbopelvic stabilization muscles. The control group followed a standard postoperative protocol, where no exercises were performed at that stage of rehabilitation. Functional outcomes and plain radiographs were evaluated at 3 weeks and subsequently at 3 and 18 months after the surgery.

Results: No hardware loosening of failure was observed in the training group. Both groups improved their walking speed after 3 months ($p < 0.01$), although improvement in the training group was significantly greater than in the control group ($p < 0.01$). Moreover, the training group significantly improved after the training period in all isometric trunk muscles measurements ($p < 0.03$), standing reach height ($p < 0.02$), and pre-activation pattern ($p < 0.05$). After 18 months, no training effects were observed.

Conclusions: The study showed that early initiation of a postoperative rehabilitation program based on principles of strength training is safe, 3 weeks after lumbar spine fusion, and enable earlier functional recovery than standard rehabilitation protocol.

Keywords: Rehabilitation, Lumbar spine fusion, Randomized controlled trial, Strength training, Early initiation, Intra-abdominal pressure

Background

Despite the significant rise in lumbar spine fusion (LSF) surgery rates in the last few decades, some 15 to 40% of lumbar fusion patients cannot expect significant improvement postoperatively according to functional ability [1–6]. The postoperative rehabilitation strategy is one of the main factors affecting the outcome. Nevertheless, only a few

studies address the effect of different protocols and timing of postoperative rehabilitation [7, 8].

The benefit of intra-abdominal pressure (IAP) on lumbar spine function is well documented [9, 10]. IAP with co-activation of the abdominal muscles provides load relief to the lumbar spine and increased stability of the trunk [10, 11]; however, IAP needs to start rising before the initiation of action to have a protective effect on the lumbar spine [12].

There is some disagreement on the optimal time to initiate a rehabilitation program after LSF. A randomized controlled trial from 2013 evaluating the impact of

* Correspondence: dejan.kernc@gmail.com
[1]Faculty of Sport, University of Ljubljana, Gortanova 22, 1000 Ljubljana, Slovenia
Full list of author information is available at the end of the article

initiating rehabilitation either 6 or 12 weeks after LSF demonstrated no difference to the patient's physical performance in terms of fitness and walking distance [8]. A study published in 2014 showed that early initiation of rehabilitation does not increase the risk of postoperative complications [13]. Conversely, Oestergaard et al. [14] showed that initiating rehabilitation after 12 weeks resulted in a significantly better clinical improvement compared to an earlier initiation.

Rehabilitation after LSF aims to improve the trunk muscles' functional capacity [7, 15]. Evaluation of LSF rehabilitation protocols should include, in addition to subjective outcomes (ODI), an objective measurement of functional ability such as strength of the stabilization muscles, physical performance, etc.

Given the above, the aim of the present study was to analyze the safety and effects in the early initiation of strength training that promote trunk stabilization through IAP and utilizing both subjective and measurable objective outcomes.

Methods

Study design, selection of subjects, surgery, and follow-up

The study was a randomized controlled trial with a baseline measurement at 3 weeks after LSF, and additionally at 3 and 18 months after LSF. The selection of subjects and surgeries were determined by three consultant spine surgeons at the Slovenian national spine center in Ljubljana.

The subjects were recruited over a 14-month period (September 2014–November 2015). The inclusion criteria for subjects were (1) a primary diagnosis of one level degenerative, low-grade isthmic spondylolisthesis or degenerative disc disease, with or without spinal stenosis; (2) age between 45 and 70 years; and (3) the absence of non-communicable diseases. The exclusion criteria for subjects were (1) previous lumbar fusion surgery, (2) degenerative or idiopathic scoliosis, (3) and inflammatory disease and history of malignancy. The National Medical Ethics Committee approved the study.

Subjects had received one level instrumented transforaminal interbody fusion. A cage of maximal feasible height was placed as anteriorly as possible to obtain segmental lordosis. Decompression was employed with respect to primary pathology, central/lateral recess stenosis in degenerative spondylolisthesis, and foramina in isthmic spondylolisthesis. No decompression was performed in patients with degenerative disc disease.

Additional control checks were employed to ensure subject safety in the exercise protocol, and subjects were examined by the managing surgeon. At 2 and 18 months postoperatively, plain radiographs were taken. Furthermore, at 18 months postoperatively, flexion/extension films were obtained to rule out hardware loosening or failure.

Sample size and randomization

All subjects received written and verbal informed consent information regarding their participation in the rehabilitation program. Subjects were required to provide signed informed consent and complete questionnaires. The method of concealed random allocation without blocking was used to form groups. As shown in a consent flow diagram (Fig. 1), 51 subjects planned for elective LSF fulfilled the study's inclusion criteria. A total of 12 subjects were excluded from the study: five due to surgery exceeding the inclusion criteria (decompression of two or more levels in four subjects, two-level fusion in one subject), four refused inclusion, one due to postoperative infection, and two due to re-hospitalization for unrelated causes. Five subjects were lost during the training period and an additional seven at latest follow-up.

By random allocation, the training group included 36% male subjects, age 60.3 (SD ± 8.1), and body mass index 27.7 (SD ± 2.7), and the control group 69% male subjects, age 61.1 (SD ± 8.1), and body mass index 30.2 (SD ± 5.6) (Table 1). For the power calculation, the ODI was used. Based on earlier studies, the standard deviation was set to 10 points [16]. A 14.1-point difference in this category was considered clinically significant. Assuming a power = 80%, a total of 32 subjects were required. For the training period, the recommended power was achieved but not for the latest follow-up.

Control group

The control group followed the hospital's standard protocols. These did not include exercises or physiotherapy prior to 3 months postoperatively.

Training group

The training group performed the rehabilitation program twice per week over 9 weeks, starting 3 weeks after the surgery. During the first training sub-period (week 1 to week 5), isometric exercises were focused on the trunk extension, flexion, and lateral flexion muscles by maintaining the lumbar spine's neutral position. Each exercise was maintained for 15 s initially, separated by 45 s' rest, and repeated three times. After each training protocol, the subjects were asked to assess the level of intensity on a 10-point Borg scale. When the level of perceived effort felt below 8, they increased the exercise duration to 20, 25, and 30 s. Interferential electrical current therapy of the trunk extensor muscles in the lumbar region, lasting 20 min, and with a frequency of 5 Hz was applied in that sub-period. During the period from week 6 to week 9, the exercises were performed with strength machines and the duration extended to 30 s. Leg adduction and hip extension exercises were added. The subjects were instructed to increase IAP with co-activation of the abdominal muscles (abdominal

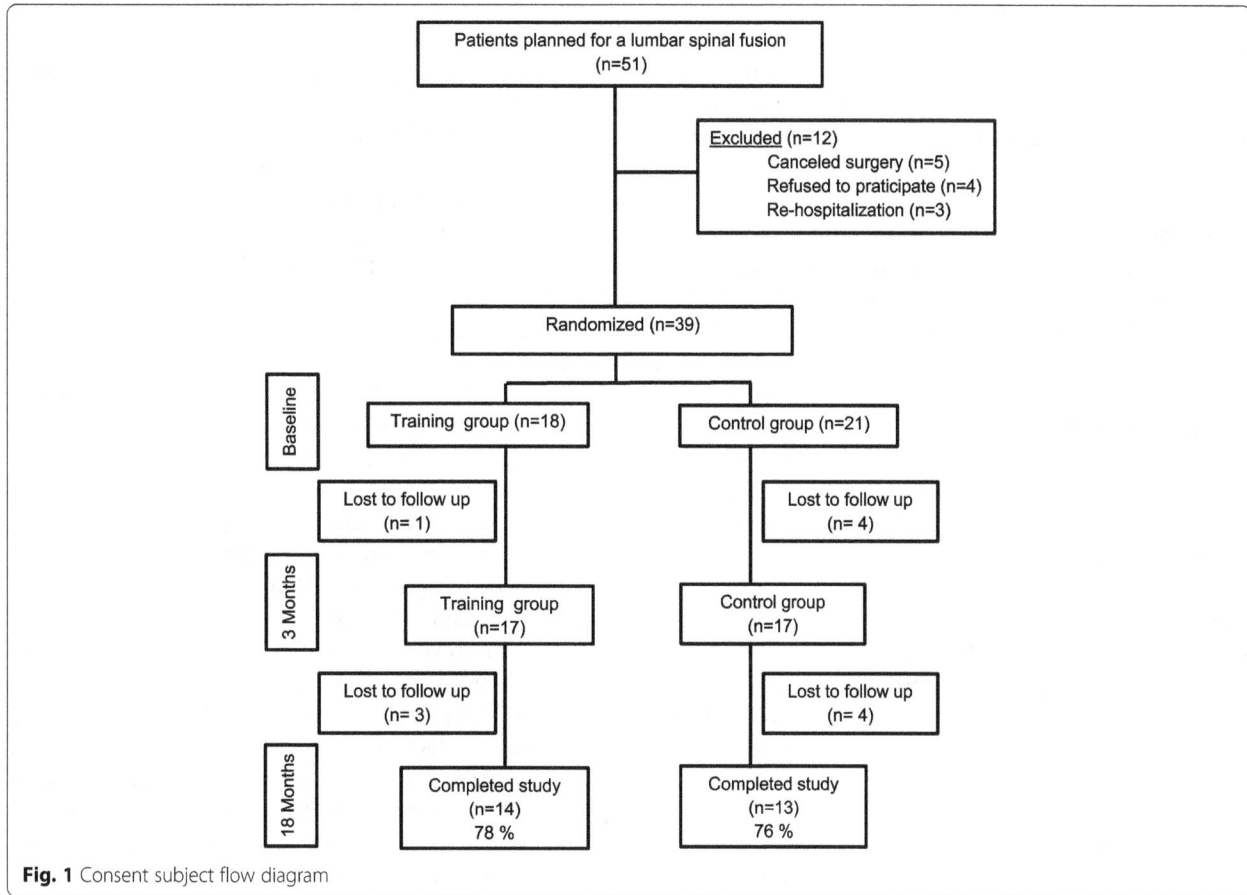

Fig. 1 Consent subject flow diagram

bracing) and maintain the neutral position of their lumbar spine before and during the exercises. Following strength training, static stretching was applied to the exercised muscle. The training sessions were supervised by the same physiotherapist.

Evaluation of the functional outcome

For each participating subject, the following background data were registered:

• Isometric trunk muscle strength

The isometric trunk muscle extension, flexion, and lateral flexion strength were measured using a strain-gauge dynamometer (Steinberg Systems, Poland). The measurements were performed in a standing position with the pelvis supported [17]. A belt was fastened around the upper body at shoulder level. Subjects gradually applied the maximal force and sustained it for 2–3 s. Maximum torque was calculated

from the force sensor data and the lever as the distance between the middle line of the belt and the iliac crest level. Three maximal efforts were performed.

• Subjects' physical performance

The physical parameters were as follows: walked distance during the 6-min walking test (6MWT) [18], number of stand-ups in 30 s during the chair stand test (CST) [19], and standing reach height test (SRH) [20].

• The IAP pre-activation pattern

To determine the initiation point of the IAP, abdominal lateral force was measured. The subjects stood in an upright position and pushed against the force plate. Time delay between the onset of lateral abdominal force rise and the onset of force rise of the force plate was calculated. Mechanical measurements were utilized rather than electromyography of m. transversus abdominis due to the confounding effect that too high skin fold may have on electromyography measurements.

• Subjects' subjective self-evaluations

○ The Oswestry disability index (ODI) presented subjects with a score index from 0 to 100 where lower scores represent lower levels of low back pain disability [14, 15].

○ The visual analogue scale (VAS) presented subjects with a back pain intensity score index from 0 to 10,

Table 1 Background subject data

Subject characteristics	Control group (n = 14)	Training group (n = 13)
Male (%)	36	69
Age (year ± SD)	60.3 ± 8.1	61.1 ± 8
Body mass index (kg/m² ± SD)	27.7 ± 2.7	30.2 ± 5.6

where 0 = "no problems" and 10 = "maximum problems" [16].

All parameters were measured at 3 weeks and 3 months following LSF. At 18 months postoperatively, all parameters, excluding IAP pre-activation pattern, were measured.

Statistical analysis

An independent t test and Wilcoxon-Mann-Whitney U tests were applied to the data using the SPSS 20.0 for Windows. The risk of type 1 error was set to 5% (a significance level of 0.05). A one-way repeated-measures ANOVA was used with the functional outcome variable as the within-subject variable and the group variable as the between-subjects factor. The Bonferroni post hoc tests were used. Spearman's rho was used to determine the correlation level between the functional outcome variables.

Results

The training group subjects (14/14) had no fusion-related complications. Two subjects out of 13 in the control group had non-union problems and were excluded from the analysis. One subject experienced no pain, despite segmental movement shown in flexion/extension films, and was treated conservatively. The other was reoperated 2 months after index surgery due to overt hardware loosening and mechanical back pain.

Analysis of baseline data showed no statistically significant difference in 6MWT between the two groups. At 3 months postoperatively, a statistically significant

training effect ($p < 0.05$) and improvement for both groups were observed. No statistically significant improvement was detected for either group at 18 months follow-up; however, the training group exceeded the expected walking distance (571 m, ± 90) when compared to age correlated normal [21]. This effect was seen to remain 18 months thereafter (Fig. 2).

Mean scores for the isometric trunk muscles strength, significant changes of differences between groups, and differences between means for each group are presented in Fig. 3. The training group significantly improved in all outcome measurements. A one-way repeated-measures ANOVA showed a significant training effect in both lateral flexions (both $p = 0.05$). In trunk extension, a tendency toward a significant improvement due to training was observed ($p = 0.06$). After 18 months, no training effects were observed in any of the trunk strength parameters.

No statistically significant differences between the groups in the progress of CST were observed after 3 and 18 months (Table 2). The training group demonstrated an initial improvement in SRH ($p < 0.04$); however, this gain was seen to reduce at further follow-up time points ($p < 0.02$). Time shift off the start with increase of IAP approached statistical significance within the training group ($p < 0.08$). ODI was reduced significantly in both groups after 3 months (both $p < 0.001$) and stayed at similar level after 18 months. VAS stayed at similar level during the follow-up time.

Correlation analysis showed that relative changes of extension and both lateral flexions were significantly correlated among themselves due to the training as well as the

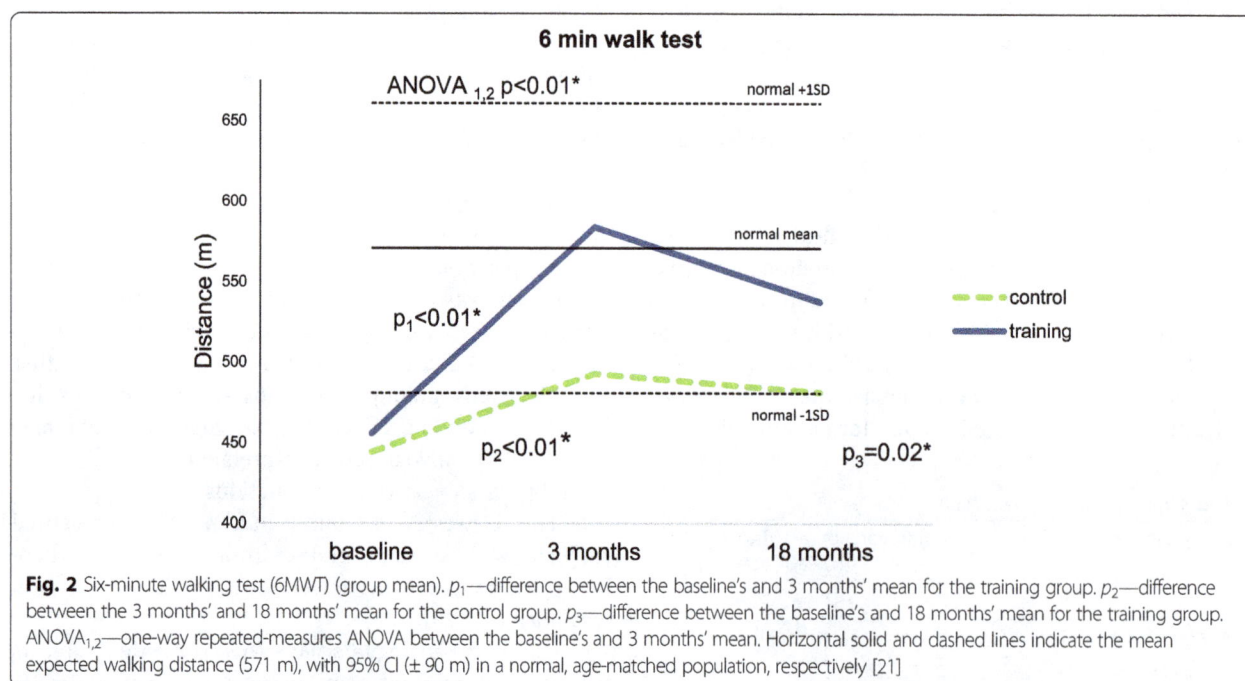

Fig. 2 Six-minute walking test (6MWT) (group mean). p_1—difference between the baseline's and 3 months' mean for the training group. p_2—difference between the 3 months' and 18 months' mean for the control group. p_3—difference between the baseline's and 18 months' mean for the training group. ANOVA$_{1,2}$—one-way repeated-measures ANOVA between the baseline's and 3 months' mean. Horizontal solid and dashed lines indicate the mean expected walking distance (571 m), with 95% CI (± 90 m) in a normal, age-matched population, respectively [21]

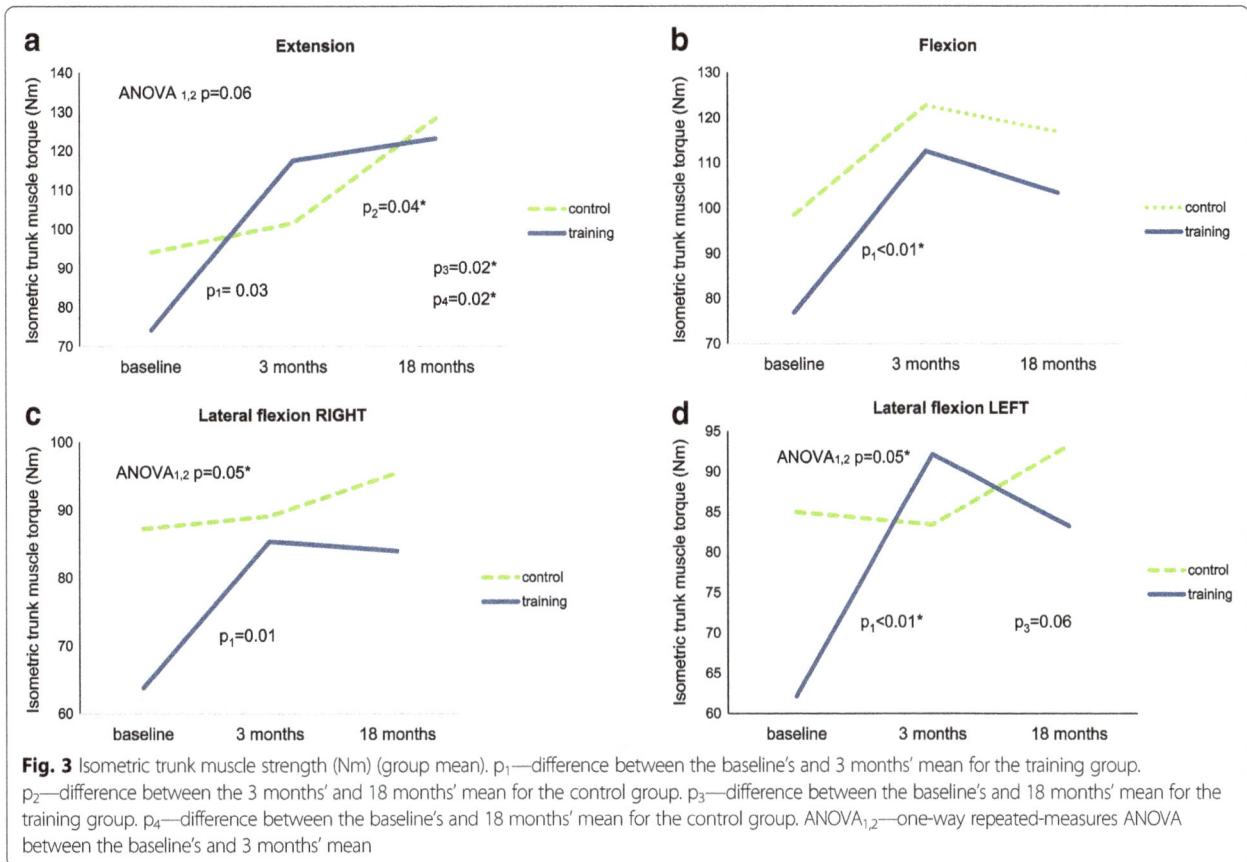

Fig. 3 Isometric trunk muscle strength (Nm) (group mean). p_1—difference between the baseline's and 3 months' mean for the training group. p_2—difference between the 3 months' and 18 months' mean for the control group. p_3—difference between the baseline's and 18 months' mean for the training group. p_4—difference between the baseline's and 18 months' mean for the control group. ANOVA$_{1,2}$—one-way repeated-measures ANOVA between the baseline's and 3 months' mean

follow-up (Table 3). In trunk flexion, a tendency toward a significant correlation was observed ($p = 0.06$–0.08). A correlation between the CST and all isometric trunk muscle strength variables was found.

Discussion

The goal of the present study was to analyze the safety and effects of early initiation of a postoperative rehabilitation program based on strength training principles supporting IAP utilization for trunk stabilization after LSF. Both groups improved their walking distance after 3 months; however, only the training group achieved and maintained normal age correlated walking distance. The training group significantly improved trunk extension, lateral flexions on both sides, SRH, and pre-activation pattern, while the control group showed no such significant improvements. A similar improvement in trunk flexion and CST was observed for both groups. Subjective self-evaluations showed a similar improvement in ODI but no changes in pain for either group. No hardware loosening or failure was observed in the training group despite commencement of rehabilitation only 3 weeks after surgery.

On analysis of early initiation of postoperative rehabilitation, Oestergaard et al. failed to show any advantages after 6 months of rehabilitation with ODI, leading the authors to conclude that starting rehabilitation early may not be advantageous for LSF patients [14]. In the present study, an earlier start point of intervention was employed. This saw both groups display improvement with ODI after only 3 months of rehabilitation. It would therefore appear that early initiation of strength training based rehabilitation does not pose any adverse effect, yet early intervention does not result in significant gain in overall rehabilitation outcomes as both groups were seen to make similar progress.

However, on examination of the functional test results of the present study, the data showed that the strength training group demonstrated superior functional gains when compared to the standard rehabilitation group. An example of such functional gains would be walking, an important everyday functional task which has previously been shown to be impaired in low-back pain patients [22, 23]. The training group exceeded the normal population's mean (571 ± 90 m), while the control group stayed beyond the area of one standard deviation [21]. The control group results are comparable to the 1-year follow-up results of Oestergaard et al. [8]. Improvement in the training group can be considered as clinically relevant, this was not shown to be the case for the control group [24]. This would lead us to conclude that early initiation of rehabilitation may not adversely affect a patient's walking ability, as stated by Oestergaard et

Table 2 Effect of rehabilitation on physical performance, pre-activation pattern and subjective self-evaluations

	Training group (n = 14)						Control group (n = 13)						ANOVA 1,2 P value	ANOVA 2,3 P value	ANOVA 1,3 P value
	Baseline	3 months	18 months	P_1 value	P_2 value	P_3 value	Baseline	3 months	18 months	P_1 value	P_2 value	P_3 value			
Physical performance															
CST (repetitions)	11.5 (±3.9)	17.1 (±4.7)	17.6 (±5.8)	0.00*	1.0	0.00*	10.5 (±4.5)	14.7 (± 5.7)	15.3 (± 6.3)	0.00*	1.0	0.01*	0.3	0.9	0.4
SRH (cm)	210.4 (±12.2)	213.6 (±13.2)	210 (±13.2)	0.02*	0.02*	1.0	212.2 (± 14.1)	211.8 (± 15)	212.5.8 (± 14.2)	1.0	1.0	1.0	0.04*	0.02*	0.6
The IAP pre-activation pattern															
Time before prime mover (s)	0.22 (±0.42)	− 0.03 (±0.22)	/	0.04*	/	/	0.22 (±0.25)	0.20 (± 0.18)	/	0.67	/	/	0.08	/	/
Subjective self-evaluations															
ODI	40.6 (± 11.9)	27.4 (±13.4)	25.7 (±15.1)	0.00*	1.0	0.02*	41.5 (±6.1)	29.5 (± 12)	27.6 (± 22)	0.00*	1.0	0.04*	0.7	0.9	0.9
VAS	2.7 (± 1)	2.7 (± 1.3)	4 (± 2.3)	1.0	0.1	0.1	3.6 (± 1.5)	3.2 (± 1.2)	3.6 (± 2.6)	1.0	0.6	1.0	0.6	0.4	0.3

Data are reported as mean (SD)

CST, chair stand test, number of stand ups; SHR, standing reach height, numbers represent centimetres; ODI, Oswestry disability index, scoring from 0 to 100, 0 = no pain; VAS, visual analogue scale, scoring from 0 to 10, 0 = "no problems" and 10 = "maximum problems"; Time before prime mover, negative numbers represent time (s) before prime mover, positive represent time (s) after prime mover; P_1-value, difference between the baseline's and 3 months' mean; P_2 value, difference between the 3 months' and 18 months' mean; P_3 value, difference between the baseline's and 18 months' mean; ANOVA, one-way repeated-measure ANOVA; ANOVA $_{1,2}$ difference between the baseline's and 3 months' mean; ANOVA $_{2,3}$ difference between the 3 months' and 18 months' mean; ANOVA $_{1,3}$ difference between the baseline's and 18 months' mean

*Significance difference between the groups, $p < 0.05$

Table 3 Correlation between initial status and changes due to training in the training group

| | | Changes | | | | | | | | | |
		6 MWT	CST	SRH	Flexion	LFR	LFL	Extension	ODI	VAS	TIME
Initial status	6 MWT	-0.81*	-0.42	0.08	-0.06	0.14	0.15	-0.06	0.25	0.26	-0.37
	CST	-0.09	-0.48	-0.29	-0.04	-0.28	-0.19	-0.33	0.27	0.32	-0.15
	SRH	-0.22	-0.46	0.02	-0.37	0.01	-0.01	-0.02	-0.38	-0.34	-0.41
	Flexion	-0.26	-0.65*	-0.07	-0.53*	-0.48	-0.51	-0.51	-0.36	-0.29	-0.44
	LFR	-0.21	-0.59*	0.03	-0.51	-0.59*	-0.65*	-0.53*	-0.33	-0.13	-0.30
	LFL	-0.28	-0.55*	-0.03	-0.45	-0.56*	-0.64*	-0.52	-0.32	-0.09	-0.42
	Extension	-0.19	-0.69*	0.03	-0.46	-0.56*	-0.56*	-0.54*	-0.34	-0.18	-0.34
	ODI	0.29	-0.05	0.25	0.01	0.06	0.14	0.06	0.08	0.12	0.23
	VAS	0.13	-0.14	0.43	-0.10	0.12	0.42	0.07	-0.24	-0.45	-0.09
	TIME	0.33	-0.04	0.20	-0.03	-0.32	-0.26	-0.23	-0.28	0.11	0.11

6MWT 6-minute walk test; *CST* chair stand test; *SHR* standing reach height; *LFR* lateral flexion right; *LFL* lateral flexion left; *ODI* Oswestry disability index; *VAS* visual analogue scale; *TIME* time before prime mover
*Significance difference, p< 0.05

al. [8]. We acknowledge that a limitation of our study is the relatively small number of patients which could add to an overestimation of positive results.

Core muscle strength evaluated by trunk extension and lateral flexion was shown to be significantly improved in the training but not in the control group, whereas trunk flexion was found to be similarly improved for both groups. One possible explanation is fear of pain during trunk extension in the control group, which had no specific training to test their pain level during maximal effort [25]. Trunk extension torques were quite low in the present study compared to some other studies involving low-back pain [26]. Even after training, they remained substantially lower than in the Kienbacher et al. study [26], where trunk extension performance was supervised by a clinical psychologist to overcome any fear-related inhibition. Therefore, the results of the trunk extension test in the present study, where no specific fear control was introduced, may be attributed mainly to improved neuromuscular function, and partly to reduced fear-related inhibition.

One important aspect included in the present strength training based rehabilitation was the use of intra-abdominal pressure [9–11]. The subjects learned to use IAP during all exercises and were advised to also do so in daily life. To support this inclusion, the activation of abdominal muscles related to IAP showed that subjects from the training group systematically shifted the initiation of IAP before starting the action and therefore afforded better protection to their lumbar spine.

Lower initial level in a specific test resulted in a greater improvement in that test after training. However, the core strength tests represented a group where subjects with the lowest general core strength improved in all these tests the most. This finding would indicate that subjects most in need of improvement would obtain it to a greater degree. The changes observed in ODI and

functional tests such as 6MWT or SRH were not shown to be related to the initial core strength level. CST was the only parameter demonstrating correlation between initial core strength and an improvement in a functional test. Thus, it may be concluded that the subjects' initial functional and strength level had an important effect on the training outcome.

The functional advantage of the training group after 3 months of rehabilitation was mostly lost at the end of the follow-up. If we assume that this plateau in functional gain represents a return to normal daily functional ability, then the data shows that 2 months engagement in the current training strategy is sufficient to achieve or even exceed normal functional performance.

Conclusions
The present study showed that early initiation of a postoperative rehabilitation program based on strength training principles supporting IAP utilization for trunk stabilization after LSF is safe and effective and enable earlier functional recovery than standard rehabilitation protocol.

Abbreviations
6MWT: 6-min walking test; CST: Chair stand test; IAP: Intra-abdominal pressure; LSF: Lumbar spine fusion; ODI: Oswestry disability index; SRH: Standing reach height test

Funding
Funding for the study was partly provided by Slovenian Research Agency Grant No. P5-142. The Slovenian Research Agency had no role in the design and conduct of the study.

Authors' contributions
All authors made substantial contribution to conception and design of the study. DK has been involved in the performance and acquisition of data,

where RV controlled the selection of patients, surgeries, and health status of individual patient. VS controlled the study performance. DK and VS analyzed and interpreted the data. All authors have been involved in writing the manuscript and approved the final version to be submitted.

Competing interests

The authors declare that they have no competing interests.

Author details

[1]Faculty of Sport, University of Ljubljana, Gortanova 22, 1000 Ljubljana, Slovenia. [2]Faculty of Medicine, University of Ljubljana, Vrazov trg 2, 1000 Ljubljana, Slovenia.

References

1. Christensen FB, Stender Hansen E, Laursen M, Thomsen K, Bunger CE. Long-term functional outcome of pedicle screw instrumentation as a support for posterolateral spinal fusion: randomized clinical study with a 5-year follow-up. Spine. 2002;27:1269–77.
2. Deyo RA, Gray DT, Kreuter W, Mirza S, Brook M. United States trends in lumbar fusion surgery for degenerative conditions. Spine. 2005;30:1441–5.
3. Fischgrund JS, Mackay M, Herkowitz HN, Brower R, Montgomery DM, Kurz LT. 1997 Volvo award winner in clinical studies: degenerative lumbar spondylolisthesis with spinal stenosis: a prospective, randomized study comparing decompressive laminectomy and arthrodesis with and without spinal instrumentation. Spine. 1997;22:2807–12.
4. France JC, Yaszemski MJ, Lauerman WC, Cain JE, Glover JM, Lawson KJ, et al. A randomized prospective study of posterolateral lumbar fusion: outcomes with and without pedicle screw instrumentation. Spine. 1999;24:553–60.
5. Möller H, Hedlund R. Instrumented and noninstrumented posterolateral fusion in adult spondylolisthesis: a prospective randomized study: part 2. Spine. 2000;25:1716–21.
6. Weinstein NJ, Lurie JD, Olson P, Bronner KK, Fisher ES, Morgan TS. United States trends and regional variations in lumbar spine surgery: 1992–2003. Spine. 2006;31:2707.
7. Christensen FB, Laurberg I, Bünger CE. Importance of the back-cafe concept to rehabilitation after lumbar spinal fusion: a randomized clinical study with a 2-year follow-up. Spine. 2003;28:2561–9.
8. Oestergaard LG, Nielsen CV, Bunger CE, Svidt K, Christensen FB. The effect of timing of rehabilitation on physical performance after lumbar spinal fusion: a randomized clinical study. Eur Spine J. 2013;22:1884–90.
9. Cholewicki J, Juluru K, McGill SM. Intra-abdominal pressure mechanism for stabilizing the lumbar spine. J Biomech. 1999;32:13–7.
10. Cholewicki J, Reeves NP. All abdominal muscles must be considered when evaluating the intra-abdominal pressure contribution to trunk extensor moment and spinal loading. J Biomech. 2004;37:953–4.
11. Hodges PW, Cresswell AG, Daggfeldt K, Thorstensson A. In vivo measurement of the effect of intra-abdominal pressure on the human spine. J Biomech. 2001;34:347–53.
12. Hodges PW, Richardson CA. Feedforward contraction of transversus abdominis is not influenced by the direction of arm movement. Exp Brain Res. 1997;114:362–70.
13. Schröter J, Lechterbeck M, Hartmann F, Gercek E. Structured rehabilitation after lumbar spine surgery: subacute treatment phase. Der Orthopade. 2014;43:1089–95.
14. Oestergaard LG, Nielsen CV, Bunger CE, Sogaaed R, Fruensgaard S, Helmig P, et al. The effect of early initiation of rehabilitation after lumbar spinal fusion: a randomized clinical study. Spine. 2012;37:1803–9.
15. Greenwood J, Mcgregor A, Jones F, Mullane J, Hurley M. Rehabilitation following lumbar fusion surgery: a systematic review and meta-analysis. Spine. 2016;41:28–36.
16. Abbott AD, Tyni-Lenné R, Hedlund R. Early rehabilitation targeting cognition, behavior, and motor function after lumbar fusion: a randomized controlled trial. Spine. 2010;35:848–57.
17. Paalanne NP, Korpelainen R, Taimela SP, Remes J, Salakka M, Karppinen JI. Reproducibility and reference values of inclinometric balance and isometric trunk muscle strength measurements in Finnish young adults. J Strength Conditioning Res. 2009;23:1618–26.
18. Laboratories A.C.o.P.S.f.C.P.F. ATS statement: guidelines for the six-minute walk test. Am J Respir Crit Care Med. 2002;166:111.
19. Bennell K, Dobson F, Hinman R. Measures of physical performance assessments: Self-Paced Walk Test (SPWT), Stair Climb Test (SCT), Six-Minute Walk Test (6MWT), Chair Stand Test (CST), Timed Up & Go (TUG), Sock Test, Lift and Carry Test (LCT), and Car Task. Arthritis Care Res. 2011;63:350–70.
20. Silfies SP, Bhattacharya A, Biely S, Smith SS, Giszter S. Trunk control during standing reach: a dynamical system analysis of movement strategies in patients with mechanical low back pain. Gait Posture. 2009;29:370–6.
21. Casanova C, Celli BR, Barria P, Casas A, Cote C, De Torres JP, et al. The 6-min walk distance in healthy subjects: reference standards from seven countries. Eur Respiratory J. 2011;37:150–6.
22. Kim CM, Eng JJ, Whittaker MW. Level walking and ambulatory capacity in persons with incomplete spinal cord injury: relationship with muscle strength. Spinal Cord. 2004;42:156–62.
23. Lamoth CJ, Meijer OG, Daffertshofer A, Wuisman P, Beek PJ. Effects of chronic low back pain on trunk coordination and back muscle activity during walking: changes in motor control. Eur Spine J. 2006;15:23–40.
24. Redelmeier DA, Bayoumi AM, Goldstein RS, Guyatt GH. Interpreting small differences in functional status: the Six Minute Walk test in chronic lung disease patients. Am J Respir Crit Care Med. 1997;155:1278–82.
25. Crombez G, Vlaeyen J, Heuts P, Lysens R. Pain-related fear is more disabling than pain itself: evidence on the role of pain-related fear in chronic back pain disability. Pain. 1999;80:329–39.
26. Kienbacher T, Fehrmann E, Habenicht R, Koller D, Oeffel C, Kollmitzer J, et al. Age and gender related neuromuscular pattern during trunk flexion-extension in chronic low back pain patients. J Neuroeng Rehabil. 2016;13(1): 16. https://doi.org/10.1186/s12984-016-0121-1. https://jneuroengrehab.biomedcentral.com/articles/10.1186/s12984-016-0121-1.

Effect of low-intensity pulsed ultrasound on distraction osteogenesis

Shenghan Lou[1,2†], Houchen Lv[2†], Zhirui Li[2], Peifu Tang[2*] and Yansong Wang[1*]

Abstract

Background: Low-intensity pulsed ultrasound (LIPUS) is a common adjunct used to promote bone healing for fresh fractures and non-unions, but its efficacy for bone distraction osteogenesis remains uncertain. This study aims to determine whether LIPUS can effectively and safely reduce the associated treatment time for patients undergoing distraction osteogenesis.

Methods: MEDLINE, EMBASE, and the Cochrane Library were searched until May 1, 2018, without language restriction. Studies should be randomized controlled trials (RCTs) or quasi-RCTs of LIPUS compared with sham devices or no devices in patients who undergo distraction osteogenesis. The primary outcome was the treatment time. The secondary outcome was the risk of complications. Treatment effects were assessed using mean differences, standardized mean differences, or risk ratios using a random-effects model. The Cochrane risk-of-bias tool was used to assess the risk of bias. The I^2 statistic was used to assess the heterogeneity. The GRADE system was used to evaluate the evidence quality.

Results: A total of 7 trials with 172 patients were included. The pooled results suggested that during the process of distraction osteogenesis, LIPUS therapy did not show a statistically significant reduction in the treatment time (mean difference, − 8.75 days/cm; 95% CI, − 20.68 to 3.18 days/cm; $P = 0.15$; $I^2 = 72\%$) or in the risk of complications (risk ratio, 0.90 in favor of LIPUS; 95% CI, 0.65 to 1.24; $I^2 = 0\%$). Also, LIPUS therapy did not show a significant effect on the radiological gap fill area (standardized mean difference, 0.48 in favor of control; 95%CI, − 1.49 to 0.52; $I^2 = 0\%$), the histological gap fill length (standardized mean difference, 0.76 in favor of control; 95%CI, − 1.78 to 0.27; $I^2 = 0\%$), or the bone density increase (standardized mean difference, 0.43 in favor of LIPUS; 95%CI, − 0.02 to 0.88; $I^2 = 0\%$).

Conclusions: Among patients undergoing distraction osteogenesis, neither the treatment time nor the risk of complications could be reduced by LIPUS therapy. The currently available evidence is insufficient to support the routine use of this intervention in clinical practice.

Keywords: Low-intensity pulsed ultrasound, Distraction osteogenesis, Fracture healing, Meta-analysis

* Correspondence: pftang301@163.com; wysgkql@163.com
†Shenghan Lou and Houchen Lv contributed equally to this work.
²Department of Orthopedics, Chinese PLA General Hospital, No. 28 Fuxing Road, Beijing 100853, People's Republic of China
¹Department of Spine Surgery, The First Affiliated Hospital of Harbin Medical University, No. 23 Youzheng Road, Harbin 150001, Heilongjiang, People's Republic of China

Background

Bone loss represents a complex set of challenges in terms of treatment and functional recovery, and management of bone defects is a challenging procedure in orthopedic surgery [1]. Autologous bone grafting along with soft tissue surgical reconstruction has been advocated for large bone defects [2]. However, there are several limitations and complications associated with this treatment, including an insufficient amount of autologous bone available for reconstruction, unavailability of autologous bone in growing children, and donor site morbidity [3, 4].

Distraction osteogenesis, developed by Ilizarov [5, 6], is a technique that creates new bone formation between opposing bone segments at the osteotomy site and activates regeneration of the soft tissue matrix surrounding the hard tissue. It overcomes the complications and limitations associated with bone grafting, providing a reliable alternative technique for the treatment of bone defects [7, 8]. Although distraction osteogenesis has a clear benefit for patients with not only skeletal defect but also any malalignment, shortening, soft tissue loss, or joint contractures, it is unfortunately associated with many complications, such as pin tract infections, soft tissue contractures, refractures, and pseudoarthrosis [8–10]. The prolonged duration of treatment is one of the major drawbacks of distraction osteogenesis, which is the primary cause for the above complications. In addition, since the length of time taken for bone union is a key factor in the patient's recovery [11], the prolonged treatment time is also harmful for the patient's recovery. Shortening the treatment time can make the technique more safe and cost-effective.

Low-intensity pulsed ultrasound (LIPUS) can cause pressure waves, converting to a biochemical signal inside the cells; stimulating signal transduction, blood flow, and angiogenesis; and promoting protein synthesis, calcium uptake, and osteogenic gene expression [12, 13]. LIPUS appears to be an effective non-invasive adjunctive therapy to promote the bone healing process, which has been approved by the US Food and Drug Administration and the National Institute of Clinical Excellence for the treatment of fresh fractures, delayed unions, and non-unions [14]. It is thought that the application of LIPUS during distraction osteogenesis can promote bone healing, reduce the treatment time, and thereby improve patient's recovery. However, the results are not totally convincing or consistent among all trials. Some trials reported a positive effect of LIPUS during the process of distraction osteogenesis [15–19], but some trials did not confirm this positive effect [20–24].

Previous systematic reviews analyzing the effect of LIPUS on fracture healing casually noted this potential [25–28], and a comprehensive meta-analysis on the topic has been available to date [29]. This meta-analysis suggests that LIPUS therapy may provide a reduction in the overall treatment time for tibial distraction osteogenesis [29]. However, owing to the limited sample sizes and the high risk of bias of the included trials, the author said that the conclusion should be considered with caution [29]. It also should be noted that this meta-analysis only focused on radiographic healing over other patient-important outcomes, such as bone density increases and the incident rate of complications. In addition, after that meta-analysis [29], a recently published trial, by far the largest trial on LIPUS treatment for distraction osteogenesis, determined that LIPUS did not influence the rate of bone healing in patients who undergo distraction osteogenesis [22].

Thus, an updated meta-analysis is necessary to provide a high-quality evidence for the use of LIPUS in patients who undergo distraction osteogenesis. The purpose of this meta-analysis of randomized controlled trials (RCTs), comparing the different effects between LIPUS treatment and sham devices or no devices, is to determine whether LIPUS can (1) reduce the associated treatment time, (2) reduce the incident rate of complications, and (3) improve bone regeneration and bone density for patients undergoing long-bone distraction osteogenesis.

Methods

This systematic review was reported according to the Preferred Reporting Item for Systematic Review and Meta-Analysis checklist [30]. A formal protocol was developed and registered on the PROSPERO international prospective register of systematic reviews (prospectively registered, CRD42017073596. Registered 11 February 2018. Https://www.crd.york.ac.uk/prospero/display_record.php?RecordID=73596).

Search strategy

MEDLINE, EMBASE, and the Cochrane Library were searched from their inception until May 1, 2018, without language restriction by two independent authors (SHL and HCL). Additionally, reference lists from retrieved trials, reports, conference abstracts, and reviews were manually scanned to further identify potentially eligible trials. The search strategy was developed using relevant text words as well as Medical Subject Headings that consisted of terms relevant to "Distraction Osteogenesis," "ultrasonic therapy," "ultrasonography," and "randomized control trial" (for the detailed search strategy, see Additional file 1: File S1).

Eligibility criteria

All RCTs of any duration assessing the association of LIPUS compared with placebo (or no additional treatment) among adults (aged ≥ 18 years) of any sex undergoing treatment with distraction osteogenesis regardless of location (long bone, short bone, flat bone, or irregular bone) of the body were potentially eligible for inclusion.

Outcome

The primary outcome was the reduction of treatment time during distraction osteogenesis, as measured by the bone healing index [31, 32], which is the time to maturation of the regenerate by the size of distraction gap, expressed in days per centimeter. The secondary outcome was the risk of complications. In addition, any other outcomes used to assess the time effect of LIPUS on bone healing were considered.

Study selection

Our search records were imported into ENDNOTE X7 reference management software, and the duplicate records were removed both electronically and manually. After excluding the duplicate and apparently irrelevant articles, the remaining studies were further reviewed by reading the full text to assess the eligibility for inclusion. Titles, abstracts, and full-text articles were screened independently by two authors (SHL and HCL) for eligibility, with discrepancies discussed with a third author (ZRL).

Data extraction

Information was carefully extracted from all the eligible publications independently by two independent reviewers (SHL and HCL), and disagreements were resolved through discussion or by seeking an independent third author (ZRL). A standard data extraction form was created using Microsoft Excel 2016 to collect data of interest. The major categories of variables to be coded were (1) study characteristics, (2) participant characteristics, (3) type of intervention (type, dose, duration), and (4) outcome characteristics. When data were only presented graphically, GetData Graph Digitizer 2.26 software was used to digitize and extract the data. When the original data were not available, we calculated the data through the available coefficients. For example, we computed the mean from median and the standard deviation (SD) from standard error (SE), interquartile range (IQR), or P values, according to the methods described in the Cochrane Handbook [33].

Risk of bias assessment

Two authors (SHL and HCL) independently assessed the risk of bias using the Cochrane risk-of-bias tool [34]. Bias was assessed across the following seven domains: (1) random sequence generation (selection bias), (2) allocation concealment (selection bias), (3) blinding of participants and personnel (performance bias), (4) blinding of outcome assessment (detection bias), (5) incomplete outcome data (attrition bias), (6) selective reporting (reporting bias), and (7) other biases. Each aspect could further be classified as a low, high, or unclear risk. Any disagreements were resolved through discussion and sometimes with another reviewer (ZRL) if necessary.

Data synthesis and analysis

The dichotomous outcomes are expressed as the risk ratios (RRs) and the 95% confidence interval (CI), using the Mantel-Haenszel method. The continuous outcomes are expressed as the mean differences (WMDs) or the standardized mean differences (SMDs) with their 95% CI, using the generic inverse variance methods.

Random-effects meta-analyses were conducted using the DerSimonian-Laird method [35], which provided more conservative estimated effects. To assess heterogeneity in results of individual studies, we used the I^2 statistic (0–40%, not important; 30–60%, moderate heterogeneity; 75–100%, considerable heterogeneity) [36]. Publication bias was assessed using the Egger regression test [37], if at least 10 trials were included in a meta-analysis, for funnel asymmetry in addition to visual inspection of the funnel plots.

When there was a significant heterogeneity ($I^2 > 50\%$) [33], both sensitivity analyses and subgroup analyses were performed to explore possible sources of heterogeneity. Sensitivity analyses were conducted using sequential omission of a single study from the total studies to evaluate the influence of each study on the pooled effect estimates. Subgroup analyses were performed based on the overall risk of bias ("low risk of bias" versus "high risk of bias").

A two-sided P value of less than or equal to .05 was deemed statistically significant. All analyses were conducted in Review Manager (version 5.3) and Comprehensive Meta-Analysis (version 2.0).

Quality of evidence

The quality of the evidence was assessed according to using the Grading of Recommendations Assessment, Development, and Evaluation (GRADE) guidelines, which uses the domains of risk of bias, inconsistency, indirectness, imprecision, and publication bias in results [38]. Each assessment result was rated as very low, low, moderate, or high. Summary tables were constructed using the GRADE Profiler (version 3.6).

Results

Study selection

Figure 1 presented the process of literature selection for this meta-analysis. A total of 538 articles were obtained through electronic and hand searches. After 392 duplicates were removed, the titles and abstracts of 146 records were reviewed, 134 records were excluded for not meeting the inclusion criteria, and, thus, the remaining 12 articles were retrieved for further assessment. Two trials were excluded because the osteotomy was treated without distraction osteogenesis [39, 40]. Three trials were excluded because the non-union was treated without distraction osteogenesis [41–43]. Finally, 7 trials

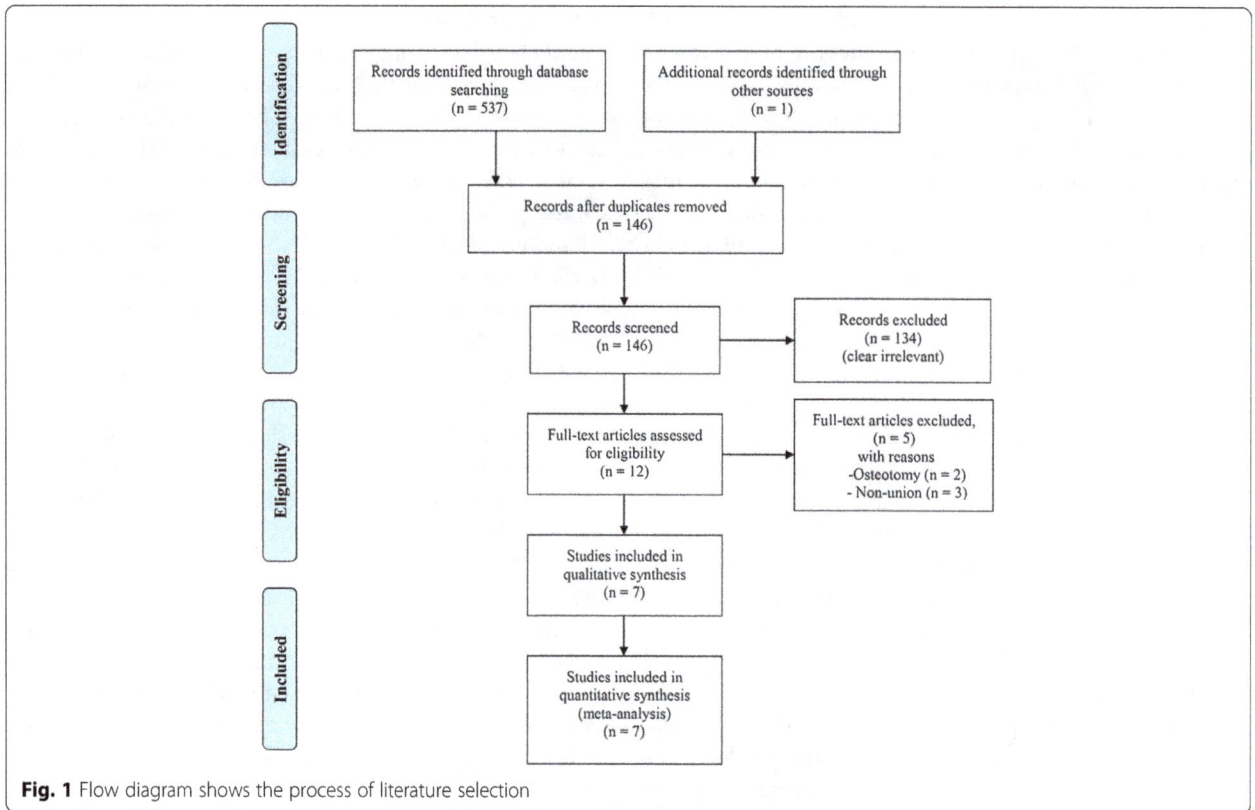

Fig. 1 Flow diagram shows the process of literature selection

fulfilled our inclusion criteria and were included in our meta-analysis [15, 18–22, 44].

Study characteristics

The study characteristics of the included trials are summarized in Table 1. All the 7 included trials were RCTs, published between 2004 and 2017 [15, 18–22, 44]. The sample sizes ranged from 8 to 62, with a total of 172 patients. Five trials performed distraction on the tibia [15, 18, 19, 22, 44], and 2 performed distraction on the mandible [20, 21]. The LIPUS treatment was used for 20 min every day for all the included trials.

Risk of bias assessment

Figure 2 summarizes the details of the risk of bias. Overall, we considered 3 trials to be at low risk of bias [20–22], and the other 4 studies to be at high risk of bias [15, 18, 19, 44]. The main limitations were failure to report method for allocation sequence generation [15, 18, 19], allocation concealment [15, 18, 19, 44], unblinded patients [15, 19, 44], and unblinded caregivers or outcome assessors [15, 18, 19, 44]. All the included trials had an unclear risk of reporting bias, because none of the included trials did have a protocol [15, 18–22, 44]. One trial had a

Table 1 Summary of study characteristics of included trials

Study	Sample size		Bone location	Mean age	Mean distraction gap (cm)	Distraction rate (mm/day)	LIPUS duration	LIPUS dose (min/day)
	LIPUS	Control						
Tsumaki N [44]	21	21	Tibia	68	0.5	1	Until healing	20
El-Mowafi HM [18]	10	10	Tibia	35	6.1	1	Until healing	20
Schortinghuis J [21]	4	4	Mandible	65	0.66	1	5 weeks	20
Schortinghuis J [20]	5	4	Mandible	56	0.51	1	7 weeks	20
Dudda M [15]	16	20	Tibia	39	6.6	Unclear	Until healing	20
Salem KH [19]	12	9	Tibia	30	7.9	1	Until healing	20
Simpson AH [22]	32	30	Tibia	37	4. cm	0.75	Until healing	20

LIPUS low-intensity pulsed ultrasound

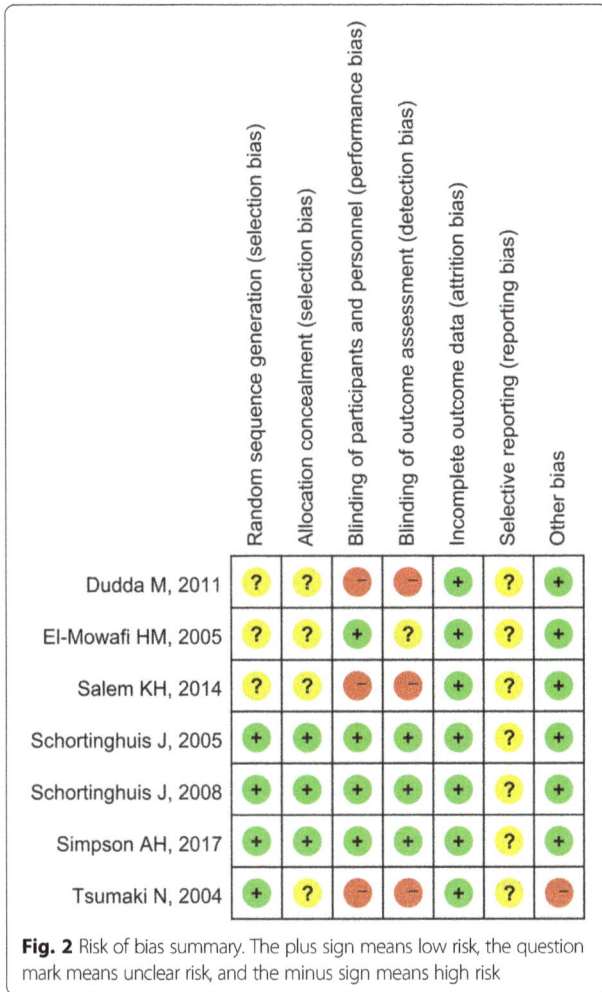

Fig. 2 Risk of bias summary. The plus sign means low risk, the question mark means unclear risk, and the minus sign means high risk

potential high risk of other biases, because of the self-control design [44].

Bone healing index

Five trials, including 152 patients, provided the available data about bone healing index [15, 18, 19, 22, 44]. The analysis did not show a statistically significant reduction

in the treatment time in favor of LIPUS (mean difference, − 8.75 days/cm; 95% CI, − 20.68 to 3.18 days/cm; $P = 0.15$; $I^2 = 72\%$; Fig. 3).

Owing to the significant heterogeneity, sensitivity analyses were performed by omitting each study in turn, and the pooled mean difference was directly affected by one trial (Additional file 2: Figure S1) [22]. Subgroup analyses suggested that the combined mean differences were 10.10 days/cm (95% CI, − 2.89 to − 23.09 days/cm; $I^2 = 0\%$) in trials with a low risk of bias and − 16.29 days/cm (95% CI, − 21.90 to − 10.68 days/cm; $I^2 = 0\%$) in trials with a high risk of bias (Fig. 3). The test for subgroup differences indicated that the findings from low risk of bias and high risk of bias subgroups were statistically significantly different from each other ($P < 0.01$ for interaction). The funnel plot suggested there was no significant publication bias (Additional file 3: Figure S2).

Risk of complications

Five trials reported the incidence rate of complications [15, 18, 20, 21, 44]. Neither the pooled risk ratio (0.90 in favor of LIPUS; 95% CI, 0.65 to 1.24; $I^2 = 0\%$; 3 trials; Fig. 4) nor the pooled risk difference (3% reduction with LIPUS, 13% reduction to 6% increase; $I^2 = 0\%$; 5 trials) showed a significant effect. There was no significant interaction with kinds of complications (risk ratio, $P = 0.35$; risk difference, $P = 0.39$; Fig. 4).

Other outcomes

Four studies reported other outcomes about bone healing [19–21, 44]. Two trials used radiological and histological methods to assess bone regeneration at the distraction gap [20, 21] and showed no significant effect of LIPUS for the radiological gap fill area (standardized mean difference, 0.48 in favor of control; 95% CI, − 1.49 to 0.52; $I^2 = 0\%$) or the histological gap fill length (standardized mean difference, 0.76 in favor of control; 95% CI, − 1.78 to 0.27; $I^2 = 0\%$) (Fig. 5). Four trials assessed bone healing with the bone density increase [19–21, 44],

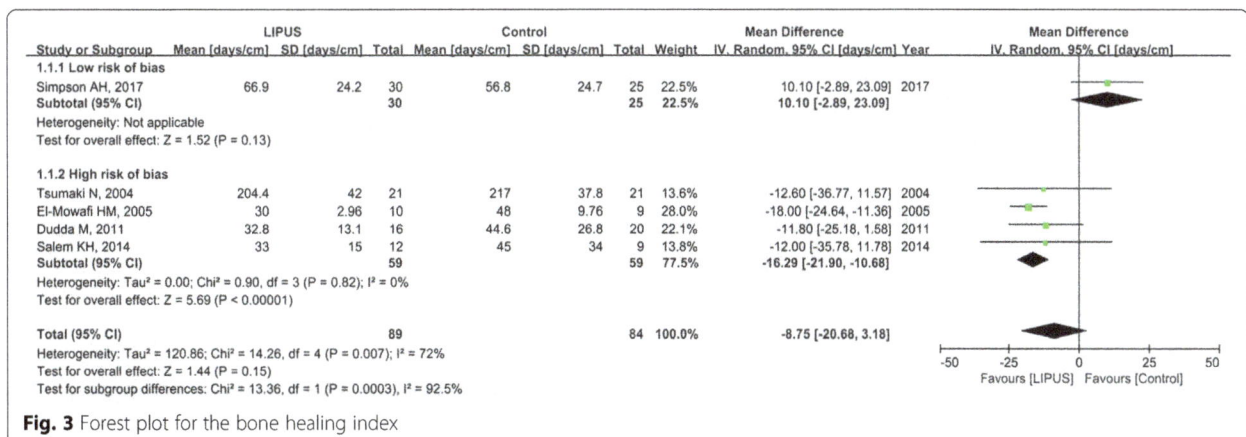

Fig. 3 Forest plot for the bone healing index

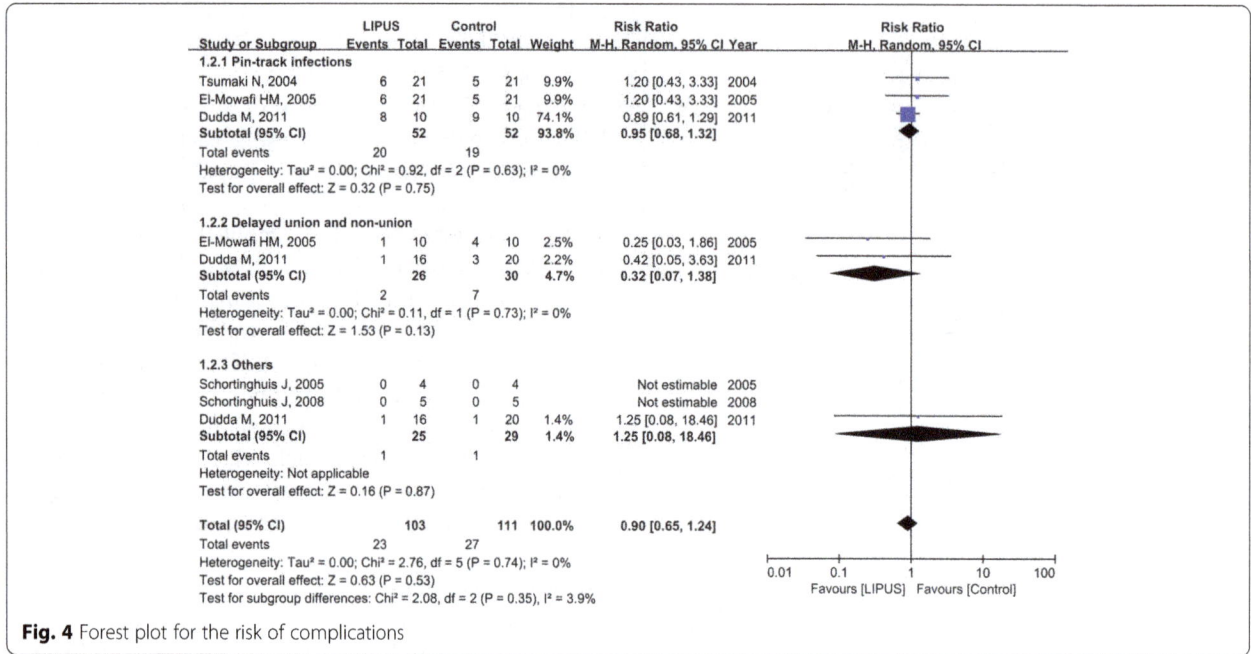

Fig. 4 Forest plot for the risk of complications

and the overall results suggested no significant effect with LIPUS (standardized mean difference, 0.43 in favor of LIPUS; 95% CI, – 0.02 to 0.88; $I^2 = 0$%) (Fig. 5).

Quality of evidence

The GRADE evidence profiles for each outcome are shown in Table 2. All the included trials were RCTs and had no significant publication bias. A risk of bias existed in each outcome except for the outcomes of the radiography gap fill area and the histology gap fill length. Inconsistency existed in the outcome of the bone healing index, which was due to the significant heterogeneity. Imprecision existed in the outcome of the radiography gap fill area, the histology gap fill length, and the bone

density increase. Although the included RCTs were considered as high-quality evidence, the available evidence of each outcome was moderate to low, which was downgraded from high due to the above limitations.

Discussion
Main findings

Our meta-analysis comprehensively and systematically reviews the current available literature, and the overall results provide low- to moderate-quality evidence that LIPUS applied to patients undergoing distraction osteogenesis has no effect on promoting the process of bone healing or reducing the risk of complications. This study also provides low-quality evidence that LIPUS treatment

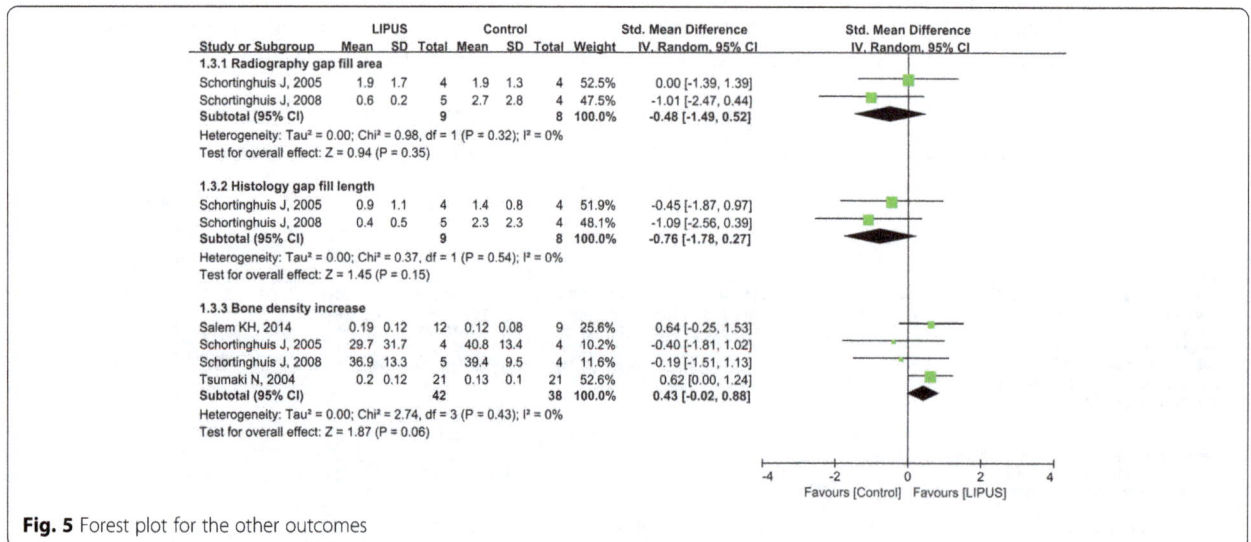

Fig. 5 Forest plot for the other outcomes

Table 2 The GRADE evidence quality for each outcome

Quality assessment							No. of patients		Effect		Quality	Importance
No. of studies	Design	Risk of bias	Inconsistency	Indirectness	Imprecision	Other considerations	New comparison	Control comparison	Relative (95% CI)	Absolute		
Bone healing index (better indicated by lower values)												
5	Randomized trials	Serious	Serious	No serious indirectness	No serious imprecision	None	89	84	N/A	MD 8.75 lower (20.68 lower to 3.18 higher)	⊕⊕OO Low	Critical
Risk of complications												
5	Randomized trials	Serious	No serious inconsistency	No serious indirectness	No serious imprecision	None	23/103 (22.3%)	27/111 (24.3%)	RR 0.90 (0.65 to 1.24)	24 fewer per 1000 (from 85 fewer to 58 more)	⊕⊕⊕O Moderate	Critical
Radiography gap fill area (better indicated by higher values)												
2	Randomized trials	No serious risk of bias	No serious inconsistency	No serious indirectness	Very serious	None	9	8	N/A	SMD 0.48 lower (1.49 lower to 0.52 higher)	⊕⊕OO Low	Important
Histology gap fill length (better indicated by higher values)												
2	Randomized trials	No serious risk of bias	No serious inconsistency	No serious indirectness	Very serious	None	9	8	N/A	SMD 0.76 lower (1.78 lower to 0.27 higher)	⊕⊕OO Low	Important
Bone density increase (better indicated by higher values)												
4	Randomized trials	Serious	No serious inconsistency	No serious indirectness	Serious	None	42	38	N/A	SMD 0.43 higher (0.02 lower to 0.88 higher)	⊕⊕OO Low	Important

N/A not applicable, *RR* risk ratio, *SMD* standardized mean difference, *MD* mean difference, *CI* confidence interval
⊕⊕⊕⊕ means high quality
⊕⊕⊕O means moderate quality
⊕⊕OO means low quality
⊕OOO means very low quality

does not have an advantage of improving the radiological gap fill area, the histological gap fill length, or the bone density increase.

Comparison with other studies

Our results are inconsistent with the previous systematic reviews, which indicate that LIPUS has a benefit for accelerating healing on distraction osteogenesis [25–29]. Our study differs from previous systematic reviews in several important aspects. First, we include the recently published trial [22], by far the largest trial on LIPUS treatment for distraction osteogenesis. Besides that, we also included one trial [21], which was missed by the previous meta-analysis [29]. Thus, eligible trials in our study were the most comprehensive. Owing to a larger sample size included in our study, we determined a different overall result from the previous meta-analysis. Second, this meta-analysis adds to the existing literature by not only assessing the outcome about bone healing, but also assessing the outcomes about the risk of complications, which is considered as a critical outcome by patients [45]. Based on this advantage, although our subgroup analyses and the previous meta-analysis [29] suggested that LIPUS had a benefit of 16 days/cm, whether LIPUS treatment could be used for all the patients is doubtful. Based on the current evidence [29, 44], a reduction of 16 days/cm, without a reduced risk of complications, might not have a clinical benefit for patients with a small bone defect (< 1 cm). Third, both sensitivity analyses and subgroup analyses were used in our study to explore the heterogeneity, and the heterogeneity of each outcome seems to get a reasonable explanation. Both the sensitivity analyses and the subgroup analyses found that the study by Simpson and colleagues [22] obviously affects the effect of LIPUS, suggesting the study design and/or sample size might be key factors. Finally, we used the GRADE approach to assess the quality of evidence, which was not used by the previous meta-analysis [29]. Since the available evidence of each outcome was only moderate to low, it is suggested that the conclusions of our study may be changed by the future studies.

Limitations

This study has limitations. First, there were some methodological limitations in the included trials, such as the unclear random method, the inadequate concealment of treatment allocation, and the open-label design. Second, the possibility of publication bias existed. Third, since not all the included trials clearly report the baseline information, it is unclear whether the age, sex, distraction rate, the size of distraction gap, and other variables could affect the effectiveness of LIPUS treatment. Given these limitations, the results of this meta-analysis should be interpreted cautiously.

Implications for further studies

Since several gaps remain regarding the LIPUS treatment for distraction osteogenesis, future trials are still needed. The design of the future trials should focus on the following points: (1) since subgroup analyses suggest that the results were significantly different between trails at low risk of bias and those at high risk of bias, and all the trials at low risk of bias suggest that LIPUS has no effect for patients undergoing distraction osteogenesis [20–22], trials should pay attention to the methodological design, and double-blinded and clearly reported randomized controlled trials are required, and (2) trials should clearly report the age, sex, and the size of distraction gap to determine whether these variables could affect the effectiveness of LIPUS treatment. Moreover, since smoking, diabetes, and soft tissue can be factors to bone healing [46, 47], the baseline of these key factors need attention; (3) trials should report more outcomes, such as the complications and the functional recovery, which are also important outcomes for patients.

Conclusion

Among patients undergoing distraction osteogenesis, neither the treatment time nor the complications could be reduced by LIPUS therapy. The currently available evidence is insufficient to support the routine use of this intervention in clinical practice.

Abbreviations
CI: Confidence interval; GRADE: Grading of Recommendations Assessment, Development, and Evaluation; LIPUS: Low-intensity pulsed ultrasound; RCT: Randomized controlled trial; RR: Risk ratio; SMD: Standardized mean difference; WMD: Mean difference

Authors' contributions
PFT and YSW were the guarantors. PFT, YSW, and SHL contributed to the conception and design of this study protocol. SHL and HCL registered the protocol with the PROSPERO database. The search strategy was developed by SHL and ZRL. SHL and HCL selected the studies for inclusion and extracted the data. ZRL, SHL, and HCL did the analyses. YSW and PFT gave advice on the data analysis and the presentation of the study results. All the authors drafted and critically reviewed this manuscript and approved the final version.

Competing interests
The authors declare that they have no competing interests.

References

1. Tsuchiya H, Tomita K. Distraction osteogenesis for treatment of bone loss in the lower extremity. J Orthop Sci. 2003;8(1):116–24.

2. Nusbickel FR, Dell PC, McAndrew MP, Moore MM. Vascularized autografts for reconstruction of skeletal defects following lower extremity trauma. A review. Clin Orthop Relat Res. 1989;243:65–70.

3. Kumar CY, BN K, Menon J, Patro DK, HB B. Calcium sulfate as bone graft substitute in the treatment of osseous bone defects, a prospective study. J Clin Diagn Res. 2013;7(12):2926–8.

4. Singh JR, Nwosu U, Egol KA. Long-term functional outcome and donor-site morbidity associated with autogenous iliac crest bone grafts utilizing a modified anterior approach. Bull NYU Hosp Jt Dis. 2009;67(4):347–51.

5. Ilizarov GA. The tension-stress effect on the genesis and growth of tissues. Part I The influence of stability of fixation and soft-tissue preservation. Clin Orthop Relat Res. 1989;238:249–81. PMID: 2910611

6. Ilizarov GA. The tension-stress effect on the genesis and growth of tissues: part II. The influence of the rate and frequency of distraction. Clin Orthop Relat Res. 1989;239:263–85. PMID: 2912628

7. Codivilla A. The classic: on the means of lengthening, in the lower limbs, the muscles and tissues which are shortened through deformity. 1905. Clin Orthop Relat Res. 2008;466:2903–9. https://doi.org/10.1007/s11999-008-0518-7. PMID: 18820986

8. Papakostidis C, Bhandari M, Giannoudis PV. Distraction osteogenesis in the treatment of long bone defects of the lower limbs: effectiveness, complications and clinical results; a systematic review and meta-analysis. Bone Joint J. 2013;95-B:1673–80. https://doi.org/10.1302/0301-620X.95B12.32385. PMID: 24293599

9. Aronson J. Limb-lengthening, skeletal reconstruction, and bone transport with the Ilizarov method. J Bone Joint Surg Am. 1997;79:1243–58. PMID: 9278087

10. Liantis P, Mavrogenis AF, Stavropoulos NA, Kanellopoulos AD, Papagelopoulos PJ, Soucacos PN, et al. Risk factors for and complications of distraction osteogenesis. Eur J Orthop Surg Traumatol. 2014;24:693–8. https://doi.org/10.1007/s00590-013-1261-7. PMID: 23793730

11. Heckman JD, Sarasohn-Kahn J. The economics of treating tibia fractures. The cost of delayed unions. Bull Hosp Jt Dis. 1997;56:63–72. PMID: 9063607

12. Harrison A, Lin S, Pounder N, et al. Mode & mechanism of low intensity pulsed ultrasound (LIPUS) in fracture repair. Ultrasonics. 2016;70:45–52.

13. Khan Y, Laurencin CT. Fracture repair with ultrasound: clinical and cell-based evaluation. J Bone Joint Surg Am. 2008;90(Suppl 1):138–44.

14. Poolman RW, Agoritsas T, Siemieniuk RA, Harris IA, Schipper IB, Mollon B, et al. Low intensity pulsed ultrasound (LIPUS) for bone healing: a clinical practice guideline. BMJ. 2017;356:j576. PMID: 28228381

15. Dudda M, Hauser J, Muhr G, Esenwein SA. Low-intensity pulsed ultrasound as a useful adjuvant during distraction osteogenesis: a prospective, randomized controlled trial. J Trauma. 2011;71:1376–80. https://doi.org/10.1097/TA.0b013e31821912b2. PMID: 22071933

16. El-Bialy TH, Elgazzar RF, Megahed EE, Royston TJ. Effects of ultrasound modes on mandibular osteodistraction. J Dent Res. 2008;87:953–7. https://doi.org/10.1177/154405910808701018. PMID: 18809750

17. El-Bialy TH, Royston TJ, Magin RL, Evans CA, Ael-M Z, Frizzell LA. The effect of pulsed ultrasound on mandibular distraction. Ann Biomed Eng. 2002;30:1251–61. PMID: 12540201

18. El-Mowafi H, Mohsen M. The effect of low-intensity pulsed ultrasound on callus maturation in tibial distraction osteogenesis. Int Orthop. 2005;29:121–4. https://doi.org/10.1007/s00264-004-0625-3. PMID: 15685456

19. Salem KH, Schmelz A. Low-intensity pulsed ultrasound shortens the treatment time in tibial distraction osteogenesis. Int Orthop. 2014;38:1477–82. https://doi.org/10.1007/s00264-013-2254-1. PMID: 24390009

20. Schortinghuis J, Bronckers AL, Gravendeel J, Stegenga B, Raghoebar GM. The effect of ultrasound on osteogenesis in the vertically distracted edentulous mandible: a double-blind trial. Int J Oral Maxillofac Surg. 2008;37:1014–21. https://doi.org/10.1016/j.ijom.2008.07.004. PMID: 18757179

21. Schortinghuis J, Bronckers AL, Stegenga B, Raghoebar GM, de Bont LG. Ultrasound to stimulate early bone formation in a distraction gap: a double blind randomised clinical pilot trial in the edentulous mandible. Arch Oral Biol. 2005;50:411–20. https://doi.org/10.1016/j.archoralbio.2004.09.005. PMID: 15748694

22. Simpson AH, Keenan G, Nayagam S, Atkins RM, Marsh D, Clement ND. Low-intensity pulsed ultrasound does not influence bone healing by distraction osteogenesis: a multicentre double-blind randomised control trial. Bone Joint J. 2017;99-B:494–502. https://doi.org/10.1302/0301-620X.99B4.BJJ-2016-0559.R1. PMID: 28385939

23. Taylor KF, Rafiee B, Tis JE, Inoue N. Low-intensity pulsed ultrasound does not enhance distraction callus in a rabbit model. Clin Orthop Relat Res. 2007;459:237–45. https://doi.org/10.1097/BLO.0b013e31803c75b4. PMID: 17545764

24. Uglow MG, Peat RA, Hile MS, Bilston LE, Smith EJ, Little DG. Low-intensity ultrasound stimulation in distraction osteogenesis in rabbits. Clin Orthop Relat Res. 2003:303–12. https://doi.org/10.1097/01.blo.0000093043.56370.5a. PMID: 14646730

25. Bashardoust TS, Houghton P, MacDermid JC, Grewal R. Effects of low-intensity pulsed ultrasound therapy on fracture healing: a systematic review and meta-analysis. Am J Phys Med Rehabil. 2012;91:349–67. https://doi.org/10.1097/PHM.0b013e31822419ba. PMID: 21904188

26. Malizos KN, Hantes ME, Protopappas V, Papachristos A. Low-intensity pulsed ultrasound for bone healing: an overview. Injury. 2006;37(Suppl 1):S56–62. https://doi.org/10.1016/j.injury.2006.02.037. PMID: 16581076

27. Rutten S, van den Bekerom MP, Sierevelt IN, Nolte PA. Enhancement of bone-healing by low-intensity pulsed ultrasound: a systematic review. JBJS Rev. 2016;4 https://doi.org/10.2106/JBJS.RVW.O.00027. PMID: 27500435

28. Watanabe Y, Matsushita T, Bhandari M, Zdero R, Schemitsch EH. Ultrasound for fracture healing: current evidence. J Orthop Trauma. 2010;24:S56–56S62. https://doi.org/10.1097/BOT.0b013e3181d2efaf PMID: 2010143405

29. Raza H, Saltaji H, Kaur H, Flores-Mir C, El-Bialy T. Effect of low-intensity pulsed ultrasound on distraction osteogenesis treatment time: a meta-analysis of randomized clinical trials. J Ultrasound Med. 2016;35:349–58. https://doi.org/10.7863/ultra.15.02043. PMID: 26782167

30. Moher D, Liberati A, Tetzlaff J, Altman DG. Preferred reporting items for systematic reviews and meta-analyses: the PRISMA statement. PLoS Med. 2009;6:e1000097. https://doi.org/10.1371/journal.pmed.1000097. PMID: 19621072

31. Aldegheri R, Renzi-Brivio L, Agostini S. The callotasis method of limb lengthening. Clin Orthop Relat Res. 1989;(241):137-45.

32. De Bastiani G, Aldegheri R, Renzi-Brivio L, Trivella G. Limb lengthening by callus distraction (callotasis). J Pediatr Orthop. 1987;7:129–34. PMID: 3558791

33. Higgins JPT, Green S. Cochrane Handbook for Systematic Reviews of Interventions Version 5.1.0 [updated March 2011]. The Cochrane Collaboration, 2011. Available from www.handbook.cochrane.org.

34. Higgins JP, Altman DG, Gøtzsche PC, et al. The Cochrane Collaboration's tool for assessing risk of bias in randomised trials. BMJ. 2011;343:d5928.

35. DerSimonian R, Laird N. Meta-analysis in clinical trials. Control Clin Trials. 1986;7:177–88. PMID: 3802833

36. Higgins JP, Thompson SG, Deeks JJ, Altman DG. Measuring inconsistency in meta-analyses. BMJ. 2003;327(7414):557–60.

37. Egger M, Davey SG, Schneider M, Minder C. Bias in meta-analysis detected by a simple, graphical test. BMJ. 1997;315(7109):629–34.

38. Atkins D, Best D, Briss PA, et al. Grading quality of evidence and strength of recommendations. BMJ. 2004;328(7454):1490.

39. Urita A, Iwasaki N, Kondo M, Nishio Y, Kamishima T, Minami A. Effect of low-intensity pulsed ultrasound on bone healing at osteotomy sites after forearm bone shortening. J Hand Surg Am. 2013;38:498–503. https://doi.org/10.1016/j.jhsa.2012.11.032. PMID: 23375786

40. Zacherl M, Gruber G, Radl R, Rehak PH, Windhager R. No midterm benefit from low intensity pulsed ultrasound after chevron osteotomy for hallux valgus. Ultrasound Med Biol. 2009;35:1290–7. https://doi.org/10.1016/j.ultrasmedbio.2009.03.008. MID: 19540659

41. Ricardo M. The effect of ultrasound on the healing of muscle-pediculated bone graft in scaphoid non-union. Int Orthop. 2006;30:123–7. https://doi.org/10.1007/s00264-005-0034-2. PMID: 16474939

42. Rutten S, Nolte PA, Korstjens CM, van Duin MA, Klein-Nulend J. Low-intensity pulsed ultrasound increases bone volume, osteoid thickness and mineral apposition rate in the area of fracture healing in patients with a delayed union of the osteotomized fibula. Bone. 2008;43:348–54. https://doi.org/10.1016/j.bone.2008.04.010. PMID: 18538648

43. Schofer MD, Block JE, Aigner J, Schmelz A. Improved healing response in delayed unions of the tibia with low-intensity pulsed ultrasound: results of a randomized sham-controlled trial. BMC Musculoskelet Disord. 2010;11:229. https://doi.org/10.1186/1471-2474-11-229. PMID: 20932272

3

Treatment of AC dislocation by reconstructing CC and AC ligaments with allogenic tendons compared with hook plates

Guheng Wang[1], Renguo Xie[1,2]* ⓘ, Tian Mao[1] and Shuguo Xing[1]

Abstract

Background: The purpose of this study was to compare outcomes between allograft reconstruction and hook plate fixation for acute dislocation of the acromioclavicular joint with a minimum 2-year follow-up.

Methods: A retrospective comparative study of patients treated for acute acromioclavicular joint dislocation from February 2010 to December 2014 in our hospital, consisting of 16 patients who were followed-up, was performed. Eight patients were treated for acute AC dislocation and underwent surgical reconstruction as follows: the coracoclavicular and acromioclavicular ligaments were reconstructed with the allogenic tendon. The other eight patients were treated with hook plates to maintain the AC joint reset. At the latest follow-up, radiographic analysis and the Constant and University of California-Los Angeles (UCLA) scores were used to evaluate shoulder function. The satisfaction of the patients in terms of the efficacy and visual analog scale (VAS) data were also recorded.

Results: After an average follow-up of 30.3 months (range 24–46 months), no patient had dislocated their joint again at the final follow-up based on X-ray examination. The Constant score was 94.4 for the allogenic tendon group and 93.8 for the hook plate group ($P = 0.57$). According to the UCLA scale ($P = 0.23$) or VAS ($P = 0.16$), we found no significant difference between the two groups. All patients reported that they were very satisfied or satisfied with the outcome of surgery, and no significant difference ($P = 0.08$) was found between the two groups.

Conclusions: The use of allogenic tendon for reconstruction of the coracoclavicular and acromioclavicular ligaments shows excellent outcomes in terms of the recovery of clinical function or radiographic outcomes for acute AC dislocation. Compared with the hook plate, the hardware did not need to be removed.

Keywords: Surgery, Acromioclavicular joint dislocation, Coracoclavicular ligaments, Acromioclavicular ligaments, Allogenic tendon, Hook plate

Background

Acromioclavicular (AC) joint dislocation is a common injury, which accounts for approximately 9% of shoulder injuries [1]. When AC joint dislocation occurs, it not only produces shoulder pain and abnormal activity symptoms but also greatly affects the strength, flexibility, and movement of the entire upper

extremity. Because previous techniques are associated with frequent complications, such as loss of reduction, fracture of the coracoids, and loosening [2–6], many studies have evaluated potential improvements in the surgical management of AC joint dislocation. Many methods exist, indicating that an ideal method still needs to be explored. Considering the possibility of vertical and anteroposterior displacement of the clavicle in AC joint dislocation, we adopted a method to reduce and maintain the reduction of the AC joint using an allogenic tendon to reconstruct the coracoclavicular and acromioclavicular ligaments in acute

* Correspondence: xrg1969@yahoo.com
[1]Department of Hand Surgery, Affiliated Hospital of Nantong University, 20# West Temple Road, Nantong 226001, People's Republic of China
[2]Department of Hand Surgery, Shanghai General Hospital, 650# Songjiang Road, Shanghai 201620, People's Republic of China

injuries. We also compared it with the clavicular hook plate treatment to assess the merits and demerits of this method.

Methods

Patients

A retrospective study of patients with acute AC joint dislocation who were treated in our hospital between February 2010 and December 2014 was performed. The institutional ethics committee approved the study, and informed consent was obtained from all study participants. In this study, eight patients (six male, two female) with an average age of 49.0 years were treated with an allogenic tendon to reconstruct the coracoclavicular and acromioclavicular ligaments after AC joint dislocation. At the same time, eight atients (five male, three female) with an average age of 41.3 years were treated with the hook plate for fixation of AC joint dislocation. Patients with chronic dislocation (≥ 3 weeks after trauma) and patients who received any operative treatment of the injured shoulder were excluded. Patients with accompanying coracoid fracture, shoulder wounds, and chronic infections were also excluded from this study.

According to the Rockwood classification, there were six cases of type III, two of type IV, and eight of type V. The mean time from injury to surgery was 2.9 (range 1–5) days. Of all injuries, 14 were caused by traffic accidents, 1 by a simple fall, and 1 by blunt trauma (Table 1).

Surgical technique
Allogenic tendon

Under interscalene regional block or general anesthesia, the patient was placed in the beach-chair position and the upper limb draped free. A saber cut incision (Fig. 1) was made in line from the coracoid process to the medial AC joint. After development of subcutaneous flaps, the deltotrapezial fascia was taken down subperiosteally, exposing the clavicle, AC joint, and coracoid process [7].

After the AC joint was exposed, the coracoclavicular (CC) and AC ligaments were identified to ensure that they were ruptured. With the deltoid flap retracted, the base of the coracoid process was exposed, and a soft tissue tunnel was made. After the AC joint was reduced, the reduction was maintained with direct pressure with assistance. Corresponding to the trapezoid ligament and conoid ligament attachment in the clavicle, two tunnels, using a 4.0 and a 3.5 mm drill bit, were drilled separately at a distance of approximately 20 and 40 mm from the distal end of the clavicle (Fig. 2a, b). Another drill tunnel (3.5 mm) was positioned on the acromion approximately 15 mm from the AC joint (Fig. 2c). This corresponds to the acromioclavicular ligament. At this time, the allogenic tendon (Tissuebank of the Orthopedic Institute of the People's Liberation Army in Beijing) was taken out of the sealed bag, washed with saline, and placed in saline with antibiotics for 30 min before use. The flexor digitorum profundus tendon was usually selected because its length and width meet the requirements.

Table 1 Data of the 16 evaluated patients

Patient	Age/sex side	Mechanism of injury	Plate removal (months)	Follow-up (months)	Type of separation[a]
Allogenic tendon					
1	34/male right	Fall from height	–	28	IV
2	43/male left	Traffic accident	–	43	V
3	59/male left	Traffic accident	–	24	V
4	64/female right	Traffic accident	–	29	IV
5	72/male left	Traffic accident	–	29	III
6	23/male left	Traffic accident	–	33	III
7	34/female right	Traffic accident	–	27	V
8	63/male left	Traffic accident	–	25	V
Hook plate					
1	56/male right	Blunt trauma	10	30	III
2	22/male left	Traffic accident	7	31	III
3	34/male left	Traffic accident	5	24	V
4	31/male left	Traffic accident	8	26	V
5	42/female right	Traffic accident	11	46	III
6	37/female right	Traffic accident	8	39	III
7	63/male right	Traffic accident	11	25	V
8	45/female left	Traffic accident	12	26	V

[a]According to the Rockwood classification [29]

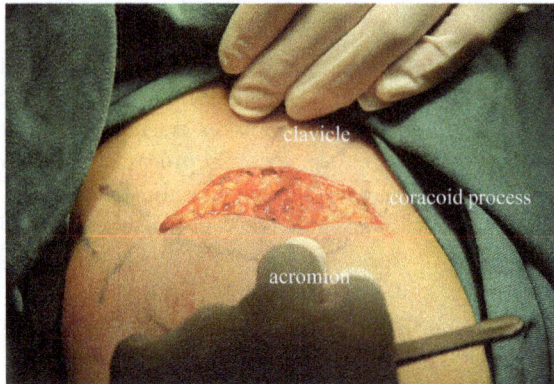

Fig. 1 Saber cut incision spanning the AC joint to just proximal to the coracoid process

(The time from tendon harvest to use was approximately 1–2 months.) Tendon donors were usually healthy and died between 20 and 50 years old. Their deaths were often caused by accidents. If one tendon was not long enough, we used two allogenic tendons to reconstruct the coracoclavicular ligament and the acromioclavicular ligament separately. Attention was paid to ensure that the graft looked firm and appeared fresh.

The prepared allogenic tendon was then pushed through the A tunnel with a curved hemostat. Next, the allogenic tendon was passed around the coracoid process and then, with the help of a passing wire, passed through the B tunnel, which was previously made. Then, the allogenic tendon was continually passed through the

C tunnel at the acromion on the clavicle. Finally, the allogenic tendon was pushed through the B tunnel again below the clavicle to reach the surface of the clavicle. Subsequently, the two free ends of the allogenic tendon were secured to each other on the surface of the clavicle with maximum manual tension between the A and B tunnels using 3-0 nonabsorbable surgical suture (Ethibond Johnson & Johnson, New Brunswick, US) (Fig. 3). Throughout the process, assistance helped to maintain the reduction of the AC joint, and both the trapezoid and conoid ligaments as well as the acromioclavicular ligament were reconstructed. Next, the trapezius-deltoid fascia was repaired and the wound closed. Before and after surgery, X-rays of the AC joint were obtained, and the dislocation is shown in Fig. 4. The X-ray after surgery confirmed that the AC joint was restored.

Hook plate

The surgical position and anesthesia were performed as in the allogenic tendon group. Centered on the AC joint, a 5- to 7-cm skin incision was made to expose the dislocation and ensure that the coracoclavicular and acromioclavicular ligaments were ruptured. The articular disc was removed if injured. The hook plate was then used to fix the dislocation (3.5 mm LCP clavicular hook plate, Synthes GmbH, Solothurn, Switzerland) as the end of the hook was inserted under the acromion. Before application of the hook plate, the depth of the acromion was measured, and the plate was pre-bent to perfectly fit the clavicle. When the hook plate was placed, 3.5-mm screws were used to fix it in place. The coracoclavicular and acromioclavicular ligaments were then repaired with #5 nonabsorbable surgical suture (Ethibond Johnson & Johnson, New Brunswick, US).

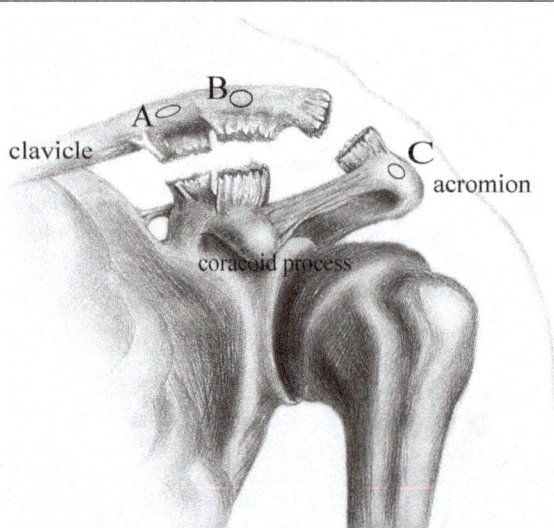

Fig. 2 Diagram of intra-operative drilling position. **a** Tunnel: approximately 40 mm from the distal end at the clavicle using a 3.5-mm drill bit. **b** Tunnel: approximately 20 mm from the distal end at the clavicle using a 4.0-mm drill bit. **c** Tunnel: approximately 15 mm to the AC joint at the acromion using a 3.5-mm drill bit

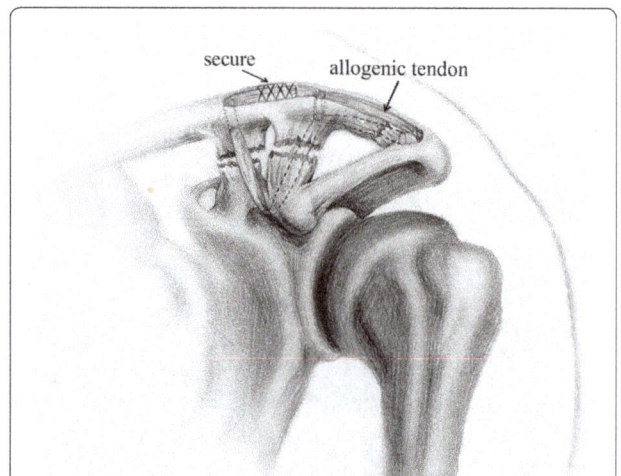

Fig. 3 Diagram of allogenic tendon used to reconstruct the coracoclavicular and acromioclavicular ligaments

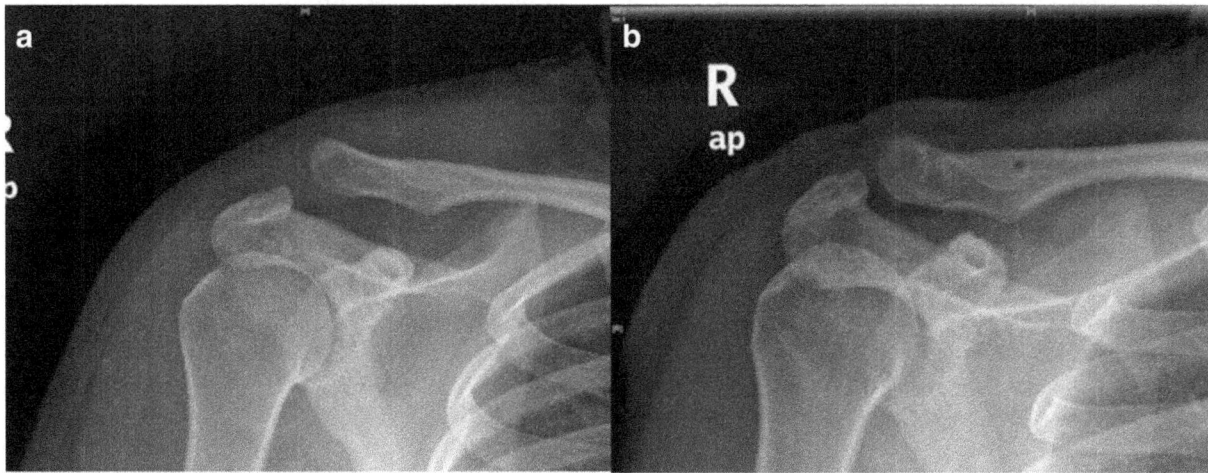

Fig. 4 a X-rays of AC joint dislocation before surgery. **b** X-rays of AC joint dislocation after surgery reconstructing the coracoclavicular and acromioclavicular ligaments with the allogenic tendon

Finally, the deltoid trapezoid fascia was closed with resorbable sutures, and the wound was closed in layers. The hook plate was removed at 9.0 (range 5–12) months after the surgery.

Postoperative management

A sandbag was used to compress the wound for 24 h after surgery. Postoperatively, the patient was placed in a shoulder immobilizer for 4 weeks, although movement of the wrist and elbow was encouraged immediately after surgery. After 4 weeks, shoulder joint motion, including the pendulum exercise, began; however, heavy physical work was not permitted until 3 months. Patients were not allowed to participate in sports activities until 6 months after the operation.

Clinical evaluation

All patients were asked to report whether they have any particular discomfort in the shoulder, which may be related to the overall surgery satisfaction (very satisfied, satisfied, partially satisfied, or not satisfied).

During follow-up, the appearance of the shoulder was assessed to determine whether there were any deformities, such as projections of the distal clavicle. At the same time, we also took X-rays and evaluated the radiographic findings, including the occurrence of osteoarthritic changes and the complete reduction degree of the AC joint. A visual analog scale (VAS: range 0–10; 0 represents no pain and 10 represents maximal imaginable pain) was used to evaluate the pain postoperatively.

Clinical evaluation of patients was performed using both the Constant [8] and University of California-Los Angeles (UCLA) [9] scoring systems. The Constant score is graded from 0 to 100, where 100 is best possible score, and consists of four dimensions: pain (0–15

points), activity level (0–20 points), range of movement (0–40 points), and power (0–25 points). We assumed that scores ≥ 90, 80–89, 70–79 and < 70 indicated excellent, good, fair, and poor, respectively. The UCLA score consisted of pain (0–10 points), function (0–10 points), range of motion (0–5 points), strength (0–5 points), and the patient's satisfaction (0–5 points). The total UCLA score is 35 points, and 34 or 35, 29–33, and ≤ 29 indicated excellent, good, and poor, respectively.

Statistical methods

The t test was used to evaluate significant differences between the two study groups for continuous variables, and the Wilcoxon test was used to evaluate significant differences for patient satisfaction during follow-up. A value of P less than 0.05 was considered as statistically significant. Statistical analysis was performed with SPSS version 16.0 software (SPSS, Chicago IL, USA).

Results

In the allogenic tendon group, the operative procedure was performed by the corresponding author, whereas all patients in the hook plate group were operated on by seniors. No patient reported any immune problems related to the allogenic tendon or hook plate.

In the allogenic tendon group, the eight patients were followed up, and the total follow-up ranged from 25 to 43 months, with a mean of 29.8 months. In the hook plate group, the total follow-up ranged from 24 to 46 months, with a mean of 30.9 months. No patients lost reduction on the final follow-up based on the X-ray results, and no patients had shoulder deformities.

All patients reported that they were very satisfied or satisfied with the outcome of the surgery. Three patients were satisfied, and five were very satisfied in the allogenic tendon group, whereas two patients were satisfied and six were very satisfied in the hook plate group. Although, there were more "very satisfied" results in the hook plate group, this difference was not significant ($P = 0.08$).

All patients returned to work without pain, and the VAS scale showed no significant difference between the two groups ($P = 0.16$).

Function

No significant differences were found between the two groups with regard to the Constant score ($P = 0.57$), with 94.4 in the allogenic tendon group (86–100, number in brackets indicates the range of the variables) compared to 93.8 in the hook plate group (84–98) (Table 2). The results for all patients were rated as excellent or good according to the score. Detailed results of the functional questionnaire are shown in Table 2.

No significant differences were found between the two groups with regard to the UCLA score, with 33.5 (30–35) for the allogenic tendon group and 34.1 (31–35) for the hook plate group ($P = 0.23$).

Discussion

The aim of our study was to introduce and evaluate the method using allogenic tendon to reconstruct the CC and AC ligaments for acute AC joint dislocation, and we also compared it with the hook plate to determine its merits and disadvantages. We believe that Rockwood types IV and V of AC joint injuries require operative treatment, and we proposed surgical treatment for patients with type III lesions involved in heavy labor or patients who participate in sports activities.

The tendon allograft played an important role in tendon and ligament reconstruction, particularly for the patients who have a shortage of autograft tendons or who do not want to use their own normally functioning tendons. Allograft tissue has many advantages over autograft tissue, including unlimited size, lack of donor site morbidity, and availability for revision surgery. The drawbacks of allogeneic tendons are that they may cause minimal immunogenicity and increase the chance of rejection compared with autograft tissues. The tendon as an allograft has low cellularity and is preserved at $-80°$ to elicit minimal immunogenicity. In our study, we did not find any adverse reactions after grafting of allogenic tendons, and the

preliminary clinical assessment did not find any significant adverse reactions [10–12]. Currently, the risk of viral transmission through allograft tissue transplantation is extremely low due to proper donor screening and tissue processing. The tendons we used were fully tested to exclude infectious diseases and sterilized to prevent the risk of infection from grafts. This documentation allowed us to use tendons from this company for recipients in our country. Therefore, we consider that reconstructing the CC and AC ligaments with allogenic tendons is a safe approach.

Up to now, more than 70 types of methods have been described for the treatment of acute AC joint dislocation, but no one method has been considered the best [13–32]. These surgical techniques can be grouped broadly into types such as fixation of the AC joint or fixation between the coracoid and clavicle and as dynamic muscle transfer or ligament reconstruction. The current literature shows the conoid ligament guarding against anterosuperior loading and the trapezoid guarding against posterior loading of the clavicle [33]. Debski et al. also clarified that the AC ligaments play an important role in constraint of horizontal motion of the distal clavicle [34]. Predicting that reconstructing the CC and AC ligaments with allogenic tendon would provide good stability of the AC joint, we designed and used this method and compared it with the hook plate procedure.

In the anatomic reconstruction method, two clavicle tunnels were used, and the allogenic tendon was passed around the base of the coracoid process (V shape), which recreated the anatomy of both the conoid and trapezoid ligaments. Based on the advantages of the V-shape technique, it was more likely that the patient would achieve greater overall stability by reducing the amount of abnormal translation. To successfully reconstruct the conoid and trapezoid ligaments using this technique, adequate exposure to the base of the coracoid is helpful and should be obtained. Subcoracoid suture placement is not completely anatomical, and poor visualization risks injury to nearby neurovascular structures; therefore, the separation and drilling should be performed with extreme care to maintain coracoid integrity and avoid potential fractures. The method we used was similar to that of Saccomanno [35] and was used at nearly the same time. The difference is that we used allogenic tendons and omitted the process of harvesting tendons.

Table 2 Clinical functional outcome of treated shoulder

	Pain (15)	Activity level (20)	Range of movement (40)	Power (25)	Constant score (100)
Allogenic tendon	14.3	19.5	37.3	23.4	94.4
Hook plate	14.4	19.4	37.8	22.3	93.8
P value	> 0.05	> 0.05	> 0.05	> 0.05	> 0.05

There are several causes of chronic pain after the surgical treatment of AC dislocations, one of which is persistent anteroposterior instability of the clavicle [36, 37]. By adding AC ligament reconstruction, the horizontal stability of the clavicle will be further strengthened. In our study, the VAS was 0.38, indicating that the results are quite good. Biomechanical studies of AC joint reconstruction with free-tissue graft for both the CC and AC ligaments provide AC joint stability similar to that of the intact AC joint and significantly better than that of the modified Weaver-Dunn procedure [38, 39]. Carofino and Mazzocca [40] used a technique that involves reconstruction of the superior AC ligament and capsule. In the presented method, we recreate the superior and inferior AC ligament and attain better stability. The results are encouraging and satisfactory.

Because of the good clinical outcomes, the hook plate remains one of the most commonly used methods for acute AC dislocations [41–44]. According to follow-up, the results confirmed that the efficacy of the clavicular hook plate was high. The advantage of the hook plate was the relatively easy implantation procedure and that it can provide immediate stability, which allows rapid healing of the torn ligaments and ensures early rehabilitation with a minimal risk of loss of reduction or implant failure. However, the implant had to be removed, which was a disadvantage and increased the rate of separation and medical costs. Compared with the hook plate, the method of allogenic tendon reconstruction did not require a second surgery and reduced the patient's pain.

We did not find any infections or other complications in either series. The hook plate is a reliable fixation tool for complete AC joint dislocations, ensuring immediate stability and allowing early mobilization with good functional and cosmetic results. With allogenic tendon grafts, the damaged anatomy can be restored without sacrificing any tendons or ligaments. Based on several in vitro biomechanical studies [38, 45–48] and our research, allogenic tendon graft reconstructions are likely to provide available alternatives for the treatment of operable AC joint dislocations. By controlling both the vertical and anteroposterior displacements of the clavicle, this technique offers strong biological reconstruction to maintain the AC joint reduction. Limitations of our study include the small number of patients and only acute injuries being studied. Further studies are necessary to confirm the reliability of this new method.

Conclusions

We prefer allografts because there is no donor site morbidity involved, and they are of adequate length to loop around the coracoid and over the clavicle. Moreover, they are readily available at our institution. Both techniques, allogenic tendon reconstruction and hook plate fixation, are effective procedures for the surgical treatment of AC joint acute dislocations of Rockwood III, IV, and V. There is no principle difference in functional outcomes between the two treatments; however, patients with allogenic tendon reconstruction do not require hardware removal and have less pain.

Abbreviations
AC: Acromioclavicular; CC: Coracoclavicular; UCLA: University of California-Los Angeles; VAS: Visual analog scale

Acknowledgements
We thank Rongrong Zhang for her help with drawing the diagram.

Authors' contributions
GHW had substantial contributions to collecting and analysis the data, assisted with operation, and was a major contributor in writing the manuscript. RGX had substantial contributions to conception and design of the study, organized the operation, and revised the manuscript. TM assisted with the operation and collected data in the study. SGX assisted with the operation and collected data in the study. All authors read and approved the final manuscript.

Competing interests
The authors declare that they have no competing interests.

References
1. Shaw MB, McInerney JJ, Dias JJ, Evans PA. Acromioclavicular joint sprains: the post-injury recovery interval. Injury. 2003;34:438–42. https://doi.org/10.1016/S0020-1383(02)00187-0.
2. Millett PJ, Braun S, Gobezie R, Pacheco IH. Acromioclavicular joint reconstruction with coracoacromial ligament transfer using the docking technique. BMC Musculoskelet Disord. 2009;14:10–6. https://doi.org/10.1186/1471-2474-10-6.
3. Boileau P, Old J, Gastaud O, Brassart N, Roussanne Y. All-arthroscopic Weaver-Dunn-Chuinard procedure with double-button fixation for chronic acromioclavicular joint dislocation. Arthroscopy. 2010;26:149–60. https://doi.org/10.1016/j.arthro.2009.08.008 . Epub 2009 Dec 30.
4. Spencer EE Jr. Treatment of grade III acromioclavicular joint injuries: a systematic review. Clin Orthop Relat Res. 2007;455:38–44.
5. Tienen TG, Oyen JF, Eggen P. A modified technique of reconstruction for complete acromioclavicular dislocation: a prospective study. Am J Sports Med. 2003;31:655–9.
6. Weinstein DM, McCann PD, McIlveen SJ, Flatow EL, Bigliani LU. Surgical treatment of complete acromioclavicular dislocations. Am J Sports Med. 1995;23:324–31.
7. Nicholas SJ, Lee SJ, Mullaney MJ, Tyler TF, McHugh MP. Clinical outcomes of coracoclavicular ligament reconstructions using tendon grafts. Am J Sports Med. 2007;35:1912–7. https://doi.org/10.1177/0363546507304715.
8. Constant CR, Murley AH. A clinical method of functional assessment of the shoulder. Clin Orthop Relat Res. 1987;214:160–4.
9. Ellman H, Hanker G, Bayer M. Repair of the rotator cuff. End-result study of factors influencing reconstruction. J Bone Joint Surg Am. 1986;68:1136–44.
10. Krocker D, Matziolis G, Pruss A, Perka C. Reconstruction of the extensor mechanism using a free, allogenic, freeze-dried patellar graft. Unfallchirurg. 2007;110:563–6.
11. Xie RG, Tang JB. Allograft tendon for second-stage tendon reconstruction. Hand Clin. 2012;28:503–9. https://doi.org/10.1016/j.hcl.2012.08.011.
12. Zhang Y, Yang K, Zhu W. Experimental research and clinical application of allogenic tendon grafting. Zhonghua Wai Ke Za Zhi. 1995;33:539–41.

13. Bannister GC, Wallace WA, Stableforth PG, Hutson MA. The management of acute acromioclavicular dislocation. A randomized prospective controlled trial. J Bone Joint Surg Br. 1989;71:848–50.

14. Boström Windhamre HA, von Heideken JP, Une-Larsson VE, Ekelund AL. Surgical treatment of chronic acromioclavicular dislocations: a comparative study of Weaver-Dunn augmented with PDS-braid or hook plate. J Shoulder Elb Surg. 2010;19:1040–8. https://doi.org/10.1016/j.jse.2010.02.006.

15. Bosworth BM. Acromioclavicular separation: new method of repair. Surg Gynecol Obstet. 1941;73:866–71.

16. Brunelli G, Brunelli F. The treatment of acromio-clavicular dislocation by transfer of the short head of the biceps. Int Orthop. 1988;12:105–8.

17. Dumontier C, Sautet A, Man M, Apoil A. Acromioclavicular dislocations: treatment by coracoacromial ligamentoplasty. J Shoulder Elb Surg. 1995;4: 130–4.

18. Ejam S, Lind T, Falkenberg B. Surgical treatment of acute and chronic acromioclavicular dislocation Tossy type III and V using the Hook plate. Acta Orthop Belg. 2008;74:441–5.

19. Jiang C, Wang M, Rong G.Proximally based conjoined tendon transfer for coracoclavicular reconstruction in the treatment of acromioclavicular dislocation. Surgical technique. J Bone Joint Surg Am. 2008;90: Suppl 2 Pt 2: 299–308. https://doi.org/10.2106/JBJS.H.00438.

20. Kappakas GS, McMaster J. Repair of acromioclavicular separation using a Dacron prosthesis graft. Clin Orthop Relat Res. 1978;31:247–51.

21. Korsten K, Gunning AC, Leenen LP. Operative or conservative treatment in patients with Rockwood type III acromioclavicular dislocation: a systematic review and update of current literature. Int Orthop. 2014;38:831–8. https://doi.org/10.1007/s00264-013-2143-7.

22. Larsen E, Bjerg-Nielsen A, Christensen P. Conservative or surgical treatment of acromioclavicular dislocation. A prospective, controlled, randomized study. J Bone Joint Surg Am. 1986;68:552–5.

23. Lemos MJ. The evaluation and treatment of the injured acromioclavicular joint in athletes. Am J Sports Med. 1998;26:137–44.

24. Luis GE, Yong CK, Singh DA, Sengupta S, Choon DS. Acromioclavicular joint dislocation: a comparative biomechanical study of the palmaris-longus tendon graft reconstruction with other augmentative methods in cadaveric models. J Orthop Surg Res. 2007;27(2):22.

25. Mlasowsky B, Brenner P, Düben W, Heymann H. Repair of complete acromioclavicular dislocation (Tossy stage III) using Balser's hook plate combined with ligament sutures. Injury. 1998;19:27–232.

26. Nüchtern JV, Sellenschloh K, Bishop N, Jauch S, Briem D, Hoffmann M, et al. Biomechanical evaluation of 3 stabilization methods on acromioclavicular joint dislocations. Am J Sports Med. 2013;41:1387–94. https://doi.org/10.1177/0363546513484892.

27. Paavolainen P, Björkenheim JM, Paukku P, Slätis P. Surgical treatment of acromioclavicular dislocation: a review of 39 patients. Injury. 1983;14:415–20.

28. Press J, Zuckerman JD, Gallagher M, Cuomo F. Treatment of grade III acromioclavicular separations. Operative versus nonoperative management. Bull Hosp Jt Dis. 1997;56:77–83.

29. Rockwood CA Jr, Williams GR Jr, Young DC. Disorders of the acromioclavicular joint. In: Rockwood Jr CA, Matsen FAIII, editors. The shoulder. 2nd ed. Philadelphia: WB Saunders; 1998. p. 483–553.

30. Salem KH, Schmelz A. Treatment of Tossy III acromioclavicular joint injuries using hook plates and ligament suture. J Orthop Trauma. 2009;23:565–9. https://doi.org/10.1097/BOT.0b013e3181971b38.

31. Weaver JK, Dunn HK. Treatment of acromioclavicular injuries, especially complete acromioclavicular separation. J Bone Joint Surg Am. 1972;54: 1187–94.

32. De Carli A, Lanzetti RM, Ciompi A, Lupariello D, Rota P, Ferretti A. Acromioclavicular third degree dislocation: surgical treatment in acute cases. J Orthop Surg Res. 2015;28:10:13. https://doi.org/10.1186/s13018-014-0150-z.

33. Debski RE, Parsons IM 3rd, Fenwick J, Vangura A. Ligament mechanics during three degree-of-freedom motion at the acromioclavicular joint. Ann Biomed Eng. 2000;28:612–8.

34. Debski RE, Parsons IM 4th, Woo SL, Fu FH. Effect of capsular injury on acromioclavicular joint mechanics. J Bone Joint Surg Am. 2001;83:1344–51.

35. Saccomanno MF, Fodale M, Capasso L, Cazzato G, Milano G. Reconstruction of the coracoclavicular and acromioclavicular ligaments with semitendinosus tendon graft: a pilot study. Joints. 2014;2:6–14.

36. Jerosch J, Filler T, Peuker E, Greig M, Siewering U. Which stabilization technique corrects anatomy best in patients with AC-separation? An experimental study. Knee Surg Sports Traumatol Arthrosc. 1999;7:365–72.

37. Taft TN, Wilson FC, Oglesby JW. Dislocation of the acromioclavicular joint. An end-result study. J Bone Joint Surg Am. 1987;69:1045–51.

38. Grutter PW, Petersen SA. Anatomical acromioclavicular ligament reconstruction: a biomechanical comparison of reconstructive techniques of the acromioclavicular joint. Am J Sports Med. 2005;33:1723–8. https://doi.org/10.1177/0363546505275646.

39. Michlitsch MG, Adamson GJ, Pink M, Estess A, Shankwiler JA, Lee TQ. Biomechanical comparison of a modified Weaver-Dunn and a free-tissue graft reconstruction of the acromioclavicular joint complex. Am J Sports Med. 2010;38:1196–203. https://doi.org/10.1177/0363546509361160.

40. Carofino BC, Mazzocca AD. The anatomic coracoclavicular ligament reconstruction: surgical technique and indications. J Shoulder Elb Surg. 2010;19:37–46. https://doi.org/10.1016/j.jse.2010.01.004.

41. De Baets T, Truijen J, Driesen R, Pittevils T. The treatment of acromioclavicular joint dislocation Tossy grade III with a clavicle hook plate. Acta Orthop Belg. 2004;70:515–9.

42. Folwaczny EK, Yakisan D, Sturmer KM. The Balser plate with ligament suture: a dependable method of stabilizing the acromioclavicular joint. Unfallchirurg. 2000;103:731–40.

43. Henkel T, Oetiker R, Hackenbruch W. Treatment of fresh Tossy III acromioclavicular joint dislocation by ligament suture and temporary fixation with the clavicular hooked plate. Swiss Surg. 1997;3:160–6.

44. Sim E, Schwarz N, Höcker K, Berzlanovich A. Repair of complete acromioclavicular separations using the acromioclavicular-hook plate. Clin Orthop Relat Res. 1995;314:134–42.

45. Costic RS, Labriola JE, Rodosky MW, Debski RE. Biomechanical rationale for development of anatomical reconstructions of coracoclavicular ligaments after complete acromioclavicular joint dislocations. Am J Sports Med. 2004; 32:1929–36. https://doi.org/10.1177/0363546504264637.

46. Harris RI, Wallace AL, Harper GD, Goldberg JA, Sonnabend DH, Walsh WR. Structural properties of the intact and the reconstructed coracoclavicular ligament complex. Am J Sports Med. 2000;28:103–8.

47. Jari R, Costic RS, Rodosky MW, Debski RE. Biomechanical function of surgical procedures for acromioclavicular joint dislocations. Arthroscopy. 2004;20: 237–45. https://doi.org/10.1016/j.arthro.2004.01.011.

48. Lee SJ, Nicholas SJ, Akizuki KH, McHugh MP, Kremenic IJ, Ben-Avi S. Reconstruction of the coracoclavicular ligaments with tendon grafts: a comparative biomechanical study. Am J Sports Med. 2003;31:648–55.

4

Optimization of parameters for femoral component implantation during TKA using finite element analysis and orthogonal array testing

Zhifang Mou[1†], Wanpeng Dong[2†], Zhen Zhang[2], Aohan Wang[2], Guanghong Hu[3], Bing Wang[4] and Yuefu Dong[4*]

Abstract

Background: Individualized and accurate implantation of a femoral component during total knee arthroplasty (TKA) is essential in achieving equal distribution of intra-articular stress and long-term survival of the prosthesis. However, individualized component implantation remains challenging. This study aimed to optimize and individualize the positioning parameters of a femoral component in order to facilitate its accurate implantation.

Methods: Using computer-simulated TKA, the positioning parameters of a femoral component were optimized individually by finite element analysis in combination with orthogonal array testing. Flexion angle, valgus angle, and external rotation angle were optimized in order to reduce the peak value of the pressure on the polyethylene liner of the prosthesis.

Results: The optimal implantation parameters of the femoral component were as follows: 1° flexion, 5° valgus angle, and 4° external rotation. Under these conditions, the peak value of the pressure on the polyethylene liner surface was minimized to 16.46 MPa. Among the three parameters, the external rotation angle had the greatest effect on the pressure, followed by the valgus angle and the flexion angle.

Conclusion: Finite element analysis in combination with orthogonal array testing can optimize the implantation parameters of a femoral component for TKA. This approach would possibly reduce the wear of the polyethylene liner and prolong the survival of the TKA prosthesis, due to its capacity to minimize stress. This technique represents a new method for preoperative optimization of the implantation parameters that can achieve the best possible TKA outcome.

Keywords: Total knee arthroplasty (TKA), Prosthesis, Implantation parameter, Optimization, Finite element analysis, Orthogonal array testing

Background

Total knee arthroplasty (TKA) is an effective therapy for terminal-stage osteoarthritis of the knee and can ameliorate pain, correct deformity, and improve the function of the joint [1]. Over 90% of implanted prostheses last approximately 10 to 15 years following TKA [2–4]. To date, TKA is a proven technique that is based on established surgical principles, among which accurate osteotomy and prosthesis implantation are fundamental requirements. TKA aims to restore the neutral mechanical alignment of the lower extremity and promote the uniform distribution of stress in the knee joint, thereby prolonging the survival of the prosthesis by reducing the wear on the polyethylene liner [5, 6]. Although a great number of factors can influence the survival of an implanted prosthesis, the surgical error that leads to implant malalignment is the most common cause of TKA failure [7–13]. The consequences of implant malalignment include an uneven distribution of intra-articular

* Correspondence: dongyuefu@163.com
[†]Zhifang Mou and Wanpeng Dong contributed equally to this work.
[4]Department of Orthopedics, The Affiliated Lianyungang Hospital of Xuzhou Medical University/the First People's Hospital of Lianyungang, Lianyungang, China
Full list of author information is available at the end of the article

load and of stress that eventually will require a revision [14]. Accurate implantation of an individualized TKA prosthesis could effectively reduce the surgical error and avoid the uneven distribution of the intra-articular load, thereby stabilizing the knee joint, reducing prosthetic loosening, and improving knee function [15–18].

The implantation of a TKA prosthesis aims to optimally restore the neutral mechanical alignment of the lower extremity, improve the therapeutic effect of the TKA, and prolong the survival of the prosthesis. Currently, the parameters used to guide the implantation of the prosthesis during TKA are usually determined by image data of the lower extremity [19]. Computer-navigated TKA can improve the accuracy of TKA prosthesis implantation and achieve a postoperative lower limb mechanical axis that is closer to the ideal position [20, 21]. Furthermore, patient-specific instrumentation has been reported to confer advantages over traditional TKA techniques with regard to the accuracy of prosthesis implantation, the efficient restoration of the neutral mechanical axis of the lower extremity, and the extension of the prosthesis survival [22, 23]. However, although a preoperative plan that is based on the anatomic features of a patient can aid the restoration of the neutral mechanical axis of the lower extremity, it cannot directly reveal the distribution of intra-articular stress and/or reliably predict the survival of the TKA prosthesis.

In the case of evenly distributed intra-articular stress, the contact surface area is increased and the stress on the polyethylene liner is decreased. This can maintain the long-term survival of the prosthesis. Therefore, an optimization of the prosthesis implantation parameters that is based on the intra-articular stress distribution in an individual patient could cause the even distribution of intra-articular stress following TKA. This strategy would be more efficient compared with a conventional preoperative planning. However, how to effectively determine the individualized optimal implantation parameters before TKA to make sure that stress of the knee joint is evenly distributed and the value is the smallest, as well as clarify the influence of different implantation parameters on stress to guide the accurate implantation of prosthesis during TKA surgery is currently a difficult problem of preoperative plan of TKA. Finite element analysis is an effective method for optimizing prosthesis implantation parameters that has been widely utilized for the design, selection, and postoperative evaluation of TKA prostheses [24, 25]. The repeatability of a finite element model allows the implantation parameters of TKA prosthesis to be effectively optimized. Using the finite element method, Cheng et al. analyzed the surface stress on the polyethylene liner caused by medial and lateral translation, anterior and posterior translation, and external rotation [26]. This study demonstrated that the peak value of the contact stress was altered by these

positioning changes, with external rotation having the greatest effect [26]. Similarly, Kang et al. highlighted that the increase in the external rotation angle resulted in a higher peak value of contact stress [13]. Although these studies demonstrated the potential clinical utility of finite element analysis for the optimization of TKA, this method has not yet been utilized to guide the implantation of an individualized TKA prosthesis. To date, a limited number of studies have described the use of finite element models in the preoperative planning of an individualized TKA prosthesis for implantation. Maybe this is due to the numerous TKA finite element models that require an extensive calculation time, which in turn limits the clinical application of this approach.

Orthogonal array testing can effectively reduce the number of TKA finite element models and improve the efficiency of the analysis prior to surgery. However, the use of orthogonal array testing for finite element modeling of TKA prosthesis has not been previously reported. We hypothesized that the implantation parameters of the femoral component could be optimized using a finite element model of the knee joint in combination with orthogonal array testing, thereby reducing the peak value of the pressure on the polyethylene liner and decreasing wear. Therefore, the main objectives of our study were (1) to determine whether finite element analysis in combination with orthogonal array testing could be used to reduce the stress on the polyethylene liner, (2) to obtain the ideal optimization, and (3) to establish which implantation parameter had the most influence on stress distribution. It was anticipated that optimization of the implantation parameters using finite element analysis and orthogonal array testing, based on the anatomy of each individual patient, could be used clinically as part of individualized preoperative planning to improve the accuracy of TKA prosthesis implantation.

Methods

Finite element model of the TKA knee joint

Three-dimensional (3D) model of the TKA prosthesis

The present study was approved by our institutional review board (No. 2016008), and informed consent was obtained from the volunteer. A cemented, posterior-stabilized knee prosthesis system (Smith and Nephew, Memphis, TN, USA) was scanned by the IMS IMPAC laser scanner (Renishaw, London, UK), and the .stl files were acquired. The .stl files were imported to the Mimics 12.0 software (Materialise, Leuven, Belgium), and 3D models of the TKA prosthetic components were generated (Fig. 1).

Simulated surgical implantation of the TKA prosthesis

The 3D models of the knee joint that were generated and validated by our previous studies were implanted by simulation surgery [27, 28]. Long-leg weight-bearing radiographs

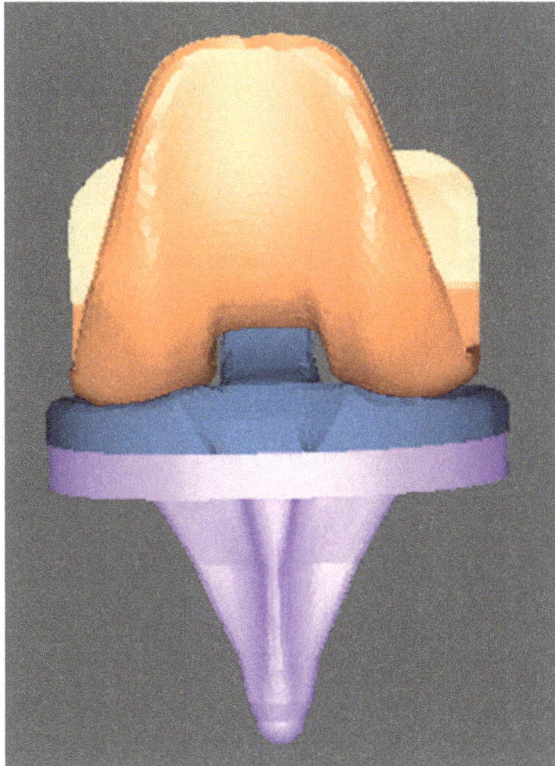

Fig. 1 3D model of the components of the prosthesis used for simulated TKA

were obtained from a 24-year-old man. Based on the anatomic characteristics of these radiographs, the valgus angle of the anatomic axis of the femur (i.e., relative to the long femoral shaft) and the mechanical axis of the femur (i.e., relative to the line connecting the center of the femoral head and the center of the knee joint) was 6°. Thus, the valgus angle of the distal femur was 6°. The femoral component implantation parameters were determined according to the conventional principles of TKA surgery: flexion 0° (i.e., the distal end of the femoral component was perpendicular to the femoral shaft axis in the sagittal plane), valgus 6° (in the coronal plane), and external rotation 3° (i.e., the posterior condylar line was rotated 3° externally with respect to the transepicondylar axis in the axial plane) (Fig. 2). These parameters were regarded as the standard parameters for positioning of the implanted femoral component and were used to construct the standard TKA model. Based on the anatomic characteristics of the lower extremities and knee joints of the volunteer as well as the principles of TKA surgery, an osteotomy was performed on the model of the femur and tibia using Mimics software. Based on the measurements obtained, No. 5 femoral and tibial component, 9-mm polyethylene liners, and 1-mm osteotomy plate were used to perform the osteotomy. A 1-mm gap was included between the prosthesis and osteotomy surface to preserve a space for implantation of a 1-mm-thick bone

cement layer. First, a distal femoral osteotomy was performed. The osteotomy surface was perpendicular to the femoral mechanical axis in the coronal plane and perpendicular to the femoral shaft axis in the sagittal plane so as to ensure a neutral implantation in the coronal and sagittal planes. The resection thickness was 11 mm to the distal articular surface of the medial condyle. The posterior condylar line was rotated 3° externally with respect to the transepicondylar axis in the axial plane. The anterior and posterior cut and the anterior and posterior oblique cut of the distal femur were obtained to complete the femoral osteotomy. Subsequently, a proximal tibial osteotomy was performed. The osteotomy surface was perpendicular to the tibial mechanical axis in the coronal plane with a posterior slope of 5° in the sagittal plane so as to ensure a neutral implantation in the coronal and sagittal planes. The thickness of the resection was 10 mm to the highest point of the lateral tibial plateau. The central line of the tibial component was aligned to the medial 1/3 of the tibial tubercle in the axial plane to complete the proximal tibial osteotomy. Finally, the femoral component, tibial component, and polyethylene liner were implanted to obtain a three-dimensional model of the knee joint after TKA (Fig. 3). After implanting the TKA prosthesis, two-dimensional and three-dimensional measurements and observations were used to confirm that the tangent surface of the most posteriorly edges of the femoral component and tibial component was aligned vertically. Posteriorly, the centerline of the femoral component was aligned to the centerline of the tibial component. Additionally, the contact areas between the femoral component and the medial and lateral compartments of the polyethylene liner were maximal and equal, ensuring matching between the components.

Finite element model of the TKA knee

The 3D models of the knee anatomic structures and TKA prosthetic components were imported into Hypermesh 15.0 software (Altair, Clifton Park, NY, USA) as .stl files; the space between the femoral component and the distal end of the femur and the space between the tibial component and the proximal end of the tibia were filled with 1-mm-thick bone cement [29]. Following generation of the mesh, the 3D finite element model of the TKA prosthesis, which we termed the standard model of the TKA knee joint, was constructed to include the femur, tibia, fibula, medial, and lateral collateral ligaments, as well as the femoral component, tibial component, polyethylene liner, and bone cement layers (Fig. 4).

Material properties, boundary conditions, and loading

The finite element analysis was carried out using the general-purpose FE code Abaqus v.6.14 (Simulia, Providence, RI, USA). The ligaments were defined as

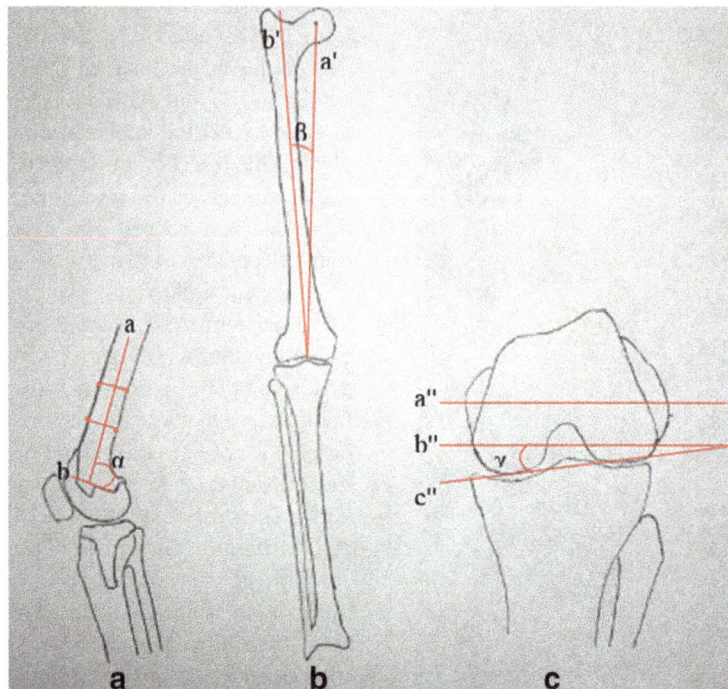

Fig. 2 Diagram illustrating the measurement of the implantation parameters for the TKA femoral component. **a** The flexion angle (in the sagittal plane) of the femoral component (α angle). Line a is the femoral shaft axis; line b lies along the bottom of the femoral implant. **b** The valgus angle (in the coronal plane) of the femoral component (β angle). Line a' is the anatomic axis of the femur; line b' is the mechanical axis of the femur. **c** The external rotation angle (in the axial plane) of the femoral component (γ angle). Line a" is the transepicondylar axis; line b" is parallel to the transepicondylar axis; and line c" is the posterior condylar line of the femur

anisotropic and hyperelastic and were modeled by an incompressible Neo-Hookean behavior with energy density function: $\psi = C_1(\widetilde{I}_1-3)$ (1), where C_1 is the initial shear modulus, and $\widetilde{I}_1$ is the first modified invariant for the right Cauchy-Green strain tensor [30]. The C_1 values of the lateral collateral ligament and medial collateral ligament were defined as 6.06 and 6.43, respectively [31]. The number of elements and the number of nodes were (964, 1620) and (1313, 2062), respectively. The remaining anatomic structures and TKA prosthetic components were modeled as isotropic linear elastic materials (Table 1). The following boundary conditions were defined:

1. The femur was limited at 0° flexion position, and all other two rotations and three translations were unconstrained. The tibia and fibula were limited in all translations and rotations.
2. Binding constraints were defined between the cortical bone and the cancellous bone, the prosthesis and the bone cement layer, and the bone cement layer and the osteotomy surface [32].
3. The lateral and medial collateral ligaments were rigidly attached to their corresponding bones, which facilitated the modeling of the ligament-bone attachment.

4. Nonlinear contact with a friction coefficient of 0.04 was assumed for the contact surfaces [33]. Two contact pairs were generated: one between the femoral component and polyethylene liner, and the other between the polyethylene liner and tibial component. The contact conditions were set as small sliding and finite sliding.

A reference vertical compressive load of 1150 N (along the Z axis, approximately twice the body weight) was applied to the midpoint of the femoral transepicondylar axis, simulating the load of the gait cycle for the 0° flexion position [27, 28, 30]. The variable in the peak value of the pressure on the polyethylene liner was observed.

Orthogonal array testing and optimization analysis
Orthogonal array testing is a design method that uses orthogonal tables to arrange and analyze multi-factor experiments. Orthogonal array testing selects some representative combinations from all the combinations of the experimental factors to perform the experiments. Through analysis of the results of these experiments, an optimal combination of experimental factors can be determined in a highly efficient and time-saving manner. Furthermore, through range analysis, the influence of

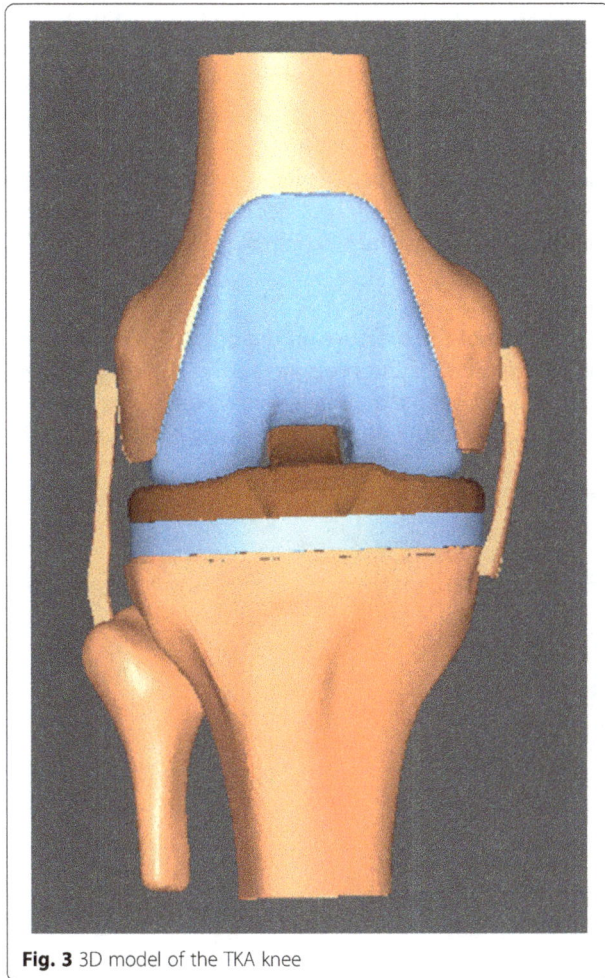

Fig. 3 3D model of the TKA knee

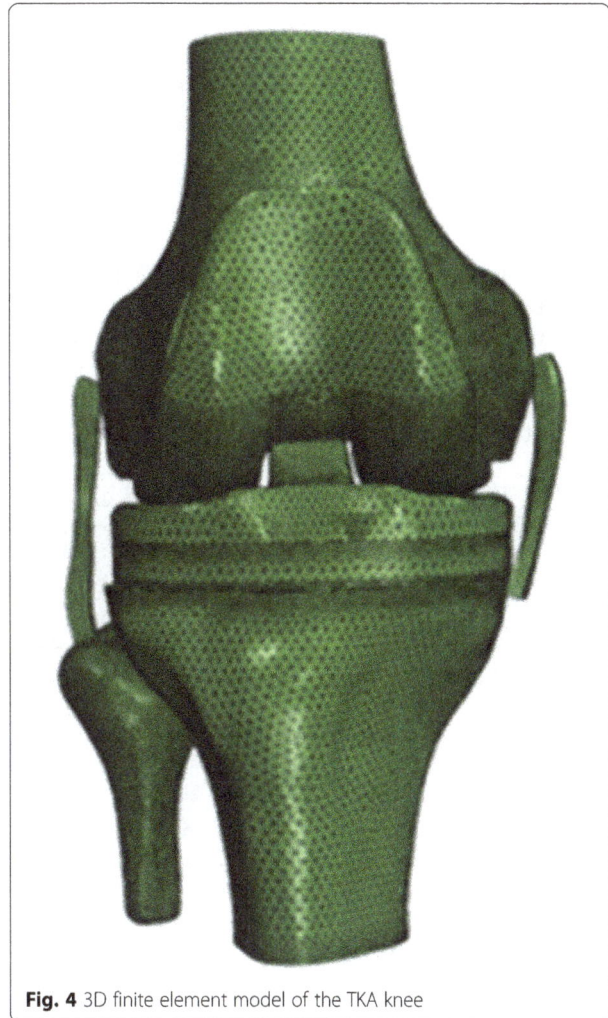

Fig. 4 3D finite element model of the TKA knee

various factors on the experimental indicators can be obtained, and the order of these factors can be determined. The advantages of orthogonal array testing and range analysis include (1) by taking advantage of the obtained experimental data, correct conclusions can be drawn based on a small number of tests rather than a comprehensive series of tests, thereby saving time; (2) the goal of optimization can be achieved; (3) the influence of various factors on the experimental indictors can be quantified; and (4) it is a straightforward technique to use, only requiring the arrangement of the experimental combinations according to the orthogonal tables.

The parameters flexion angle (A), valgus angle (B), and rotation angle (C) that were related to the positioning of the implanted femoral component were selected for optimization. Three levels were specified for each factor: the flexion angle of the femoral component was set at 0°, 1°, or 2°; the valgus angle was set at 5°, 6°, or 7°; and the rotation angle was set at 3°, 4°, or 5°. An orthogonal table, $L_9(3^4)$, was selected (Table 2). The standard TKA model was re-adjusted in Hypermesh software to

construct different TKA models that fulfilled the requirement of the orthogonal array testing.

According to the orthogonal array testing, nine TKA finite element models were generated (using different combinations of position parameters of the femoral component). The definition of the material properties, boundary conditions, and loading was identical for each model. The peak values of the pressure induced by

Table 1 Material properties, element number, and node for the TKA knee

	Elastic modulus (MPa)	Poisson's ratio	Element number	Node number
Cortical bone	16,600	0.3	23,117	7865
Cancellous bone	2400	0.3	53,675	12,024
Femoral component	210,000	0.3	84,796	21,431
Tibial component	117,000	0.3	37,532	9551
Polyethylene liner	685	0.4	28,248	7917
Bone cement layer	3000	0.3	32,852	11,144

Table 2 Design of the orthogonal array testing

Plane	Experimental factors		
	Flexion angle A (°)	Valgus angle B (°)	External rotation C (°)
1	0	5	3
2	1	6	4
3	2	7	5

different implantation parameters were compared and ranked using finite element analysis and orthogonal array testing. Subsequently, the minimal peak value of the pressure was obtained, and the corresponding implantation parameters were considered to be the optimal parameters of the femoral component.

Validation of the optimized parameters derived from the orthogonal array testing

A finite element model of the TKA knee was re-constructed using the implantation parameters optimized by the orthogonal array testing. The distribution of the peak pressure of the pressure on the polyethylene liner was analyzed and compared with that of all the other models in order to validate the optimized parameters (Fig. 5).

Results

Distribution of the pressure on the polyethylene liner

The distribution of the pressure on the polyethylene liner was acquired, and the peak value of the stress for each model is shown in Table 3. The highest peak value of the

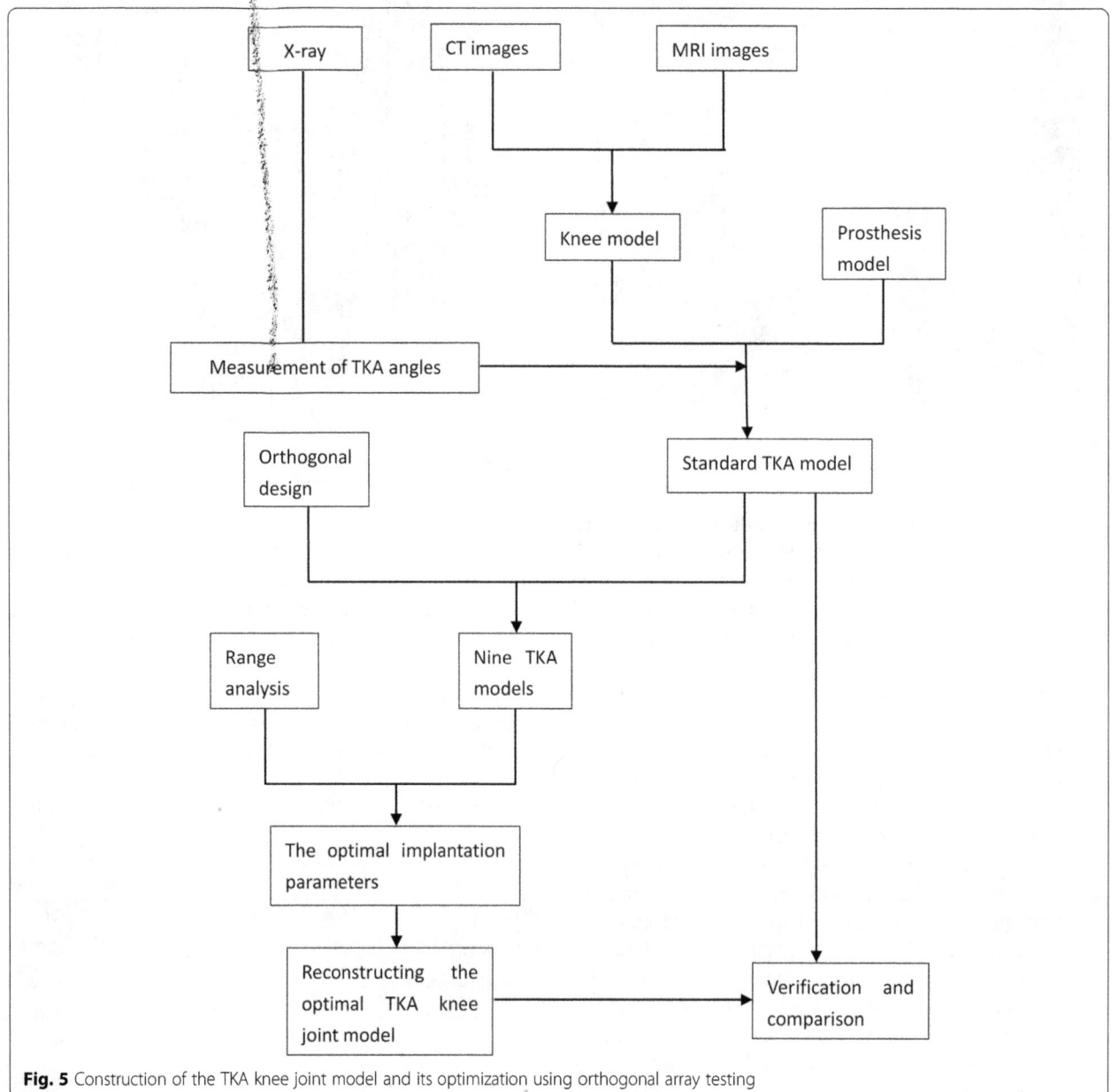

Fig. 5 Construction of the TKA knee joint model and its optimization using orthogonal array testing

Table 3 Experimental level combinations of the orthogonal array testing

Model	Experimental level combination	Flexion angle (°)	Valgus angle (°)	External rotation (°)	Peak value of the pressure (MPa)
1	$A_1B_1C_1$	0	5	3	21.29
2	$A_1B_2B_2$	0	6	4	19.82
3	$A_1B_3C_3$	0	7	5	30.83
4	$A_2B_1C_2$	1	5	4	16.46
5	$A_2B_2C_3$	1	6	5	27.25
6	$A_2B_3C_1$	1	7	3	24.49
7	$A_3B_1C_3$	2	5	5	24.07
8	$A_3B_2C_1$	2	6	3	30.22
9	$A_3B_3C_2$	2	7	4	23.68

pressure among the nine models was 30.83 MPa (group $A_1B_3C_3$, Fig. 6c), which occurred in the medial compartment; the lowest peak value of the pressure was 16.46 MPa (group $A_2B_1C_2$, Fig. 6d), which was also observed in the medial compartment. The findings indicated that minor variations in the implantation parameters could result in

relatively large changes in the stress, highlighting the importance of accurate prosthesis implantation. The standard model of the TKA knee was not included in the nine constructed models but was also examined: the peak value of the pressure on the polyethylene liner was 18.14 MPa (Fig. 6j) and was localized in the medial compartment.

Parameter optimization by orthogonal array testing

Using the orthogonal array experimental design, the range analysis of the peak values of the pressure from the nine models was carried out. The results of this analysis are shown in Table 4, in which K_{ji} represents the mean of the peak value of the stress for the experimental factor j at level i.

The range was calculated using the following formula: $R_j = \max_{1 \le i \le m} k_{ji} - \min_{1 \le i \le m} k_{ji}$ (2), where R_j represents the range of experimental factor j, and m represents the number of the level. For example, the maximum K_{13} was 25.99 and the minimum K_{12} was 22.73 under the first factor; thus, the range R_1 (K_{13}-K_{12}) was 3.26. The range analysis suggested that among the three factors studied,

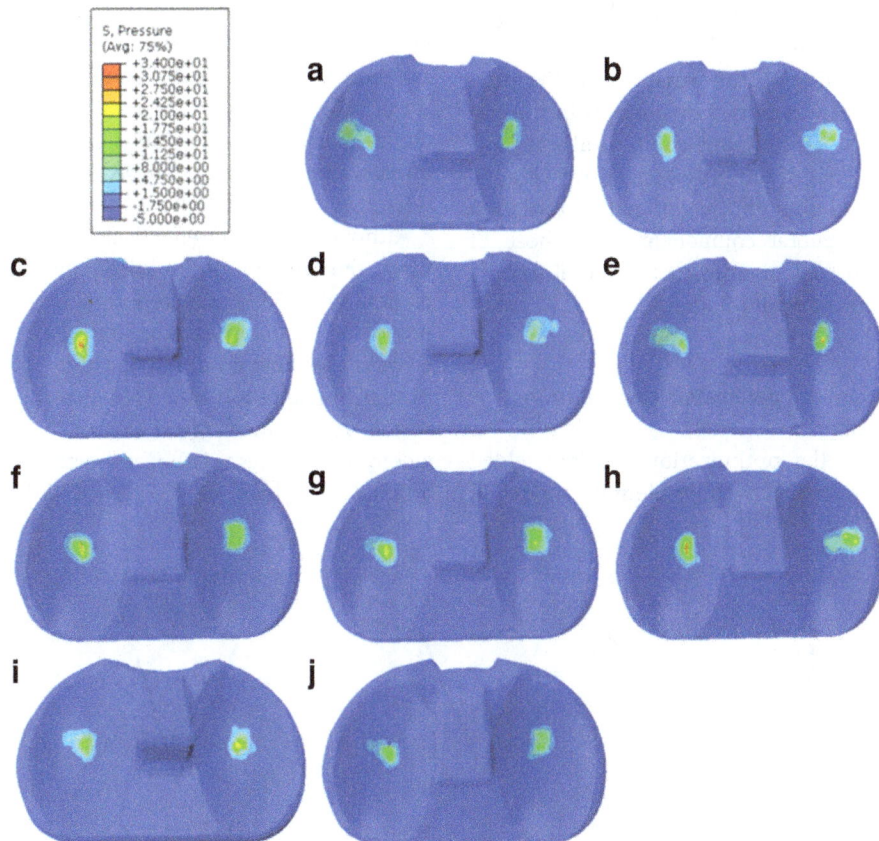

Fig. 6 Distribution of the pressure on the polyethylene liner. **a**: model of group $A_1B_1C_1$. **b**: model of group $A_1B_2C_2$. **c**: model of group $A_1B_3C_3$. **d**: model of group $A_2B_1C_2$. **e**: model of group $A_2B_2C_3$. **f**: model of group $A_2B_3C_1$. **g**: model of group $A_3B_1C_3$. **h**: model of group $A_3B_2C_1$. **i**: model of group $A_3B_3C_2$. **j**: standard model

Table 4 Optimization of the results of the orthogonal array testing

Model	Experimental factor j (j = 1, 2, 3, 4)				Peak value of the pressure (MPa)
	A	B	C	D	
1	1	1	1	1	21.29
2	1	2	2	2	19.82
3	1	3	3	3	30.83
4	2	1	2	3	16.46
5	2	2	3	1	27.25
6	2	3	1	2	24.49
7	3	1	3	2	24.07
8	3	2	1	3	30.22
9	3	3	2	1	23.68
K_{j1}	23.98	20.61	25.33	24.07	
K_{j2}	22.73	25.76	19.99	22.79	
K_{j3}	25.99	26.33	27.38	25.84	
Rang R_j	3.26	5.72	7.39	3.05	
Ranking	C > B > A				
Optimal level	A_2	B_1	C_2		

the external rotation angle exhibited the highest pressure effect on the polyethylene liner, followed by the valgus angle and the flexion angle.

A trend diagram indicating the variations in the peak value of the stress that was caused by changes in the implantation parameters of the femoral component was plotted by the range analysis of the orthogonal array (Fig. 7). According to the trend diagram, the optimal implantation parameters for the femoral component were those of group $A_2B_1C_2$, which corresponded to 1° femoral flexion, 5° valgus angle, and 4° external rotation.

Validation of the optimized parameters derived from orthogonal array testing

In order to validate the optimization results yielded by orthogonal array testing, a finite element model of

the TKA knee was constructed based on the optimized implantation parameters, namely $A_2B_1C_2$. The minimal peak value of the pressure was 16.46 MPa, which was 46.6% lower than the maximal peak value (30.83 MPa) and 9.3% lower than that of the standard model.

Discussion

The methods that enable accurate implantation of the TKA prosthesis for each patient can ensure that intra-articular stress is evenly distributed across the liner. The minimization of stress would be expected to reduce the wear of the polyethylene liner and prolong the survival of the TKA prosthesis. In the current study, the optimized implantation parameters for the TKA prosthesis were obtained using finite element analysis in combination with orthogonal array testing. The lowest pressure on the polyethylene liner was achieved with femoral component implantation parameters that included 1° flexion, 5° valgus angle, and 4° external rotation. The present findings indicate that among the three factors that influence the pressure on the polyethylene liner, the external rotation angle had the greatest effect followed by the valgus and the flexion angles. This suggests that both the external rotation angle and the valgus angle are important parameters during TKA surgery that are required to ensure accurate implantation of the prosthesis. We envisage that our technique could be used clinically during preoperative planning to optimize the implantation parameters based on the anatomic characteristics of each individual patient.

Although TKA can effectively ameliorate pain and improve the function of the knee joint, the post-TKA satisfaction rate (90%) was reported to be lower than that noted for total hip arthroplasty [34]. Surgical technical error is the most common cause of TKA failure [7]. Improper implantation of a TKA prosthesis leading to loss of the neutral mechanical axis of the lower extremity is a common technical issue, and orthopedic surgeons have attempted various approaches in order to improve the

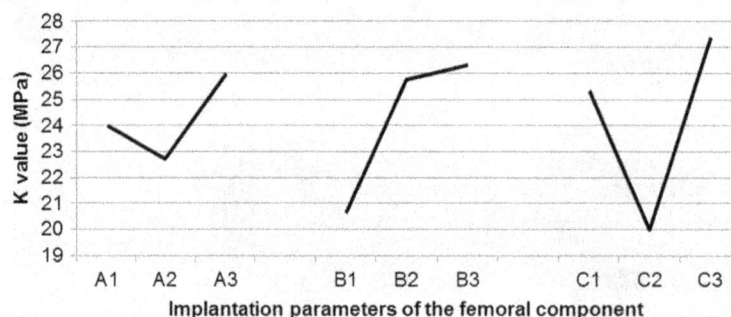

Fig. 7 Trend diagram showing the variations in the peak value of the pressure (K value) caused by changes in the implantation parameters of the femoral component

accuracy of implantation, the therapeutic efficacy, and the post-TKA satisfaction. A detailed preoperative planning can aid the optimization of the accuracy of prosthesis implantation and restore the neutral alignment of the mechanical axis. Currently, prosthesis implantation parameters are usually obtained from preoperative imaging studies of the patient's lower extremities [19]. In the current study, the TKA prosthesis implantation parameters were determined through finite element analysis in combination with orthogonal array testing. This is a technique that has shown great promise in the improvement of the accuracy of prosthesis implantation and the reduction of the surgical technical error. The present study utilized computer simulations that allowed preoperative prediction of the distribution of the intra-articular stress. Using finite element analysis and orthogonal array testing, it was possible to reduce the peak value of the pressure on the polyethylene liner by 9.3% compared with conventional preoperative measurements. Such a reduction in peak pressure would be predicted to reduce the wear of the polyethylene liner and decrease the rate of prosthesis loosening, thereby increasing the survival time of the prosthesis. The current method that was developed for the determination of the prosthesis implantation parameters differs from that used conventionally and has not been described previously. Although the research objectives differed between the present study and previous investigations, the distribution of stress in the standard model of our study was similar to that of models described in the published literature [6, 35, 36]. Moreover, the peak value of the stress in the medial compartment was higher than that in the lateral compartment [6, 35, 36].

Accurate implantation of a prosthesis can lead to a neutral mechanical axis of the lower extremity, longer prosthesis survival, amelioration of pain, and improved function [37, 38]. Previous studies have suggested that a deviation in the mechanical axis of the lower extremity of equal to and/or less than 3° (≤ 3°) can achieve optimal clinical efficacy and longer survival. Huijbregts et al. demonstrated that the prognosis of patients was poor when the deviation of the mechanical axis of the lower extremity was larger than 3° in the coronal plane, implying that the distal femoral osteotomy angle in the coronal plane was an essential factor that contributed to the efficacy of the prosthesis [39]. Kim et al. determined that longer stability could be achieved when the mechanical axis of the femoral component in the sagittal plane ranged between 0° and 3° [40]. In addition, Gromov et al. reported that the clinical results were optimal and the survival period was increased to its maximum when the external rotation angle that was relative to the posterior condylar axis, ranged between 2° and 5° in the axial plane [41]. Consistent with previous investigations, we determined that the optimized implantation of a femoral

component could reduce stress in the liner, with the key parameters for accurate implantation being the femoral flexion, the valgus, and external rotation angles. A notable finding of the present study was that the peak value of the pressure on the polyethylene liner varied greatly from a maximal value of 30.83 MPa to a minimal value of 16.46 MPa, corresponding to a difference of 14.37 MPa (87.3%). This variation was evident even within the conventionally accepted range of parameters for the implantation of the femoral component. It was reported by Matsuda et al. that a 5° alteration of the valgus angle in the coronal plane led to a 50% increase in the contact stress on the polyethylene liner of a femoral component [42]. By comparison, we found that a 2° alteration of the valgus angle, from 1° valgus to 1° varus, led to an 87.3% increase in the stress on the polyethylene liner. Moreover, additional alterations in the sagittal plane and in the axial rotation synergistically amplified this effect. Therefore, alterations in the implantation parameters of a femoral component can greatly affect the peak value of the pressure on the polyethylene liner, even when the surgical technical error is within the clinically accepted range. This highlights the potential benefits of developing new techniques in order to refine the accuracy of TKA prosthesis implantation.

Previous studies have shown that neutral mechanical alignment (0° ± 3°) of the lower extremities after TKA surgery can obtain a better long-term prosthesis survival rate [37–39]. However, it is still possible that aseptic loosening can occur after TKA surgery [43]. Lee et al. reported that 13 of 687 TKA knee joints in the neutral position had aseptic loosening within 8 years [44]. In this study, compressive stress in the medial or lateral compartment was not evenly distributed even when the positional alignment of the lower extremities was controlled at 0° ± 1°. The uneven distribution of stress in the medial and lateral compartments may eventually lead to the occurrence of aseptic loosening of TKA knee joints with a neutral mechanical alignment. In 7 of the 10 constructed models of the TKA knee joint, the peak value of the compressive stress was higher in the medial compartment than in the external compartment. Moreover, the highest peak value of compressive stress (30.83 MPa) was in the medial compartment, which is consistent with the clinical phenomenon that the internal tibial plateau of the TKA knee joint is susceptible to bone resorption and collapse [45]. These findings further suggest that we should pay attention to maintaining good rotation, flexion alignment, and soft tissue balance of the prosthesis as well as ensure alignment of the lower extremities in the neutral alignment after TKA surgery.

Previous studies have utilized finite element analyses in order to elucidate the effects of implantation parameters on the stress of the femoral component. These investigations have suggested that different parameters exert varying effects. One study determined that the internal-external rotation, the medial-lateral translation, and the anterior-posterior translation could change the stress on a polyethylene liner by 27.1, 23.3, and 7.63%, respectively [26]. Among these parameters, the angle of the external rotation had the greatest effect [26]. Similarly, it was found by Liau et al. that alterations in the internal translation, internal rotation, and varus angle of a femoral component could induce changes in the stress of 67.6, 14.3, and 145.9%, respectively; the varus angle exerted the largest effect on contact stress [46]. In the current study, the flexion, valgus, and external rotation angles of the TKA prosthesis were analyzed by orthogonal array testing in order to investigate their effects on the pressure on the polyethylene liner. The current method resulted in the determination of the optimal parameters that could be used for preoperative planning and during the surgery in order to achieve accurate implantation. The optimal parameters for femoral component implantation were 1° flexion, 5° valgus angle, and 4° external rotation, which minimized the peak value of the stress on the polyethylene liner to 16.46 MPa. These parameters differed from the parameters obtained by conventional anatomic measurements based on radiography, i.e., 0° flexion, 6° valgus, and 3° external rotation [41]. Using the conventional parameters, the peak value of the pressure on the polyethylene liner was 18.14 MPa (i.e., 9.3% higher than that for the optimal parameters), implying that an implanted femoral component with a little bit of flexion, reduced valgus, and increased external rotation could decrease the stress on the liner. An optimal match between the femoral component and the polyethylene liner was obtained and resulted in a maximum increase in the contact surface area and a minimum decrease in the stress on the liner [26]. In the current study, the variation of the three factors was within the clinically acceptable range and this revealed that the external rotation angle exhibited the greatest effect on the stress, followed by the valgus and the flexion angles. It is likely that the external rotation and the valgus angles exhibited a greater effect on the matching between the femoral component and the polyethylene liner compared with the flexion angle. This indicated that the suboptimal values used for the external rotation and the valgus angles could contribute notably to increased wear damage to the liner. Therefore, during TKA, attention should be paid with regard to the correct external rotation and valgus angles.

A notable feature of the current study was that the orthogonal array testing was utilized in order to reduce the number of TKA models and enhance the efficiency of the analysis. A total of 27 finite element models of the TKA knee would be required in order to include three implantation parameters as well as three different levels

in the analysis; the orthogonal array testing effectively reduced the workload to only nine models. Therefore, the orthogonal array testing simplified the preoperative analysis and was far less time-consuming compared with the use of the 27 models. To the best of our knowledge, this is the first study to demonstrate that the combination of finite element analysis and orthogonal array testing can enhance the efficiency of preoperative planning with regard to the optimization of the implantation of the TKA prosthesis. We suggest that this approach could be applied in clinical practice to improve the accuracy of TKA.

The method of femoral component implantation optimization used in this study and the results obtained are not applicable to kinematically aligned TKA because the surgical ideas and principles of mechanically aligned TKA are completely different to those of kinematically aligned TKA. The principle of mechanically aligned TKA surgery is to correct lower extremity deformity and restore the neutral mechanical alignment of the lower extremities (achieved through varying amounts of resection of the medial and lateral condyles and through soft tissue balance, etc.) in order to distribute the load evenly in the knee joint [15, 18]. However, the idea of kinematically aligned TKA is to restore the natural physiological state and mechanical alignment of the lower extremity, using techniques such as equal amounts of resection of the medial and lateral condyles, and to reduce the release of soft tissues as much as possible [47, 48]. For the knee joint in our case, the optimal implantation parameters for the femoral component were 1° flexion, 5° valgus, and 4° external rotation. However, if kinematically aligned TKA was applied, the implantation parameters for the femoral component would need to be 0° flexion (to maintain a good patellar tracking), 8° valgus (through measurement, to ensure equal amounts of resection of the distal femur), and 0° external rotation (to ensure equal amounts of resection of the posterior femoral condyle). Furthermore, kinematically aligned TKA usually uses a cruciate-retaining knee prosthesis rather than a posterior-stabilized knee prosthesis.

The present study has some limitations. Firstly, the cortical and cancellous bones of the knee joint are nonlinear materials, and their properties would be even more complex under pathological conditions such as osteoporosis. However, the bones of the knee joint were simplified into isotropic linear elastic materials. Nonetheless, we believe this simplification is acceptable when the elastic modulus of the femoral and tibial prosthesis is considered. Furthermore, for patients with severe osteoporosis, the elastic moduli of the femur and tibia could be reduced during the process of finite element analysis. Secondly, the study was conducted under the simulated condition of a static, straight position. The results would be more reliable if the intra-articular stress distribution was analyzed under dynamic conditions, for example if the changes in stress in the knee joint were examined under different flexion angles. Thirdly, only the femoral component was optimized, whereas optimization of the tibial component was not considered. Optimization of the tibial component as well as the femoral component would likely yield results that were closer to the clinically accepted targets. Lastly, the emphasis of the study was the accuracy of femoral component implantation and the soft tissue balance was not considered. In future studies, the effect of soft tissue balance on intra-articular stress should be explored.

Conclusions

In summary, the current study demonstrated that the implantation of a TKA femoral component could be optimized using finite element analysis in combination with orthogonal array testing in order to minimize the peak value of the pressure on the polyethylene liner. Furthermore, the effects of various implantation parameters on the stress were determined. Notably, even minor alterations of the implantation parameters within the clinically acceptable range resulted in substantial changes in the peak value of the pressure on the polyethylene liner. The orthopedic surgeon should pay particular attention to the external rotation and valgus angles in order to ensure accurate implantation of a femoral component. The method based on finite element analysis of femoral component implantation could also be used for tibial component implantation. Our novel technique represents a new approach for preoperative planning and optimization of the implantation parameters in order to achieve the best possible TKA results.

Abbreviations

3D: Three-dimensional; TKA: Total knee arthroplasty

Funding

This work was supported by the National Natural Science Foundation of China (grant number 31670956).

Authors' contributions

ZFM and WPD conceived and coordinated the study, designed, performed, and analyzed the experiments, and wrote the paper. ZZ, AHW, GHH, BW, and YFD carried out the data collection and data analysis, and revised the paper. All authors reviewed the results and approved the final version of the manuscript.

Competing interests

The authors declare that they have no competing interests.

Author details

[1]Department of Critical Care Medicine, The Affiliated Lianyungang Hospital of Xuzhou Medical University/the First People's Hospital of Lianyungang, Lianyungang, China. [2]School of Materials Engineering, Shanghai University of Engineering Science, Shanghai, China. [3]Institute of Plasticity Forming Technology & Equipment, Shanghai Jiao Tong University, Shanghai, China. [4]Department of Orthopedics, The Affiliated Lianyungang Hospital of Xuzhou Medical University/the First People's Hospital of Lianyungang, Lianyungang, China.

References

1. Allen CL, Hooper GJ, Oram BJ, Wells JE. Does computer-assisted total knee arthroplasty improve the overall component position and patient function? Int Orthop. 2014;38:251–7.
2. Colizza WA, Insall JN, Scuderi GR. The posterior stabilized total knee prosthesis. Assessment of polyethylene damage and osteolysis after a ten-year-minimum follow-up. J Bone Joint Surg Am. 1995;77:1713–20.
3. Emmerson KP, Moran CG, Pinder IM. Survivorship analysis of the kinematic stabilizer total knee replacement: a 10- to 14-year follow-up. J Bone Joint Surg Br. 1996;78:441–5.
4. Sharkey PF, Hozack WJ, Rothman RH, Shastri S, Jacoby SM. Insall award paper. Why are total knee arthroplasties failing today? Clin Orthop Relat Res. 2002;(404):7–13.
5. Berend ME, Ritter MA, Meding JB, Faris PM, Keating EM, Redelman R, et al. Tibial component failure mechanisms in total knee arthroplasty. Clin Orthop Relat Res. 2004;(428):26–34.
6. Innocenti B, Bellemans J, Catani F. Deviations from optimal alignment in TKA: is there a biomechanical difference between femoral or tibial component alignment? J Arthroplast. 2016;31:295–301.
7. Incavo SJ, Wild JJ, Coughlin KM, Beynnon BD. Early revision for component malrotation in total knee arthroplasty. Clin Orthop Relat Res. 2007;458:131–6.
8. Jacobs MA, Hungerford DS, Krackow KA, Lennox DW. Revision total knee arthroplasty for aseptic failure. Clin Orthop Relat Res. 1988;(226):78–85.
9. Akagi M, Matsusue Y, Mata T, Asada Y, Horiguchi M, Iida H, et al. Effect of rotational alignment on patellar tracking in total knee arthroplasty. Clin Orthop Relat Res. 1999;(366):155–63.
10. Berger RA, Crossett LS, Jacobs JJ, Rubash HE. Malrotation causing patellofemoral complications after total knee arthroplasty. Clin Orthop Relat Res. 1998;(356):144–53.
11. Hakki S, Coleman S, Saleh K, Bilotta VJ, Hakki A. Navigational predictors in determining the necessity for collateral ligament release in total knee replacement. J Bone Joint Surg Br. 2009;91:1178–82.
12. Ghosh KM, Merican AM, Iranpour F, Deehan DJ, Amis AA. The effect of femoral component rotation on the extensor retinaculum of the knee. J Orthop Res. 2010;28:1136–41.
13. Kang KT, Koh YG, Son J, Kwon OR, Baek C, Jung SH, et al. Measuring the effect of femoral malrotation on knee joint biomechanics for total knee arthroplasty using computational simulation. Bone Joint Res. 2016;5:552–9.
14. Wong J, Steklov N, Patil S, Flores-Hernandez C, Kester M, Colwell CW Jr, et al. Predicting the effect of tray malalignment on risk for bone damage and implant subsidence after total knee arthroplasty. J Orthop Res. 2011;29:347–53.
15. Fang DM, Ritter MA, Davis KE. Coronal alignment in total knee arthroplasty: just how important is it? J Arthroplast. 2009;24:39–43.
16. Parratte S, Pagnano MW, Trousdale RT, Berry DJ. Effect of postoperative mechanical axis alignment on the fifteen-year survival of modern, cemented total knee replacements. J Bone Joint Surg Am. 2010;92:2143–9.
17. Bonner TJ, Eardley WG, Patterson P, Gregg PJ. The effect of post-operative mechanical axis alignment on the survival of primary total knee replacements after a follow-up of 15 years. J Bone Joint Surg Br. 2011;93:1217–22.
18. Sikorski JM. Alignment in total knee replacement. J Bone Joint Surg Br. 2008;90:1121–7.
19. Tanzer M, Makhdom AM. Preoperative planning in primary total knee arthroplasty. J Am Acad Orthop Surg. 2016;24:220–30.
20. Todesca A, Garro L, Penna M, Bejui-Hugues J. Conventional versus computer-navigated TKA: a prospective randomized study. Knee Surg Sports Traumatol Arthrosc. 2017;25:1778–83.
21. Tingart M, Luring C, Bathis H, Beckmann J, Grifka J, Perlick L. Computer-assisted total knee arthroplasty versus the conventional technique: how

precise is navigation in clinical routine? Knee Surg Sports Traumatol Arthrosc. 2008;16:44–50.

22. Anderl W, Pauzenberger L, Kolblinger R, Kiesselbach G, Brandl G, Laky B, et al. Patient-specific instrumentation improved mechanical alignment, while early clinical outcome was comparable to conventional instrumentation in TKA. Knee Surg Sports Traumatol Arthrosc. 2016;24:102–11.

23. Ferrara F, Cipriani A, Magarelli N, Rapisarda S, De Santis V, Burrofato A, et al. Implant positioning in TKA: comparison between conventional and patient-specific instrumentation. Orthopedics. 2015;38:e271–80.

24. D'Lima DD, Chen PC, Colwell CW Jr. Polyethylene contact stresses, articular congruity, and knee alignment. Clin Orthop Relat Res. 2001;(392):232–8.

25. Thompson JA, Hast MW, Granger JF, Piazza SJ, Siston RA. Biomechanical effects of total knee arthroplasty component malrotation: a computational simulation. J Orthop Res. 2011;29:969–75.

26. Cheng CK, Huang CH, Liau JJ, Huang CH. The influence of surgical malalignment on the contact pressures of fixed and mobile bearing knee prostheses—a biomechanical study. Clin Biomech (Bristol, Avon). 2003;18:231–6.

27. Dong Y, Hu G, Dong Y, Hu Y, Xu Q. The effect of meniscal tears and resultant partial meniscectomies on the knee contact stresses: a finite element analysis. Comput Methods Biomech Biomed Engin. 2014;17:1452–63.

28. Dong Y, Hu G, Yang H, Zhang L, Hu Y, Dong Y, et al. Accurate 3D reconstruction of subject-specific knee finite element model to simulate the articular cartilage defects. J Shanghai Jiaotong Univ (Sci). 2011;16:620–7.

29. Perillo-Marcone A, Taylor M. Effect of varus/valgus malalignment on bone strains in the proximal tibia after TKR: an explicit finite element study. J Biomech Eng. 2007;129:1–11.

30. Pena E, Calvo B, Martinez MA, Palanca D, Doblare M. Finite element analysis of the effect of meniscal tears and meniscectomies on human knee biomechanics. Clin Biomech (Bristol, Avon). 2005;20:498–507.

31. Weiss JA, Gardiner JC. Computational modeling of ligament mechanics. Crit Rev Biomed Eng. 2001;29:303–71.

32. Chang TW, Yang CT, Liu YL, Chen WC, Lin KJ, Lai YS, et al. Biomechanical evaluation of proximal tibial behavior following unicondylar knee arthroplasty: modified resected surface with corresponding surgical technique. Med Eng Phys. 2011;33:1175–82.

33. Halloran JP, Easley SK, Petrella AJ, Rullkoetter PJ. Comparison of deformable and elastic foundation finite element simulations for predicting knee replacement mechanics. J Biomech Eng. 2005;127:813–8.

34. Zihlmann MS, Stacoff A, Romero J, Quervain IK, Stussi E. Biomechanical background and clinical observations of rotational malalignment in TKA: literature review and consequences. Clin Biomech (Bristol, Avon). 2005;20:661–8.

35. Sharma A, Komistek RD, Ranawat CS, Dennis DA, Mahfouz MR. In vivo contact pressures in total knee arthroplasty. J Arthroplast. 2007;22:404–16.

36. Werner FW, Ayers DC, Maletsky LP, Rullkoetter PJ. The effect of valgus/varus malalignment on load distribution in total knee replacements. J Biomech. 2005;38:349–55.

37. Banerjee S, Cherian JJ, Elmallah RK, Jauregui JJ, Pierce TP, Mont MA. Robotic-assisted knee arthroplasty. Expert Rev Med Devices. 2015;12:727–35.

38. Song EK, Seon JK, Yim JH, Netravali NA, Bargar WL. Robotic-assisted TKA reduces postoperative alignment outliers and improves gap balance compared to conventional TKA. Clin Orthop Relat Res. 2013;471:118–26.

39. Huijbregts HJ, Khan RJ, Fick DP, Hall MJ, Punwar SA, Sorensen E, et al. Component alignment and clinical outcome following total knee arthroplasty: a randomised controlled trial comparing an intramedullary alignment system with patient-specific instrumentation. Bone Joint J. 2016; 98-B:1043–9.

40. Kim YH, Park JW, Kim JS, Park SD. The relationship between the survival of total knee arthroplasty and postoperative coronal, sagittal and rotational alignment of knee prosthesis. Int Orthop. 2014;38:379–85.

41. Gromov K, Korchi M, Thomsen MG, Husted H, Troelsen A. What is the optimal alignment of the tibial and femoral components in knee arthroplasty? Acta Orthop. 2014;85:480–7.

42. Matsuda S, Whiteside LA, White SE. The effect of varus tilt on contact stresses in total knee arthroplasty: a biomechanical study. Orthopedics. 1999;22:303–7.

43. Li Z, Esposito CI, Koch CN, Lee YY, Padgett DE, Wright TM. Polyethylene damage increases with varus implant alignment in posterior-stabilized and constrained condylar knee arthroplasty. Clin Orthop Relat Res. 2017;475: 2981–91.

44. Lee BS, Cho HI, Bin SI, Kim JM, Jo BK. Femoral component varus malposition is associated with tibial aseptic loosening after TKA. Clin Orthop Relat Res. 2018;476:400–7.

45. Innocenti B, Truyens E, Labey L, Wong P, Victor J, Bellemans J. Can medio-lateral baseplate position and load sharing induce asymptomatic local bone resorption of the proximal tibia? A finite element study. J Orthop Surg Res. 2009;17(4):26.

46. Liau JJ, Cheng CK, Huang CH, Lo WH. The effect of malalignment on stresses in polyethylene component of total knee prostheses—a finite element analysis. Clin Biomech (Bristol, Avon). 2002;17:140–6.

47. Ji HM, Han J, Jin DS, Seo H, Won YY. Kinematically aligned TKA can align knee joint line to horizontal. Knee Surg Sports Traumatol Arthrosc. 2016;24: 2436–41.

48. Howell SM, Papadopoulos S, Kuznik KT, Hull ML. Accurate alignment and high function after kinematically aligned TKA performed with generic instruments. Knee Surg Sports Traumatol Arthrosc. 2013;21:2271–80.

5

Epidemiology of distal radius fracture in Akershus, Norway, in 2010–2011

Håkon With Solvang[1†], Robin Andre Nordheggen[1*†] (iD), Ståle Clementsen[1,2], Ola-Lars Hammer[1,2] and Per-Henrik Randsborg[1]

Abstract

Background: Several studies published over the last decade indicate an increased incidence of distal radius fractures (DRF). With Norway having one of the highest reported incidence of DRFs, we conducted a study to assess the epidemiology of DRFs and its treatment in the catchment area of Akershus University Hospital (AHUS).

Methods: Patients 16 years or older who presented to AHUS with an acute DRF during the years 2010 and 2011 were prospectively recorded and classified according to the AO fracture classification system. The mechanism of injury and treatment modality were noted.

Results: Overall, 1565 patients with an acute DRF presented to the institution in 2010–2011, of which 1134 (72%) were women. The overall annual incidence was 19.7 per 10,000 inhabitants 16 years or older. Women had an exponential increase in incidence after the age of 50, though the incidence for both genders peaked after the age of 80 years. There was an even distribution between extra- and intra-articular fractures. Falling while walking outside was the most common mechanism of injury. Of the 1565 registered, 418 (26.7%) patients underwent surgery, with a volar locking plate being the preferred surgical option in 77% of the cases.

Conclusion: The overall incidence of distal radius fractures was lower in our study than earlier reports from Norway. Postmenopausal women had a higher risk of fracture than the other groups, and low-energy injuries were most dominant. 26.7% were treated operatively, which is higher than earlier reports, and might reflect an increasing preference for surgical treatment.

Keywords: Distal radius fracture, Epidemiology, Volar locking plate, AO classification

Background

Distal radius fracture (DRF) is one of the most common fractures in the human body. It has a bimodal distribution, with a peak incidence among young patients with high-energy traumas and elderly patients with low-energy falls [1–4]. In addition to the individual morbidity, considerable financial resources are spent investigating and treating this injury [5]. Absence from work adds to this socioeconomic load. From the 1950s, a continuous increase in the incidence of DRFs has been described. However, some recent studies describe a stabilizing trend [2, 6], or even a decline in incidence [1, 7], especially in young postmenopausal women [2, 4, 8].

Treatment of DRFs varies, not only between countries but also between national regions and individual hospitals. Following the introduction of volar locking plates (VLP) in the early 2000s, surgical management seems to increase at the cost of conservative treatment [7].

The purpose of the current study is to map the incidence of DRFs among the adult population in the catchment area of Akershus University Hospital (AHUS). Moreover, we studied the distribution between genders, the mechanism of injury, the type of fracture, and the choice of treatment.

Methods

AHUS is a level 2-university hospital covering suburban and urban regions in and outside Oslo, Norway. Patients

* Correspondence: robin.nordheggen@studmed.uio.no
Håkon With Solvang and Robin Andre Nordheggen are co-first authors
[†]Håkon With Solvang and Robin Andre Nordheggen contributed equally to this work.
[1]The Department of Orthopedic Surgery, Akershus University Hospital, 1478 Lørenskog, Norway
Full list of author information is available at the end of the article

16 years or older who presented to AHUS with an acute DRF between January 1, 2010, and December 31, 2011, were eligible for inclusion. A DRF was defined as a fracture of the radius within 3 cm from the radiocarpal joint [9]. To be included in the study, patients had to live within the catchment area of AHUS. Patients primarily treated in another hospital but who had their follow-up appointments at AHUS were also included in this study. All data were registered prospectively in a database. Patient demographics (gender and age), the mechanism of injury, and time of injury were registered. The fractures were classified according to the *Arbeitsgemeinschaft fur Osteosyntesefragen* (AO) fracture classification system by a senior orthopedic consultant, to either a type A (extra-articular), type B (partial articular), or type C (complete intra-articular) fracture. To verify the total number of patients and type of treatment, a search was made in the hospital's electronic files by entering the diagnosis code. The medical records and the radiographs for each registered patient in the prospective database were then retrospectively reviewed and verified from the electronic files.

The age and gender distribution in the catchment area of AHUS were available from Statistics Norway [10]. In January 2011 (halfway in the study period), the catchment area included 398,094 adults 16 years and older. The annual incidence, specified per 10,000 person years, could then be calculated.

The statistical analysis was performed using the Statistical Package for Social Sciences version 22.0 (Armonk, NY: IBM Corp.). Comparison between categorical variables was compared with the X^2 test. T tests were used to compare groups with normally distributed continuous variables, while nonparametric variables were analyzed using Mann-Whitney U test. Statistical significance was considered for p values < 0.05, and all tests were two sided. The data are reported with 95% confidence interval (95% CI) where applicable.

Results

One thousand five hundred sixty-five patients with a distal radius fracture were included in the study. One thousand one hundred thirty-four (72%) of them were women. Median age in men was 47 (16–93) years and 63 (16–98) years in women. Four hundred eighteen (26.7%) fractures were operated. The incidence among women had an exponential growth after the age of 50, with the highest incidence over the age of 80. The incidence in men peaked between the ages 16–19 and above 80 (Fig. 1).

The overall annual fracture incidence was 19.7 (95% CI 18.7–20.7) per 10,000 inhabitants 16 years or older. The incidence was higher among women than men (Table 1).

Complete data were available for 854 (54.5%) of the 1565 patients where mechanism of injury, fracture classification, and operational method were noted. The most common mechanism of injury was falling while walking outdoors, affecting 447 (52%) patients (Table 2). Ice or snow contributed to 294 (66%) of these injuries. Of all the fractures, walking outdoors contributed to 360 (60%) in women and 87 (34%) in men.

Women were more often injured indoors while men sustained more injuries at work, in traffic, and during sports.

In our material of 854 wrist fractures, 822 (96.3%) were classified according to the AO system. The remaining 32 fractures were children's fractures with open growth plates (despite being older than 16 years). These fractures were included in the epidemiological calculations, but could not be classified according to the AO classification system. We found 430 (52%) type A fractures, 97 (12%) type B fractures, and 295 (36%) type C fractures (Table 3).

One hundred fifty-nine (37%) of the type A fractures were operated, mostly (121, 76%) with a VLP. One hundred forty-two (36%) of the intra-articular fractures were operated. Among the 97 type B simple intra-articular fractures, 38 (39%) were operated, 30 (79%) of them with

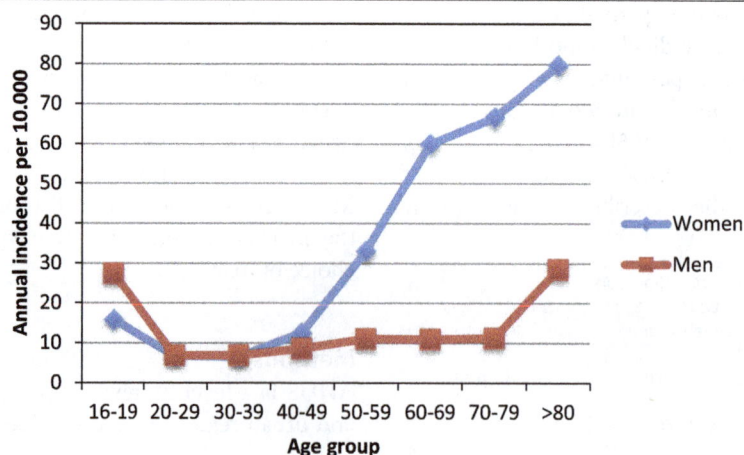

Fig. 1 Annual incidence of distal radius fractures per 10,000 persons, 16 years or older

Table 1 Annual incidence of distal radial fractures per 10,000 inhabitants 16 years or older

Gender	Age	Population January 1, 2011	Number of fractures	Annual incidence (95% CI)
Women	16–19	12,908	41	15.9 (9.0–22.8)
	20–29	28,782	40	6.9 (3.9–9.9)
	30–39	36,097	48	6.6 (4.0–9.9)
	40–49	39,223	99	12.6 (9.1–16.1)
	50–59	30,789	204	33.1 (26.7–39.5)
	60–69	27,203	324	60 (50.9–69.1)
	70–79	15,156	202	66.6 (53.7–68.5)
	>80	11,023	176	79.8 (63.2–96.4)
	Total	201,181	1134	28.2 (25.9–30.5)
Men	16–19	13,639	75	27.5 (18.7–36.3)
	20–29	29,263	41	7.0 (4.0–10.0)
	30–39	35,728	50	7.0 (4.2–9.8)
	40–49	41,261	72	8.7 (5.9–11.5)
	50–59	31,619	70	11.1 (7.4–14.8)
	60–69	26,339	58	11.0 (7.0–15.0)
	70–79	12,780	29	11.3 (5.5–17.1)
	>80	6284	36	28.6 (15.4–41.8)
	Total	196,913	431	10.9 (9.5–12.3)

a volar locking plate. Finally, of the 295 type C-classified (intra-articular) fractures, 104 (35%) were operated, 79 (76%) with a VLP (Fig. 2).

The difference in number of operations between extra-articular (159 of 430) and intra-articular (142 of 392) fractures was not statistically significant ($p = 0.8$). Seventy-four of the 301 (24.6%) operated patients were primarily considered for conservative treatment.

One hundred seventy-two (80%) of the operated women and 72 (72%) of the operated men were treated with a VLP. This difference was not statistically significant ($p = 0.1$). The rest of the operated patients were treated either with external fixation (EF), with or without additional pins, or by closed reduction and percutaneous pinning (CRPP).

Table 2 Mechanism of injury of 854 distal radius fractures treated during 2010 and 2011

Mechanism	Men (%)	Women (%)	Total (%)
Home accidents	24 (9)	106 (18)	130 (15)
Traffic	14 (6)	13 (2)	27 (3)
Walking	87 (34)	360 (60)	447 (52)
Accidents at work	40 (16)	6 (1)	46 (5)
Sports	60 (24)	74 (12)	134 (16)
Playing	4 (1)	8 (1)	12 (2)
Other	25 (10)	33 (6)	58 (7)
Total	254 (100)	600 (100)	854 (100)

Table 3 Classification of 822 distal radius fractures presenting to Akershus University Hospital during 2010 and 2011

AO type	Women (%)	Men (%)	Total (%)
A	308 (53)	122 (50)	430 (52)
B	76 (13)	21 (9)	97 (12)
C	195 (34)	100 (41)	295 (36)
Total	579 (100)	243 (100)	822 (100)

AO Arbeitsgemeinschaft fur Osteosynytesefragen

Discussion

The main finding in this study is the overall incidence of DRFs of 19.7 (95% CI 18.7–20.7) per 10,000 inhabitants 16 years or older. This is lower than what has been seen in other Nordic countries where the incidence has been between 26 [4] and 38 [9] per 10,000 inhabitants.

The incidence among men in our study is relatively close to the findings in both Sweden [4] and the UK [11]. Higher incidences are however described in studies from the Norwegian cities of Bergen [9] and Oslo [2] (Fig. 3).

In women older than 50 years of age, the annual incidence lies relatively close to the reports from the Netherlands [12] and Switzerland [13]. In addition, our findings are just below the reported results from Sweden [4, 14] and the southern part of Norway [1]. Our results are however considerably lower than the Norwegian studies from Oslo and Bergen [2, 9] (Fig. 4).

The studies from Oslo and Bergen were conducted several decades ago. More recent studies show a considerably lower incidence and are closer to our findings [1, 8, 15]. The present study might therefore indicate a true decline in incidence in DRFs. The study population, criteria of inclusion, and study design differ however between the various studies, making comparison challenging. The studies from Bergen and Oslo started their inclusion in patients above the age of 20 years. The incidence of distal radius fractures among children is high, but decreases towards the age of 15–16 years in both genders [16]. In our study, the incidence among women aged 16–19 years is relatively low compared to the other age groups. This will give a low total incidence among women compared to studies not including this group. The incidence in males of the same age group is the second highest, which will increase the total incidence among men.

Elderly are more physically active now than in previous decades, potentially improving both bone mass and neuromuscular control. This could partly explain why our results are lower than previous reports. Geographical differences, as well as snow and ice conditions during the particular winters of our study, may also have reduced the fracture incidence compared to older studies.

We found that the majority (72%) of wrist fractures affect women, which is supported by other studies [1, 2, 4, 8, 9]. As ours and other studies suggest, the

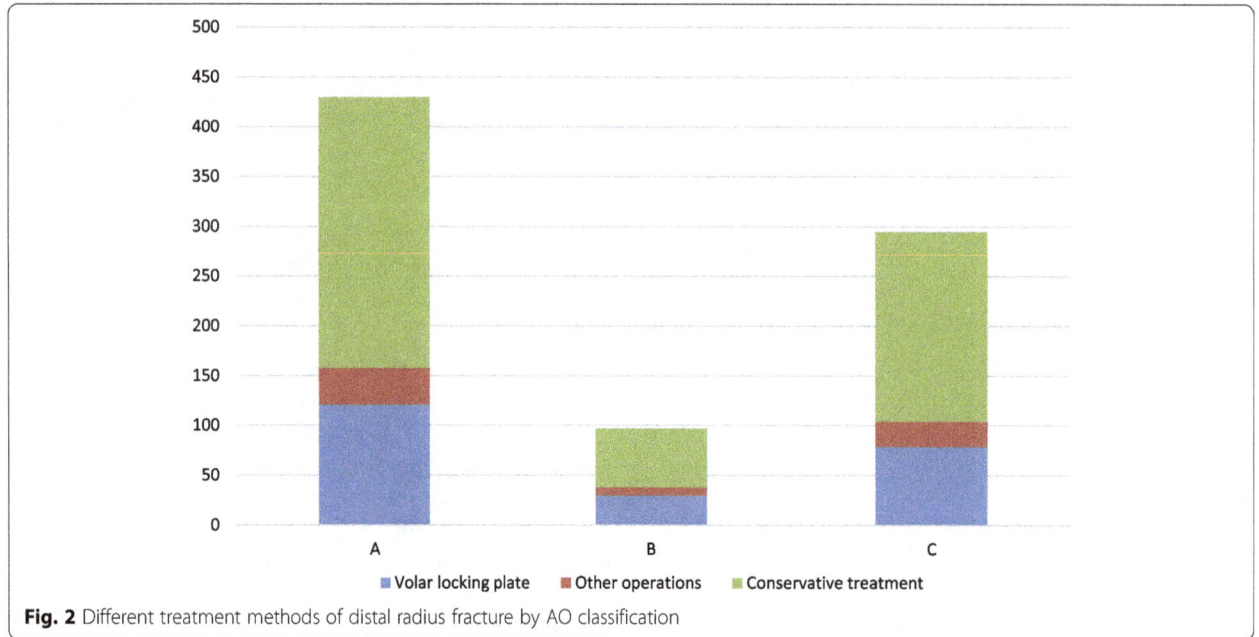

Fig. 2 Different treatment methods of distal radius fracture by AO classification

distribution was more even among men in the different age groups, with a peak between 16–19 years and above 80 [1, 2, 9] (Fig. 1). Among women, however, we found an exponential increase in incidence between the ages of 50 and 69. It is well established that postmenopausal women have an increased risk of distal radius fractures [1, 2, 4, 8, 9]. This might be explained by reduced bone density and the increased risk of osteoporosis after the menopause [17]. The prevalence of osteoporosis and the risk of fracture is also especially high in the Nordic countries [18, 19] where risk factors such as snow, ice, and slippery roads increase the risk of injury [2, 9, 20].

The exponential growth in our study was followed by a linear increase until the age of 80 (Fig. 1). Similar results have been described in other studies [2, 4, 8, 11];

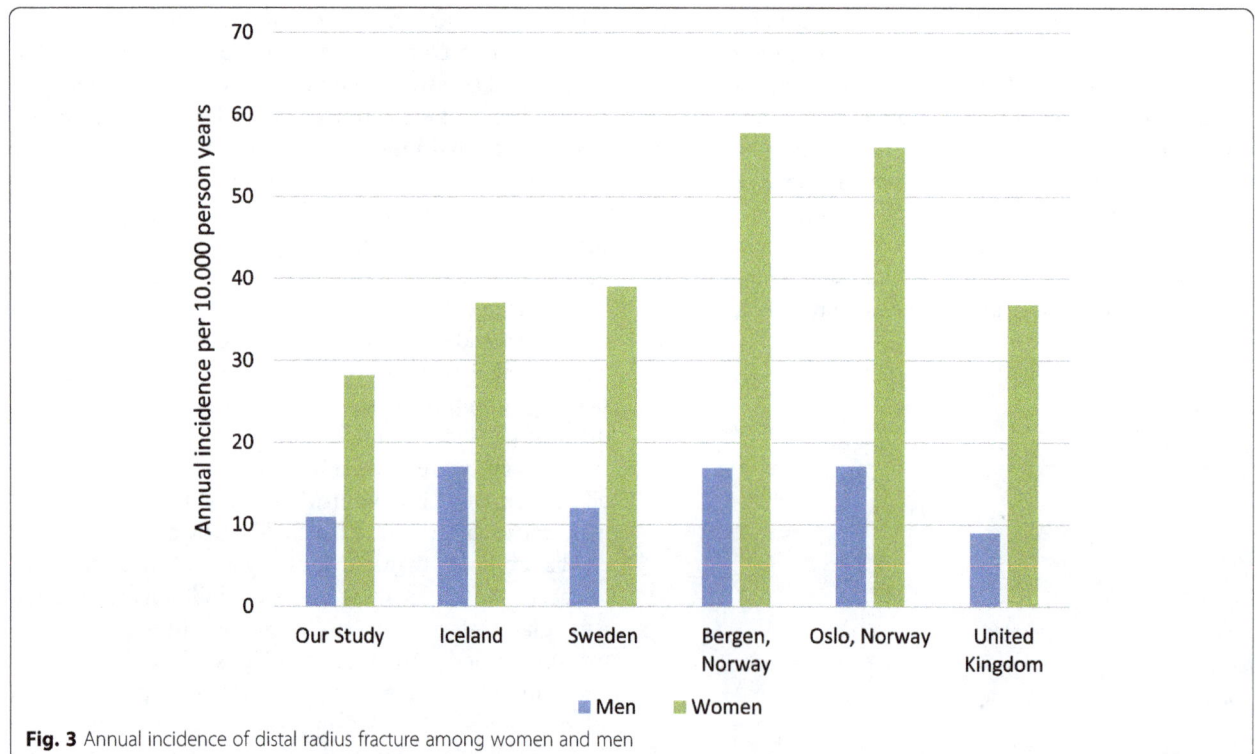

Fig. 3 Annual incidence of distal radius fracture among women and men

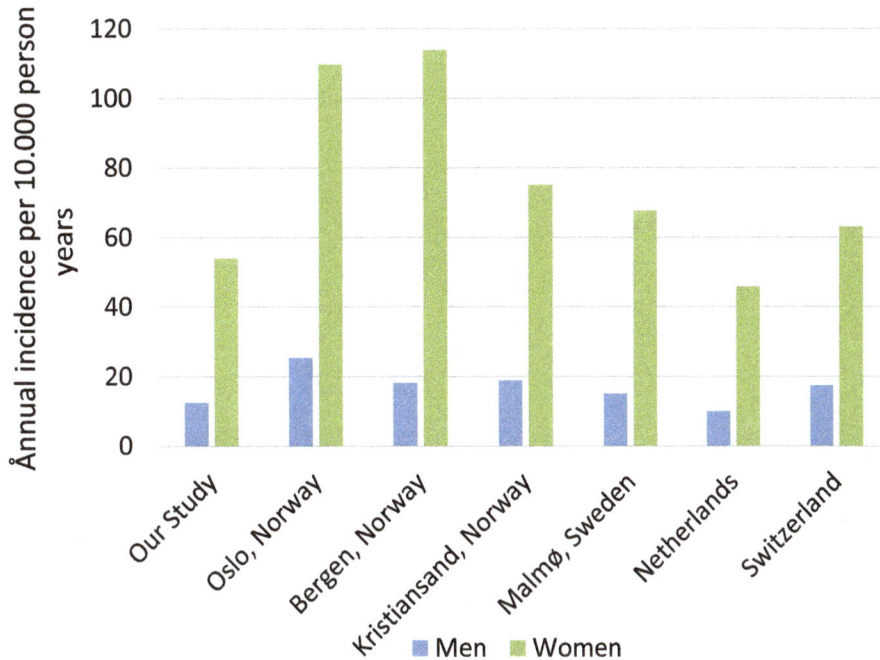

Fig. 4 Annual incidence of distal radius fracture among women and men over the age of 50

however, a decrease after the age of 70 has also been suggested [9, 21].

Older people have a tendency to sustain central fractures when falling, such as fractures of the hip and vertebrae, perhaps because of their reduced neuromuscular control. Younger people are more able to protect themselves with their arms and legs and therefore sustain more distal fractures [3, 22]. Recent studies have found the incidence of DRFs to increase also after the age of 70 [2, 4, 8, 11], indicating that older people are living a more active lifestyle, causing fracture of the distal parts of their body more often than before.

The AO type A fracture constituted the majority of the fractures, followed by type C and type B. Our review shows an equal distribution of extra-articular and intra-articular fractures, both genders combined. This tendency was similar to a Dutch report [23]. The results differ from a study from Iceland where 32% of the fractures in patients above the age of 18 involved the articular surface of the distal radius [8]. In Sweden, the results were even lower with 22% [4].

Among males, we found that 50% of the fractures were intra-articular. Similar results are described in the Icelandic study (42%); however, lower results are found in Sweden (29%) [4, 8]. Among Norwegian females, the results were similar, with a small predominance of extra-articular fractures (53%). The prevalence was however lower than the comparing results from Iceland and Sweden, where the extra-articular fractures were more dominating [4, 8]. This difference may be explained by

different criteria of inclusion. Both the Swedish and Icelandic studies also included forearm fractures, which will affect the intra- and extra-articular fraction.

Several international studies suggest an increasing tendency for operative treatment [7, 14, 24–26]. Even though most patients were conservatively treated in our study, 418 (26.7%) underwent surgery (Fig. 2). This is a higher percentage than what is found in Sweden (20%) [14] and USA (17%) [24], but comparable to what is previously found in Norway (28%) [25]. We found that the preferred type of surgery was the volar locking plate in 77% of the patients. From 2005 to 2010 in Sweden, the use of VLP tripled and peaked at 67% [14]. A Finnish study found a 108% increased use of VLP over a 10-year period [26]. In Norway, the use of VLP increased from 53% in 2009 to 81% in 2014, while the amount of EF and CRPP went down [25].

Even though the volar locking plate has been increasingly popular and studies have demonstrated good results, there are few randomized controlled trials on this subject. The conclusions are not homogenous regarding what is the optimal surgical treatment [14, 27–33].

The Norwegian Orthopaedic Association published in 2013 guidelines that propose VLP as the preferred implant in most cases. This might explain the increased use in Norway [25].

Our study has some limitations. There is a possibility that not all distal radius fractures have been registered with the code S52.5 (distal radius fracture) or been miscoded. Furthermore, some of the patients belonging to

AHUS might have been treated elsewhere. However, AHUS is the only hospital in this area that treats acute injuries and the loss of patients to neighboring hospitals has previously been found to be insignificant [16].

Regarding mechanism of injury, fracture classification, and operational method, there might be a certain selection bias, as the total number of patients with the diagnosis was 1565 and our material consisted of 854 (54.5%) registered patients.

The strengths in our study are the prospective design of the study.

Conclusions

Compared to earlier Norwegian reports, we found a lower incidence of distal radius fracture. Our numbers are comparable to more recent European studies and might be due to a real decrease in incidence of DRFs.

Postmenopausal women had a higher risk of fractures than the other groups, and low-energy injuries were most dominant. 26.7% of the patients were treated operatively, which is higher than earlier reports, and might reflect an increasing trend for surgical treatment. VLP was the preferred choice of treatment in 77% of the cases.

Abbreviations
AHUS: Akershus University Hospital; CRPP: Closed reduction and percutaneous pinning; DRF: Distal radius fracture; EF: External fixation; VLP: Volar locking plate

Authors' contributions
HWS and RAN collected and analyzed the data and wrote the first and final draft. Both authors contributed equally to the work. SC collected the data, analyzed the radiographs, and revised the manuscript. OLH contributed to the study design, analyzed the radiographs, and supervised and critically revised the manuscript. PHR contributed to the study design and statistical analysis and supervised and critically revised the manuscript. All authors approved the final manuscript.

Competing interests
The authors declare that they have no competing interests.

Author details
[1]The Department of Orthopedic Surgery, Akershus University Hospital, 1478 Lørenskog, Norway. [2]The Faculty of Medicine, The University of Oslo, Oslo, Norway.

References
1. Diamantopoulos AP, et al. The epidemiology of low- and high-energy distal radius fracture in middle-aged and elderly men and women in Southern Norway. PLoS One. 2012;7(8):e43367.
2. Lofthus C, et al. Epidemiology of distal forearm fractures in Oslo, Norway. Osteoporos Int. 2008;19(6):781–6.
3. Nellans KW, Kowalski E, Chung KC. The epidemiology of distal radius fractures. Hand Clin. 2012;28(2):113–25.
4. Brogren E, Petranek M, Atroshi I. Incidence and characteristics of distal radius fractures in a southern Swedish region. BMC Musculoskelet Disord. 2007;8(1):48.
5. Shauver MJ, et al. Current and future national costs to medicare for the treatment of distal radius fracture in the elderly. J Hand Surg. 2011;36(8): 1282–7.
6. Melton L III, et al. Long-term trends in the incidence of distal forearm fractures. Osteoporos Int. 1998;8(4):341–8.
7. Wilcke MK, Hammarberg H, Adolphson PY. Epidemiology and changed surgical treatment methods for fractures of the distal radius: a registry analysis of 42,583 patients in Stockholm County, Sweden, 2004–2010. Acta Orthop. 2013;84(3):292–6.
8. Sigurdardottir K, Halldorsson S, Robertsson J. Epidemiology and treatment of distal radius fractures in Reykjavik, Iceland, in 2004: comparison with an Icelandic study from 1985. Acta Orthop. 2011;82(4):494–8.
9. Hove LM, et al. Fractures of the distal radius in a Norwegian city. Scand J Plast Reconstr Surg Hand Surg. 1995;29(3):263–7.
10. Statistisk sentralbyrå. Available from: https://www.ssb.no/en/. Accessed 3 Jan 2018.
11. Thompson PW, Taylor J, Dawson A. The annual incidence and seasonal variation of fractures of the distal radius in men and women over 25 years in Dorset, UK. Injury. 2004;35(5):462–6.
12. De Putter C, et al. Epidemiology and health-care utilisation of wrist fractures in older adults in The Netherlands, 1997–2009. Injury. 2013; 44(4):421–6.
13. Lippuner K, et al. Remaining lifetime and absolute 10-year probabilities of osteoporotic fracture in Swiss men and women. Osteoporos Int. 2009;20(7): 1131–40.
14. Mellstrand-Navarro C, et al. The operative treatment of fractures of the distal radius is increasing. Bone Joint J. 2014;96(7):963–9.
15. Hoff M, Torvik IA, Schei B. Forearm fractures in Central Norway, 1999–2012: incidence, time trends, and seasonal variation. Arch Osteoporos. 2016;11(1):7.
16. Randsborg P-H, et al. Fractures in children: epidemiology and activity-specific fracture rates. JBJS. 2013;95(7):e42.
17. Cawthon PM. Gender differences in osteoporosis and fractures. Clin Orthop Relat Res. 2011;469(7):1900–5.
18. Gjesdal CG, et al. Femoral and whole-body bone mineral density in middle-aged and older Norwegian men and women: suitability of the reference values. Osteoporos Int. 2004;15(7):525–34.
19. Kanis JA, et al. International variations in hip fracture probabilities: implications for risk assessment. J Bone Miner Res. 2002;17(7):1237–44.
20. Diamantopoulos AP, et al. Short-and long-term mortality in males and females with fragility hip fracture in Norway. A population-based study. Clin Interv Aging. 2013;8:817.
21. Falch J. Epidemiology of fractures of the distal forearm in Oslo, Norway. Acta Orthop Scand. 1983;54(2):291–5.
22. Vogt MT, et al. Distal radius fractures in older women: a 10-year follow-up study of descriptive characteristics and risk factors. The study of osteoporotic fractures. J Am Geriatr Soc. 2002;50(1):97–103.
23. Bentohami A, et al. Incidence and characteristics of distal radial fractures in an urban population in The Netherlands. Eur J Trauma Emerg Surg. 2014; 40(3):357–61.
24. Fanuele J, et al. Distal radial fracture treatment: what you get may depend on your age and address. J Bone Joint Surg Am. 2009;91(6):1313.
25. Kvernmo HD, Otterdal P, Balteskard L. Treatment of wrist fractures 2009–14. Tidsskr Nor Laegeforen. 2017;137(19):1501–05.
26. Mattila VM, et al. Significant change in the surgical treatment of distal radius fractures: a nationwide study between 1998 and 2008 in Finland. J Trauma Acute Care Surg. 2011;71(4):939–43.

27. Abramo A, et al. Open reduction and internal fixation compared to closed reduction and external fixation in distal radial fractures: a randomized study of 50 patients. Acta Orthop. 2009;80(4):478–85.

28. Day CS, Maniwa K, Wu WK. More evidence that volar locked plating for distal radial fractures does not offer a functional advantage over traditional treatment options: commentary on an article by Alexia Karantana, FRCS (Orth), et al. "Surgical treatment of distal radial fractures with a volar locking plate versus conventional percutaneous methods. A randomized controlled trial". JBJS. 2013;95(19):e147.

29. Rozental TD, Blazar PE. Functional outcome and complications after volar plating for dorsally displaced, unstable fractures of the distal radius. J Hand Surg. 2006;31(3):359–65.

30. Leung F, et al. Comparison of external and percutaneous pin fixation with plate fixation for intra-articular distal radial fractures: a randomized study. JBJS. 2008;90(1):16–22.

31. Wei DH, et al. Unstable distal radial fractures treated with external fixation, a radial column plate, or a volar plate: a prospective randomized trial. JBJS. 2009;91(7):1568–77.

32. Westphal T, et al. Outcome after surgery of distal radius fractures: no differences between external fixation and ORIF. Arch Orthop Trauma Surg. 2005;125(8):507–14.

33. Williksen JH, et al. Volar locking plates versus external fixation and adjuvant pin fixation in unstable distal radius fractures: a randomized, controlled study. J Hand Surg. 2013;38(8):1469–76.

6

A meta-analysis of unicompartmental knee arthroplasty revised to total knee arthroplasty versus primary total knee arthroplasty

Xuedong Sun[1] and Zheng Su[2*]

Abstract

Background: This study was performed to compare the clinical outcomes of unicompartmental knee arthroplasty (UKA) revised to total knee arthroplasty (TKA) versus primary TKA.

Methods: Relevant trials were identified via a search of the Cochrane Central Register of Controlled Trials and PubMed from inception to 17 June 2017. A meta-analysis was performed to compare postoperative outcomes between revised UKA and primary TKA with respect to the Western Ontario and McMaster Universities Osteoarthritis Index (WOMAC) score, Knee Society Score (KSS), mean polyethylene thickness, hospital stay, revision rate, range of motion (ROM), and complications.

Results: Five of 233 studies involving 536 adult patients (revised UKA group, $n = 209$; primary TKA group, $n = 327$) were eligible for inclusion in the meta-analysis. The primary TKA group had better WOMAC scores, KSS, and ROM than the revised UKA group ($P < 0.05$). Compared with primary TKA, revision of UKA to TKA required more augments, stems, and bone grafts and a thicker polyethylene component ($P < 0.05$). There were no significant differences between the two groups in the revision rate, hospital stay, or complications ($P > 0.05$).

Conclusion: Conversion of UKA to TKA is associated with poorer clinical outcomes than primary TKA. Furthermore, we believe that conversion of UKA to TKA is more complicated than performing primary TKA. Revision UKA often requires more augments, stems, and bone grafts and thicker polyethylene components than primary TKA. However, patients who undergo conversion of UKA to TKA have similar hospital stay, complications, and revision rate as patients who undergo primary TKA.

Keywords: Knee osteoarthritis, Unicompartmental knee arthroplasty, Total knee arthroplasty, Meta-analysis

Background

The best treatment options for patients with unicompartmental osteoarthritis of the knee are still controversial [1]. Total knee arthroplasty (TKA) and unicompartmental knee arthroplasty (UKA) are both used to treat osteoarthritis of the knee. Because of the continuous development of surgical techniques and component design since the early 1970s [2, 3], UKA has become a more successful and reliable treatment method for unicompartmental knee

osteoarthritis. When UKA failure occurs, TKA is an alternative treatment for many patients. However, some authors have reported poor outcomes of conversion of UKA to TKA [4–6], whereas others have reported more favorable outcomes [7, 8]. Hence, it is important for patients to understand the potential clinical outcomes of revision surgery during their preoperative deliberation. No previous meta-analysis has compared the clinical outcomes of revised UKA versus primary TKA. Therefore, we performed a meta-analysis of clinical studies to compare revised UKA and primary TKA by evaluating knee pain, knee function, and other parameters.

* Correspondence: asue1006@sina.com
[2]Department of Medical Oncology, Weifang People's Hospital, no. 151 Guangwen Road, Weifang 260041, China
Full list of author information is available at the end of the article

Table 1 Newcastle–Ottawa scale

Study	Selection				Comparability		Exposure			Quality score
	Cases definition	Cases representativeness	Controls selection	Controls definition	Comparable for a, b, c*	Comparable for d, e, f*	Exposure ascertainment	Controls ascertainment	Non-response rate	
Järvenpää J [5]	1	0	0	1	a, b, c	d, f	1	1	1	7
Rancourt MF [9]	1	0	0	1	a, b, c	f	1	1	1	7
Becker R [10]	1	0	0	1	a, b, c	f	1	1	1	7
Lunebourg A [11]	1	0	0	1	a, b, c	e	1	1	1	7
Cross MB [12]	1	0	0	1	a, b, c	NA	1	1	1	6

NA data not available

Comparability ^{variables}: a = age; b = sex; c = body mass index; d = operation time point; e = single surgeon; f = the same compartment

*If all characteristics of a, b, and c were comparable, 1 point was assigned; if one, two, or three characteristics of d, e, and f were comparable, 1 point was assigned; otherwise, 0 points were assigned

Methods

Search strategy

The Cochrane Central Register of Controlled Trials and PubMed databases were searched to identify relevant studies published in English from inception to 17 June 2017. The following search strategy was used to maximize search specificity and sensitivity: [(revision uka) OR (revised uka) OR (revised unicompartmental knee) OR (revision unicompartmental knee) OR (revised ukr) OR (revision ukr)] AND [(total knee) OR tka OR tkr], where "ukr" stands for unicompartmental knee replacement and "tkr" stands for total knee replacement.

Selection of studies

Two independent authors (X.D.S. and Z.S.) initially selected studies based on their titles and abstracts. Full

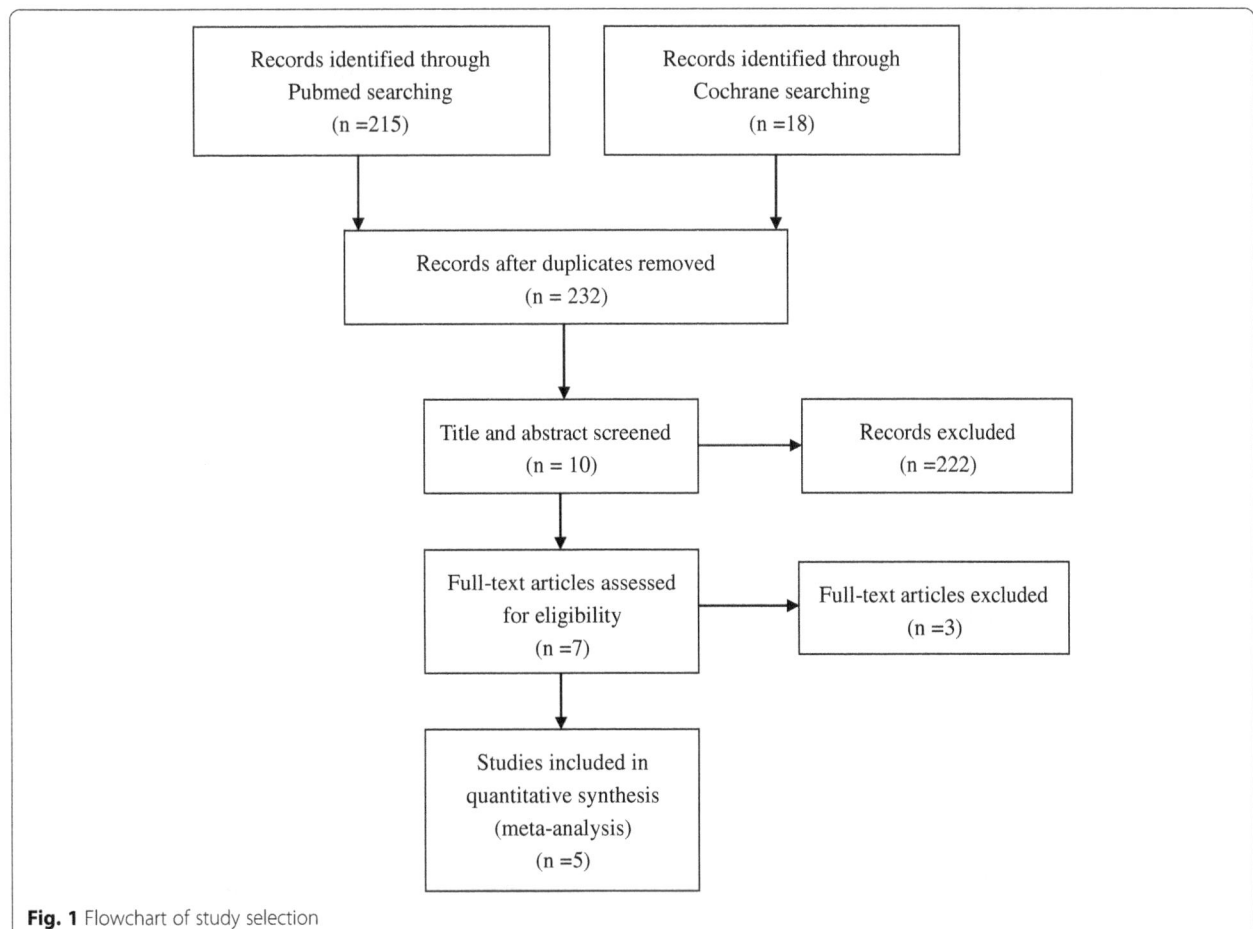

Fig. 1 Flowchart of study selection

Table 2 Characteristics of included studies

References	Years	Patients (n) rUKA/pTKA	Mean age (years) rUKA/ pTKA	Female rUKA/ pTKA	Mean follow-up (years)	Mean BMI (kg/m^2) rUKA/ pTKA	Outcome
Järvenpää J [5]	2010	21/28	74.9(7.4)/ 75.2(7.2)	12/17	10.5	28.5(4)/ 30.5(4.4)	Hospital stay, ROM, WOMAC scores, revisions, complications, requirement of augments, stems, and bone grafts
Rancourt MF [9]	2012	63/126	67.49(10.24)/ 66.71(9.77)	45/90	3	31.6(6.15)/ 32.53(6.57)	Hospital stay, WOMAC scores, mean polyethylene thickness, requirement of augments, stems, and bone grafts
Lunebourg A [11]	2015	48/48	71(9)/72(12)	36/32	7	28(4)/28(4)	ROM, KSS, mean polyethylene thickness, revisions, complications, requirement of augments, stems, and bone grafts
Becker R [10]	2004	28/28	71.5(6.8)/ 71.5(6.6)	23/23	4.6	31.2(3.2)/ 31.1(4.4)	ROM, WOMAC scores, KSS
Cross MB [12]	2014	49/97	61.5/58.9	30/50	4.8	31.65/32.76	hospital stay, ROM, KSS, revisions, complications, requirement of augments, stems, and bone grafts

rUKA revised unicompartmental knee arthroplasty, *pTKA* primary total knee arthroplasty, *BMI* body mass index, *ROM* range of motion, *WOMAC* Western Ontario and McMaster Universities Osteoarthritis Index, *KSS* Knee Society Score

papers were retrieved if a decision could not be made from the abstracts. Any disagreement between the two authors was resolved by consensus.

The inclusion criteria were

- Comparison of clinical outcomes between revised UKA and primary TKA
- Prospective study or retrospective study
- Cohort study, case control study, or randomized controlled trial
- Mean follow-up duration of at least 2 years
- Comparison of at least one of the following outcomes: Western Ontario and McMaster Universities Osteoarthritis Index (WOMAC) score, Knee Society Score (KSS), mean polyethylene thickness, hospital stay, range of

motion (ROM), postoperative complications (nerve injury, hematoma, deep vein thrombosis, patellar tendon disruption, fractures, infection, component loosening, stiffness), and revision rates
- Sufficient data for extraction and pooling (i.e., reporting of the mean, standard deviation, and number of subjects for continuous outcomes and the number of subjects for dichotomous outcomes)

The exclusion criteria were

- Revision of infectious loosening after UKA
- Review articles or case reports
- Revision of patellofemoral replacement
- Performance of bilateral TKA or UKA

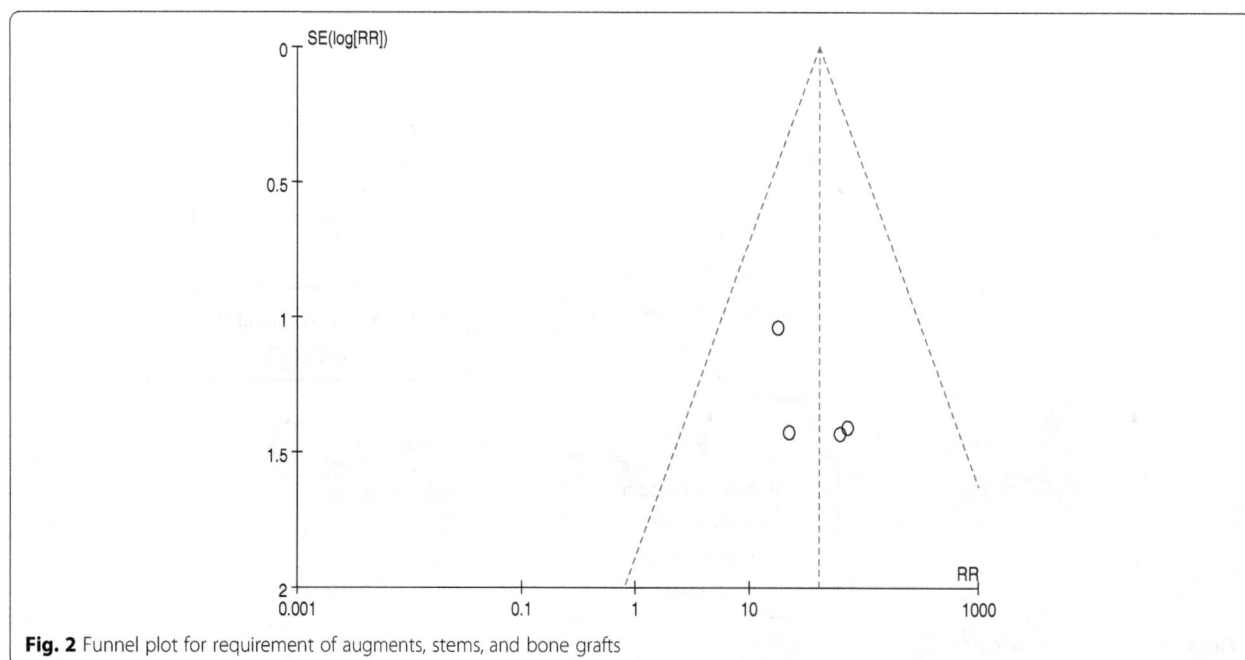

Fig. 2 Funnel plot for requirement of augments, stems, and bone grafts

Study or Subgroup	Revised UKA Mean	SD	Total	Primary TKA Mean	SD	Total	Weight	Mean Difference IV, Random, 95% CI
Cross MB 2014	3.2	1.7	49	1.84	1.5	97	34.7%	1.36 [0.80, 1.92]
Järvenpää J 2010	8.3	1.05	21	7.9	1.83	28	31.1%	0.40 [-0.41, 1.21]
Rancourt MF 2012	4.67	1.9	63	4.89	2.17	126	34.2%	-0.22 [-0.82, 0.38]
Total (95% CI)			133			251	100.0%	0.52 [-0.48, 1.53]

Heterogeneity: Tau² = 0.68; Chi² = 14.35, df = 2 (P = 0.0008); I² = 86%
Test for overall effect: Z = 1.02 (P = 0.31)

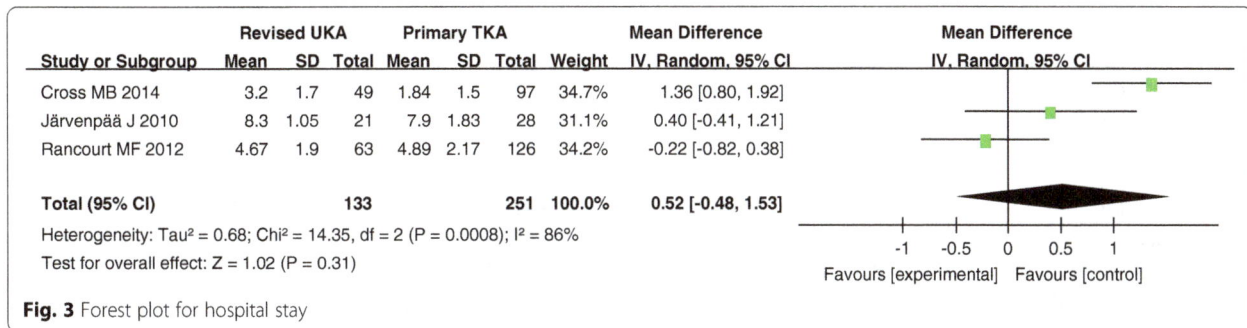

Fig. 3 Forest plot for hospital stay

Data extraction

Two reviewers (X.D.S. and Z.S.) independently performed data extraction using standardized data extraction forms. The general characteristics of each study were extracted [i.e., mean age, sex, body mass index (BMI), ROM, mean polyethylene thickness, hospital stay, postoperative complications, revision rate, KSS, and WOMAC score]. Any disagreement between the two reviewers was resolved by consensus.

Quality assessment

Both authors (X.D.S. and Z.S.) independently assessed the risk of bias for each study in accordance with the Newcastle–Ottawa scale (Table 1). Three domains were assessed, and the total possible score was 9 points. Disagreements between the two authors were resolved by consensus.

Statistical analysis

Dichotomous outcomes are expressed as the risk ratio (RR) with 95% confidence interval (CI), while continuous outcomes are expressed as the mean difference (MD) with 95% CI. Heterogeneity is expressed as P and I^2. This value of I^2 ranges from 0% (complete consistency) to 100% (complete inconsistency). If the P value of the heterogeneity test was < 0.1 or $I^2 > 50\%$, a random-effects model was used in place of the fixed modality. Publication bias was tested using funnel plots. Forest plots were used to graphically present the results of individual studies and the respective pooled estimate of effect size. All statistical analyses were performed with Review Manager (version 5.3.0 for Windows; Cochrane Collaboration, Nordic Cochrane Centre, Copenhagen, Denmark).

Results

Search results

A flowchart of the studies considered for inclusion in our review is shown in Fig. 1. We identified 233 potential citations (215 from PubMed, 18 from the Cochrane Library) comparing the clinical outcomes of revised UKA and primary TKA. After reading the articles, 5 of the 233 citations were selected for the meta-analysis. The characteristics of these five studies [5, 9–12] are shown in Table 2.

Meta-analysis results

The meta-analysis included five studies, involving a total of 536 patients [5, 9–12]. The revised UKA group included 209 patients, while the primary TKA group included 327 patients. The MD for age and BMI were 0.43 (P = 0.61; 95% CI, – 1.24–2.10) and – 0.67 (P = 0.13; 95% CI, – 1.56–0.21), respectively; there were no significant differences between groups in age or BMI. There was also no significant difference between groups in the proportion of female patients (RR = 1.06; P = 0.36; 95% CI, 0.94–1.19). Thus, the age, sex, and BMI of the two groups were comparable. A funnel plot based on the

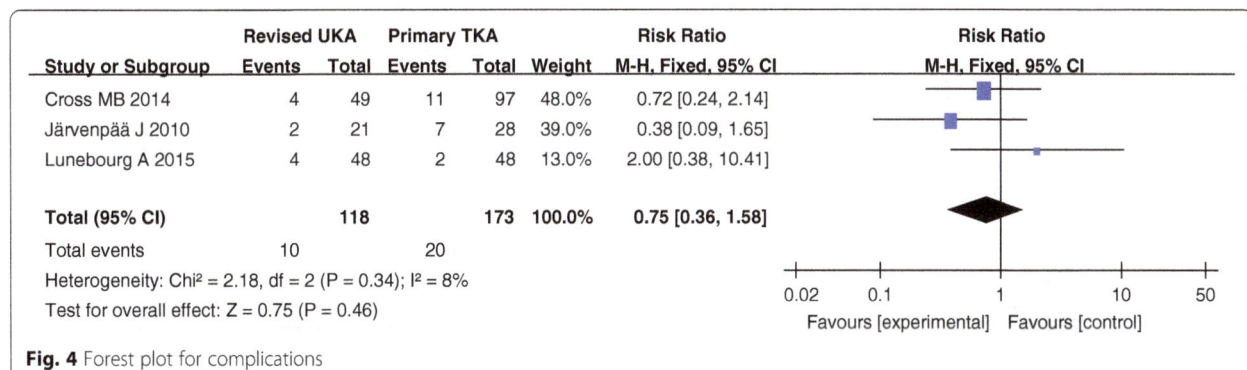

Study or Subgroup	Revised UKA Events	Total	Primary TKA Events	Total	Weight	Risk Ratio M-H, Fixed, 95% CI
Cross MB 2014	4	49	11	97	48.0%	0.72 [0.24, 2.14]
Järvenpää J 2010	2	21	7	28	39.0%	0.38 [0.09, 1.65]
Lunebourg A 2015	4	48	2	48	13.0%	2.00 [0.38, 10.41]
Total (95% CI)		118		173	100.0%	0.75 [0.36, 1.58]
Total events	10		20			

Heterogeneity: Chi² = 2.18, df = 2 (P = 0.34); I² = 8%
Test for overall effect: Z = 0.75 (P = 0.46)

Fig. 4 Forest plot for complications

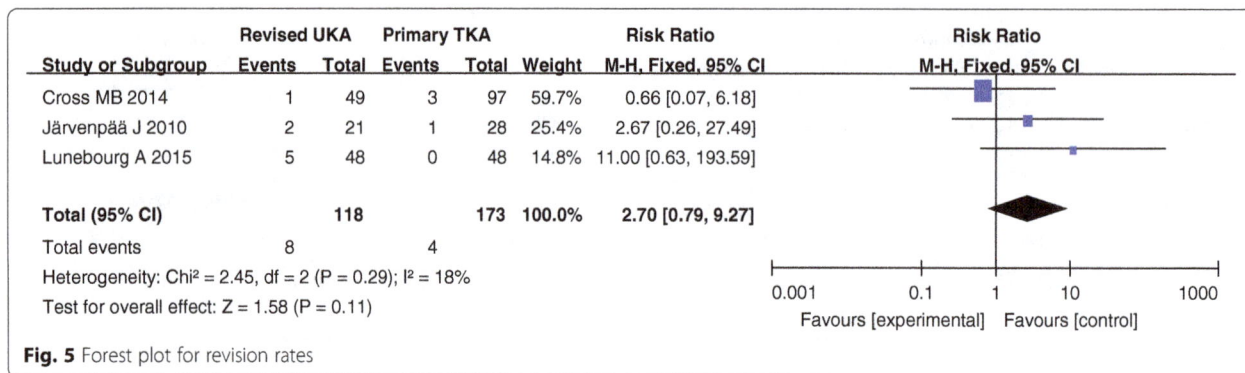

Fig. 5 Forest plot for revision rates

most frequently cited outcome was broadly symmetrical, indicating minimal publication bias (Fig. 2).

Hospital stay, complications, and revision rates

The hospital stay, complications, and revision rates are summarized in Figs. 3, 4, and 5. There were no significant differences between these variables in the primary TKA group versus the revised UKA group ($P > 0.05$).

WOMAC scores, KSS, and ROM

The WOMAC score (0–100) encompasses evaluation of the knee as well as patients' symptoms and functional disability. The score has three main categories: pain, stiffness, and function. The KSS consists of the Knee Society Knee Score (KKS 0–100) and the Knee Society Function Score (KFS 0–100).

The MD of the WOMAC function, pain, and stiffness scores (0–100) for revised UKA were 6.66 ($P = 0.005$; 95% CI, 2.05–11.28), 6.55 ($P = 0.004$; 95% CI, 2.12–10.99), and 10.03 ($P = 0.01$; 95% CI, 2.05–18.01), respectively, all of which were higher than those for primary TKA. The WOMAC scores were significantly different between the two groups (Figs. 6, 7, and 8).

The MD of the KFS for revised UKA was – 12.74 ($P = 0.03$; 95% CI, – 24.26 to – 1.21), which was lower than that for primary TKA. There was a significant difference in the KFS was observed between the two groups (Fig. 9).

The MD of the KKS and ROM for revised UKA were – 8.12 ($P = 0.05$; 95% CI, – 16.14 to – 0.09) and – 6.93 ($P = 0.05$; 95% CI, – 13.87–0.01), respectively. These results imply that the ROM and KKS tended to be better in the primary TKA group than that in revised UKA group, but the differences between the two groups were not statistically significant (Figs. 10 and 11).

Polyethylene thickness and requirement for augments, stems, and bone grafts

Three studies involving 341 patients provided data on polyethylene thickness. The polyethylene thickness used for the revised UKA group was significantly thicker than that used for the primary TKA group (MD = 2.13; 95% CI, 1.68–2.58; $P < 0.00001$) (Fig. 12).

Four studies involving 480 patients provided data on the requirements for augments, stems, and bone grafts. There was a significantly greater proportion of usage of augments, stems, and bone grafts in the revised UKA group than in the primary TKA group (RR = 40.12; $P < 0.00001$; 95% CI 10.90–147.60) (Fig. 13).

Discussion

The most important finding of the present meta-analysis was that the primary TKA group showed better outcomes than the revised UKA group in terms of WOMAC scores, KSS, and ROM. There was a greater proportion of usage of augments, stems, and bone grafts in the revised UKA group than in the primary TKA

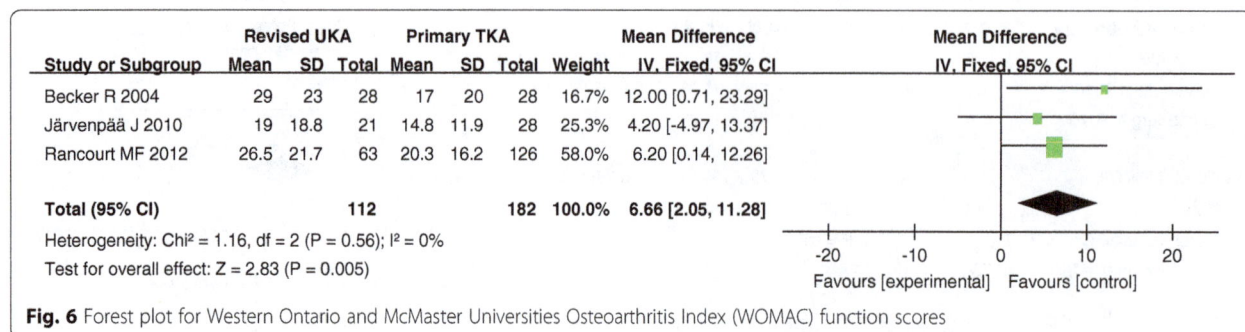

Fig. 6 Forest plot for Western Ontario and McMaster Universities Osteoarthritis Index (WOMAC) function scores

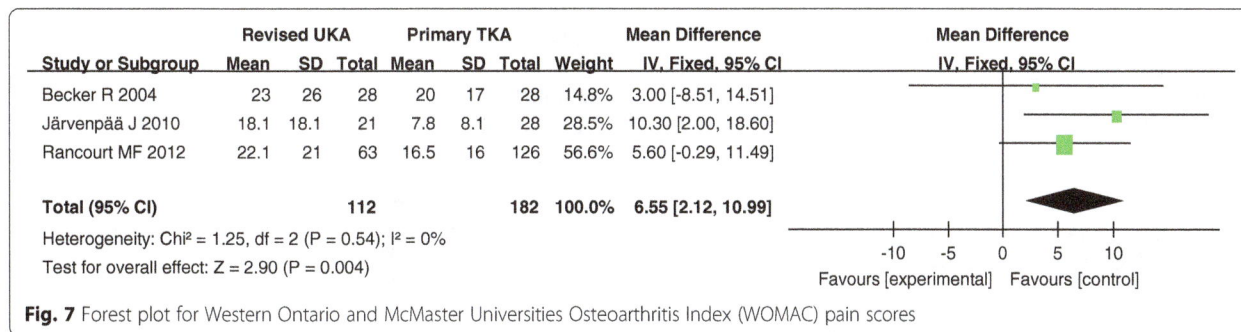

Fig. 7 Forest plot for Western Ontario and McMaster Universities Osteoarthritis Index (WOMAC) pain scores

group, and the polyethylene thickness used for the revised UKA group was thicker than that used for the primary TKA group. However, there were no significant differences between the revised UKA group and the primary TKA group in the hospital stay, complications, and revision rates.

In our review, the primary TKA group yielded superior KSS and WOMAC pain, stiffness, and function scores compared with the revised UKA group. Lunebourg et al [11] and Miller et al [6] reported that the mean KSS was significantly worse in the revised UKA group than that in the primary TKA group, whereas Cross et al [12] did not favor this view. Järvenpää et al [5] stated that the outcomes of WOMAC pain and stiffness scores were better in the primary TKA group, and the WOMAC function scores did not significantly differ between the revised UKA group and the primary TKA group; however, Becker et al [10] reported the opposite. These studies only used a single questionnaire to evaluate each patient. The KSS only evaluates walking and stair-climbing activities, whereas the self-assessed WOMAC scores assess the ability of the patient to perform activities of daily living in more detail. Therefore, the results of the two groups were able to be evaluated more comprehensively with the combination of objective and subjective outcome systems used in our study.

ROM is one of the most important clinical outcomes that reflects the function of the knee. The revised UKA group had decreased ROM compared with

the primary TKA group in the present study, which is in accordance with other studies [10–12]. Scarring or thickening of the joint capsule is more likely after revision surgery, and this may be partially responsible for the decreased knee flexion. Therefore, early recognition and enhanced recovery after surgery are critical for successful outcomes.

Bone loss is reportedly experienced by 77% of patients who undergo conversion of UKA [8]. Bone defects reportedly occur in 60.6% of the cases [13], and bone loss can also occur at the time of component removal [14]. Some studies have also verified this view from other aspects; 34% of patients required conversion to a revision type of TKA with augments, stems, or bone grafts [15], and 33% of cases reportedly require revision components (with the majority on the tibial side) [16]. Furthermore, UKA to TKA conversion was often accompanied by the use of thicker polyethylene [9, 10, 17]. Wynn Jones et al. [18] reported that UKA to TKA conversion with a thicker polyethylene was related to the initial polyethylene thickness of the UKA, and that these cases with thicker polyethylene more often needed an augment or a stem. In the present meta-analysis, we found a greater proportion of usage of augments, stems, and bone grafts and a thicker polyethylene component in the revised UKA group than in the primary TKA group; this indicates that the revised operations were more complicated, and thus required excellent surgical technique. Therefore, we believe that converting UKA to TKA is more difficult than performing primary TKA. In UKA revision, surgeons should

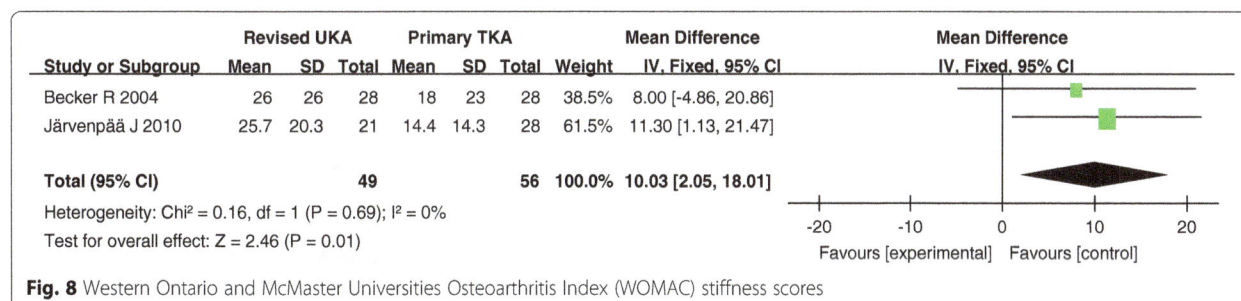

Fig. 8 Western Ontario and McMaster Universities Osteoarthritis Index (WOMAC) stiffness scores

Study or Subgroup	Revised UKA Mean	SD	Total	Primary TKA Mean	SD	Total	Weight	Mean Difference IV. Random. 95% CI
Becker R 2004	56.1	15	28	64.1	19	28	32.2%	-8.00 [-16.97, 0.97]
Cross MB 2014	79	24	49	85	19	97	33.9%	-6.00 [-13.71, 1.71]
Lunebourg A 2015	66	26	48	90	9	48	33.8%	-24.00 [-31.78, -16.22]
Total (95% CI)			125			173	100.0%	-12.74 [-24.26, -1.21]

Heterogeneity: Tau² = 86.34; Chi² = 12.03, df = 2 (P = 0.002); I² = 83%
Test for overall effect: Z = 2.17 (P = 0.03)

Favours [experimental]   Favours [control]

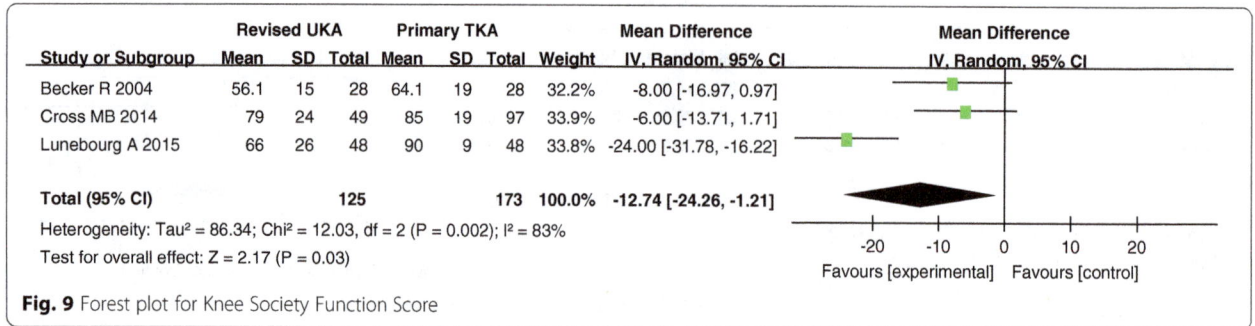

Fig. 9 Forest plot for Knee Society Function Score

perform adequate preoperative preparation to ensure successful operation.

UKA is still a successful and reliable treatment method for unicompartmental knee osteoarthritis. Previous studies have revealed that UKA results in less perioperative blood loss, a shorter hospital stay, fewer complications, better ROM, greater level of activity, more normal gait, and a subsequently quicker recovery compared with TKA [19–21]. Moreover, one retrospective series of patients undergoing UKA reported an 11-year survival rate of 92% [22], and another study reported a 12-year survival rate of 94% among patients aged ≤ 60 years [23]. However, with the widespread use of UKA, a greater early revision rate of UKA has been reported. Two previous studies reported that patients undergoing UKA were at greater risk of early revision than those undergoing primary TKA [24, 25]; however, these studies did not account for surgeon proficiency. Surgeon experience is essential for the attainment of good results in UKA [26]. The reported revision rates for UKA are 0.99% for UKA conducted by surgeons performing > 12 UKAs per year, 4.6% for those performing 8 to 11 UKAs per year, 6.4% for those performing 2 to 7 UKAs per year, and 8.3% for those performing 1 UKA per year [27]. In addition, a study evaluating the published long-term outcomes of > 8000 medial Oxford Phase 3 UKAs reported that very good outcomes were achieved by both designer and non-designer

surgeons, and that the annual revision rate was 0.74% [28]. In conclusion, UKA has a greater long-term survival rate because of improved surgical techniques and modern implant designs along with increased experience with the procedure. Therefore, higher-volume surgeons can achieve better UKA outcomes and a revision rate comparable with that of TKA, but TKA may be a wiser choice for less experienced surgeons.

The strengths of the study are the compatibility of the patient populations in terms of age, sex, and BMI, and the use of both objective and subjective data. The limitations include the insufficient sample size, different types of prostheses used, and lack of survival rate calculation. Future studies with large sample sizes could provide enhanced analyses, and additional evaluation criteria are needed.

Conclusion

The present meta-analysis has shown that conversion of UKA to TKA is associated with poorer clinical outcomes than primary TKA. Furthermore, we believe that converting UKA to TKA is more complicated than performing primary TKA. Surgeons should be aware that revision UKA more often requires augments, stems, and bone grafts and thicker polyethylene components than primary TKA. However, there are no statistically significant differences between the two groups in the hospital stay, complications, or revision rates.

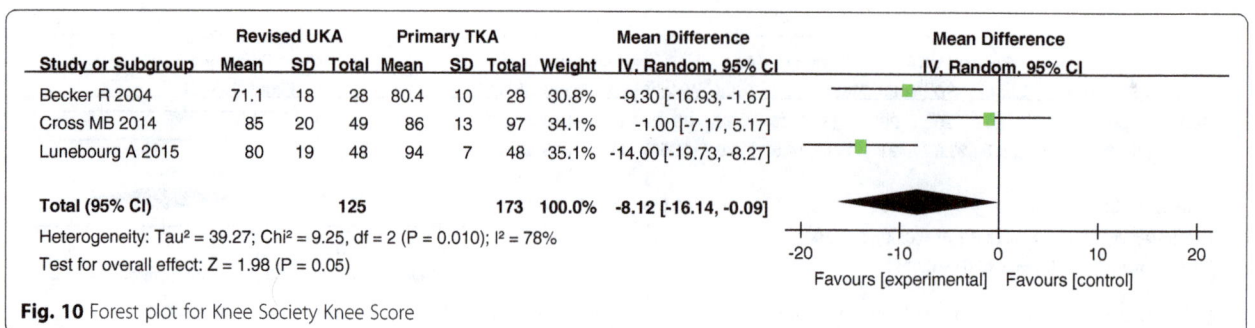

Study or Subgroup	Revised UKA Mean	SD	Total	Primary TKA Mean	SD	Total	Weight	Mean Difference IV. Random. 95% CI
Becker R 2004	71.1	18	28	80.4	10	28	30.8%	-9.30 [-16.93, -1.67]
Cross MB 2014	85	20	49	86	13	97	34.1%	-1.00 [-7.17, 5.17]
Lunebourg A 2015	80	19	48	94	7	48	35.1%	-14.00 [-19.73, -8.27]
Total (95% CI)			125			173	100.0%	-8.12 [-16.14, -0.09]

Heterogeneity: Tau² = 39.27; Chi² = 9.25, df = 2 (P = 0.010); I² = 78%
Test for overall effect: Z = 1.98 (P = 0.05)

Favours [experimental]   Favours [control]

Fig. 10 Forest plot for Knee Society Knee Score

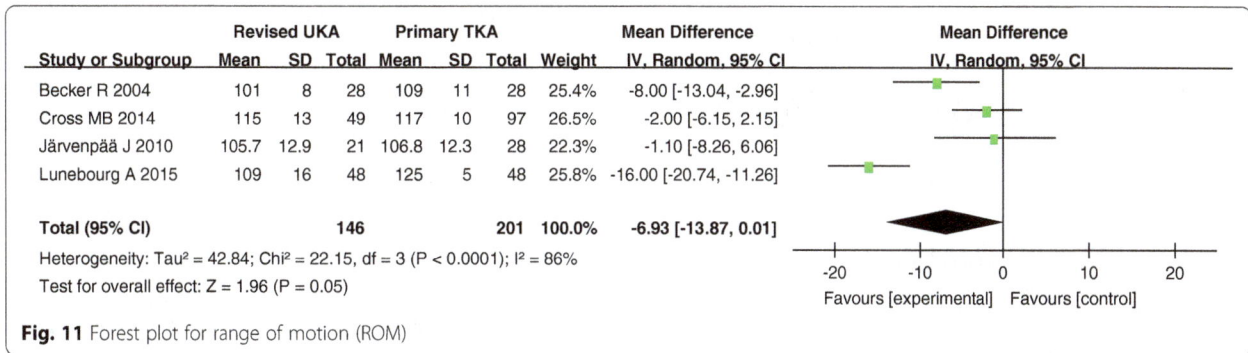

Fig. 11 Forest plot for range of motion (ROM)

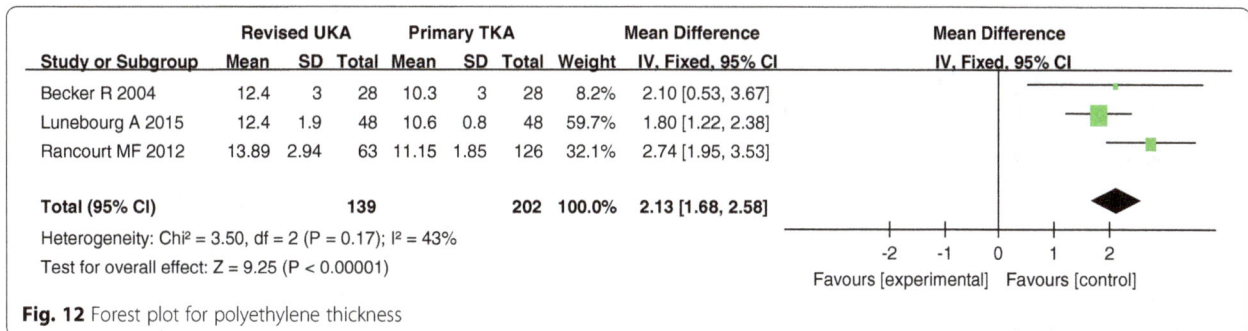

Fig. 12 Forest plot for polyethylene thickness

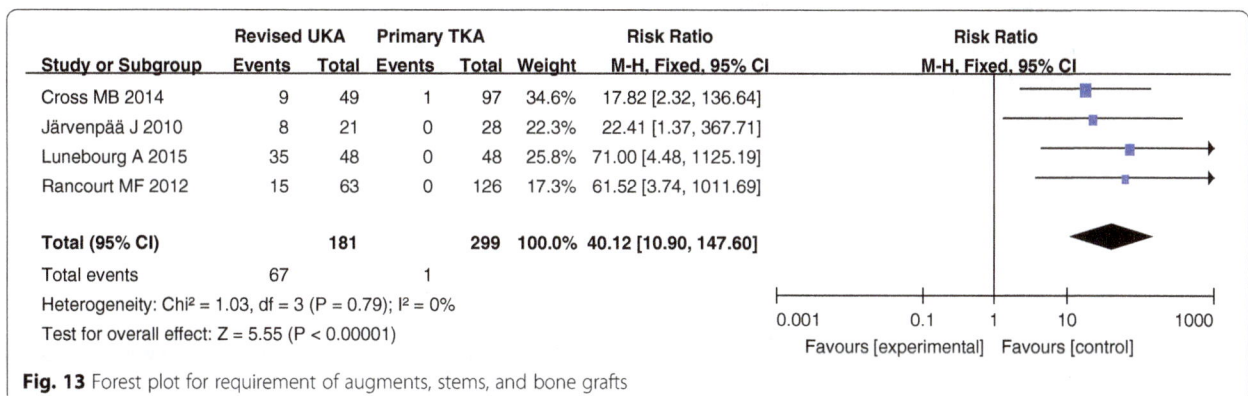

Fig. 13 Forest plot for requirement of augments, stems, and bone grafts

Abbreviations

BMI: Body mass index; CI: Confidence interval; KFS: Knee Society Function Score; KKS: Knee Society Knee Score; KSS: Knee Society Score; MD: Mean difference; ROM: Range of motion; RR: Risk ratio; TKA: Total knee arthroplasty; UKA: Unicompartmental knee arthroplasty; WOMAC: Western Ontario and McMaster Universities Osteoarthritis Index

Authors' contributions

XDS collected important background information and data. ZS performed the statistical analyses. XDS and ZS drafted the manuscript. Both authors read and approved the final manuscript.

Competing interests

The authors declare that they have no competing interests.

Author details

[1]Department of Orthopaedics, Weifang People's Hospital, no. 151 Guangwen Road, Weifang 260041, China. [2]Department of Medical Oncology, Weifang People's Hospital, no. 151 Guangwen Road, Weifang 260041, China.

References

1. Mont MA, Stuchin SA, Paley D, Sharkey PF, Parvisi J, Tria AJ Jr, Bonutti PM, Etienne G. Different surgical options for monocompartmental osteoarthritis of the knee: high tibial osteotomy versus unicompartmental knee arthroplasty versus total knee arthroplasty: indications, techniques, results, and controversies. Instr Course Lect. 2004;53:265–83.
2. Insall J, Walker P. Unicondylar knee replacement. Clin Orthop Relat Res. 1976;120:83–5.
3. Skolnick MD, Bryan RS, Peterson LF. Unicompartmental polycentric knee arthroplasty: description and preliminary results. Clin Orthop Relat Res. 1975; 112:208–14.
4. Pearse A, Hooper G, Rothwell A, et al. Survival and functional outcome after revision of a unicompartmental to a total knee replacement: the new Zealand National Joint Registry. J Bone Joint Surg Br. 2010;92(4):508–12.
5. Järvenpää J, Kettunen J, Miettinen H, et al. The clinical outcome of revision knee replacement after unicompartmental knee arthroplasty versus primary total knee arthroplasty: 8-17 years follow-up study of 49 patients. Int Orthop. 2010;34(5):649–53.
6. Miller M, Benjamin JB, Marson B, Hollstien S. The effect of implant constrainton results of conversion of unicompartmental knee arthroplasty to total knee arthroplasty. Orthopedics. 2002;25(12):1353–7.
7. Johnson S, Jones P, Newman J. The survivorship and results of total knee replacements converted from unicompartmental knee replacements. Knee. 2007;14(2):154–7.
8. Springer BD, Scott RD, Thornhill TS. Conversion of failed unicompartmental knee arthroplasty to TKA. Clin Orthop Relat Res. 2006;446:214–20.
9. Rancourt MF, Kemp KA, Plamondon SM, et al. Unicompartmental knee arthroplasties revised to total knee arthroplasties compared with primary total knee arthroplasties. J Arthroplast. 2012;27(8 Suppl):106–10.
10. Becker R, John M, Neumann WH. Clinical outcomes in the revision of unicondylar arthoplasties to bicondylar arthroplasties. A matched-pair study. Arch Orthop Trauma Surg. 2004;124(10):702–7.
11. Lunebourg A, Parratte S, Ollivier M, et al. Are revisions of unicompartmental knee arthroplasties more like a primary or revision TKA? J Arthroplast. 2015; 30(11):1985–9.
12. Cross MB, Yi PY, Moric M, et al. Revising an HTO or UKA to TKA: is it more like a primary TKA or a revision TKA? J Arthroplast. 2014;29(9 Suppl):229–31.
13. Saragaglia D, Estour G, Nemer C, Colle PE. Revision of 33 unicompartmental knee prostheses using total knee arthroplasty: strategy and results. Int Orthop. 2009;33(4):969–74.
14. Cerciello S, Morris BJ, Lustig S, Visonà E, Cerciello G, Corona K, Neyret P. Lateral tibial plateau autograft in revision surgery for failed medial unicompartmental knee arthroplasty. Knee Surg Sports Traumatol Arthrosc. 2017;25(3):773–8.
15. Craik JD, El Shafie SA, Singh VK, Twyman RS. Revision of unicompartmental knee arthroplasty versus primary total knee arthroplasty. J Arthroplast. 2015; 30(4):592–4.
16. Robb CA, Matharu GS, Baloch K, Pynsent PB. Revision surgery for failed unicompartmental knee replacement: technical aspects and clinical outcome. Acta Orthop Belg. 2013;79(3):312–7.
17. Sarraf KM, Konan S, Pastides PS, Haddad FS, Oussedik S. Bone loss during revision of unicompartmental to total knee arthroplasty: an analysis of implanted polyethylene thickness from the National Joint Registry data. J Arthroplasty. 2013;28(9):1571–4.
18. Wynn Jones H, Chan W, Harrison T, Smith TO, Masonda P, Walton NP. Revision of medial Oxford unicompartmental knee replacement to a total knee replacement: similar to a primary? Knee. 2012;19(4):339–43.
19. Berger RA, Meneghini RM, Jacobs JJ, Sheinkop MB, Della Valle CJ, Rosenberg AG, Galante JO. Results of unicompartmental knee arthroplasty at a minimum of 10 years of follow-up. J Bone Joint Surg Am. 2005;87(5):999–1006.
20. Van der List JP, Chawla H, Villa JC, Pearle AD. The role of patient characteristics on the choice of unicompartmental versus total knee arthroplasty in patients with medial osteoarthritis. J Arthroplast. 2017;32(3): 761–6.
21. Siman H, Kamath AF, Carrillo N, Harmsen WS, Pagnano MW, Sierra RJ. Unicompartmental knee arthroplasty vs total knee arthroplasty for medial compartment arthritis in patients older than 75 years: comparable reoperation, revision, and complication rates. J Arthroplast. 2017;32(6):1792–7.
22. Swienckowski JJ, Pennington DW. Unicompartmental knee arthroplasty in patients sixty years of age or younger. J Bone Joint Surg Am. 2004;86(A Suppl 1(Pt 2)):131–42.
23. Felts E, Parratte S, Pauly V, Aubaniac JM, Argenson JN. Function and quality of life following medial unicompartmental knee arthroplasty in patients 60 years of age or younger. Orthop Traumatol Surg Res. 2010;96:861–7.
24. Robertsson O, Bizjajeva S, Fenstad A, et al. Knee arthroplasty in Denmark, Norway and Sweden. A pilot study from the Nordic Arthroplasty Register Association. Acta Orthop. 2010;81(1):82–9.
25. Koskinen E, Eskelinen A, Paavolainen P, et al. Comparison of survival and cost-effectiveness between unicondylar arthroplasty and total knee arthroplasty in patients with primary osteoarthritis: a follow-up study of 50,493 knee replacements from the Finnish arthroplasty register. Acta Orthop. 2008;79(4):499–507.
26. Zambianchi F, Digennaro V, Giorgini A, Grandi G, Fiacchi F, Mugnai R, Catani F. Surgeon's experience influences UKA survivorship: a comparative study between all-poly and metal back designs. Knee Surg Sports Traumatol Arthrosc. 2015;23(7):2074–80.
27. Tregonning R, Rothwell A, Hobbs T, Hartnett N. Early failure of the Oxford phase 3 cemented medial uni-compartmental knee joint arthroplasty. J Bone Joint Surg Br. 2009;91-B(Supp II):339.
28. Mohammad HR, Strickland L, Hamilton TW, Murray DW. Long-term outcomes of over 8,000 medial Oxford phase 3 unicompartmental knees-a systematic review. Acta Orthop. 2018;89(1):101–7.

7

The etiology of idiopathic congenital talipes equinovarus

Vito Pavone, Emanuele Chisari, Andrea Vescio, Ludovico Lucenti, Giuseppe Sessa and Gianluca Testa[*]

Abstract

Background: Also known as clubfoot, idiopathic congenital talipes equinovarus (ICTEV) is the most common pediatric deformity and occurs in 1 in every 1000 live births. Even though it has been widely researched, the etiology of ICTEV remains poorly understood and is often described as being based on a multifactorial genesis. Genetic and environmental factors seem to have a major role in the development of this disease. Thus, the aim of this review is to analyze the available literature to document the current evidence on ICTEV etiology.

Methods: The literature on ICTEV etiology was systematically reviewed using the following inclusion criteria: studies of any level of evidence, reporting clinical or preclinical results, published in the last 20 years (1998–2018), and dealing with the etiology of ICTEV.

Results: A total of 48 articles were included. ICTEV etiology is still controversial. Several hypotheses have been researched, but none of them are decisive. Emerging evidence suggests a role of several pathways and gene families associated with limb development (HOX family; PITX1-TBX4), the apoptotic pathway (caspases), and muscle contractile protein (troponin and tropomyosin), but a major candidate gene has still not been identified. Strong recent evidence emerging from twin studies confirmed major roles of genetics and the environment in the disease pathogenesis.

Conclusions: The available literature on the etiology of ICTEV presents major limitations in terms of great heterogeneity and a lack of high-profile studies. Although many studies focus on the genetic background of the disease, there is lack of consensus on one or multiple targets. Genetics and smoking seem to be strongly associated with ICTEV etiology, but more studies are needed to understand the complex and multifactorial genesis of this common congenital lower-limb disease.

Keywords: Clubfoot, ICTEV, Pathogenesis, Genetics, Risk factors, Etiology

Background

Congenital talipes equinovarus (CTEV) is a foot deformity characterized by hindfoot varus, forefoot (metatarsus) adductus, an augmented midfoot arch (cavus), and equinus. This pediatric malformation can be classified according to its clinical presentation. It can be secondary or syndromic when its presentation is associated with another congenital disease (20% of cases). However, it may also occur as an isolated birth defect with no other malformations (80% of cases), which introduces the concept of idiopathic CTEV (ICTEV). The etiology of CTEV is largely unknown. Secondary CTEV is usually a manifestation of distal arthrogryposis (DA), congenital myotonic dystrophy, myelomeningocele, or other congenital diseases. While the clinical presentation may be similar to the idiopathic form, secondary CTEV seems to derive from neuromuscular [1] and fetal abnormalities [2] involved in its etiopathogenesis, thus making ICTEV and syndromic CTEV rather different in clinical presentation, treatment, and proposed etiopathogenetic mechanism [3, 4].

ICTEV is one of the most common pediatric deformities. The epidemiological studies published over the last 55 years suggest a birth prevalence in the range of 0.5 to 2.0 cases/1000 live births, which results in an estimated 7–43 cases of clubfoot/year/million population, depending mainly on the birth rate [5]. The higher prevalence

* Correspondence: gianpavel@hotmail.com
Department of General Surgery and Medical Surgical Specialties, Section of Orthopaedics and Traumatology, University Hospital Policlinico-Vittorio Emanuele, University of Catania, Via Plebiscito, 628, 95124 Catania, Italy

seems to be associated with social-demographic, genetic, and environmental risk factors, which explain its prevalence among low- and middle-income countries [5] and closed societies like the Maori population [6]. It affects males more than females [7] with a male-to-female ratio of 2:1, which is similar across different ethnic groups [8–11]. Kruse et al. proposed a reason for the gender difference in 2008 [12], but the phenotypic variability in affected individuals is still unknown.

Several treatments have been proposed throughout the centuries, but today, the gold-standard treatment is the Ponseti method [13, 14]. In syndromic cases, current evidence supports the Ponseti method or other more invasive surgical procedures [15]. The aim of this review is to analyze the available literature to provide an update on the evidence related to ICTEV etiology.

Materials and methods

We conducted this systematic review according to the guidelines of the Preferred Reporting Items for Systematic Reviews and Meta-Analyses (PRISMA) [16]. Two medical electronic databases (PubMed and Science Direct) were searched by a single author (CE) on March 20, 2018. The research string used was "(clubfoot OR congenital talipes equinovarus OR clubfeet) AND (pathology OR embryology OR etiology OR etiopathogenesis OR genetics OR pathophysiology)." A

total of $n = 1590$ articles were found. After excluding duplicates, $n = 974$ articles were selected.

The initial titles and abstracts were screened using the following inclusion criteria: studies of any level of evidence reporting clinical or preclinical results published in the last 20 years (1998–2018) and dealing with the etiology of ICTEV. Exclusion criteria were articles written in other languages or studies with a focus on secondary/syndromic CTEV, such as distal arthrogryposis, myelomeningocele, and Moebius syndrome. We also excluded all the remaining duplicates, articles dealing with other topics, with poor scientific methodology, or without an accessible abstract.

At the end of the first screening, we selected $n = 76$ articles that were eligible for full-text reading. After reading the full text, we ultimately selected $n = 48$ articles that satisfy the criteria. A PRISMA [16] flowchart of the selection and screening method is provided in Fig. 1. Reference lists from the selected papers were also screened.

Results

The included articles [3, 4, 12, 17–62] mainly focus on genetic research [17, 21–23, 25, 27, 29–31, 37–50, 52, 54–56, 58, 60, 61], epidemiological studies [12, 19, 20, 24, 32, 33, 35, 36, 53], MRI analysis [26, 51, 59], and histological histochemical analysis [18, 24, 28, 57] in ICTEV patients. Two

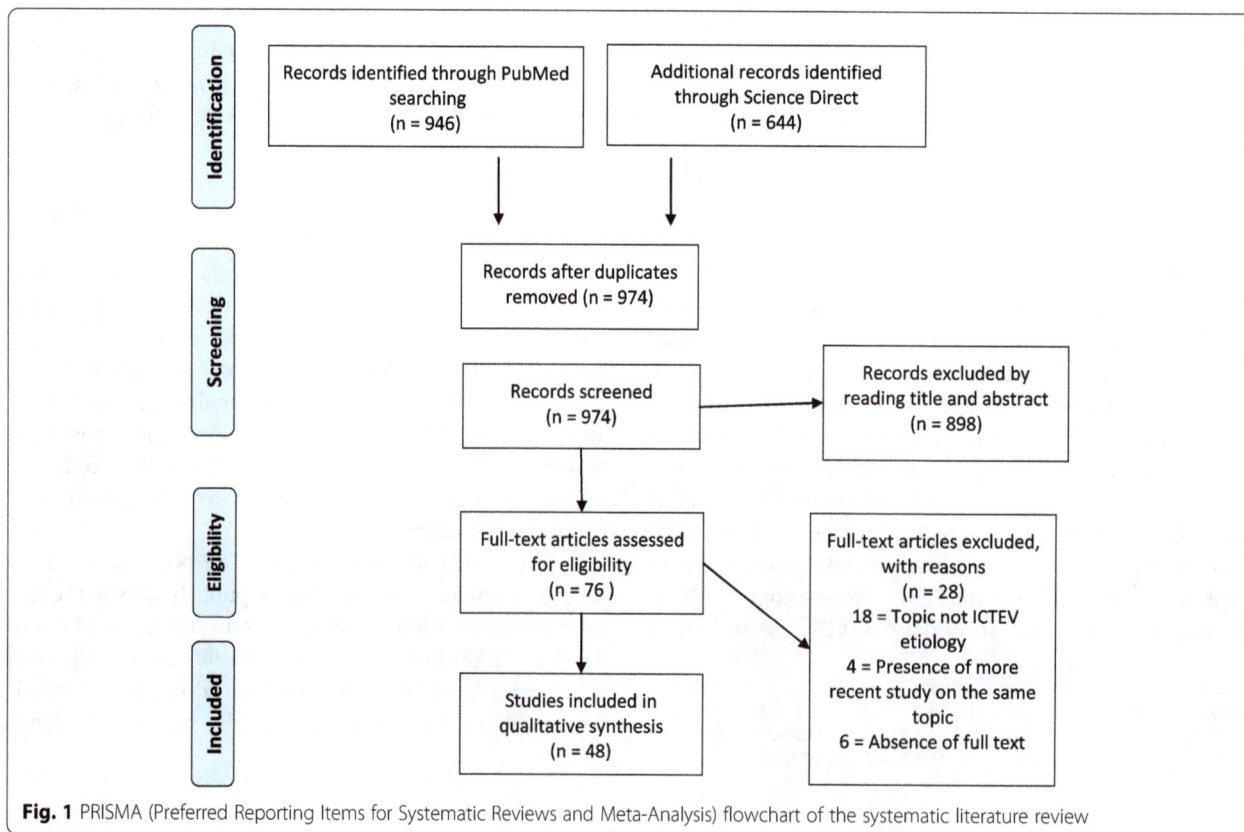

Fig. 1 PRISMA (Preferred Reporting Items for Systematic Reviews and Meta-Analysis) flowchart of the systematic literature review

previous reviews [3, 4, 62] reporting a significant analysis of the current evidence and research prospective were also included since they are part of the present evidence of the topic. The main findings of the included articles except for the two reviews were summarized (Table 1.)

ICTEV has historically been linked to several risk factors: oligohydramnios, smoking, parental age, parental education, parity, maternal anxiety or depression, alcohol use, and season of birth. A previous epidemiological study based on the difference in prevalence in different communities suggested that environmental factors have a role in pathogenesis. In 2014, a twin study done in Denmark surveyed 34,485 twins and found evidence of a role of environmental factors. The authors concluded that the presence of a genetic role in the development of the disease was not enough to explain the results. Therefore, they reported strong evidence of the presence of environmental factors to explain the statistical analysis [32]. Another study from 2013 [20] was conducted in a rural area of Turkey and showed that parental consanguineous marriage was associated with a higher risk of ICTEV. Even though the sample investigated was small, this result may support an etiology based on multiple genes and environmental factors.

Even though the role of environmental factors has been confirmed by several studies, all the proposed factors except for smoking were not significantly associated with ICTEV, which was linked to DNA oxidative damage caused by tobacco smoking [33–36]. A meta-analysis examined 172 reports containing cumulative data for 173,687 individuals and 11,674,332 unaffected controls published from 1959 to 2010. The analysis looked at the effects of smoking during pregnancy and showed that 15,673 individuals with CTEV and maternal smoking had an OR of 1.28 (95% CI 1.10–1.47) [34].

Genes involved in the metabolism of smoke-derived products may also contribute to the development of birth defects. Therefore, N-acetylation genes including NAT1, NAT2, and other related genes were screened for association analysis. Polymorphisms in the NAT2 gene cause decreased acetylation activity and have been associated with TEV. This suggests a deficit in the biotransformation of aromatic amines and the accumulation of DNA adducts, leading to a potential toxic effect and the development of TEV [27].

Hecht et al. [27] examined the variants of the NAT2 gene in 56 ICTEV multiplex families, 57 trios with a positive family history, and 160 simplex individuals. They reported a slight decrease in the expected number of homozygotes for the normal NAT2 allele in the Hispanic simplex trios. Significantly, a slow NAT2 acetylator phenotype was detected among the ICTEV patients, suggesting that slow acetylation may be a risk factor for ICTEV.

Genetic factors

Genetics has a crucial role in the development of ICTEV, even though no major gene candidate has been identified [3]. There is evidence of a family history of TEV in 24–50% of cases [22]. Results from twin studies showed concordance in monozygotic twins (32%) compared to dizygotic twins (2.9%), and a frequency of recurrence in 10–20% of families supports a role for genes in ICTEV [19, 32, 63]. There is also reported a unique case of bilateral ICTEV in preterm triplets, which provides even further support for a genetic etiology [19]. Many different families of genes were identified to play a role in the disease and a prospective role in the development of personalized conservative and surgical approaches [64]. Several families of genes and pathways were identified and investigated using mainly the candidate gene approach.

Homeobox family genes

The homeobox genes represent a family of transcription factors that play a central role in the morphogenesis processes of embryonic development. In particular, this family determines the correct genesis of the axial skeleton and limbs, which is why they were proposed as candidate genes for ICTEV pathogenesis [65]. Several candidate gene studies found a locus of genetic susceptibility associated with ICTEV in the HOX domain and the caspase domain [25, 37].

In 2009 and 2016, two large studies showed that ICTEV was associated with alteration in the regulator domain of HoxA and HoxD [38, 39]. Higher activity of the promotor was also reported as a result of promotor variation [40]. Based on the emerging evidence, we can assume that perturbation to the HOXA, HOXC, and HOXD clusters of genes may play a role in the etiology and pathogenesis of ICTEV [66].

Caspases pathway genes

Cysteine-dependent aspartate-directed proteases (caspases) are part of a family of cysteine proteases that play essential roles in apoptosis, necrosis, and inflammation processes. This family was investigated since caspase activity seems to be related to correct limb development, and related genes were first associated with ICTEV in 2005 by Heck et al. [50].

A CASP10 gene variant was found in simplex ICTEV in white and Hispanic trios. In 2007, Ester et al. [58] researched other alterations in three caspase genes. They genotyped SNPs of three different genes (Casp8, Casp10, and CFLAR) to investigate their association with ICTEV. One SNP in each of the genes was associated with the disease. Several haplotypes constructed from these SNPs displayed altered transmission, suggesting that genetic

Table 1 Main findings of the included article

Ref	Author	Subjects	Pathway/molecule involved	Results
[12]	Kruse et al. (2008)	1093 individuals: 291 with clubfoot and 802 unaffected relatives	Polygenic threshold model with sex dimorphism	This study demonstrates the presence of the Carter effect in idiopathic clubfoot. A polygenic inheritance of clubfoot can explain this effect, with females requiring a greater genetic load to be affected.
[17]	Gurnett et al. (2008)	A five-generation family with asymmetric right-sided predominant idiopathic clubfoot	PITX1	A single missense mutation (c.388G → A) was identified in PITX1 through Genome-wide linkage analysis.
[18]	Poon (2009)	Primary cell culturefrom the medial aspect of the talonavicular joint and from the plantar surface of the calcaneocuboid joint (around 10 ft)	Beta-catenin	There was a more than twofold increase in the beta-catenin protein in the contracted tissues.
[19]	Pagnotta et al. (2011)	Three homozygous preterm triplets	Presence of Bilateral ICTEV	Such a presentation had not been previously described and supports a genetic etiology of congenital idiopathic talipes equinovarus deformity.
[20]	Sahin et al. (2013)	28 cases (infants with idiopathic CTEV) and 575 controls (healthy infants) were recruited	Case-control study	Significant risk factors for idiopathic CTEV were work status (employed), consanguineous marriage, sex (male), and gestational age (> 42 weeks).
[21]	Alvarado et al.(2013)	413 isolated talipes equinovarus patients	PITX1, TBX4, HOXC13, UTX, CHD1, and RIPPLY2	A genome-wide screening found 12 rare copy number variants segregated with talipes equinovarus in multiplex pedigrees, containing the developmentally expressed transcription factors and transcriptional regulators PITX1, TBX4, HOXC13, UTX, CHD (chromodomain protein)1, and RIPPLY2
[22]	Shyy et al. (2009)	CAND2 gene was sequenced in 256 clubfoot patients, and 75 control patients, while WNT7a was screened using 56 clubfoot patients and 50 control patients	CAND2 and WNT7	Polymorphism was found in each gene, but the single nucleotide change in CAND2 was a silent mutation that did not alter the amino acid product, and the single nucleotide change in WNT7a was in the upstream, non-coding or promoter region before the start codon.
[23]	Shyy et al. (2010)	24 bilateral congenital idiopathic clubfoot patients and 24 matched controls and screened an additional 76 patients in each discovered SNP	MYH 1, 2, 3, and 8	Many single-nucleotide polymorphisms were found; none proved to be significantly associated with the phenotype of congenital idiopathic clubfoot.
[24]	Herceg et al. (2006)	95 ft in 68 ICTEV patients yielded a total of 431 muscle specimens	Histological and histochemical muscle specimens analysis	This study does not support the theory that a neuromuscular abnormality may be significant in the etiology of idiopathic talipes equinovarus because of the absence of significant alteration.
[25]	Wang et al. (2008)	Rat embryo	HOXD13 – FHL1	The findings suggest that HOXD13 may regulate the expression of FHL1 in the development of ICTEV.
[26]	Ippolito et al. (2009)	MR of both legs was taken in three cohorts of patients with unilateral ICTEV: 8 untreated new-borns (age range 10 days to 2 weeks); 8 children who had been treated with the Ponseti method (age range 2–4 years); 8 adults whose deformity had been corrected (age range 19–23 years)	Muscular atrophy	The study shows that leg muscular atrophy is a primitive pathological component of CCF which is already present in the early stages of fetal CCF development.
[27]	Hecht et al. (2007)	56 multiplex ITEV families, 57 trios with a positive family history and 160 simplex trios with ITEV	NAT 1 and NAT 2	The result suggests that slow NAT2 acetylation may be a risk factor for ITEV.
[28]	Ošťádal et al. (2015)	13 relapsed ICTEV	Proteomic analysis of the extracellular matrix	The major result of the present study was the observation that the extracellular matrix in clubfoot is composed of an additional 16 proteins, including collagens V, VI, and XII, as well as the previously described collagen types I and III and transforming growth factor beta.
[29]	Gurnett et al. (2009)	31 patients (five with familial vertical talus, 20 with familial clubfoot, and six with DA1	TNNT3, MYH3, TPM2	Although mutations in MYH3, TNNT3, and TPM2 are frequently associated with distal arthrogryposis syndromes, they were not present in patients with familial vertical talus or clubfoot.

Table 1 Main findings of the included article *(Continued)*

Ref	Author	Subjects	Pathway/molecule involved	Results
[30]	Wang et al. (2013)	Abductor hallucis muscle samples were obtained from 15 ICTEV patients. Peripheral blood samples were obtained from 84 ICTEV patients	SOX 9	mRNA and protein expression levels of SOX9 were detected through real-time polymerase chain reaction and western blot analysis, respectively and were found to be significantly higher in ICTEV muscle samples compared with those in control samples
[31]	Cao et al. (2009)	Rat ICTEV model	HOXD13 – Gli3	Findings suggest that *HoxD13* directly interacts with the promoter of *Gli3*. The increase of *Gli3* expression in the ICTEV model animal might result from the low expression of *HoxD13*.
[32]	Engell et al. (2014)	46,418 twin individuals	Twin study	The study found an overall self-reported prevalence of congenital clubfoot of 0.0027. They concluded that non-genetic factors must play a role, and a genetic factor might contribute, in the etiology of congenital clubfoot.
[33]	Parker et al. (2009)	6139 cases of clubfoot from 2001 through 2005 plus 10 controls per case.	Risk factors and prevalence	The overall prevalence of clubfoot was 1.29 per 1000 in live births. Maternal smoking and diabetes showed significant associations.
[34]	Hackshaw et al. (2011)	15,673 clubfoot cases	Smoking	Significant positive associations with maternal smoking were found for clubfoot (OR 1.28, 95% CI 1.10–1.47)
[35]	Dickinson et al (2008)	443 cases of clubfoot and 4492 randomly sampled controls	Smoking	This study is consistent with the hypothesis that smoking during pregnancy is associated with a slightly increased risk of an infant being born with clubfoot.
[36]	Honein (2000)	346 infants with isolated clubfoot and 3029 infants without defects	Smoking	This study confirms the importance of familial factors and smoking in the etiology of clubfoot and identifies a potentially important interaction.
[37]	Wang et al. (2005)	84 idiopathic congenital talipes equinovarus nuclear pedigrees	HOXD10, HOXD12 and HOXD13	HOXD12 andHOXD13 are important susceptible genes of idiopathic congenital talipes equinovarus.
[38]	Ester et al. (2009)	179 extended families and 331 simplex families and 88 trios with a positive family history. The validation population consisted of 144 NHW simplex trios	HOXA and HOXD gene clusters	These results suggest a biologic model for clubfoot in which perturbation of HOX and apoptotic genes together affect muscle and limb development, which may cause the downstream failure of limb rotation into a plantar grade position.
[39]	Alvarado et al. (2016)	1178 probands with clubfoot or verticaltalus and 1775 controls	HOXC	Since HOXD10 has been implicated in the etiology of congenital vertical talus, variation in its expression may contribute to the lower limb phenotypes occurring with 5′ HOXC microdeletions.
[40]	Weymouth et al. (2016)	Nuclear extracts isolated from undifferentiated and differentiated C2C12 mouse muscle cells	HOXA9, TPM1, and TPM2	Results show that associated promoter variants in HOXA9, TPM1, and TPM2, alter promoter expression suggesting that they have a functional role.
[41]	Liu et al. (2011)	25 children with ICTEV and 5 normal controls	COL9A1	COL9A1 protein is highly expressed in patients with ICTEV and rs1135056, which is located in the coding region of COL9A1 gene, may be associated with the pathogenesis of ICTEV.
[42]	Zhao et al. (2016)	87 children with congenital talipes equinovarus and 174 control subjects	COL9A1	In conclusion, our results indicate that the COL9A1 rs35470562 variant may contribute to congenital talipes equinovarus susceptibility in the Chinese population examined.
[43]	Zhang et al. (2006)	84 idiopathic congenital talipes equinovarus nuclear pedigree	GLI3	There is an association between GLI3 gene and ICTEV, and exons 9,10,11,12 are not its mutation hot spots.
[44]	Lu et al. (2012)	605 probands (from 148 multiplex and 457 simplex families) with non-syndromic clubfoot	*TBX4* and chromosome 17q23.1q23.2	These results demonstrate that variation in and around the *TBX4* gene and the 17q23.1q23.2 microduplication are not a frequent cause of this common orthopedic birth defect and narrows the 17q23.1q23.2 non-syndromic clubfoot-associated region.

Table 1 Main findings of the included article *(Continued)*

Ref	Author	Subjects	Pathway/molecule involved	Results
[45]	Peterson et al. (2014)	One family: mother, daughter, and two sons	TBX4	Although TBX4 remains the candidate gene for congenital clubfoot involving 17q23.1–q23.2 duplications, the explanation for variable expressivity and penetrance remains unknown.
[46]	Alvarado et al. (2011)	Mice model	Pitx1	Morphological data suggest that PITX1 haplo insufficiency may cause a developmental field defect preferentially affecting the lateral lower leg, a theory that accounts for similar findings in human clubfoot.
[47]	Alvarado et al. (2010)	66 isolated idiopathic clubfoot probands with at least one affected first-degree relative	TBX4	Our result suggests that this chromosome 17q23.1q23.2 microduplication is a relatively common cause of familial isolated clubfoot and provides strong evidence linking clubfoot etiology to abnormal early limb development.
[48]	Dobbs et al. (2006)	21 affected individuals and 17 unaffected individuals	HOXD10	This mutation was recently described in a family of Italian descent with congenital vertical talus (CVT) and Charcot-Marie-Tooth deformity HOXD10 gene mutations were not identified in any of the other families or sporadic patients with CVT, suggesting that genetic heterogeneity underlies this disorder.
[49]	Shrimpton et al. (2004)	36 members of a single family	HOXD10	In the study family, this mutation was fully penetrant and exhibited significant evidence of linkage (LOD 6.33; $\theta = 0$), and it very likely accounts for congenital vertical talus in heterozygotes.
[50]	Heck et al. (2005)	57 multiplex ITEV families and 83 simplex trios	CASP8, CASP10	Genotyping of SNPs throughout the genes in this sample of ITEV families has revealed positive linkage with association to the major allele of a variant in CASP10 in simplex ITEV white and Hispanic trios.
[51]	Duce et al. (2013)	The lower legs of six CTEV (2 bilateral, 4 unilateral) and five control young adults (ages 12–28)	3D MRI and MRA	The proportion of muscle in affected CTEV legs was significantly reduced compared with control and unaffected CTEV legs, while proportion of muscular fat increased. No spatial abnormalities in the location or branching of arteries were detected, but hypoplastic anomalies were observed.
[52]	Zhang et al. (2016)	29 individuals of the same family	ANXA3 and MTHFR	Following whole genome sequencing and comparative analysis, several differential gene variants were identified to enable a further distinction from clubfoot.
[53]	Lochmiller et al. (1998)	A total of 285 propositi were ascertained, with detailed family history information available in 173 cases and medical records on the remaining 112 propositi	Genetic and environmental risk factor	A family history of ITEV was noted in 24.4% of all propositi studied. These findings, in addition to the detailed analysis of 53 pedigrees with ITEV history, suggest that the potential role of a gene or genes operating in high-risk families produces this foot deformity.
[54]	Yang et al. (2016)	three-generation pedigree and 53 sporadic patients with CTEV	FLNB	The results provide evidence for the involvement of FLNB in the pathogenesis of isolated CTEV and have expanded the clinical spectrum of FLNB mutations.
[55]	Zhang et al. (2014)	96 isolated clubfoot patients and 1000 controls	NCOR2, ZNF664 FOXN3, SORCS1, and MMP7/ TMEM123	The study suggests a potential role for common genetic variation in several genes that have not previously been implicated in clubfoot pathogenesis.
[56]	Weymouth et al. (2011)	The discovery dataset was comprised of 224 multiplex families, which include 137 non Hispanic white (NHW) and 87 Hispanic families, and 357 simplex families, which includes 139 NHW and 218 Hispanic families	TNNC2 and TPM1	The results reported suggest that variation in genes that encode contractile proteins of skeletal myofibers may play a role in the etiology of clubfoot.
[57]	Gilbert et al. (2001)	Two normal feet from a 40-week-old stillborn fetus, and samples from six calcanei from children with relapsed CTEV, aged 2, 3, 4, and 5 years, were studied	Histological analysis of the calcaneum	The process of ossification in CTEV was retarded. The talipes cartilage matrix contained fewer cartilage canals and chondrocytes

Table 1 Main findings of the included article *(Continued)*

Ref	Author	Subjects	Pathway/molecule involved	Results
[58]	Ester et al. (2007)	210 simplex trios and 139 multiplex families	SNPs spanning seven apoptotic genes-Casp3, Casp8, Casp9, Casp10, Bid, Bcl-2, and Apaf1	One SNP in each of the genes provided impressive evidence of association with idiopathic talipes equinovarus
[60]	Sharp et al (2006).	375 case-parent triads	C677T polymorphism in MTHFR	DNA synthesis may be relevant in clubfoot development
[61]	Bonafe et al. (2002)	125 ITEV probands and their parents	DTDST	The R279W mutation is no more frequent in this population of ITEV probands than in controls.

variation in apoptotic genes may play a role in the development of ICTEV.

Collagen family genes

The collagen family genes were also linked to ICTEV. The focus of related genetic research has been on the COL9A1 and COL1A1 genes. COL9A1 encodes for one of the three alpha chains of type IX collagen, a component of the hyaline cartilage, while COL1A1 encodes for pro-alpha 1 chains of type I collagen, a component of most connective tissue that is abundant in bone and tendons. In 2008, COL1A1 was investigated in healthy and ICTEV patients. The study reported a higher expression of COL1A1 in patients with ICTEV than in healthy patients. A − 161(T → C) heterozygous mutation and a + 274(C → G) homozygous mutation were also identified in the COL1A1 gene in patients with ICTEV, suggesting that COL1A1 variants could be linked to the onset of ICTEV [37].

Based on previous studies, Wang et al. [30] investigated genes that regulate COL91A1 expression (SOX9) in 2012. They reported no mutations of the gene but a higher expression of SOX9 in the muscular cells of ICTEV patients. COL9A1 polymorphism seems to modulate the gene expression and influence the protein function. Three studies reported a role of these polymorphisms in ICTEV in the populations examined [41, 42, 67].

GLI3 gene

The GLI3 gene encodes for a C2H2-type zinc finger protein of the GLI family. In 2005, a study showed how a mutation of this gene was associated with the occurrence of ICTEV [43]. In 2009, another study [31] reported how HoxD13 directly interacts with the promoter of GLI3. They observed that GLI3 mRNA and protein expression levels were increased in ICTEV-model rats. This may mean that HOXD13 is a transcription factor of GLI3. Low expression of HOXD13 might lead to increased GLI3 expression level during limb formation, which likely plays a key role in ICTEV pathogenesis.

T-box family

The T-box family comprises transcription factors that play a crucial role in embryogenesis and morphogenesis.

Like other genes with a similar role, they are candidates for possible genetics inducers of ICTEV. TBX3 and TBX4 are the main family members studied. The TBX3 protein is a transcriptional factor of the T-box family. A 2014 study reported that mutations in this gene affect limb development were proven to have transmission disequilibrium in ICTEV patients, suggesting susceptibility to ICTEV [65].

PITX1-TBX4 pathway

TBX4 protein is a transcriptional factor that is mainly expressed in the hindlimb and is thus associated with ICTEV pathogenesis [68]. It was further studied in association with another transcriptional factor, PITX1, which is part of the same pathway. The PITX1-TBX4 pathway is responsible for early limb development. Numerous studies report that mutations in the genes encoding the transcription factors PITX1 and TBX4 lead to a reduction in lower-limb musculature and classic clubfoot phenotypes in both humans and mice [17, 44–46]. Studies support a role of the PITX1-TBX4 developmental pathway in TEV etiology.

Gurnett et al. [17] researched these pathway alterations in a five-generation family with asymmetric ICTEV segregating as an autosomal dominant condition. A single missense mutation (E130K) located in a highly conserved domain of the PITX1 gene has been identified. Another study showed that PITX1 downregulation causes a clubfoot-like phenotype in mice, thus providing evidence of the involvement of PITX in ICTEV pathogenesis [46].

TBX4 microdeletions and microduplications have been reported in patients affected by ICTEV, suggesting that chromosome 17q23.1q23.2 microduplication is a relatively common cause of familial isolated clubfoot [47]. However, in 2012, Lu et al. [44] examined the possible correlation between the hindfoot-specific gene TBX4 and ICTEV. They concluded that the microduplication is a rare cause of familial isolated clubfoot and can be segregated as an autosomal dominant phenotype. Significant variations were not present in the two known TBX4 hindlimb enhancers sequenced in 95 patients from simplex families.

A recent study conducted in 2017 reported that the PITX1-TBX4 pathway can be associated with HOXC alteration in vertical talus. They identified a HOXC13 deletion that segregated with clubfoot in a three-generation family [21]. Deletions of part of the HOXC gene cluster were later identified in two of five families with autosomal dominant isolated congenital vertical talus, suggesting that it is a possible cause of familial vertical talus [39]. Interestingly, HOXD10 mutations were previously identified in two families with vertical talus [48, 49], which strongly supports a role of homeobox gene mutations in the etiology of isolated vertical talus. However, because mutations in the PITX1-TBX4-HOXC pathway are infrequent in patients with clubfoot, other genetic mechanisms remain to be discovered and investigated [64].

Troponin and tropomyosin genes

The troponin (Tn) family is a protein complex involved in striated muscle contraction and has three subunits: Tn-I, Tn-T, and Tn-C. The Tn-I subunit inhibits actomyosin ATPase, while the Tn-T subunit binds tropomyosin and Tn-C. The Tn-C subunit binds calcium and overcomes the inhibitory action of the troponin complex on actin filaments.

A 2011 study analyzed 15 genes encoding proteins that control myofiber contractility in a cohort of both non-Hispanic white (NHW) and Hispanic families. They reported an association between ICTEV patients and multiple SNPs of two genes regulating troponin activity, TNNC2 and TPM1, suggesting a possible role in the etiology [56].

TPM1 is a member of the tropomyosin family, which comprises actin-binding proteins involved in the contraction of both striated and smooth muscles and the cytoskeleton of non-muscular cells. The associations of multiple SNPs in the TPM1 gene with ICTEV suggest a potential role of genes that encode contractile proteins of skeletal myofibers in the etiology of ICTEV [23]. ICTEV patients present a clinically evident alteration of the calf muscle at birth, which usually resituates after treatment [26, 69, 70]. This suggests the involvement of genes that play a role in muscle morphogenesis.

Distal arthrogryposis is a cause of syndromic TEV that is characterized by variations in genes that encode for components of the muscle contractile complex (MYH3, TPM2, TNNT3, TNNI2, and MYH8), resulting in muscle contractures. The similar phenotype suggests that these genes could be candidate genes. However, one study found that the development of the disease was different in ICTEV and in DA, even though it suggested a potential role of many regulatory candidate genes that could cause developmental defects in the hypaxial musculature that is invariably observed in clubfoot [24].

In contrast to other studies, Gurnett et al. [29] investigated 39 patients in 2009 to find mutations in the TNNT3, MYH3, and TPM2 genes in patients with ICTEV. The results showed an absence of correlation of these mutations in ICTEV patients. Recent evidence showed an absence of significant histological and cytological alteration of muscles after treatment [24]. Another work proposed an innovative 3D RM study of the muscle morphology to show how intramuscular fat distribution plays an important role in the morphology of the leg [51]. The potential of using MRI has also been suggested to better understand the clinical severity of an affected patient [71].

CAND2 and Wnt7a

In 2009, a study investigated two candidate genes, CAND2 and Wnt7a, and tested their role in the pathogenesis of ICTEV. They genotyped the CAND2 gene in 256 clubfoot patients and 75 control patients, while Wnt7a was screened using 56 clubfoot patients and 50 control patients. The study reported a polymorphism in each gene. However, the association results indicated that CAND2 and WNT7a are not major genes involved in the etiology of ICTEV [22].

In 2009, Poon et al. [18] showed that foot tissues were related to higher beta catenin levels. This was probably related to the Wnt signaling pathway and the synthesis of type III collagen. In particular, a higher amount of type III collagen was reported in studies analyzing the extracellular matrix of ICTEV tissues [28, 57]. More research is needed to understand the interactions of these growth factors with other proteins and their role in ICTEV etiology.

Dysplasia sulfate transporter gene

The dysplasia sulfate transporter (DTDST) gene was suggested to cause ICTEV and investigated by Bonafé et al. [61]. They tested whether R279 W mutations are responsible for the occurrence, but alterations in the coding region were not identified in 10 probands with ICTEV and a positive family history. The authors concluded that the R279 W mutation is no more frequent in this population of ICTEV probands than in controls.

Methylenetetrahydrofolate reductase gene

In 2006, Sharp et al. found that children who carry the 677T variant of the methylenetetrahydrofolate reductase gene (MTHFR) have a lower risk of ICTEV [60]. Another study later used whole genome sequencing to investigate the variants of MTHFR and the annexin A3 gene (ANXA3). They reported an MTHFR variant that is different from the variant associated with clubfoot in the study by Sharp et al. [52]. Bioinformatic analysis showed that the protein-binding region could be altered by this mutation (a sequence shift: the wild type is 264, while the mutant type is 267). Despite sharing some similar symptoms, these findings imply that the variant was associated with another genetic disease and not ICTEV. Furthermore, specific CNV profiles were identified in association with the diseased samples, thus further demonstrating the complexity of this multigenerational disorder [52].

Discussion

The etiology of ICTEV remains unknown as stated in recent reviews [3, 4, 72]. Many theories have been developed, but no one has clarified the major roles in the pathogenesis of idiopathic clubfoot. Recent studies have focused on the interaction between genetics and environmental factors, showing a multifactorial identity of the disease. Today, this remains the most validated theory.

A recent paper [73] reported a genetic analysis on a spontaneous autosomal recessive mouse model of peroneal muscular atrophy (PMA). It was used to understand the underlying developmental causes of ICTEV. The PMA mutation was mapped, and several candidate genes were identified, of which LIMK1 was upregulated in mutant mice. Collison et al. also reported that in chickens, LIMK1 upregulation can cause sciatic nerve defects and a TEV phenotype [73]. Further studies should be conducted using these models.

The years of research using the candidate gene approach has provided us more knowledge on the possible pathways involved in ICTEV pathogenesis, but it has failed to find a major gene causing the disease. The literature illustrates the great heterogeneity of the genetic causes of ICTEV. The candidate approach has probably not recognized the real amount of various causative variants and has likely underestimated the phenotypical and genotypical variants. The reported studies were also done using also different technical approaches, such as genome-wide association analysis (GWAS), linkage analysis, the technique of copy number variation, and whole exome sequencing. These next-generation genetic analyses should lead future studies on ICTEV etiology. Collaborative multicenter studies involving large populations might be a necessary step to shed light on the etiology of this complex disease. ICTEV inheritance is most often considered complex, with more than 75% of all cases reporting no family history [17, 53]. Thus, a large-scale GWAS study might reveal interesting results.

The filamin B (FLNB) gene encodes a member of the filamin family. The encoded protein interacts with glycoprotein Ib alpha as part of the process of repairing vascular injuries. The platelet glycoprotein Ib complex includes glycoprotein Ib alpha and binds the actin cytoskeleton. In 2016, Yang et al. performed WES sequencing and Sanger sequencing to identify and validate disease-causing mutations in a three-generation pedigree and 53 sporadic patients with ICTEV, respectively. A c.4717G>T (p.D1573Y) mutation in the FLNB gene, which co-segregated with ICETV, was identified in the pedigree. Two additional novel missense mutations in the same gene, c.1897A>G (p.M633V) and c.2195A>G (p.Y732C), were identified in the 53 sporadic patients, thus providing evidence of the involvement of the FLNB gene in ICTEV [54].

In 2014, Zhang et al. performed a GWAS study of the DNA of 396 isolated clubfoot patients and 1000 controls of European descent. The DNA was genotyped for > 600,000 single nucleotide polymorphisms (SNPs) to identify novel genes for ICTEV. The variants selected were then replicated with an independent cohort of 370 isolated clubfoot cases and 363 controls of European descent. The study found a strong association with the disease for an intergenic SNP on chromosome 12q24.31 between NCOR2 and ZNF664 (rs7969148, OR = 0.58, $p = 1.25 \times 10^{-5}$), which was significant on replication (combined OR = 0.63, $p = 1.90 \times 10^{-7}$). However, additional suggestive SNPs (Hox Genes, PITX1, TBX4, FOXN3, SORCS1, and MMP7/TMEM123) in the identified pathways were not significant in the replication phase [55]. With the aid of a new animal model, next-generation studies may have the potential to identify genes underlying the phenotype and elucidate the inheritance pattern and penetrance of the disorder [3].

Conclusions

The available literature on the etiology of ICTEV presents major limitations in terms of great heterogeneity and lack of high-profile studies. Although many studies have focused on the genetic background of the disease, there is a lack of consensus on one or multiple targets. Recent evidence shows a major role of both genetic and environmental factors. Thus far, smoking is the major environmental factor supported by recent evidence. The etiology of ICTEV is probably multifactorial and associated with multiple gene alterations, and large multi-center studies are required to investigate them. Further large international collaborative studies using next-generation sequencing technology in ICTEV patients are strongly encouraged.

Abbreviations
DTDST: Dysplasia sulphate transporter; FLNB: Filamin B; GWAS: Genome wide association analysis; ICTEV: Idiopathic congenital talipes equinovarus; MTHFR: Methylenetetrahydrofolate reductase; PMA: Peroneal muscular atrophy; PRISMA: Preferred Reporting Items for Systematic Reviews and Meta-Analyses

Authors' contributions
The design of the study was made by VP, EC, and GT. EC wrote the manuscript. EC searched the literatures and analyzed and collected the data. VP and GT assisted in the critical revision of the manuscript for important intellectual content. Editing was made by VP, GT, and EC. VP provided financial funding. All authors read and approved the final manuscript.

Competing interests
The authors declare that they have no competing interests.

References
1. Lovell ME, Morcuende JA. Neuromuscular disease as the cause of late clubfoot relapses: report of 4 cases. Iowa Orthop J. 2007;27:82–4.
2. Hester TW, Parkinson LC, Robson J, Misra S, Sangha H, Martin JE. A hypothesis and model of reduced fetal movement as a common pathogenetic mechanism in clubfoot. Med Hypotheses. 2009;73:986–8.
3. Basit S, Khoshhal KI. Genetics of clubfoot; recent progress and future perspectives. Eur J Med Genet. 2018;61(2):107–13.
4. Yong BC, Xun FX, Zhao LJ, Deng HW, Xu HW. A systematic review of association studies of common variants associated with idiopathic congenital talipes equinovarus (ICTEV) in humans in the past 30 years. Springerplus. 2016;5(1):896.
5. Smythe T, Kuper H, Macleod D, Foster A, Lavy C. Birth prevalence of congenital talipes equinovarus in low- and middle-income countries: a systematic review and meta-analysis. Trop Med Int Heal. 2017;22(3):269–85.
6. Chapman C, Stott NS, Port RV, Nicol RO. Genetics of club foot in Maori and Pacific people. J Med Genet. 2000;37(9):680–3.
7. Zionts LE, Jew MH, Ebramzadeh E, Sangiorgio SN. The influence of sex and laterality on clubfoot severity. J Pediatr Orthop. 2017;37(2):e129–33.
8. Pavone V, Bianca S, Grosso G, Pavone P, Mistretta A, Longo MR, et al. Congenital talipes equinovarus: an epidemiological study in Sicily. Acta Orthop. 2012;83(3):294–8.
9. Wijayasinghe SR, Abeysekera WYM, Dharmaratne TSS. Descriptive epidemiology of congenital clubfoot deformity in Sri Lanka. J Coll Physicians Surg Pak. 2018;28(2):166–8.
10. McConnell L, Cosma D, Vasilescu D, Morcuende J. Descriptive epidemiology of clubfoot in Romania: a clinic-based study. Eur Rev Med Pharmacol Sci. 2016;20(2):220–4.
11. Palma M, Cook T, Segura J, Pecho A, Morcuende JA. Descriptive epidemiology of clubfoot in Peru: a clinic-based study. Iowa Orthop J. 2013;33:167–71.
12. Kruse LM, Dobbs MB, Gurnett CA. Polygenic threshold model with sex dimorphism in clubfoot inheritance: the Carter effect. J Bone Joint Surg Am. 2008;90(12):2688–94.
13. Shabtai L. Worldwide spread of the Ponseti method for clubfoot. World J Orthop. 2014;5(5):585.
14. Pavone V, Testa G, Costarella L, Pavone P, Sessa G. Congenital idiopathic talipes equinovarus: an evaluation in infants treated by the Ponseti method. Eur Rev Med Pharmacol Sci. 2013;17(19):2675–9.
15. Hosseinzadeh P, Kelly DM, Zionts LE. Management of the relapsed clubfoot following treatment using the Ponseti method. J Am Acad Orthop Surg. 2017;25(3):195–203.
16. Moher D, Liberati A, Tetzlaff J, Altman DG, PRISMA Group. Preferred Reporting Items for systematic reviews and meta-analyses: the PRISMA statement. PLoS Med. 2009;6(7):e1000097.
17. Gurnett CA, Alaee F, Kruse LM, Desruisseau DM, Hecht JT, Wise CA, et al. Asymmetric lower-limb malformations in individuals with homeobox PITX1 gene mutation. Am J Hum Genet. 2008;83(5):616–22.
18. Poon R, Li C, Alman BA. Beta-catenin mediates soft tissue contracture in clubfoot. Clin Orthop Relat Res. 2009;467(5):1180–5.
19. Pagnotta G, Boccanera F, Rizzo G, Agostino R, Gougoulias N, Maffulli N. Bilateral clubfoot in three homozygous preterm triplets. J Foot Ankle Surg. 2011;50(6):718–20.
20. Sahin O, Yildirim C, Akgun RC, Haberal B, Yazici AC, Tuncay IC. Consanguineous marriage and increased risk of idiopathic congenital talipes equinovarus: a case-control study in a rural area. J Pediatr Orthop. 2013;33(3):333–8.
21. Alvarado DM, Buchan JG, Frick SL, Herzenberg JE, Dobbs MB, Gurnett CA. Copy number analysis of 413 isolated talipes equinovarus patients suggests role for transcriptional regulators of early limb development. Eur J Hum Genet. 2013;21(4):373–80.
22. Shyy W, Dietz F, Dobbs MB, Sheffield VC, Morcuende JA. Evaluation of CAND2 and WNT7a as candidate genes for congenital idiopathic clubfoot. Clin Orthop Relat Res. 2009;467(5):1201–5.
23. Shyy W, Wang K, Sheffield VC, Morcuende JA. Evaluation of embryonic and perinatal myosin gene mutations and the etiology of congenital idiopathic clubfoot. J Pediatr Orthop. 2010;30(3):231–4.
24. Herceg MB, Weiner DS, Agamanolis DP, Hawk D. Histologic and histochemical analysis of muscle specimens in idiopathic talipes equinovarus. J Pediatr Orthop. 2006;26(1):91–3.
25. Wang LL, Fu WN, Li-Ling J, Li ZG, Li LY, Sun KL. HOXD13 may play a role in idiopathic congenital clubfoot by regulating the expression of FHL1. Cytogenet Genome Res. 2008;121(3–4):189–95.
26. Ippolito E, De Maio F, Mancini F, Bellini D, Orefice A. Leg muscle atrophy in idiopathic congenital clubfoot: is it primitive or acquired? J Child Orthop. 2009;3(3):171–8.
27. Hecht JT, Ester A, Scott A, Wise CA, Iovannisci DM, Lammer EJ, et al. NAT2 variation and idiopathic talipes equinovarus (clubfoot). Am J Med Genet Part A. 2007;143A(19):2285–91.
28. Ošťádal M, Eckhardt A, Herget J, Mikšík I, Dungl P, Chomiak J, et al. Proteomic analysis of the extracellular matrix in idiopathic pes equinovarus. Mol Cell Biochem. 2015;501(1–2):133–9.
29. Gurnett CA, Alaee F, Desruisseau D, Boehm S, Dobbs MB. Skeletal muscle contractile gene (TNNT3, MYH3, TPM2) mutations not found in vertical talus or clubfoot. Clin Orthop Relat Res. 2009;467(5):1195–200.
30. Wang Z, Yan N, Liu L, Cao D, Gao M, Lin C, Jin C. SOX9 overexpression plays a potential role in idiopathic congenital talipes equinovarus. Mol Med Rep. 2013;7(3):821–5.
31. Cao D, Jin C, Ren M, Lin C, Zhang X, Zhao N. The expression of Gli3, regulated by HOXD13, may play a role in idiopathic congenital talipes equinovarus. BMC Musculoskelet Disord. 2009;10(1):142.
32. Engell V, Nielsen J, Damborg F, Kyvik KO, Thomsen K, Pedersen NW. Heritability of clubfoot: a twin study. J Child Orthop. 2014;8(1):37–41.
33. Parker SE, Mai CT, Strickland MJ, Olney RS, Rickard R, Marengo L, et al. Multistate study of the epidemiology of clubfoot. Birth Defects Res A Clin Mol Teratol. 2009;85(11):897–904.
34. Hackshaw A, Rodeck C, Boniface S. Maternal smoking in pregnancy and birth defects: a systematic review based on 173 687 malformed cases and 11.7 million controls. Hum Reprod Update. 2011;17(5):589–604.
35. Dickinson KC, Meyer RE, Kotch J. Maternal smoking and the risk for clubfoot in infants. Birth Defects Res A Clin Mol Teratol. 2008;82(2):86–91.
36. Honein MA, Paulozzi LJ, Moore CA. Family history, maternal smoking, and clubfoot: an indication of a gene-environment interaction. Am J Epidemiol. 2000;152(7):658–65.
37. Wang L, Jin C, Liu L, Zhang X, Ji S, Sun K. Analysis of association between 5' HOXD gene and idiopathic congenital talipes equinovarus. Zhonghua Yi Xue Yi Chuan Xue Za Zhi. 2005;22(6):653–6.
38. Ester AR, Weymouth KS, Burt A, Wise CA, Scott A, Gurnett CA. Altered transmission of HOX and apoptotic SNPs identify a potential common pathway for clubfoot. Am J Med Genet A. 2009;149A(12):2745–52.
39. Alvarado DM, McCall K, Hecht JT, Dobbs MB, Gurnett CA. Deletions of 5' HOXC genes are associated with lower extremity malformations, including clubfoot and vertical talus. J Med Genet. 2016;53(4):250–5.
40. Weymouth KS, Blanton SH, Powell T, Patel CV, Savill SA, Hecht JT. Functional assessment of clubfoot associated HOXA9, TPM1, and TPM2 variants suggests a potential gene regulation mechanism. Clin Orthop Relat Res. 2016;474(7):1726–35.
41. Liu LY, Jin CL, Jiang L, Lin CK. Expression of COL9A1 gene and its polymorphism in children with idiopathic congenital talipes equinovarus. Zhongguo Dang Dai Er Ke Za Zhi. 2011;13(6):478–81.

42. Zhao XL, Wang YJ, Wu YL, Han WH. Role of COL9A1 genetic polymorphisms in development of congenital talipes equinovarus in a Chinese population. Genet Mol Res. 2016;15(4).

43. Zhang X, Jin CL, Liu LY, Zhao N, Zhang LJ, Ji SJ. Association and mutation analysis of GLI3 gene in idiopathic congenital talipes equinovarus. Zhonghua Yi Xue Yi Chuan Xue Za Zhi. 2006;23(5):551–4.

44. Lu W, Bacino CA, Richards BS, Alvarez C, VanderMeer JE, Vella M, et al. Studies of TBX4 and chromosome 17q23.1q23.2: an uncommon cause of nonsyndromic clubfoot. Am J Med Genet A. 2012;158(7):1620–7.

45. Peterson JF, Ghaloul-Gonzalez L, Madan-Khetarpal S, Hartman J, Surti U, Rajkovic A, et al. Familial microduplication of 17q23.1-q23.2 involving TBX4 is associated with congenital clubfoot and reduced penetrance in females. Am J Med Genet A. 2014;164(2):364–9.

46. Alvarado DM, McCall K, Aferol H, Silva MJ, Garbow JR, Spees WM, et al. Pitx1 haploinsufficiency causes clubfoot in humans and a clubfoot-like phenotype in mice. Hum Mol Genet. 2011;20(20):3943–52.

47. Alvarado DM, Aferol H, McCall K, Huang JB, Techy M, Buchan J, et al. Familial isolated clubfoot is associated with recurrent chromosome 17q23.1q23.2 microduplications containing TBX4. Am J Hum Genet. 2010;87: 154–60.

48. Dobbs MB, Gurnett CA, Pierce B, Exner GU, Robarge J, Morcuende JA, et al. HOXD10 M319K mutation in a family with isolated congenital vertical talus. J Orthop Res. 2006;24(3):448–53.

49. Shrimpton AE, Levinsohn EM, Yozawitz JM, Packard DS Jr, Cady RB, Middleton FA, et al. A HOX gene mutation in a family with isolated congenital vertical talus and Charcot-Marie-Tooth disease. Am J Hum Genet. 2004;75(1):92–6.

50. Heck AL, Bray MS, Scott A, Blanton SH, Hecht JT. Variation in CASP10 gene is associated with idiopathic talipes equinovarus. J Pediatr Orthop. 2005; 25(5):598–602.

51. Duce SL, D'Alessandro M, Du Y, Jagpal B, Gilbert FJ, Crichton L, et al. 3D MRI analysis of the lower legs of treated idiopathic congenital talipes equinovarus (clubfoot). PLoS One. 2013;8(1):e54100.

52. Zhang Z, Kong Z, Zhu M, Lu W, Ni L, Bai Y. Whole genome sequencing identifies ANXA3 and MTHFR mutations in a large family with an unknown equinus deformity associated genetic disorder. Mol Biol Rep. 2016;43(10): 1147–55.

53. Lochmiller C, Johnston D, Scott A, Risman M, Hecht JT. Genetic epidemiology study of idiopathic talipes equinovarus. Am J Med Genet. 1998;79(2):90–6.

54. Yang H, Zheng Z, Cai H, Li H, Ye X, Zhang X. Three novel missense mutations in the filamin B gene are associated with isolated congenital talipes equinovarus. Hum Genet. 2016;135(10):1181–9.

55. Zhang TX, Haller G, Lin P, Alvarado DM, Hecht JT, Blanton SH, et al. Genome-wide association study identifies new disease loci for isolated clubfoot. J Med Genet. 2014;51(5):334–9.

56. Weymouth KS, Blanton SH, Bamshad MJ, Beck AE, Alvarez C, Richards S. Variants in genes that encode muscle contractile proteins influence risk for isolated clubfoot. Am J Med Genet A. 2011;155(9):2170–9.

57. Gilbert JA, Roach HI, Clarke NMP. Histological abnormalities of the calcaneum in congenital talipes equinovarus. J Orthop Sci. 2001;6(6):519–26.

58. Ester AR, Tyerman G, Wise CA, Blanton SH, Hecht JT. Apoptotic gene analysis in idiopathic talipes equinovarus (clubfoot). Clin Orthop Relat Res. 2007;462(462):32–7.

59. Ippolito E, Dragoni M, Antonicoli M, Farsetti P, Simonetti G, Masala S. An MRI volumetric study for leg muscles in congenital clubfoot. J Child Orthop. 2012;6(5):433–8.

60. Sharp L, Miedzybrodzka Z, Cardy AH, Inglis J, Madrigal L, Barker S. The C677T polymorphism in the methylenetetrahydrofolate reductase gene (MTHFR), maternal use of folic acid supplements, and risk of isolated clubfoot: a case-parent-triad analysis. Am J Epidemiol. 2006;164(9):852–61.

61. Bonafe L, et al. DTDST mutations are not a frequent cause of idiopathic talipes equinovarus (club foot). J Med Genet. 2002;39(4):e20.

62. Chesney D, Barker S, Miedzybrodzka Z, Haites N, Maffulli N. Epidemiology and genetic theories in the etiology of congenital talipes equinovarus. Bull Hosp Jt Dis. 1999;58(1):59–64.

63. Barker S, Chesney D, Miedzybrodzka Z, Maffulli N. Genetics and epidemiology of idiopathic congenital talipes equinovarus. J Pediatr Orthop. 2003; 23(2):265–72.

64. Dobbs MB, Gurnett CA. The 2017 ABJS Nicolas Andry award: advancing personalized medicine for clubfoot through translational research. Clin Orthop Relat Res. 2017;475(6):1716–25.

65. Raines AM, Magella B, Adam M, Potter SS. Key pathways regulated by HoxA9,10,11/HoxD9,10,11 during limb development. BMC Dev Biol. 2015; 15(1):28.

66. Dobbs MB, Gurnett CA. Genetics of clubfoot. J Pediatr Orthop B. 2012;21(1):7–9.

67. Brachvogel B, Zaucke F, Dave K, Norris EL, Stermann J, Dayakli M, et al. Comparative proteomic analysis of normal and collagen IX null mouse cartilage reveals altered extracellular matrix composition and novel components of the collagen IX interactome. J Biol Chem. 2013;288(19): 13481–92.

68. Menke DB, Guenther C, Kingsley DM. Dual hindlimb control elements in the Tbx4 gene and region-specific control of bone size in vertebrate limbs. Development. 2008;135(15):2543–53.

69. Irani RN, Sherman MS. The pathological anatomy of idiopathic clubfoot. Clin Orthop Relat Res. 2012;84:14–20.

70. Isaacs H, Handelsman JE, Badenhorst M, Pickering A. The muscles in club foot--a histological histochemical and electron microscopic study. J Bone Joint Surg Br. 1977;59–B(4):465–72.

71. Moon DK, Gurnett CA, Aferol H, Siegel MJ, Commean PK, Dobbs MB. Soft-tissue abnormalities associated with treatment-resistant and treatment-responsive clubfoot. J Bone Jt Surg. 2014;96(15):1249–56.

72. Cardy A, Barker S, Chesney D, Sharp L, Maffulli N, Miedzybrodzka Z. Pedigree analysis and epidemiological features of idiopathic congenital talipes equinovarus in the United Kingdom: a case-control study. BMC Musculoskelet Disord. 2007;8(1):62.

73. Collinson JM, Lindström NO, Neves C, Wallace K, Meharg C, Charles RH, et al. The developmental and genetic basis of 'clubfoot' in the peroneal muscular atrophy mutant mouse. Development. 2018;145(3):dev160093.

8

Rotator cuff tear healing process with graft augmentation of fascia lata in a rabbit model

Takeshi Kataoka, Takeshi Kokubu, Tomoyuki Muto, Yutaka Mifune[*], Atsuyuki Inui, Ryosuke Sakata, Hanako Nishimoto, Yoshifumi Harada, Fumiaki Takase, Yasuhiro Ueda, Takashi Kurosawa, Kohei Yamaura and Ryosuke Kuroda

Abstract

Background: Fascia lata augmentation of massive rotator cuff tears has shown good clinical results. However, its biological effect during the early healing process is not clearly understood. The purpose of the study was to evaluate the biological efficacy of fascia lata augmentation during the early healing process of rotator cuff tears using a rabbit rotator cuff defect model.

Methods: The infraspinatus tendon was resected from the greater tuberosity of a rabbit to create a rotator cuff tear. The tendon edge was directly sutured to the humeral head. The rotator cuff repaired site was augmented with a fascia lata autograft (augmentation group, group A). The rotator cuff defect in the contralateral shoulder was repaired without augmentation (reattachment group, group R). A group with intact rotator cuff was set as the control group. Histological examinations and mechanical analysis were conducted 4 and 8 weeks postoperatively.

Results: In the HE staining, the tendon maturing score of group A was higher than that of group R at 4 weeks postoperatively. In the safranin O staining, proteoglycan staining at the repaired enthesis in group A at 4 weeks postoperatively was stronger than that in group R. Picrosirius red staining showed that type III and type I collagen in group A was more strongly expressed than that in group R at 4 weeks postoperatively. The ultimate failure load of the infraspinatus tendon–humeral head complex in group A was statistically higher than that in group R at 4 weeks postoperatively. The ultimate failure load of group A was similar to that of the control group.

Conclusion: The biological and mechanical contribution of fascia lata augmentation for massive rotator cuff tears was analyzed in this study. Type III collagen was reported to be expressed during the tendon healing process. Although the biological action similar to natural ligament healing occurred around the fascia lata grafts, type III collagen was gradually replaced by type I collagen as the tissue matured. Our results suggest that fascia lata augmentation could stimulate biological healing and provide initial fixation strength of the repaired rotator cuff.

Keywords: Large and massive rotator cuff tear, Fascia lata augmentation, Type III collagen, Ultimate failure load

* Correspondence: m-ship@kf7.so-net.ne.jp
Department of Orthopaedic Surgery, Kobe University Graduate School of Medicine, 7-5-1 Kusunoki-cho, Chuo-ku, Kobe, Hyogo 650-0017, Japan

Background

Rotator cuff tears have been reported to occur in > 50% of patients aged > 60 years [1]. They cause chronic pain and severe dysfunction, leading to degenerative changes in the glenohumeral joint [2, 3]. Excellent outcomes of arthroscopic rotator cuff repair for small and medium tears have been recently reported [4, 5]. In contrast, large and massive rotator cuff tears are challenging for surgeons. Various surgical procedures, such as musculotendinous transfer [6], autograft augmentation [7], or synthetic materials [8] are available for the repair of massive rotator cuff tears. However, retears have been a common complication after surgical repair of such tears. The retear rates have been reported to be 14–66% for large or massive tears [9–13]. Shoulders without cuff retear had better function during daily activities and better range of motion than shoulders with retears [3]. Retears are presumed to result from high tension and insufficient initial biological healing at the repair site [14]. We have performed a single-row repair with graft augmentation of the fascia lata for large and massive rotator cuff tears to reduce tension at the tendon–bone repair site [15]. However, its biological effect during the early healing period has not been clearly understood. The purpose of the study was to evaluate the biological efficacy of fascia lata augmentation during the early healing process of rotator cuff tears using a rabbit rotator cuff defect model.

Methods

Animal model of rotator cuff repair

This investigation was approved by the Institutional Animal Care and Use Committee and carried out according to the Kobe University Animal Experimentation Regulations (permission number P140102). Twenty-four skeletally mature female Japanese white rabbits were used in this study. Their age was 16 weeks, and their mean weight was 3.1 kg (range, 2.7–3.5 kg). Intravenous pentobarbital (30 mg/kg; Kyoritsu Seiyaku, Tokyo, Japan) was administered to rabbits. Lidocaine (1%, 10 mg/kg; AstraZeneca, London, UK) was subcutaneously injected. Rabbits were placed in a lateral position, a 3-cm skin incision was made over the lateral border of the acromion on both shoulders, and the infraspinatus tendons were exposed. The infraspinatus tendons (5 × 5 mm) were resected from the greater tuberosity to create rotator cuff defects, and decortication was subsequently performed at the greater tuberosity of the humeral head (1 × 5 mm) to remove normal enthesis and expose the cancellous bone. Two bone tunnels were created from the footprint in the left shoulder using a 1.0-mm Kirschner wire, and tendon edge was sutured directly to the humeral head using a 4-0 nylon suture (reattachment group, group R). Tendons in the right shoulder were repaired similarly, and the repaired site was augmented with a fascia lata autograft (5 × 5 mm) (augmentation group, group A) (Fig. 1). A fascia lata autograft was harvested from the lateral aspect of the right thigh. The fascia lata was transplanted on the repair site and sutured using two simple stitches with a 4-0 nylon. All rabbits were mobilized postoperatively and were immediately allowed to move freely within their cages. The rabbits were euthanized using overdose of pentobarbital sodium at 4 and 8 weeks postoperatively. Four rabbits did not undergo surgery and were examined mechanically as normal controls.

Histological analysis

The infraspinatus tendon–humeral head complexes were fixed in 4% paraformaldehyde, decalcified with 0.25 mol/l ethylenediaminetetraacetic acid in a phosphate-buffered saline (pH 7.5), and embedded in paraffin. Continuous sections (7 μm in thickness) were cut in the sagittal plane in the middle of the tendons. Tissue sections were stained

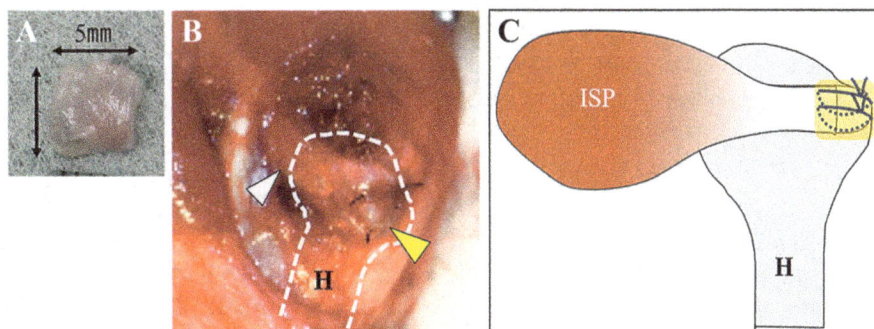

Fig. 1 Animal model of rotator cuff repair. **a** Macrography of the fascia lata autograft (5 × 5 mm). **b** Fascia lata autograft was transplanted on the rotator cuff repaired site (white arrow head, infraspinatus tendon; yellow arrow head, transplanted fascia lata; H, humeral head). **c** Scheme of ISP (infraspinatus tendon) repair with fascia lata. Yellow square is transplanted fascia lata

with hematoxylin–eosin (HE) and safranin O for the histologic characterization of tissue composition, and the histological findings were evaluated at two points: the tendon proper and tendon insertion using light microscopy. Watkins et al. reported the tendon maturing scoring system to quantitatively evaluate the regenerated tendon [16]. Six histologic parameters, including cellularity, fibrocytes, vascularity, fiber diameter, parallel cells, and parallel fibers, were evaluated to identify the characteristics of the maturity of cellular and intercellular constituents. The sections were stained by the picrosirius red method with 0.2% phosphomolybdic acid hydrate, 0.4% direct red 80, and 1.3% 2,4,6-trinitrophenol (Polysciences, Inc., Warrington, PA, USA) to evaluate collagen fiber localization and analyzed using Zeiss AxioSkop2 and polarizing microscope (Carl Zeiss, Jena, Germany). Picrosirius red staining shows type I and III collagen fibers as yellow and green, respectively, under the polarizing microscope. The collagen content was calculated as a percentage of the pixels of each tendon–bone interface (green/total pixels or yellow/total pixels) using Adobe Photoshop CC 2015 software (Adobe Systems Incorporated, San Jose, USA).

Mechanical analysis

The infraspinatus tendon–humeral head complexes were harvested from each shoulder, and all soft tissues, except for the infraspinatus tendon, were removed. The humerus was placed in specially designed devices using polymethyl methacrylate resin, the tendon was wrapped with a cotton gauze sponge, and the sponge was sutured to the tendon 10 times using a 1-0 nylon at 5-mm intervals and subsequently clamped to the device [17]. The complex was placed vertically to a tensile sensor (AG-I SHIMAZU Co, Kyoto, Japan) (Fig. 2). Before conduction of the tensile test, the infraspinatus tendon–humeral head complexes were preconditioned with a static preload of 0.5 N for 5 min, followed by 10 cycles of loading and unloading at a strain amplitude of approximately 0.5% at a rate of 20 mm/min. The ultimate failure load was immediately recorded after preconditioning in uniaxial tension at 20 mm/min [18]. The ultimate failure load and stiffness were measured from the load–deformation curve.

Statistical analysis

Data are presented as the mean ± standard deviation. The Steel-Dwass test was performed to compare the mechanical property and collagen content in the three groups.

Statistical analyses of the tendon maturing score were performed using Student's *t* test between groups A and R.

p values of < 0.05 were considered statistically significant.

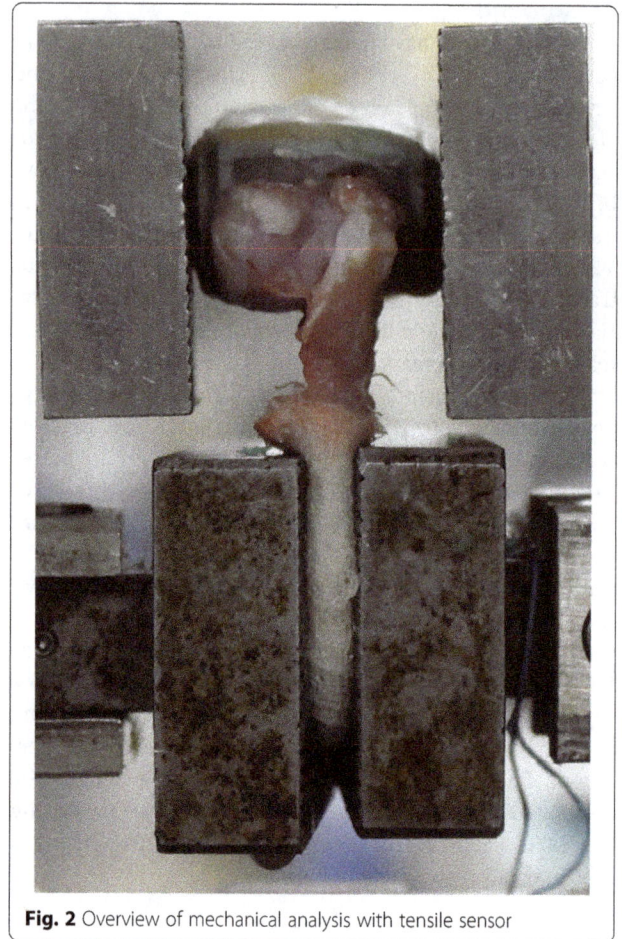

Fig. 2 Overview of mechanical analysis with tensile sensor

Results

Histological examination

In group A, the fibers were thicker and more parallel and cell alignment was more parallel compared with that in group R at 4 weeks postoperatively. A perfect score in the tendon maturing score system is 24 points. At 4 weeks, the tendon maturing scores were 13.8 ± 0.9 and 10.0 ± 1.2 in groups A and R, respectively. A statistically significant difference was found between groups A and R (Fig. 3), (Table 1).

In the safranin O staining, proteoglycan staining at the repaired enthesis in group A at 4 weeks postoperatively was stronger than that in group R (Fig. 4).

Picrosirius red staining showed different collagen fiber localizations at the enthesis. Type I and III collagen fibers were observed as yellow and green, respectively, with a polarizing microscope (Fig. 5). Type III collagen in group A (46.9 ± 9.9%) was more strongly expressed than that in group R (32.3 ± 5.3%) at 4 weeks postoperatively. However, the type III collagen expression of group R (46.0 ± 5.0%) was significantly higher than that of group A (37.6 ± 2.4%) at 8 weeks postoperatively. Type III collagen expressions in both operative groups were

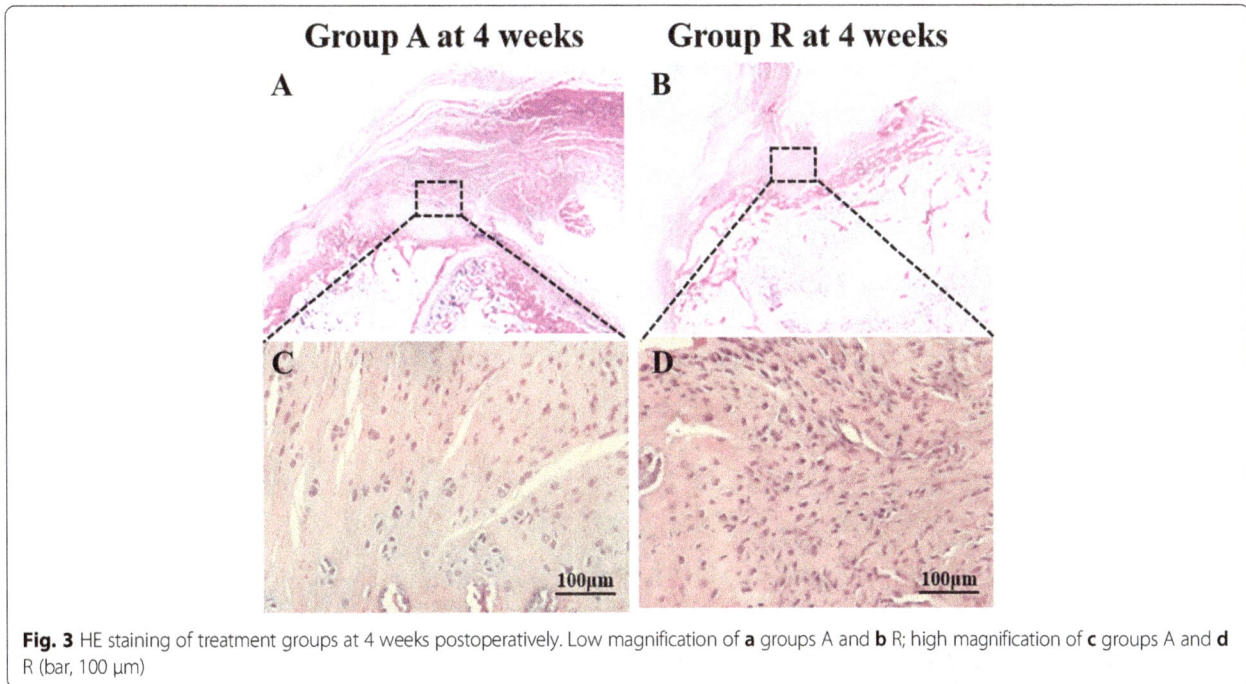

Fig. 3 HE staining of treatment groups at 4 weeks postoperatively. Low magnification of **a** groups A and **b** R; high magnification of **c** groups A and **d** R (bar, 100 μm)

significantly higher than those in the control group $(20.2 \pm 4.9\%)$ at 4 and 8 weeks postoperatively (Fig. 6).

Type I collagen in group A $(21.7 \pm 7.0\%)$ was more strongly expressed than that in group R $(8.0 \pm 1.6\%)$ at 4 weeks postoperatively. However, there was no significant difference between group A $(31.5 \pm 7.7\%)$ and group R $(24.0 \pm 6.8\%)$ at 8 weeks postoperatively. Type I collagen expression in the control group $(56.6 \pm 7.6\%)$ was statistically higher than that in both operative groups at 4 and 8 weeks postoperatively (Fig. 7).

Biomechanical testing

The ultimate failure load of the tendon–humeral head complex was 79.7 ± 4.9 N and 66.7 ± 8.3 N in groups A and R, respectively, at 4 weeks postoperatively, which showed a statistically significant difference $(p < 0.05)$. The failure load of group A at 4 weeks postoperatively was similar to that of the control group $(85.6 \pm 11.3$ N). However, the ultimate failure load of groups A and R was 88.2 ± 20.4 N and 77.3 ± 17.2 N, respectively, at 8 weeks postoperatively, and no significant difference was found among the three groups (Fig. 8).

In contrast, the stiffness of groups A and R was 7.6 ± 2.9 N/mm and 7.8 ± 3.7 N/mm, and 8.0 ± 1.9 N/mm and 11.0 ± 4.3 N/mm at 4 and 8 weeks postoperatively,

respectively. The stiffness of the control group was 16.9 ± 3.7 N/mm. The stiffness did not show a significant difference between groups A and R, but the stiffness of both groups was significantly lower than that of the control group at 4 weeks postoperatively. A significant difference was observed only between group A and the control group at 8 weeks postoperatively (Fig. 9).

Discussion

Repair site retear is a common complication of large or massive rotator cuff repairs. Several factors are considered as causes of retear, such as blood circulation disorder due to rotator cuff repair, rotator cuff degeneration, and rotator cuff retraction [12, 19]. Furthermore, when the tear size increases, the traction force applied to the repaired site also increases, leading to weakness of initial fixation force and repaired cuff retear. Alternative therapies, such as tendon transfers, autografts, allografts, and synthetic materials, have been reported to reduce stress with the repair site after repair of massive rotator cuff tears.

We have performed fascia lata augmentation for large or massive rotator cuff tears [15]. In a cadaveric model, rotator cuff repair with augmentation with a fascia lata patch significantly had less gap formation at the tendon–

Table 1 Results of the tendon maturing score in groups A and R at 4 weeks postoperatively ($^*p < 0.05$)

	Cellularity	Fibrocytes	Vascularity	Fiber diameter	Cells parallel	Fibers parallel	Total
Group A	2.00 ± 0.58	2.00 ± 0.58	2.00 ± 0.58	$2.50 \pm 0.50^*$	$2.67 \pm 0.47^*$	$2.67 \pm 0.47^*$	$13.8 \pm 0.90^*$
Group R	1.33 ± 0.47	1.83 ± 0.37	2.00 ± 0.58	1.83 ± 0.37	1.50 ± 0.50	1.50 ± 0.50	10.0 ± 1.15

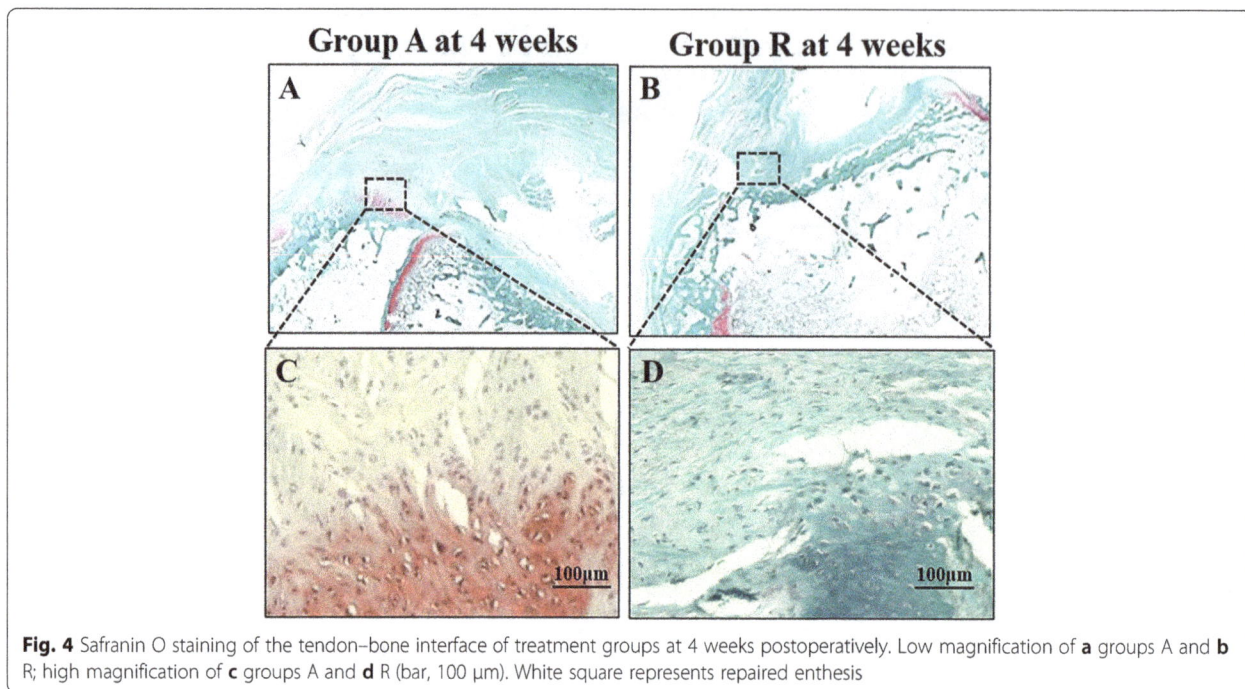

Fig. 4 Safranin O staining of the tendon–bone interface of treatment groups at 4 weeks postoperatively. Low magnification of **a** groups A and **b** R; high magnification of **c** groups A and **d** R (bar, 100 μm). White square represents repaired enthesis

bone interface with cyclic loading compared with non-augmented repair, indicating the possibility of reducing the incidence of rotator cuff repair failure due to addition of the fascia lata patch [20]. In our study, the mechanical strength of fascia lata augmentation was higher than that of the repaired group at 4 weeks postoperatively. Fascia lata augmentation has been suggested to provide the initial fixation strength of the repaired rotator cuff.

The main structural component of the tendon is type I collagen. However, in the early phase of tendon healing, type III collagen increases and gradually replaces type I

collagen as the tissue matures. This process is essential for maintaining the structure and function of the tendon [21, 22]. Hirose et al. found that a similar healing process occurs during the healing of rotator cuff tears. In the early phase of healing, repair tissue predominantly produces type III collagen, and type I collagen subsequently increases and replaces type III collagen [23].

In a rat anterior cruciate ligament repair model, Mifune et al. showed that an increase in cellularity and angiogenesis was observed in augmented grafts compared with conventionally reconstructed grafts. Rat-specific type III

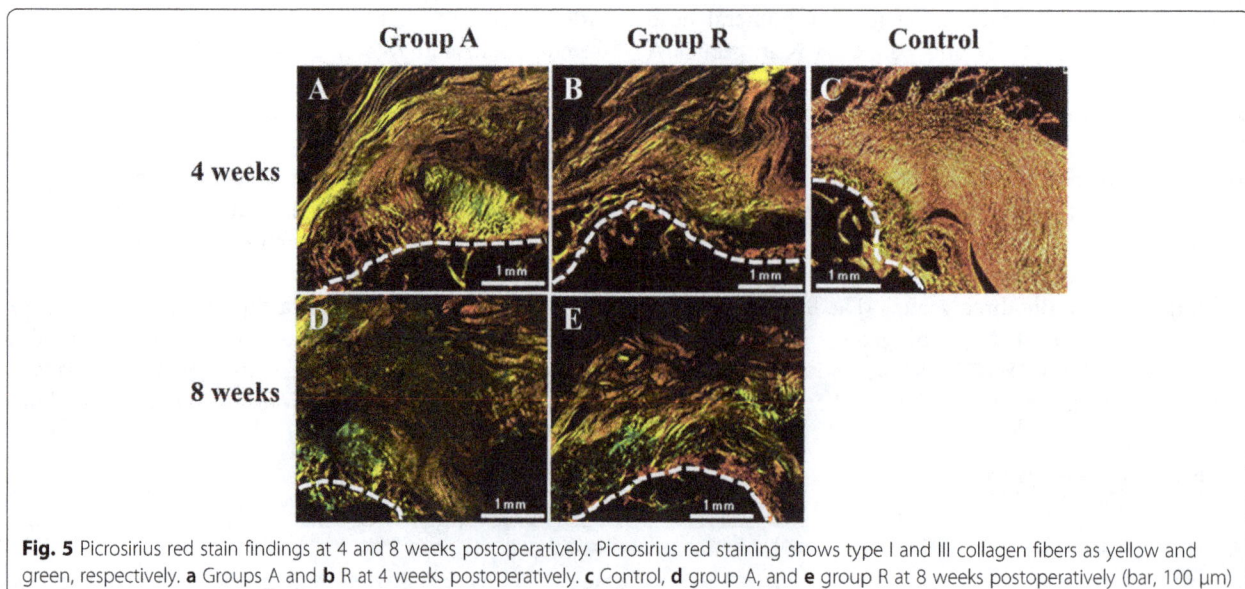

Fig. 5 Picrosirius red stain findings at 4 and 8 weeks postoperatively. Picrosirius red staining shows type I and III collagen fibers as yellow and green, respectively. **a** Groups A and **b** R at 4 weeks postoperatively. **c** Control, **d** group A, and **e** group R at 8 weeks postoperatively (bar, 100 μm)

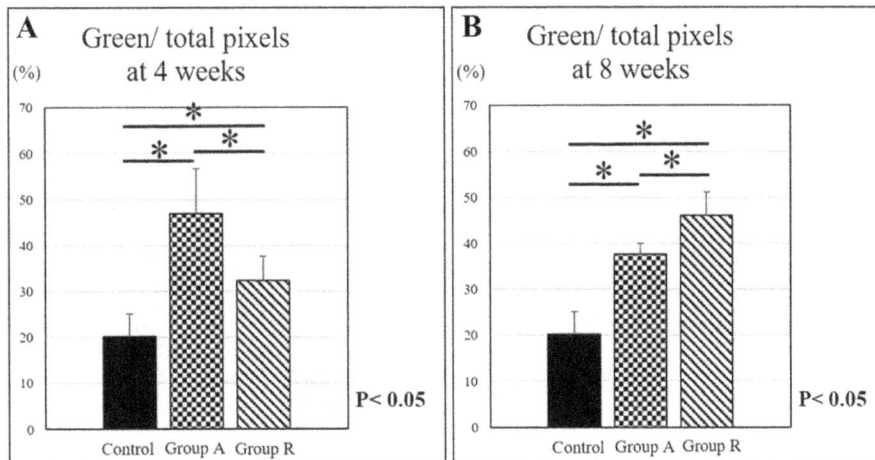

Fig. 6 Type III collagen content was calculated as a percentage of the pixels of each image (green/total pixels) in picrosirius red staining at **a** 4 and **b** 8 weeks postoperatively (*$p < 0.05$)

collagen expression and biomechanical strength in augmented grafts were also significantly higher than that in the conventional reconstruction group [24].

In the present study, picrosirius red staining was used to evaluate collagen fiber localization. In this method, the color of the collagen fiber changes depending on its thickness. As fiber thickness increases, the color changes from green to yellow to orange to red [25]. Because type III collagen fibers are usually thinner than type I collagen fibers, type I and III collagen fibers are stained yellow and green, respectively. Picrosirius red staining revealed type I and III collagen expression in the enthesis. Type III collagen expression in the fascia lata augmentation group at 4 weeks postoperatively was higher than that in the reattachment group. The expression of type III collagen rapidly decreased in

augmentation group at 8 weeks. In contrast, type I collagen expression in augmentation group at 4 weeks was higher than that in reattachment group.

Tendon maturation score of augmentation group was higher than that of reattachment group. These results suggested that fascia lata augmentation could stimulate type III collagen expression and type I collagen replacement and promote enthesis healing process in early phase. However, type I collagen expressions of both operative group at 4 and 8 weeks were lower than that of control group. The less expression of type I collagen in the operative group caused lower stiffness compared to the normal tendon.

Strong proteoglycan staining at the enthesis in the fascia lata augmentation group was observed, whereas less staining was observed in the control group in

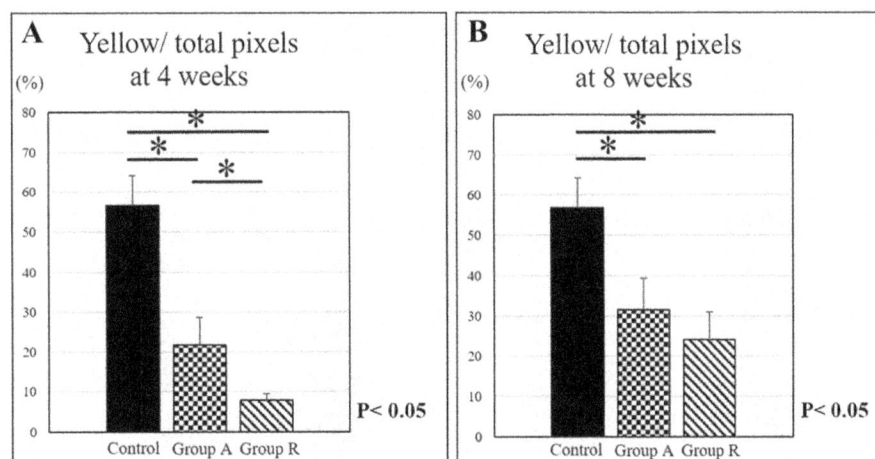

Fig. 7 Type I collagen content was calculated as a percentage of the pixels of each image (yellow/total pixels) in picrosirius red staining at **a** 4 and **b** 8 weeks postoperatively (*$p < 0.05$)

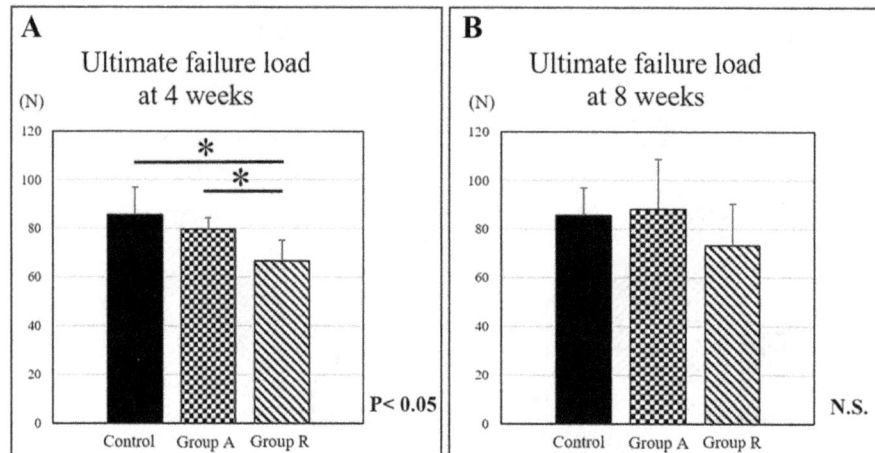

Fig. 8 Ultimate failure load of the tendon–humeral head complex at **a** 4 and **b** 8 weeks postoperatively (*$p < 0.05$)

safranin O staining. Proteoglycan is a cartilage matrix produced by chondrocytes. Increased proteoglycan at the repaired enthesis has been reported to lead to increased chondrocytes at the enthesis [26]. The anatomical structure of the enthesis consists of fibrocartilage with the following four zones: ligament substance, unmineralized fibrocartilage, mineralized fibrocartilage, and bone. Because the material properties of the special insertion zone are intermediate between the ligament and bone, a new cartilage transmits loads and decreases stress concentration at the attachment site [18]. Leung et al. reported that new cartilage formation during the healing process was associated with the mechanical property of the tendon–bone interface [27]. Fascia lata augmentation might promote fibrocartilage regeneration at the enthesis and contribute superior mechanical strength compared with the repair without augmentation.

Another possibility of the effectivity of fascia lata graft is its function as a scaffold. Decortication of the footprint was performed to stimulate the bone marrow after rotator cuff repair. Bone marrow stimulation is caused by the migration of bone marrow-derived mesenchymal stem cells (MSCs) [28]. The presence of MSCs in the bone marrow provides a potential for differentiation into tendon tissues [29]. We speculate that the fascia lata autograft over the repaired site might prevent MSCs to spread from the footprint.

The present study has several limitations. First, this rabbit model was an acute rotator cuff injury model. The animal models may differ from chronic human rotator cuff injury. Second, the anatomy between the rabbit shoulder and that of humans are different, and the short rotator cuff muscles of rabbits do not form a rotator cuff that is similar to humans. Third, because

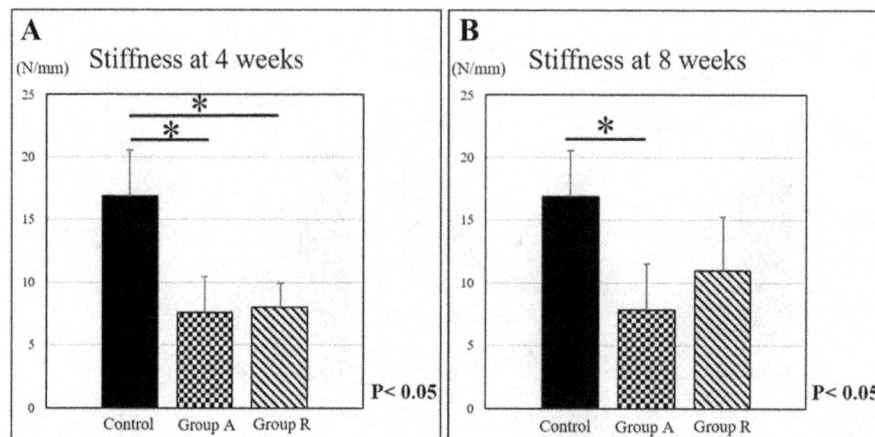

Fig. 9 Stiffness of regenerated tissues at **a** 4 and **b** 8 weeks postoperatively (*$p < 0.05$)

rabbits have a greater healing capacity than humans, the tendon–bone healing process in the rabbits progressed faster than that in humans.

In clinical situations, some problems such as hematoma, discomfort, and pain of donor site might be caused after graft harvest. However, Mihata et al. reported that they made autograft for arthroscopic superior capsule reconstruction (SCR) from fascia lata because the tissue is stiff enough to obtain superior shoulder stability after SCR, and no patients had any dysfunction with the harvest site at the final follow-up [30]. Furthermore, autograft has no concern of an immune reaction, zoonosis, or foreign body reaction [15].

The results from the present study suggest that fascia lata augmentation could stimulate biological healing and provide initial fixation strength of the repaired rotator cuff.

Conclusion

The fascia lata augmentation for massive rotator cuff tears could stimulate type III collagen expression and type I collagen replacement and promote enthesis healing process in early phase. Mechanically, the fascia lata augmentation provided initial fixation strength of the repaired rotator cuff.

Abbreviations
MSCs: Bone marrow-derived mesenchymal stem cells; HE: Hematoxylin–eosin; ISP: Infraspinatus; SCR: Superior capsule reconstruction

Acknowledgements
The authors would like to give their special thanks to Minako Nagata, Maya Yasuda, and Kyoko Tanaka for their skilled technical assistance.

Authors' contributions
Setting up the research was done by TKO. Animal surgery was done by TKA, TM, YH, FT, YU, TKU, and KY. Data analysis (histological, mechanical analysis) was done by TKA, YM, and AI. Statistical analysis was done by TKA, RS, and HN. Manuscript preparation was done by TKA, YM, and AI. Supervising was done by RK. All authors read and approved the final manuscript.

Competing interests
The authors declare that they have no competing interests.

References
1. Sher JS, Uribe JW, Posada A, Murphy BJ, Zlatkin MB. Abnormal findings on magnetic resonance images of asymptomatic shoulders. J Bone Joint Surg Am. 1995;77(1):10–5.
2. Konno N, Itoi E, Kido T, Sano A, Urayama M, Sato K. Glenoid osteophyte and rotator cuff tears: an anatomic study. J Shoulder Elb Surg. 2002;11(1):72–9.
3. Harryman DT 2nd, Mack LA, Wang KY, Jackins SE, Richardson ML, Matsen FA 3rd. Repairs of the rotator cuff. Correlation of functional results with integrity of the cuff. J Bone Joint Surg Am. 1991;73(7):982–9.
4. Sugaya H, Maeda K, Matsuki K, Moriishi J. Functional and structural outcome after arthroscopic full-thickness rotator cuff repair: single-row versus dual-row fixation. Arthroscopy. 2005;21(11):1307–16.
5. Morse K, Davis AD, Afra R, Kaye EK, Schepsis A, Voloshin I. Arthroscopic versus mini-open rotator cuff repair: a comprehensive review and meta-analysis. Am J Sports Med. 2008;36(9):1824–8.
6. Gavriilidis I, Kircher J, Magosch P, Lichtenberg S, Habermeyer P. Pectoralis major transfer for the treatment of irreparable anterosuperior rotator cuff tears. Int Orthop. 2010;34(5):689–94.
7. Sano H, Kumagai J, Sawai T. Experimental fascial autografting for the supraspinatus tendon defect: remodeling process of the grafted fascia and the insertion into bone. J Shoulder Elb Surg. 2002;11(2):166–73.
8. Labbe MR. Arthroscopic technique for patch augmentation of rotator cuff repairs. Arthroscopy. 2006;22(10):1136. e1131–1136
9. Zumstein MA, Jost B, Hempel J, Hodler J, Gerber C. The clinical and structural long-term results of open repair of massive tears of the rotator cuff. J Bone Joint Surg Am. 2008;90(11):2423–31.
10. Koh KH, Kang KC, Lim TK, Shon MS, Yoo JC. Prospective randomized clinical trial of single- versus double-row suture anchor repair in 2- to 4-cm rotator cuff tears: clinical and magnetic resonance imaging results. Arthroscopy. 2011;27(4):453–62.
11. Toussaint B, Schnaser E, Bosley J, Lefebvre Y, Gobezie R. Early structural and functional outcomes for arthroscopic double-row transosseous-equivalent rotator cuff repair. Am J Sports Med. 2011;39(6):1217–25.
12. Kim JR, Cho YS, Ryu KJ, Kim JH. Clinical and radiographic outcomes after arthroscopic repair of massive rotator cuff tears using a suture bridge technique: assessment of repair integrity on magnetic resonance imaging. Am J Sports Med. 2012;40(4):786–93.
13. Tashjian RZ, Hollins AM, Kim HM, et al. Factors affecting healing rates after arthroscopic double-row rotator cuff repair. Am J Sports Med. 2010;38(12):2435–42.
14. Yamamoto N, Itoi E, Tuoheti Y, et al. Glenohumeral joint motion after medial shift of the attachment site of the supraspinatus tendon: a cadaveric study. J Shoulder Elb Surg. 2007;16(3):373–8.
15. Kokubu T, Mifune Y, Inui A, Kuroda R. Arthroscopic rotator cuff repair with graft augmentation of fascia lata for large and massive tears. Arthrosc Tech. 2016;5(6):e1235–8.
16. Watkins JP, Auer JA, Gay S, Morgan SJ. Healing of surgically created defects in the equine superficial digital flexor tendon: collagen-type transformation and tissue morphologic reorganization. Am J Vet Res. 1985;46(10):2091–6.
17. Inui A, Kokubu T, Mifune Y, et al. Regeneration of rotator cuff tear using electrospun poly(d,l-Lactide-Co-Glycolide) scaffolds in a rabbit model. Arthroscopy. 2012;28(12):1790–9.
18. Inui A, Kokubu T, Fujioka H, et al. Application of layered poly (L-lactic acid) cell free scaffold in a rabbit rotator cuff defect model. Sports Med Arthrosc Rehabil Ther Technol. 2011;3:29.
19. Kim SJ, Kim SH, Lee SK, Seo JW, Chun YM. Arthroscopic repair of massive contracted rotator cuff tears: aggressive release with anterior and posterior interval slides do not improve cuff healing and integrity. J Bone Joint Surg Am. 2013;95(16):1482–8.
20. McCarron JA, Milks RA, Mesiha M, et al. Reinforced fascia patch limits cyclic gapping of rotator cuff repairs in a human cadaveric model. J Shoulder Elb Surg. 2012;21(12):1680–6.
21. Dahlgren LA, Mohammed HO, Nixon AJ. Temporal expression of growth factors and matrix molecules in healing tendon lesions. J Orthop Res. 2005;23(1):84–92.
22. Williams IF, McCullagh KG, Silver IA. The distribution of types I and III collagen and fibronectin in the healing equine tendon. Connect Tissue Res. 1984;12(3–4):211–27.

23. Hirose K, Kondo S, Choi HR, Mishima S, Iwata H, Ishiguro N. Spontaneous healing process of a supraspinatus tendon tear in rabbits. Arch Orthop Trauma Surg. 2004;124(6):374–7.

24. Mifune Y, Ota S, Takayama K, et al. Therapeutic advantage in selective ligament augmentation for partial tears of the anterior cruciate ligament: results in an animal model. Am J Sports Med. 2013;41(2):365–73.

25. Whittaker P, Kloner RA, Boughner DR, Pickering JG. Quantitative assessment of myocardial collagen with picrosirius red staining and circularly polarized light. Basic Res Cardiol. 1994;89(5):397–410.

26. Harada Y, Mifune Y, Inui A, et al. Rotator cuff repair using cell sheets derived from human rotator cuff in a rat model. J Orthop Res. 2016;35(2):289–96.

27. Leung KS, Chong WS, Chow DH, et al. A comparative study on the biomechanical and histological properties of bone-to-bone, bone-to-tendon, and tendon-to-tendon healing: an Achilles tendon-calcaneus model in goats. Am J Sports Med. 2015;43(6):1413–21.

28. Jo CH, Shin JS, Park IW, Kim H, Lee SY. Multiple channeling improves the structural integrity of rotator cuff repair. Am J Sports Med. 2013;41(11):2650–7.

29. Taniguchi N, Suenaga N, Oizumi N, et al. Bone marrow stimulation at the footprint of arthroscopic surface-holding repair advances cuff repair integrity. J Shoulder Elb Surg. 2015;24(6):860–6.

30. Mihata T, Lee TQ, Fukunishi K, et al. Return to sports and physical work after arthroscopic superior capsule reconstruction among patients with irreparable rotator cuff tears. Am J Sports Med. 2018;46(5):1077–83.

9

Standardisation of basal medium for reproducible culture of human annulus fibrosus and nucleus pulposus cells

Ann-Kathrin Schubert[1,2]* (iD), Jeske J. Smink[2], Matthias Pumberger[3], Michael Putzier[3], Michael Sittinger[1] and Jochen Ringe[1]

Abstract

Background: The lifetime prevalence of degenerative disc disease is dramatically high. Numerous investigations on disc degeneration have been performed on cells from annulus fibrosus (AF) and nucleus pulposus (NP) of the intervertebral disc (IVD) in cell culture experiments utilising a broad variety of basal culture media. Although the basal media differ in nutrient formulation, it is not known whether the choice of the basal media itself has an impact on the cell's behaviour in vitro. In this study, we evaluated the most common media used for monolayer expansion of AF and NP cells to set standards for disc cell culture.

Methods: Human AF and NP cells were isolated from cervical discs. Cells were expanded in monolayer until passage P2 using six different common culture media containing alpha-Minimal Essential Medium (alpha-MEM), Dulbecco's Modified Eagle's Medium (DMEM) or Ham's F-12 medium (Ham's F-12) as single medium or in a mixture of two media (alpha/F-12, DMEM/alpha, DMEM/F-12). Cell morphology, cell growth, glycosaminoglycan production and quantitative gene expression of cartilage- and IVD-related markers aggrecan, collagen type II, forkhead box F1 and keratin 18 were analysed. Statistical analysis was performed with two-way ANOVA testing and Bonferroni compensation.

Results: AF and NP cells were expandable in all tested media. Both cell types showed similar cell morphology and characteristics of dedifferentiation known for cultured disc cells independently from the media. However, proceeding culture in Ham's F-12 impeded cell growth of both AF and NP cells. Furthermore, the keratin 18 gene expression profile of NP cells was changed in alpha-MEM and Ham's F-12.

Conclusion: The impact of the different media itself on disc cell's behaviour in vitro was low. However, AF and NP cells were only robust, when DMEM was used as single medium or in a mixture (DMEM/alpha, DMEM/F-12). Therefore, we recommend using these media as standard medium for disc cell culture. Our findings are valuable for the harmonisation of preclinical study results and thereby push the development of cell therapies for clinical treatment of disc degeneration.

Keywords: Annulus fibrosus, Nucleus pulposus, Basal medium, Cell growth, Dedifferentiation, Disc marker

* Correspondence: ann-kathrin.schubert@charite.de
[1]Tissue Engineering Laboratory and Berlin-Brandenburg Center for Regenerative Therapies, Charité - Universitätsmedizin Berlin, corporate member of Freie Universität Berlin, Humboldt-Universität zu Berlin and Berlin Institute of Health, Augustenburger Platz 1, Südstraße 2, 13353 Berlin, Germany
[2]CO.DON AG, Teltow, Germany
Full list of author information is available at the end of the article

Background

The lifetime prevalence of degenerative disc disease (DDD) is very high. Over 90% of over age 50 show radiographic signs of DDD in magnetic resonance imaging studies [1]. Degeneration of the intervertebral disc (IVD) is a natural process occurring during ageing and is under continuous investigation [2]. The IVD is a cartilage-like tissue and consists of two compartments, the inner nucleus pulposus (NP) and the surrounding annulus fibrosus (AF). Both contain specific cells that maintain the extracellular matrix (ECM) through synthesis and degradation of ECM proteins. Cellular activity and metabolism is dependent on nutrient supply. The IVD is an avascular tissue, and thus nutrients are only supplied by the blood system of the adjacent vertebral bodies via a physical barrier, the cartilage endplate (CEP). In mature discs, the distance between an AF or NP cell and CEP is up to 6–8 mm and can only be overcome by free diffusion of fluids through the IVD tissue [3]. Although disc cells are adapted to the limited nutrient supply, an imbalance in the ECM maintenance occurs with age. The resulting impaired distribution of matrix degrading enzymes causes the DDD. To treat DDD, cell-based therapeutic approaches are of increasing clinical importance [4]. In disc cell therapy, cells are isolated from the disc and are expanded ex vivo before they are implanted into the impaired disc. Cell expansion is necessary to obtain a sufficient cell number for implantation. These strategies aim to slow down the degeneration process and are predominantly tested in preclinical studies using cell culture experiments [5].

Reviewing the literature of the two last decades, we found no common protocol available for disc cell expansion. Although cell growth and maintenance of disc cell viability is affected by nutrition [6], the cell culture medium differs with respect to serum and glucose concentration, as well as in supplementation of ascorbic acid, growth factors and non-essential amino acids. Studies even utilise a variety of basal cell culture media: alpha-Minimal Essential Medium (alpha-MEM), Dulbecco's Modified Eagle's Medium (DMEM) or Ham's F-12 medium (Ham's F-12). These synthetic culture media were originally developed for different cell types, and nutrition is changed by the medium itself. Harry Eagle found the minimal nutritional requirements to support growth and multiplication of adherent mammalian cells in vitro [7]. For more demanding cell types such as primary embryonic cells, Renato Dulbecco increased the concentration of amino acids and vitamins and added trace elements and bicarbonates resulting in DMEM [8]. DMEM has been established as universal medium for various cell types of primary source and immortalised cell lines. Another modification of Eagle's medium, alpha-MEM, is enriched with non-essential amino acids

and further vitamins for cell-lines of mouse and hamster hybrid cells [9]. Richard G. Ham, another pioneer in the field of nutritional biochemistry, defined different basal media for fibroblast cells, e.g. Ham's F-12. Ham's F-12 was the first medium that was used for chondrocyte expansion in cell culture [10]. In addition, alpha-MEM supports cell growth and stimulation of collagen synthesis in primary osteogenic and chondrogenic cells [11]. However, only few studies use Ham's F-12 or alpha-MEM to culture the chondrocyte-like disc cells. For disc cell culture, DMEM is predominantly used as single medium or in a mixture with Ham's F-12 (DMEM/F-12).

It is well known, that cell growth of primary disc cells is affected by the choice of serum and glucose concentration [12]. Furthermore, cells are altered by supplementation of growth factors or change in oxygen concentration [13, 14]. However, not much is known about the impact of the different basal media itself on human disc cells. Since nutrition is altered by the basal medium itself, we hypothesised that the choice of medium would influence the behaviour of cultured disc cells. Cells used for cell therapy could thus possibly show different characteristics, when cultured with different media. As cell expansion is the inevitable step in the manufacturing process of a cell therapeutic product, we put the focus on simple cell expansion rather than complex tissue engineering. Hence, the aim of our study was to set standards for 2D culture of human AF and NP cells with respect to the used basal medium. Therefore, we exposed human AF and NP cells to the different basal media and evaluated the cell's response regarding cell morphology, cell growth, glycosaminoglycan (GAG) production and expression of cartilage and IVD-related genes. Although Ham's F-12 and alpha-MEM are not commonly used as single medium for disc cell culture besides DMEM, we tested each medium separately and in a mixture of two media to see individual impacts. In order to prevent any bias by other culture conditions, we used consistent culture conditions (5% CO_2, 95% humidity, normoxia), and all samples from all donors were exactly treated the same way regarding seeding density, time point of media exchange and subcultivation, as well as media and serum batch.

Methods

Tissue source and sample preparation

IVD tissue was obtained from five patients (female/male ratio 3/2) during anterior cervical fusion. All patients showed only mild radiographic degenerative changes of the IVD but failed conservative treatment (Miyazaki degeneration grade ≤ 3, Modic change ≤ 2) [15]. The mean age was 49 years (range 42–52 years).

AF and NP were macroscopically resected from the IVD tissue using lamellae appearance and tissue colour as criteria. Other tissues such as CEP were discarded. Only tissue parts with clear assignment to either AF or NP in macroscopic evaluation were used for this study. In addition, no IVD tissue with macroscopic signs of degeneration, e.g. a greyish colour or sclerotic parts, were used for this study.

Histological analysis

To confirm correct separation of AF and NP in macroscopic preparation, we performed standard histological staining of each AF and NP sample. A representative small tissue part was embedded in Tissue-Tek® O.C.T. Compound (Sakura Finetek, Staufen, Germany), frozen in liquid nitrogen and stored at −80 °C until sectioning. Samples were cryosectioned at a thickness of 6 µm. To show tissue morphology, sections were fixed with methanol/acetone (1:1 v/v %) and stained with Mayer's haematoxylin (Dako, Germany) and eosin-G solution (Roth, Karlsruhe, Germany). To analyse sulphated GAGs, the sections were fixed with 4% formaldehyde (Herbeta, Germany) and stained with 1% alcian blue 8GS solution (Roth) and counterstained with nuclear fast red-aluminium sulphate solution (Roth). To demonstrate acidic GAGs, the sections were fixed with 92% ethanol and stained with 0.7% safranin O solution (Sigma-Aldrich) and subsequently counterstained with 0.2% fast green solution (Sigma-Aldrich).

Cell isolation and cell culture

AF and NP samples were washed with phosphate-buffered saline (PBS, Biochrom, Berlin, Germany), and wet weight was determined, separately. Samples were minced, and cells were released by enzymatically treating with 3333 U/mL collagenase CLS II (Biochrom), 1 U/mL collagenase P (Sigma-Aldrich, Taufkirchen, Germany) and 333 U/mL hyaluronidase (Sigma-Aldrich) in a spinner flask under gentle stirring for 4 h at 37 °C (5% CO_2, 95% humidity, normoxia) [16]. After cellular release, the cell solution was put through a 100 µm nylon cell strainer (BD Falcon, Franklin Lakes, NJ, USA), centrifuged at 600×g, and supernatant was discarded. The viable cell number was determined using trypan blue (Sigma-Aldrich) dye exclusion. From cellular release, three NP and five AF samples of all five donors had a sufficient cell yield to perform all experiments with all media and were thus included in this study.

Cells were cultured in 12-well plates with the different media in duplicates until passage P2 under consistent culture conditions (37 °C, 5% CO_2, 95% humidity, normoxia). Medium was replaced every second day. For subcultivation, the cells were detached with trypsin/ethylenediaminetetraacetic acid (Biochrom) at day 6 of passage P0 and day 3 of passage P1 and P2, respectively. Seeding density was always 9000 cells/cm².

Cell culture media

AF and NP cells were cultured using six different media (all from Biochrom): (1) alpha-MEM, (2) DMEM, (3) Ham's F-12, (4) 1:1 (v/v %) alpha-MEM and Ham's F-12 (alpha/F-12), (5) 1:1 (v/v %) DMEM and alpha-MEM (DMEM/alpha) and (6) 1:1 (v/v %) DMEM and Ham's F-12 (DMEM/F-12). The original formulation of alpha-MEM, DMEM and Ham's F-12 is shown in Table 1. As the distributor only provided alpha-MEM without L-glutamine, stable L-glutamine (Biochrom) was added to alpha-MEM to achieve the glutamine concentration of the original alpha-MEM formulation (4 mM). All media were supplemented with 10% human serum (HS) (German Red Cross, Berlin, Germany) and 1% antibiotics (100 U/mL penicillin, 100 mg/mL streptomycin, Biochrom). To avoid donor variability, serum was pooled from eight donors (German Red Cross), and serum batch was not changed in this study.

Cell growth analysis

The cell growth of AF and NP cells was studied based on the population doubling (PD) in each passage P0, P1 and P2 and the cumulative population doubling level (cPDL) at the end of passage P2. The PD was calculated at each subcultivation with the equation PD = 3.32*(log(final cell number)−log(initial cell number)). Adding up PDs of all passages resulted in cPDL [17]. The growth rate was studied using the population doubling rate (PDR) in each passage with the equation PDR = PD/culture time [days] [18]. PD, cPDL and PDR are parameters to describe the proliferation capacity and growth rate of cell expansion, respectively.

Glycosaminoglycan analysis

GAG deposition was analysed by alcian blue and nuclear fast red staining (see above) of the cell layer. Cells were seeded on 8-well chamber slides (BD Falcon) and cultured like the main culture. Before cells reached 100% confluency, slides were washed with PBS, fixed with acetone and stored at −20 °C until staining.

GAG secretion was analysed with standard 1,9-dimethylmethylene blue assay using chondroitin sulphate sodium salt from shark (Sigma-Aldrich) to generate standard curves as described before [19]. Standard and samples of each donor were measured in triplicates. Culture supernatants were collected from all media exchanges and pooled within same passage. Total sample volume was determined for calculation of total amount of secreted GAGs.

Gene expression analysis

Gene expression analysis was performed for standard cartilage marker aggrecan (ACAN), collagen type I (COL1A1), collagen type II (COL2A2) and IVD-related genes keratin 18 (KRT18) and forkhead box F1 (FOXF1).

Table 1 Original formulation of alpha-MEM, DMEM and Ham's F-12

Substance		alpha-MEM	DMEM	Ham's F-12
Nutrients	D-Glucose	5.6×10^0	5.6×10^0	1.0×10^1
	Sodium pyruvate	1.0×10^0	1.0×10^0	1.0×10^0
	Sodium bicarbonate	2.4×10^1	4.4×10^1	1.4×10^1
	Lipoic acid	9.7×10^{-4}	–	1.0×10^{-3}
	Linoleic acid	–	–	3.0×10^{-4}
	NaCl	1.2×10^2	1.1×10^2	1.3×10^2
	KCl	5.4×10^0	5.4×10^0	3.0×10^0
	$MgSO_4 \cdot 7H_2O$	8.1×10^{-1}	8.1×10^{-1}	–
	$MgCl_2 \cdot 6H_2O$	–	–	6.0×10^{-1}
	$Na_2HPO_4 \cdot H_2O$	1.1×10^0	8.7×10^{-1}	1.0×10^0
	$CaCl_2 \cdot 2H_2O$	1.8×10^0	1.8×10^0	3.0×10^{-1}
	$Fe(NO_3)_3 \cdot 9H_2O$	–	2.5×10^{-4}	–
	$FeSO_4 \cdot 7H_2O$	–	–	3.0×10^{-3}
	$CuSO_4 \cdot 5H_2O$	–	–	1.0×10^{-5}
	$ZnSO_4 \cdot 7H_2O$	–	–	3.0×10^{-3}
	Hypoxanthine	–	–	3.0×10^{-2}
	Thymidine	–	–	3.0×10^{-3}
Vitamins	Folic acid	2.3×10^{-3}	9.1×10^{-3}	2.9×10^{-3}
	Vitamin B_{12}	1.0×10^{-3}	–	1.0×10^{-3}
	Pyridoxal·HCl	4.9×10^{-3}	2.0×10^{-2}	–
	Pyridoxine·HCl	–	–	3.0×10^{-4}
	Niacinamid	8.0×10^{-3}	3.3×10^{-2}	3.0×10^{-4}
	D-Ca-pantothenate	2.1×10^{-3}	8.4×10^{-3}	1.0×10^{-3}
	Biotin	4.1×10^{-4}	–	3.0×10^{-5}
	Riboflavin	2.7×10^{-4}	1.1×10^{-3}	1.0×10^{-4}
	Thiamine·HCl	3.0×10^{-3}	1.2×10^{-2}	1.0×10^{-3}
	Ascorbic acid	2.8×10^{-1}	–	–
Amino acids essential	L-Isoleucine	4.0×10^{-1}	8.0×10^{-1}	3.0×10^{-2}
	L-Leucine	4.0×10^{-1}	8.0×10^{-1}	9.9×10^{-2}
	L-Lysine HCl	4.0×10^{-1}	8.0×10^{-1}	2.0×10^{-1}
	L-Methionine	1.0×10^{-1}	2.0×10^{-1}	3.0×10^{-2}
	L-Phenylalanine	2.0×10^{-1}	4.0×10^{-1}	3.0×10^{-2}
	L-Threonine	4.0×10^{-1}	8.0×10^{-1}	1.0×10^{-1}
	L-Tryptophan	5.0×10^{-2}	7.8×10^{-2}	9.8×10^{-3}
	L-Valine	4.0×10^{-1}	8.0×10^{-1}	1.0×10^{-1}
Semi-essential	L-Cysteine·H_2O	2.2×10^{-1}	–	2.3×10^{-1}
	L-Tyrosine	2.0×10^{-1}	4.0×10^{-1}	3.0×10^{-2}
	L-Arginine·HCl	6.0×10^{-1}	4.0×10^{-1}	1.0×10^0
	L-Histidine·HCl·H_2O	2.0×10^{-1}	2.0×10^{-1}	1.0×10^{-1}
Non-essential	L-Alanine	2.8×10^{-1}	–	1.0×10^{-1}
	L-Asparagine·H_2O	3.3×10^{-1}	–	8.8×10^{-2}
	L-Aspartic acid	2.3×10^{-1}	–	1.0×10^{-1}
	L-Glutamine	$4.0 \times 10^{0}*$	4.0×10^0	1.0×10^0
	L-Glutamic acid	5.1×10^{-1}	–	1.0×10^{-1}

Table 1 Original formulation of alpha-MEM, DMEM and Ham's F-12 *(Continued)*

Substance		alpha-MEM	DMEM	Ham's F-12
	Glycine	6.7×10^{-1}	4.0×10^{-1}	1.0×10^{-1}
	L-Proline	3.5×10^{-1}	–	3.0×10^{-1}
	L-Serine	2.4×10^{-1}	4.0×10^{-1}	1.0×10^{-1}
	L-Cystine	4.2×10^{-1}	2.0×10^{-1}	–
Vitaminoids	Inositol	1.1×10^{-2}	4.0×10^{-2}	1.0×10^{-1}
	Choline chloride	7.2×10^{-3}	2.9×10^{-2}	1.0×10^{-1}
Supplements	Putrescine·2HCl	–	–	1.0×10^{-3}
	Phenol red	2.8×10^{-2}	4.2×10^{-2}	2.8×10^{-2}

Concentration is shown in mM. *As the distributor only provided alpha-MEM without L-glutamine, the user supplemented L-glutamine to achieve the original concentration in alpha-MEM

No common marker genes were available to analyse the human NP and AF phenotype, separately.

For isolation of total RNA, samples were treated with TriReagent (Sigma-Aldrich), 1-bromo-3-chloropropane extraction (Sigma-Aldrich) and purified using the RNeasy Mini Kit with on-column DNase I digestion (Qiagen, Hilden, Germany) according to the manufacturer's instructions. The cDNA was synthesised using the Transcriptor First Strand cDNA Synthesis Kit (Roche, Mannheim, Germany) according to the manufacturer's instructions. The gene expression analysis was performed by quantitative PCR using the primer-UPL probe system of Roche and conducted on the LightCycler® 480 (Roche). Expression of housekeeping genes ATP5F1B and RPL13A was used to normalise the individual mRNA expression level. The data are expressed as relative gene expression levels and calculated using the E-method developed by Roche (https://lifescience.roche.com). Primer and probes are shown in Table 2. The samples were measured in triplicates.

Statistical analysis

Data are expressed as mean with standard deviation. Statistical analysis between groups (media 1–6) was performed with two-way ANOVA and Bonferroni compensation (GraphPad PRISM 6.0). A p value of less than 0.05 was considered statistically significant.

Results

Characterisation of AF and NP tissue samples

AF and NP tissue from cervical IVD were macroscopically distinguishable using lamellae appearance and colour as criteria (Fig. 1a). AF tissue was dense and showed its typical fibrous structure in the outer region (oAF). In the inner region of the AF (iAF), the lamellae were rather distant. NP region was white in appearance and had a soft and loose appearance. The successful separation of AF from NP was confirmed by histological evaluation. Histological staining showed the fibrillary character of the AF, whereas the NP did not contain lamellae (Fig. 1b). Furthermore, the typical zonal difference of GAG expression in oAF and iAF could be observed in alcian blue and safranin O staining (Fig. 1c

Table 2 Primer and probes

Gene title	Accession number[#]	Primer sequence		UPL probe
		forward	reverse	
ACAN	NM_001135.3 NM_013227.3	ctggaagtcgtggtgaaagg	tcgagggtgtagcgtgtaga	21
COL1A1	NM_000088.3	gggattccctggacctaaag	ggaacacctcgctctcca	67
COL2A1	NM_001844.4 NM_033150.2	ccctggtcttggtggaaa	cattggtccttgcattactcc	19
FOXF1	NM_001451.2	cagcctctccacgcactc	cctttcggtcacacatgct	5
KRT18	NM_000224.2 NM_199187.1	aagctggaggctgagatcg	tccaaggcatcaccaagatta	70
ATP5FB1*	NM_001686.3	agaggtcccatcaaaaccaa	tcctgctcaacactcatttcc	50
RPL13A*	NM_012423.3 NM_00127049.1	caagcggatgaacaccaac	tgtggggcagcatacctc	28

*Housekeeping genes used as reference genes in normalisation for calculation of mRNA expression level
[#]Includes all transcript variants of this gene covered by the chosen primers

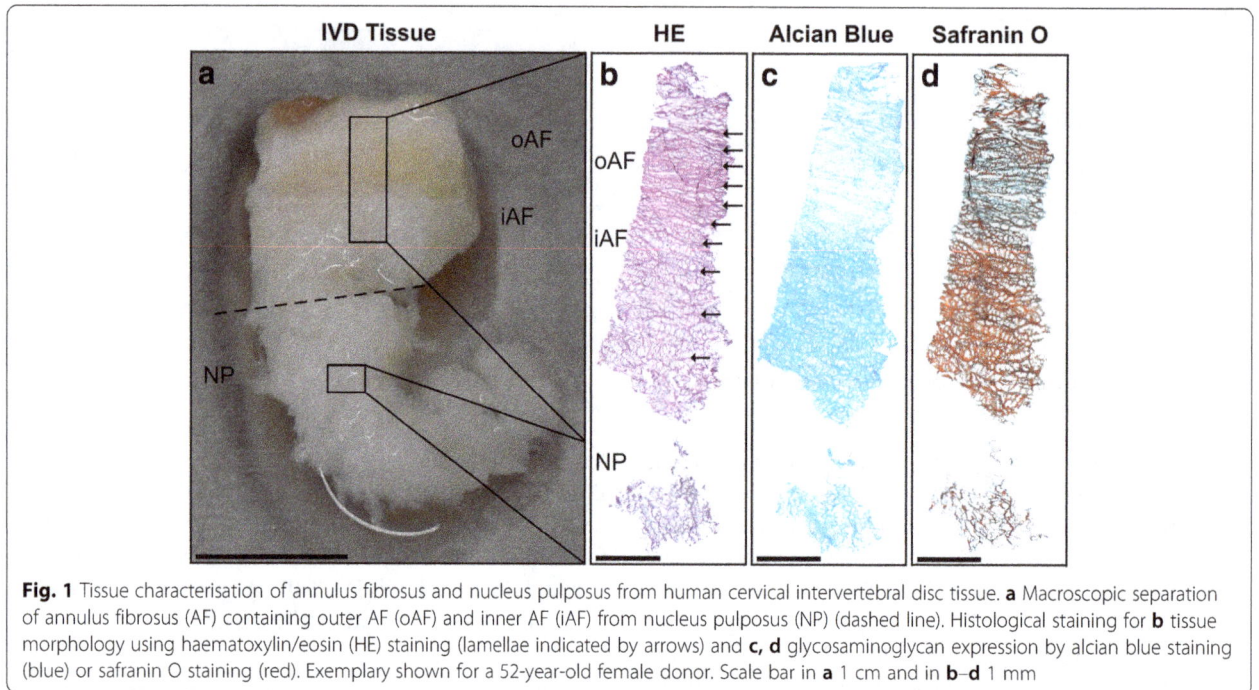

Fig. 1 Tissue characterisation of annulus fibrosus and nucleus pulposus from human cervical intervertebral disc tissue. **a** Macroscopic separation of annulus fibrosus (AF) containing outer AF (oAF) and inner AF (iAF) from nucleus pulposus (NP) (dashed line). Histological staining for **b** tissue morphology using haematoxylin/eosin (HE) staining (lamellae indicated by arrows) and **c, d** glycosaminoglycan expression by alcian blue staining (blue) or safranin O staining (red). Exemplary shown for a 52-year-old female donor. Scale bar in **a** 1 cm and in **b–d** 1 mm

and d). The GAG expression in the NP was similar to the iAF, and only appeared to be stained less strongly due to its looser tissue organisation.

After enzymatic release of the cells from the two different tissues, 860.3 ± 279.3 AF cells and 491.5 ± 120.3 NP cells per milligramme of wet tissue could be recovered on average. Hence, the cellularity in AF tissue was 1.7 as high as in NP tissue.

Cell morphology and cell growth of primary AF and NP cells in different cell culture media

There was no difference in cell morphology visible between cultured AF cells and NP cells. In passage P0, the cells showed isodiametric cell morphology and turned into a spindle-shaped, fibroblastic morphology through passaging. Both cell types arranged typically honeycombed at low confluency and were crowded reaching high cell density resulting in a more elongated shape (Fig. 2a–f). However, in Ham's F-12 NP cells did not reach same confluency compared to the other media at

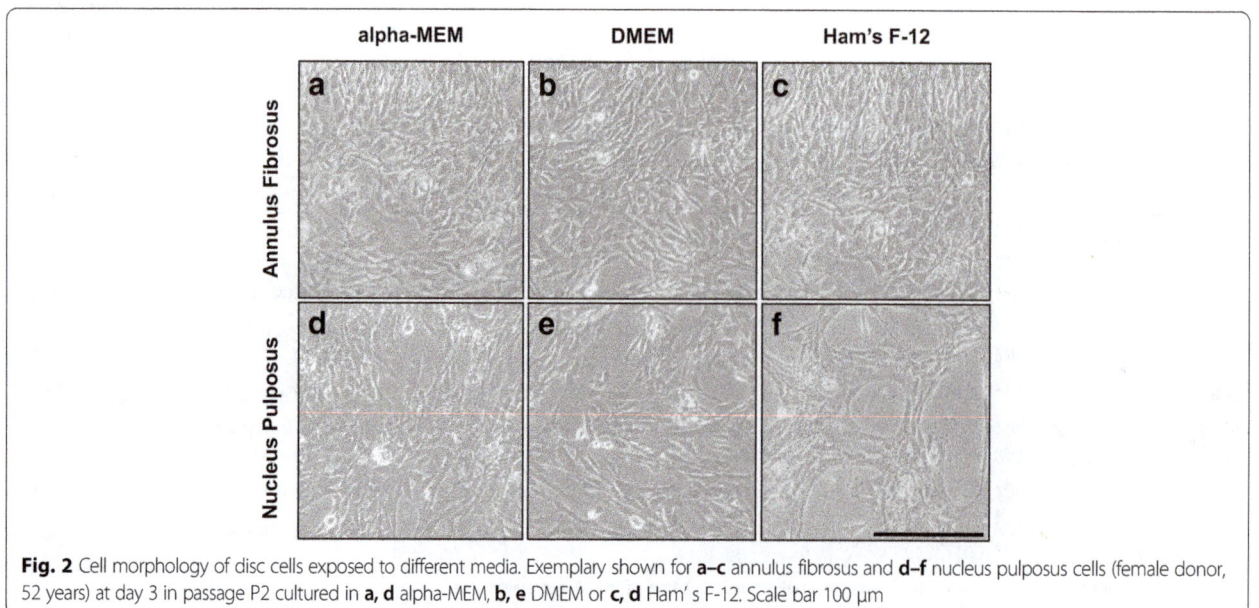

Fig. 2 Cell morphology of disc cells exposed to different media. Exemplary shown for **a–c** annulus fibrosus and **d–f** nucleus pulposus cells (female donor, 52 years) at day 3 in passage P2 cultured in **a, d** alpha-MEM, **b, e** DMEM or **c, d** Ham's F-12. Scale bar 100 μm

the same culture day and detained in the honeycombed arrangement (Fig. 2f).

Nevertheless, both AF and NP cells were expandable in all tested media. Cell viability was always higher than 95%. The cell population of both AF and NP cells doubled around three times per passage (Table 3). Comparing the tested media, there was no significant difference in PD within the single passages. Nevertheless, at the end of passage P2, the cPDL of AF cells was significantly higher when cultured in alpha-MEM compared to Ham's F-12 and alpha/F-12, as well as in DMEM/alpha compared to Ham's F-12. In NP cells, cPDL was also significantly higher when cultured in alpha-MEM compared to Ham's F-12 and all three media mixtures. This effect on cPDL was also significant when NP cells were cultured in DMEM compared to Ham's F-12 or alpha/F-12.

After seeding in passage P0, AF cells adhered to the cell culture surface within several hours, whereas NP cells took 1 to 2 days for initial attachment, independently from the medium. Furthermore, the freshly isolated cells needed some time to adapt to the cell culture conditions in vitro. This was clearly shown for both cell types in all media since the growth rate, calculated as PDR per day, was lower in passage P0 compared to the subsequent passages P1 and P2 (Table 4). Ham's F-12 was the only medium showing both a drop in PDR of NP cells in passage P2 compared to P1 (Table 4), and a constant decrease of PDs through passaging of NP cells (Table 3). In all other media, cell growth was similar for both AF and NP cells.

Glycosaminoglycan production in AF and NP cells cultured with different media

Although GAGs were produced in both cell types in passage P0, GAGs could not be detected anymore in passage P1 and P2 (Fig. 3). This was independent from the tested medium and was seen in all donors. GAG deposition in AF and NP cells was only visible in passage P0 (Fig. 3a), but showed no clear trend for the different tested media. However, GAG secretion in passage P0 was significantly lower in Ham's F-12 for AF cells, but not for NP cells (Fig. 3b).

Gene expression profile of cartilage and IVD-related markers in AF and NP cells cultured with different media

The overall gene expression profile of the cartilage markers was independent from the tested media in both AF and NP cells. Through passaging, the standard cartilage markers ACAN and COL2A1 diminished, whereas COL1A1 slightly increased (Fig. 4). Differences between the media were only seen in ACAN and COL2A1 expression in cells of passage P0. ACAN was significantly lower expressed in AF cells cultured in Ham's F-12 compared to DMEM and DMEM/alpha (Fig. 4a). This was also seen for NP cells but without statistical significance (Fig. 4b). COL2A1 expression was significantly lower in AF cells cultured in alpha-MEM and alpha/F-12 compared to DMEM (Fig. 4c), and in NP cells cultured in alpha-MEM compared to DMEM/alpha (Fig. 4d). COL1A1 expression showed no significant difference between the tested media in both cell types (Fig. 4e and f).

FOXF1 and KRT18 are IVD-related marker genes and thus gene expression was analysed to the see a possible impact of the tested media on the disc phenotype of cultured disc cells (Fig. 5). KRT18 and FOXF1 should have a stable expression in disc cells regardless of the passage number [20, 21]. In both AF and NP cells, FOXF1 expression was not changed by the different media (Fig. 5a and b). In AF cells,

Table 3 Population doubling level of disc cells cultured in different culture media

PD		alpha-MEM	DMEM	Ham's F-12	alpha/F-12	DMEM/alpha	DMEM/F-12
AF	P0	3.5 ± 0.1	3.3 ± 0.4	2.9 ± 0.1	3.3 ± 0.1	3.5 ± 0.3	3.4 ± 0.2
	P1	3.3 ± 0.4	3.1 ± 0.8	2.6 ± 0.6	2.6 ± 0.4	3.0 ± 0.5	2.8 ± 0.6
	P2	3.3 ± 0.5	3.1 ± 0.0	3.1 ± 0.6	3.1 ± 0.6	3.4 ± 0.3	3.1 ± 0.6
	cPDL	10.2 ± 0.2 *#	9.5 ± 0.4	8.5 ± 0.8	9.0 ± 0.7	9.9 ± 0.7 *	9.3 ± 0.7
NP	P0	3.7 ± 0.4	3.3 ± 0.5	3.1 ± 0.4	2.9 ± 0.2	2.7 ± 0.7	2.8 ± 0.5
	P1	3.0 ± 0.1	2.8 ± 0.3	2.5 ± 0.3	2.5 ± 0.4	2.7 ± 0.2	2.8 ± 0.0
	P2	2.9 ± 0.2	2.9 ± 0.2	2.1 ± 0.3	2.5 ± 0.2	2.8 ± 0.3	2.8 ± 0.3
	cPDL	9.6 ± 0.3*#+§	9.1 ± 0.6*#	7.7 ± 0.5	7.8 ± 0.6	8.2 ± 0.2	8.3 ± 0.5

PD Population doubling in each passage P0, P1 and P2; *cPDL* cumulated PD level at the end of passage P2; *AF* annulus fibrosus; *NP* nucleus pulposus. Data is shown as mean ± SD (AF *n* = 5, NP *n* = 3).
*Significant (p value < 0.05) compared to Ham's F-12
#Significant (p value < 0.05) compared to alpha/F-12
+Significant (p value < 0.05) compared to DMEM/alpha
§Significant (p value < 0.05) compared to DMEM/F-12

Table 4 Population doubling rate of disc cells cultured in different culture media in each passage

PDR		alpha-MEM	DMEM	Ham's F-12	alpha/F-12	DMEM/alpha	DMEM/F-12
AF	P0	0.6 ± 0.1	0.6 ± 0.1	0.5 ± 0.1	0.5 ± 0.1	0.6 ± 0.1	0.6 ± 0.1
	P1	1.1 ± 0.0	1.0 ± 0.2	0.8 ± 0.2	0.9 ± 0.1	1.0 ± 0.1	1.0 ± 0.1
	P2	1.1 ± 0.2	1.1 ± 0.0	1.1 ± 0.2	1.1 ± 0.2	1.2 ± 0.1	1.1 ± 0.2
NP	P0	0.6 ± 0.1	0.5 ± 0.0	0.5 ± 0.1	0.4 ± 0.1	0.4 ± 0.1	0.4 ± 0.1
	P1	1.0 ± 0.0	1.0 ± 0.1	0.9 ± 0.1	0.9 ± 0.2	1.0 ± 0.0	1.0 ± 0.0
	P2	1.0 ± 0.0	1.0 ± 0.1	0.7 ± 0.1	0.8 ± 0.1	0.9 ± 0.1	0.9 ± 0.1

PDR Population doubling rate (per day) in each passage P0, P1, P2; *AF* annulus fibrosus; *NP* nucleus pulposus. Data is shown as mean ± SD (AF $n = 5$, NP $n = 3$)

KRT18 expression was also not significantly changed through passaging or the choice of medium (Fig. 5c). Furthermore, KRT18 expression was stable in NP cells when cultured in DMEM, DMEM/alpha, DMEM/F-12 and alpha/F-12 (Fig. 5d). In contrast, KRT18 expression increased in NP cells with proceeding culture in Ham's F-12 and alpha-MEM, and KRT18 was significantly higher expressed after two passages in Ham's F-12 compared to all other media. Interestingly, the mRNA expression level of both FOXF1 and KRT18 was similar in AF and NP cells.

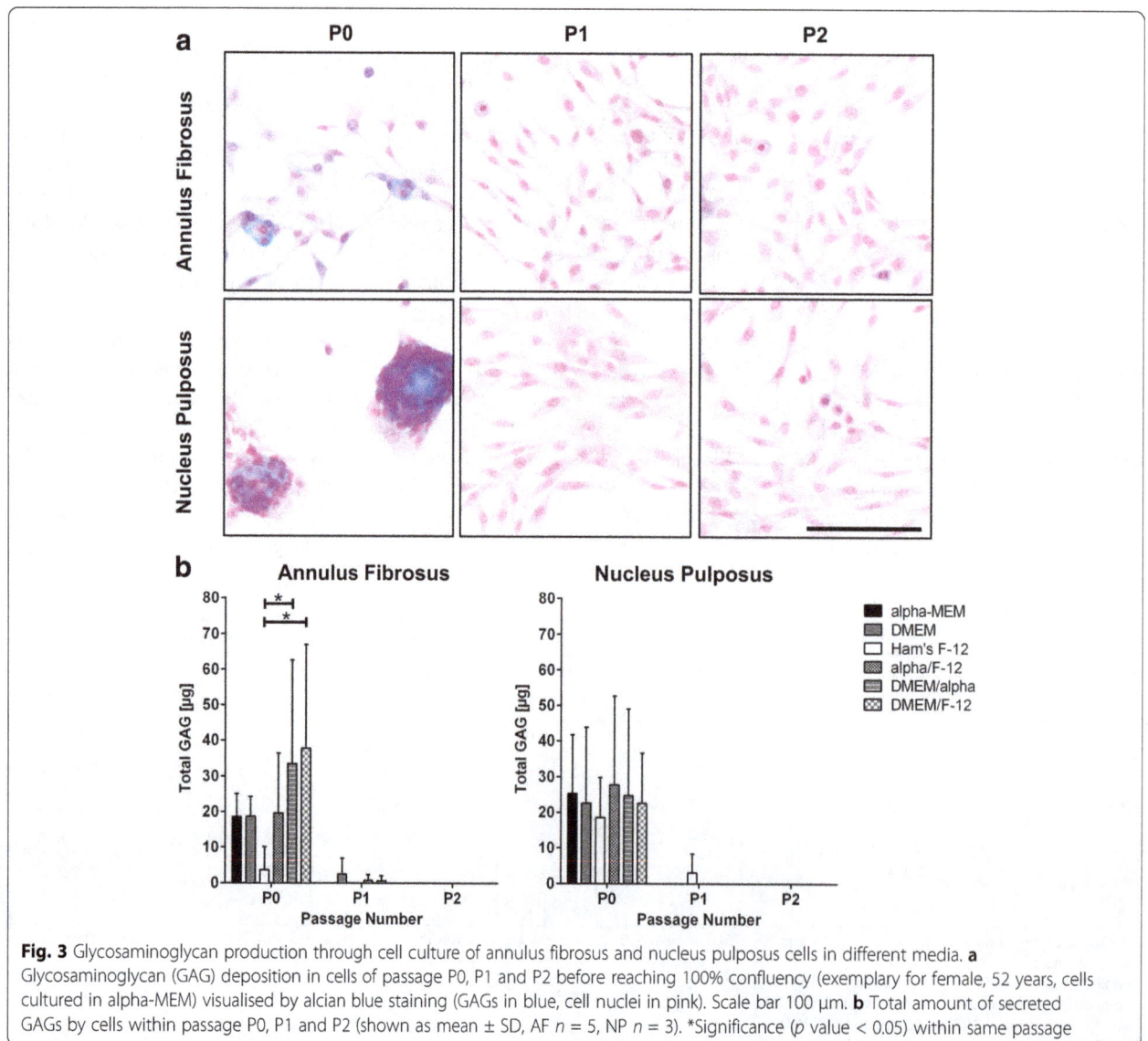

Fig. 3 Glycosaminoglycan production through cell culture of annulus fibrosus and nucleus pulposus cells in different media. **a** Glycosaminoglycan (GAG) deposition in cells of passage P0, P1 and P2 before reaching 100% confluency (exemplary for female, 52 years, cells cultured in alpha-MEM) visualised by alcian blue staining (GAGs in blue, cell nuclei in pink). Scale bar 100 μm. **b** Total amount of secreted GAGs by cells within passage P0, P1 and P2 (shown as mean ± SD, AF $n = 5$, NP $n = 3$). *Significance (p value < 0.05) within same passage

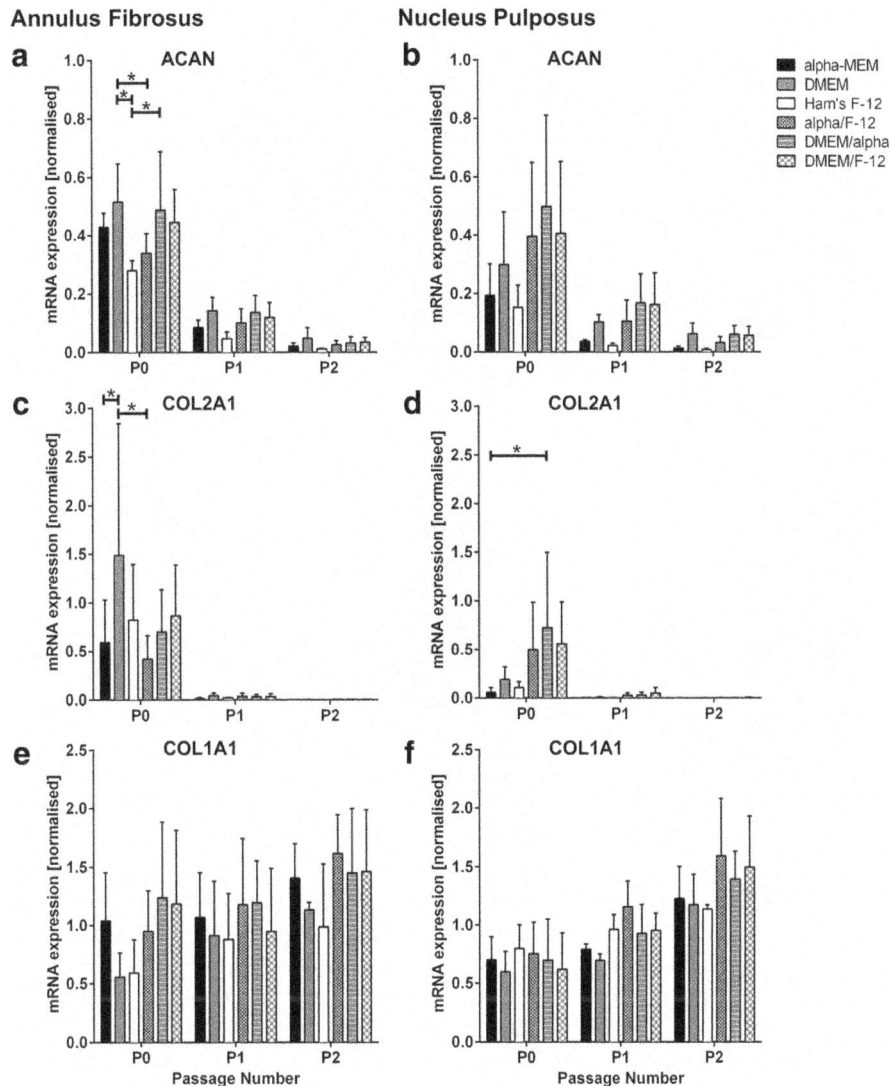

Fig. 4 Gene expression of cartilage-related markers. **a, b** ACAN, **c, d** COL2A1 and **e, f** COL1A1 is shown for **a, c, e** annulus fibrosus and **b, d, f** nucleus pulposus cells of passage P0, P1 and P2 cultured in different media. Data is presented as mRNA expression level (normalised to reference genes ATP5FB1 and RPL13A) and shown as mean ± SD (AF $n = 5$, NP $n = 3$). *Significance (p value < 0.05) compared to all other media within same passage

Discussion

Only few studies are available comparing the basal media regarding cell growth, cell morphology and proteoglycan synthesis of disc cells isolated from young rats and rabbits [22, 23]. In this study, we analysed for the first time the impact of different culture media on the in vitro behaviour of primary cells isolated from AF and NP from human IVD.

The visual description of AF and NP tissue and the different AF and NP cellularity was consistent with other studies [24, 25]. In addition, initial cell attachment was delayed for cells isolated from the NP [26]. Furthermore, the histological examination of the AF and NP starting material suggested a successful separation of AF and NP during

sample preparation. Hence, we exclude mixing-up of AF and NP cells, even though both cell types behaved very similar in cell culture.

As expected, both AF and NP cells showed proliferation in all tested media that are commonly used for disc cell expansion. Both AF and NP cells underwent a morphological change from an isodiametric to a spindle-shaped appearance through passaging. Furthermore, cells lost the ability to produce GAGs, as well as to express ACAN and COL2A1 after passaging, whereas COL1A1 was still present. These are typical characteristics of dedifferentiation, a process that is known for 2D culture of high specialised cells such as disc cells or cartilage cells [25, 27, 28]. The primary cells switch from

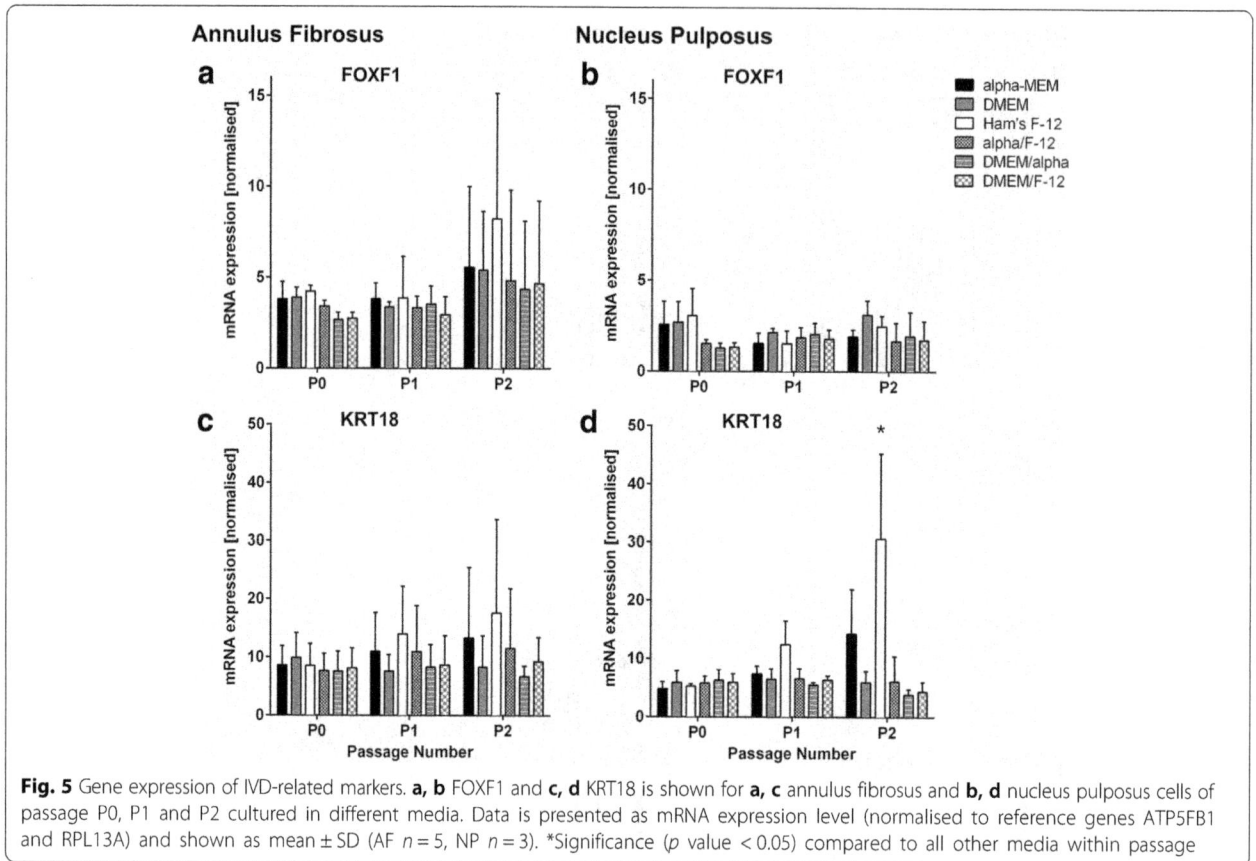

Fig. 5 Gene expression of IVD-related markers. **a, b** FOXF1 and **c, d** KRT18 is shown for **a, c** annulus fibrosus and **b, d** nucleus pulposus cells of passage P0, P1 and P2 cultured in different media. Data is presented as mRNA expression level (normalised to reference genes ATP5FB1 and RPL13A) and shown as mean ± SD (AF $n = 5$, NP $n = 3$). *Significance (p value < 0.05) compared to all other media within passage

their native state into a proliferative state, triggered by their attachment to the cell culture surface. Thereby, cells stop synthesising ECM molecules, e.g. GAGs and aggrecan, and switch their collagen expression from type II to type I. This was seen in all media and confirmed previous results [22]. Hence, the presence of different media did not affect dedifferentiation of cultured disc cells.

Nevertheless, our results showed that the choice of medium affected cell growth and gene expression of the IVD-related marker KRT18. The proliferation capacity of both AF and NP cells was impaired in Ham's F-12 compared to alpha-MEM and DMEM. A lower cell growth in Ham's F-12 compared to DMEM and a similar cell growth between alpha-MEM and DMEM was reported before for rat AF and rabbit NP cells, respectively [22, 23]. Although cell growth was highest in alpha-MEM and lowest in Ham's F-12, both media increased the KRT18 expression in NP cells. This is a major change in the cell's behaviour in vitro, because disc cells should typically show a stable expression of the IVD-related marker KRT18 through 2D expansion [20, 21]. As the differences between the media were only seen after proceeding culture in passage P2 but not in P0 or P1, the change in cell's behaviour cannot be simply explained by dedifferentiation processes, but was indeed driven by the culture media and its different

nutrient supply. In addition, all differences seen between the single media were compensated when the media were used in a mixture.

Comparing the media formulations, the glucose concentration is two times higher in Ham's F-12 than in alpha-MEM and DMEM (Table 1). As glycolysis is the main energy source in disc cells [29] and glucose consumption increases with higher glucose concentration [30], we would have expected a higher performance of the cells in Ham's F-12 compared to alpha-MEM or DMEM. However, cell growth and GAG production was lower in Ham's F-12, and expression of cartilage-related genes was unaffected by the different media. Disc cells are used to glucose concentrations in vivo comparable to alpha-MEM, DMEM (0.56 mM) and Hams' F-12 (1 mM). Furthermore, cell growth of human NP cells is not variant with glucose levels of either 1.8 or 2.5 mM [12]. Hence, the difference in glucose supplied by the different media was too low to have an impact that was previously described for human NP cells when cultured with either 0.5 mM or 5 mM glucose [6, 31]. This indicates that glucose was not the most important factor triggering the different performance of AF and NP cells observed in the different media.

The glutamine concentration is apparently four times higher in alpha-MEM and DMEM (4 mM) than in Ham's

F-12 (1 mM). Cell growth was higher in alpha-MEM and DMEM compared to Ham's F-12. Other studies showed that proliferation capacity is more dependent on glutamine rather than glucose [32]. Glutamine is an alternative energy source for rapidly dividing cells that have a high demand on energy, especially when glucose level is low. So, if both glutamine and glucose are present in vitro, cells might prefer glutamine as it is faster metabolised. Nevertheless, glucose is mandatory in cell culture as the stimulatory effect of glutamine is only seen in presence of glucose [33]. The higher concentration of glucose in Ham's F-12, however, appeared to be insufficient to compensate its lower glutamine concentration. Therefore, the continuous low glutamine level could be one reason for the lower cell growth of AF and NP cells in Ham's F-12.

In passage P2, when decrease in cell growth was observed for NP cells in Ham's F'12, NP cells detained in a honeycombed orientation and did not spread into free spaces between cells. A similar stratification pattern is described for immortalised AF cells when cultured in Ham's F-12 [34]. Another study associates the cell's behaviour with a low calcium concentration [35], comparable to the level existing in Ham's F-12 (0.3 mM). Furthermore, calcium mediates cell attachment and cell–cell interaction through adhesion molecules, and is a major regulator in cell proliferation [36]. At a calcium concentration lower than 0.5 mM, cell proliferation is retarded [37]. Hence, AF and NP cells showed higher cell growth in alpha-MEM and DMEM compared to Ham's F-12, because alpha-MEM and DMEM contain more calcium (1.8 mM) that is comparable to the physiological range in the blood [38]. In addition, a calcium concentration like in Ham's F-12 was found to be more favourable for the expansion of other cell types like keratinocytes [39].

The presence of other components, for example ascorbic acid, could further have affected the cell's behaviour in the different media. Ascorbic acid functions as a cofactor in collagen assembling and therefore facilitates ECM development. Despite the other media, alpha-MEM contains ascorbic acid (280 µM). However, both AF and NP cells were not stimulated in collagen expression on mRNA level or in GAG protein expression when cultured in alpha-MEM. By comparing with the literature, 280 µM ascorbic acid has a visible effect on GAG synthesis by disc cells [40], whereas supplementation of 1000 µM is necessary to increase collagen synthesis [41, 42]. Hence, ascorbic acid at a low concentration as used here or commonly supplemented in literature (100–280 µM) might not be relevant for disc cell culture.

We assume that low levels of other media components that are additionally present in Ham's F-12 or rather missing in either alpha-MEM or DMEM were introduced to the cell culture as a component of the added

serum. Therefore, trace elements, fatty acids, vitamins or other amino acids with slightly different concentration in the basal medium are not discussed here. In this study, we used the same serum batch constantly for all experiments. However, serum obtained from different donors contains variant concentrations of growth factors [43]. Furthermore, growth factor concentration is different in serum obtained from different origins (autologous, allogeneic, xenogeneic) and serum-replacements (like platelet rich plasma) [13, 43]. This is of importance, as the disc cell's behaviour is altered when growth factors are supplemented to the cell culture medium [44, 45]. Hence, both the serum batch and serum origin could possibly have a greater impact on disc cells in vitro than has been seen here between the different basal media.

The overall observed difference between the tested media in passage P0 to P2 was lower than expected. It would be interesting to see the cell's response in higher passages. However, we decided to stop cell culture in passage P2, when AF and NP cells reached a cPDL of 9.4 ± 0.8 and 8.5 ± 0.8 on average, respectively, to avoid a bias by general cell culture effects. It is known from other cartilage cells that the genetic stability is altered, when cells are cultured higher than a cPDL of 10 [46].

In agreement with other studies, the cultured AF cells were indistinguishable from NP cells regarding cell morphology and cell growth [2, 25, 47]. Furthermore and in line with literature, AF and NP cells showed similar mRNA expression level of the IVD-related marker FOXF1 and KRT18 [48, 49]. The higher KRT18 expression level in NP cells compared to AF cells was triggered by the proceeding culture in Ham's F-12, as this was not seen for the other media. Hence, the KRT18 expression was influenced by the choice of medium and therefore nutrient supply. A previous study showed that KRT18 is down-regulated in cultured NP cells when cells are obtained from degenerated human IVD tissue [50]. An increase in KRT18 expression is only reported for NP cells, when the cell culture system is changed from 2D to 3D or throughout prolonged culture in a 3D environment [51, 52]. This further suggests that KRT18 expression in NP cells is sensitive to environmental conditions. A high ratio of aggrecan and collagen type II is another characteristic for human NP tissue [20]. Apparently, this is only true for native tissue at protein level, because we and others could not recover that ratio in primary NP cells on mRNA level [53, 54]. In addition, there was no difference between AF and NP cells in overall gene expression of ACAN, COL2A1 and COL1A1 [55]. Therefore, the common cartilage and IVD-related markers used in this study were not suitable to discriminate AF and NP cells in vitro.

Nevertheless, our results indicate that the choice of medium has an impact on the behaviour of disc cells in vitro. Furthermore, AF and NP cells were influenced differently. Ham's F-12 impaired cell growth in NP but not in AF cells. In addition, the proceeding culture in Ham's F-12 changed the KRT18 expression only in NP cells. Hence, it is possible that different culture media are required for AF and NP cells in order to preserve their individual cell characteristics. This is of relevance as cell-based therapeutic approaches often utilise herniated IVD tissue as starting tissue material for cell isolation [56, 57]. The herniated tissue contains a heterogeneous cell population as it originates either in the NP or AF compartment of the disc depending on the hernia location [58, 59]. Therefore, as long as no marker is available to separate human AF and NP cells, the choice of medium is important for the development of cell-therapeutic products targeted for either AF or NP repair.

Conclusion

AF and NP cells were expandable in all tested media. The different media did not affect the typical process of dedifferentiation known for cultured disc cells. Furthermore, both cell types showed same proliferation capacity and expression of IVD-related markers when cultured in DMEM as single medium or in a mixture. In contrast, the proceeding culture in Ham's F-12 impeded cell growth. In addition, Ham's F-12 and alpha-MEM changed the KRT18 gene expression profile in NP cells. The observed differences between the basal media were based on its different content of glutamine and calcium rather than glucose. Therefore, the choice of medium influenced the disc cell's behaviour in vitro as hypothesised. In conclusion, we recommend using DMEM, DMEM/alpha or DMEM/F-12 for standardised expansion of AF and NP cells in vitro. Using standardised media will generate preclinical research results with higher comparability and thus accelerate the development of cell-therapeutic approaches for disc regeneration.

Abbreviations

2D: Two-dimensional; ACAN: Aggrecan; AF: Annulus fibrosus; alpha-MEM: Alpha-Minimal Essential Medium; ATP5F1B: ATP synthase F1 subunit beta; CEP: Cartilage endplate; COL2A1: Collagen type I; COL2A2: Collagen type II; cPDL: Cumulative population doubling level; DDD: Degenerative disc disease; DMEM: Dulbecco's Modified Eagle's Medium; ECM: Extracellular matrix; F-12: Ham's F-12 medium; FOXF1: Forkhead box F1; GAG: Glycosaminoglycan; HS: Human serum; IVD: Intervertebral disc; KRT18: Keratin 18; mRNA: Messenger ribosomal nucleic acid; NP: Nucleus pulposus; PD: Population doubling; PDR: Population doubling rate; RPL13A: Ribosomal protein L13a

Acknowledgments
We acknowledge the assistance of the BCRT Cell Harvesting Core Unit.

Funding
This study was supported by the Berlin-Brandenburg Center for Regenerative Therapies (BCRT) funded by Bundesministerium für Bildung und Forschung (grant 13GW0099) and the CO.DON AG.

Authors' contributions
AS designed and performed the experiments, was responsible for data acquisition, analysis and interpretation and wrote the paper. JJS contributed to research design, data interpretation and improved the manuscript. MP and MP contributed the disc material and data acquisition in a clinical context. MS and JR were responsible for original research design and improved the manuscript. All authors read and approved the final manuscript.

Competing interests
AS and JJS were employees at CO.DON AG. All other authors declare that they have no competing interests.

Author details
¹Tissue Engineering Laboratory and Berlin-Brandenburg Center for Regenerative Therapies, Charité - Universitätsmedizin Berlin, corporate member of Freie Universität Berlin, Humboldt-Universität zu Berlin and Berlin Institute of Health, Augustenburger Platz 1, Südstraße 2, 13353 Berlin, Germany. ²CO.DON AG, Teltow, Germany. ³Center for Musculoskeletal Surgery, Department of Orthopaedics, Charité - Universitätsmedizin Berlin, corporate member of Freie Universität Berlin, Humboldt-Universität zu Berlin and Berlin Institute of Health, Berlin, Germany.

References
1. Cheung KM, Karppinen J, Chan D, Ho DW, Song YQ, Sham P, Cheah KS, Leong JC, Luk KD. Prevalence and pattern of lumbar magnetic resonance imaging changes in a population study of one thousand forty-three individuals. Spine (Phila Pa 1976). 2009;34(9):934–40.
2. Wang F, Cai F, Shi R, Wang XH, Wu XT. Aging and age related stresses: a senescence mechanism of intervertebral disc degeneration. Osteoarthr Cartil. 2016;24(3):398–408.
3. Urban JP. The role of the physicochemical environment in determining disc cell behaviour. Biochem Soc Trans. 2002;30(Pt 6):858–64.
4. Oehme D, Goldschlager T, Ghosh P, Rosenfeld JV, Jenkin G. Cell-based therapies used to treat lumbar degenerative disc disease: a systematic review of animal studies and human clinical trials. Stem Cells Int. 2015; https://doi.org/10.1155/2015/946031
5. Mern DS, Beierfuss A, Thome C, Hegewald AA. Enhancing human nucleus pulposus cells for biological treatment approaches of degenerative intervertebral disc diseases: a systematic review. J Tissue Eng Regen Med. 2014;8(12):925–36.
6. Bibby SR, Urban JP. Effect of nutrient deprivation on the viability of intervertebral disc cells. Eur. Spine J. 2004;13(8):695–701.
7. Eagle H. Nutrition needs of mammalian cells in tissue culture. Science. 1955; 122(3168):501–14.
8. Dulbecco R, Freeman G. Plaque production by the polyoma virus. Virology. 1959;8(3):396–7.
9. Stanners CP, Eliceiri GL, Green H. Two types of ribosome in mouse-hamster hybrid cells. Nat New Biol. 1971;230(10):52–4.
10. Ham RG, Sattler GL. Clonal growth of differentiated rabbit cartilage cells. J Cell Physiol. 1968;72(2):109–14.
11. Pinnell SR. Regulation of collagen biosynthesis by ascorbic acid: a review. Yale J Biol Med. 1985;58(6):553–9.

12. Turner SA, Wright KT, Jones PN, Balain B, Roberts S. Temporal analyses of the response of intervertebral disc cells and mesenchymal stem cells to nutrient deprivation. Stem Cells Int. 2016; https://doi.org/10.1155/2016/5415901.

13. Wang SZ, Chang Q, Lu J, Wang C. Growth factors and platelet-rich plasma: promising biological strategies for early intervertebral disc degeneration. Int Orthop. 2015;39(5):927–34.

14. Gorth DJ, Lothstein KE, Chiaro JA, Farrell MJ, Dodge GR, Elliott DM, Malhotra NR, Mauck RL, Smith LJ. Hypoxic regulation of functional extracellular matrix elaboration by nucleus pulposus cells in long-term agarose culture. J Orthop Res. 2015;33(5):747–54.

15. Miyazaki M, Hong SW, Yoon SH, Morishita Y, Wang JC. Reliability of a magnetic resonance imaging-based grading system for cervical intervertebral disc degeneration. J Spinal Disord Tech. 2008;21(4):288–92.

16. Stich S, Stolk M, Girod PP, Thome C, Sittinger M, Ringe J, Seifert M, Hegewald AA. Regenerative and immunogenic characteristics of cultured nucleus pulposus cells from human cervical intervertebral discs. PLoS One. 2015;10(5):e0126954.

17. Cristofalo VJ, Allen RG, Pignolo RJ, Martin BG, Beck JC. Relationship between donor age and the replicative lifespan of human cells in culture: a reevaluation. Proc Natl Acad Sci U S A. 1998;95(18):10614–9.

18. Kaji K, Matsuo M. Aging of chick embryo fibroblasts in vitro--I. Saturation density and population doubling rate. Exp Gerontol. 1978;13(6):439–45.

19. Bartz C, Meixner M, Giesemann P, Roel G, Bulwin GC, Smink JJ. An ex vivo human cartilage repair model to evaluate the potency of a cartilage cell transplant. J Transl Med. 2016;14(1):317.

20. Risbud MV, Schoepflin ZR, Mwale F, Kandel RA, Grad S, Iatridis JC, Sakai D, Hoyland JA. Defining the phenotype of young healthy nucleus pulposus cells: recommendations of the spine research interest group at the 2014 annual ORS meeting. J Orthop Res. 2015;33(3):283–93.

21. van den Akker GG, Surtel DA, Cremers A, Rodrigues-Pinto R, Richardson SM, Hoyland JA, van Rhijn LW, Welting TJ, Voncken JW. Novel immortal human cell lines reveal subpopulations in the nucleus pulposus. Arthritis Res Ther. 2014;16(3):R135.

22. Ichimura K, Tsuji H, Matsui H, Makiyama N. Cell culture of the intervertebral disc of rats: factors influencing culture, proteoglycan, collagen, and deoxyribonucleic acid synthesis. J Spinal Disord. 1991;4(4):428–36.

23. Rastogi A, Thakore P, Leung A, Benavides M, Machado M, Morschauser MA, Hsieh AH. Environmental regulation of notochordal gene expression in nucleus pulposus cells. J Cell Physiol. 2009;220(3):698–705.

24. Chou AI, Bansal A, Miller GJ, Nicoll SB. The effect of serial monolayer passaging on the collagen expression profile of outer and inner anulus fibrosus cells. Spine (Phila Pa 1976). 2006;31(17):1875–81.

25. Kluba T, Niemeyer T, Gaissmaier C, Grunder T. Human anulus fibrosis and nucleus pulposus cells of the intervertebral disc: effect of degeneration and culture system on cell phenotype. Spine (Phila Pa 1976). 2005;30(24):2743–8.

26. Horner HA, Roberts S, Bielby RC, Menage J, Evans H, Urban JP. Cells from different regions of the intervertebral disc: effect of culture system on matrix expression and cell phenotype. Spine (Phila Pa 1976). 2002;27(10):1018–28.

27. von der Mark K, Gauss V, von der Mark H, Muller P. Relationship between cell shape and type of collagen synthesised as chondrocytes lose their cartilage phenotype in culture. Nature. 1977;267(5611):531–2.

28. Gorensek M, Jaksimovic C, Kregar-Velikonja N, Gorensek M, Knezevic M, Jeras M, Pavlovcic V, Cor A. Nucleus pulposus repair with cultured autologous elastic cartilage derived chondrocytes. Cell Mol Biol Lett. 2004; 9(2):363–73.

29. Urban JP, Winlove CP. Pathophysiology of the intervertebral disc and the challenges for MRI. J Magn Reson Imaging. 2007;25(2):419–32.

30. Bibby SR, Jones DA, Ripley RM, Urban JP. Metabolism of the intervertebral disc: effects of low levels of oxygen, glucose, and pH on rates of energy metabolism of bovine nucleus pulposus cells. Spine (Phila Pa 1976). 2005; 30(5):487–96.

31. Rinkler C, Heuer F, Pedro MT, Mauer UM, Ignatius A, Neidlinger-Wilke C. Influence of low glucose supply on the regulation of gene expression by nucleus pulposus cells and their responsiveness to mechanical loading. J Neurosurg Spine. 2010;13(4):535–42.

32. Slivac I, Gaurina Srcek V, Radosevic K, Porobic I, Bilic K, Fumic K, Kniewald Z. Growth characteristics of channel catfish ovary cells-influence of glucose and glutamine. Cytotechnology. 2008;57(3):273–8.

33. Slivac I, Blajic V, Radosevic K, Kniewald Z, Gaurina Srcek V. Influence of different ammonium, lactate and glutamine concentrations on CCO cell growth. Cytotechnology. 2010;62(6):585–94.

34. van den Akker GG, Surtel DA, Cremers A, Richardson SM, Hoyland JA, van Rhijn LW, Voncken JW, Welting TJ. Novel immortal cell lines support cellular heterogeneity in the human annulus fibrosus. PLoS One. 2016;11(1): e0144497.

35. Hennings H, Michael D, Cheng C, Steinert P, Holbrook K, Yuspa SH. Calcium regulation of growth and differentiation of mouse epidermal cells in culture. Cell. 1980;19(1):245–54.

36. Ko KS, Arora PD, Bhide V, Chen A, McCulloch CA. Cell-cell adhesion in human fibroblasts requires calcium signaling. J Cell Sci. 2001;114(Pt 6): 1155–67.

37. Boynton AL, Whitfield JF, Isaacs RJ, Morton HJ. Control of 3T3 cell proliferation by calcium. In Vitro. 1974;10:12–7.

38. Goldstein DA. Serum calcium. In: Walker HK, Hall WD, Hurst JW, editors. Clinical Methods: The History, Physical, and Laboratory Examinations. 3rd ed. Boston: Butterworths; 1990. Available from: https://www.ncbi.nlm.nih.gov/books/NBK201/.

39. Dahm AM, de Bruin A, Linat A, von Tscharner C, Wyder M, Suter MM. Cultivation and characterisation of primary and subcultured equine keratinocytes. Equine Vet J. 2002;34(2):114–20.

40. Lee YJ, Kong MH, Song KY, Lee KH, Heo SH. The relation between Sox9, TGF-beta1, and proteoglycan in human intervertebral disc cells. J Korean Neurosurg Soc. 2008;43(3):149–54.

41. Flagler DJ, Huang CY, Yuan TY, Lu Z, Cheung HS, Intracellular Flow GWY. Cytometric measurement of extracellular matrix components in porcine intervertebral disc cells. Cell Mol Bioeng. 2009;2(2):264–73.

42. Kim MH. Effect of L-ascorbic acid on collagen synthesis in 3T6 fibroblasts and primary cultured cells of chondrocytes. J Korean Soc Food Sci Nutr. 2006;35:42–7.

43. Tallheden T, van der Lee J, Brantsing C, Mansson JE, Sjogren-Jansson E, Lindahl A. Human serum for culture of articular chondrocytes. Cell Transplant. 2005;14(7):469–79.

44. Gruber HE, Fisher EC Jr, Desai B, Stasky AA, Hoelscher G, Hanley EN Jr. Human intervertebral disc cells from the annulus: three-dimensional culture in agarose or alginate and responsiveness to TGF-beta1. Exp Cell Res. 1997; 235(1):13–21.

45. Hegewald AA, Cluzel J, Kruger JP, Endres M, Kaps C, Thome C. Effects of initial boost with TGF-beta 1 and grade of intervertebral disc degeneration on 3D culture of human annulus fibrosus cells. J Orthop Surg Res. 2014;9:73.

46. Wallenborn M, Petters O, Rudolf D, Hantmann H, Richter M, Ahnert P, Rohani L, Smink JJ, Bulwin GC, Krupp W, et al. Comprehensive high-resolution genomic profiling and cytogenetics of human chondrocyte cultures by GTG-banding, locus-specific FISH, SKY and SNP array. Eur Cell Mater. 2018;35:225–41.

47. Chen YF, Zhang YZ, Zhang WL, Luan GN, Liu ZH, Gao Y, Wan ZY, Sun Z, Zhu S, Samartzis D, et al. Insights into the hallmarks of human nucleus pulposus cells with particular reference to cell viability, phagocytic potential and long process formation. Int J Med Sci. 2013;10(13):1805–16.

48. van den Akker GGH, Koenders MI, van de Loo FAJ, van Lent P, Blaney Davidson E, van der Kraan PM. Transcriptional profiling distinguishes inner and outer annulus fibrosus from nucleus pulposus in the bovine intervertebral disc. Eur Spine J. 2017;26(8):2053–62.

49. Rutges J, Creemers LB, Dhert W, Milz S, Sakai D, Mochida J, Alini M, Grad S. Variations in gene and protein expression in human nucleus pulposus in comparison with annulus fibrosus and cartilage cells: potential associations with aging and degeneration. Osteoarthr Cartil. 2010;18(3):416–23.

50. Lv FJ, Peng Y, Lim FL, Sun Y, Lv M, Zhou L, Wang H, Zheng Z, Cheung KM, Leung VY. Matrix metalloproteinase 12 is an indicator of intervertebral disc degeneration co-expressed with fibrotic markers. Osteoarthr Cartil. 2016; 24(10):1826–36.

51. Sun Y, Lv M, Zhou L, Tam V, Lv F, Chan D, Wang H, Zheng Z, Cheung KM, Leung VY. Enrichment of committed human nucleus pulposus cells expressing chondroitin sulfate proteoglycans under alginate encapsulation. Osteoarthr Cartil. 2015;23(7):1194–203.

52. Wan S, Borland S, Richardson SM, Merry CL, Saiani A, Gough JE. Self-assembling peptide hydrogel for intervertebral disc tissue engineering. Acta Biomater. 2016;46:29–40.

53. Park JY, Kuh SU, Park HS, Kim KS. Comparative expression of matrix-associated genes and inflammatory cytokines-associated genes according

to disc degeneration: analysis of living human nucleus pulposus. J Spinal Disord Tech. 2011;24(6):352–7.

54. Choi EH, Park H, Park KS, Park KS, Kim BS, Han IB, Shin DA, Lee SH. Effect of nucleus pulposus cells having different phenotypes on chondrogenic differentiation of adipose-derived stromal cells in a coculture system using porous membranes. Tissue Eng Part A. 2011;17(19–20):2445–51.

55. Sive JI, Baird P, Jeziorsk M, Watkins A, Hoyland JA, Freemont AJ. Expression of chondrocyte markers by cells of normal and degenerate intervertebral discs. Mol Pathol. 2002;55(2):91–7.

56. Meisel HJ, Siodla V, Ganey T, Minkus Y, Hutton WC, Alasevic OJ. Clinical experience in cell-based therapeutics: disc chondrocyte transplantation a treatment for degenerated or damaged intervertebral disc. Biomol Eng. 2007;24(1):5–21.

57. Tschugg A, Diepers M, Simone S, Michnacs F, Quirbach S, Strowitzki M, Meisel HJ, Thome C. A prospective randomized multicenter phase I/II clinical trial to evaluate safety and efficacy of NOVOCART disk plus autologous disk chondrocyte transplantation in the treatment of nucleotomized and degenerative lumbar disks to avoid secondary disease: safety results of phase I-a short report. Neurosurg Rev. 2017;40(1):155–62.

58. Moore RJ, Vernon-Roberts B, Fraser RD, Osti OL, Schembri M. The origin and fate of herniated lumbar intervertebral disc tissue. Spine (Phila Pa 1976). 1996;21(18):2149–55.

59. Rajasekaran S, Babu JN, Arun R, Armstrong BR, Shetty AP, Murugan S. ISSLS prize winner: a study of diffusion in human lumbar discs: a serial magnetic resonance imaging study documenting the influence of the endplate on diffusion in normal and degenerate discs. Spine (Phila Pa 1976). 2004;29(23): 2654–67.

10

5-year clinical and radiographic follow-up of the uncemented Symax hip stem in an international study

Dennis Silvester Maria Gerardus Kruijntjens[1]* ⓘD, Per Kjaersgaard-Andersen[2], Peter Revald[2], Jane Schwartz Leonhardt[2], Jacobus Johannes Chris Arts[1] and René Hendrikus Maria ten Broeke[1]

Abstract

Background: The uncemented Symax hip stem is developed through optimization of the uncemented Omnifit hip stem. The Symax stem design combines an anatomical anteverted proximal geometry with a straight distal section. The proximal part is coated with a biomimetic hydroxyapatite (HA) coating for improved osseointegration to enhance load transfer and to minimize proximal bone loss. The distal part is treated with an anodization surface treatment in order to prevent distal bone apposition, which is expected to prevent distal loading and reduce proximal stress shielding. Aim of this study is to report mid-term clinical performance and evaluate whether the radiographic features are in line with the design principles of the Symax hip.

Methods: The biomimetic hydroxyapatite-coated uncemented Symax hip stem was evaluated in 80 patients during a 5-year prospective clinical international study. Harris Hip Score (HHS), Oxford Hip Score (OHS), and Western Ontario and McMaster Universities Arthritis Index (WOMAC) were performed preoperatively and postoperatively at 6 months and 1, 2, 3 and 5 years. Anteroposterior radiographs of the pelvis and axial radiographs of the operated hips were evaluated immediately postoperative and at follow-up 6 months and 1, 2, 3, and 5 years. Wilcoxon signed-rank test was used to analyse whether clinical outcome scores changed statistically significant over time. The overall percentage of agreement between two radiology assessment teams was used to evaluate observer agreement of radiology results. The Cohen's Kappa was evaluated as a measure of reliability to quantify the agreement between raters, corrected for chance agreement.

Results: Clinical outcome scores were excellent at 5 years with mean HHS of 98.1, mean OHS of 16.2 and mean WOMAC of 6.9. Only 2.7% of the patients had pain at rest or on weight-bearing, and mid-thigh pain was reported by 1.4% of the patients after 5 years. The percentage of agreement between radiology assessment teams was 94 to 100%, except for distal line formation (48%). Radiographic evaluation showed stable stems and signs of excellent progressive proximal fixation and favourable bone remodeling.

Conclusions: The excellent mid-term clinical and radiographic performances are in line with the design principles and coating properties of this new implant and earlier published results.

Keywords: Symax, Uncemented hip stem, Clinical, Radiographic, Total hip arthroplasty

* Correspondence: d.kruijntjens@gmail.com
[1]Department of Orthopaedic Surgery, Research School Caphri, Maastricht University Medical Centre, P. Debyelaan 25, P.O. Box 5800, 6202 AZ Maastricht, the Netherlands
Full list of author information is available at the end of the article

Background

New designs of uncemented hip stems focus on enhancing osseointegration, improved interface sealing, optimized load transfer, diminishing the rate of loosening, and on improving clinical outcomes. For these purposes, optimizations can be realized in the geometry of the stem, the choice of material, surface texture, and the type and extent of the osseointegrative coating [1–6]. These considerations resulted in the development of the uncemented Symax stem design (Stryker Orthopaedics, Amsterdam, the Netherlands) as an optimization of the well-documented, second-generation uncemented Omnifit hip stem [3, 7, 8]. Histological and histomorphometric analyses on retrieved implanted Symax hip stems have already proven early proximal ingrowth as a result of the new BONIT-hydroxyapatite (HA) coating (DOT GmbH, Rostock, Germany) and the distal DOTIZE surface treatment (DOT GmbH, Rostock, Germany) [9]. Furthermore, improved bone remodeling was already established in a 2-year follow-up dual-energy X-ray absorptiometry (DEXA) study compared to the Omnifit hip stem [10]. This international study is part of a stepwise clinical introduction of the Symax hip stem according to Malchau et al. [11], illustrating the 'phased innovation' of this new implant. As part of this clinical introduction also, a prospective radiostereometric analysis (RSA) study and a large prospective clinical cohort study are ongoing. The aim of this study is to report mid-term clinical performance and evaluate whether the radiographic features are in line with the design principles of the Symax hip stem in an international setting during 5 years of clinical follow-up in a cohort of 80 patients.

It was hypothesized that the new BONIT-HA coating and the distal DOTIZE surface treatment, together with an optimized geometrical design, would generate both a mechanically stable stem with mid-term radiographic features of consistent and progressive excellent proximal fixation and radiographic signs that would also underline the effects of the distal surface treatment. The combination of these would anticipate a superior bone remodeling that is highly recognizable on conventional radiographs.

Methods

Between September 2004 and November 2005, 80 patients were included in this prospective international study performed at the Maastricht University Medical Centre (MUMC), the Netherlands (centre 1, $n = 30$), and the Vejle Hospital, Denmark (centre 2, $n = 50$). Eligibility criteria were patients requiring primary uncemented total hip arthroplasty (THA), age older than 18 years, and BMI less or equal to 35. Exclusion criteria were bilateral hip complaints, impaired cognitive function, and use of medication or illness influencing bone metabolism. Baseline demographic data were similar for both study centres (Table 1).

Ethical board approval was obtained from the local Institutional Review Board (centre 1: METC 04-112; centre 2: S-VF-20040133), and informed consent was obtained from each patient prior to surgery. This study was conducted according to the ethical standards of the Declaration of Helsinki of 1975, as revised in 2013 in Fortaleza (Brasil), and following the ISO 14155 Good Clinical Practice (GCP) guidelines.

Surgical protocol

The posterolateral approach to the hip was used by four senior hip surgeons. Patients received 24-h intravenous antibiotic prophylaxis and deep venous thrombosis prophylaxis with low molecular weight heparins. Full weight-bearing was allowed from the first postoperative day. In this study, complete excision of the joint capsule was performed in 86.7% of the patients in centre 1 compared to 2.0% in centre 2. Non-steroidal anti-inflammatory drug (NSAIDs) prescription to prevent heterotopic bone formation also varied; 96.7% of the patients in centre 1 received NSAIDs, compared to only 4.0% of patients in centre 2.

Implant

The Symax hip stem is an uncemented design forged from Ti6Al4V alloy. Primary mechanical stability is provided by anatomical metaphyseal geometry, based on CT-analysis of the proximal femur (data on file at Stryker). The hip stem features a size-dependent anteversion, neck length, and offset, with a centrum-collum-diaphyseal (CCD) angle of 128° (data on file at Stryker). Axial stability is pursued by the straight distal section in the femoral canal (Fig. 1). Secondary biological stability is accomplished by fast osseous integration due to the BONIT-HA coating on the metaphyseal part of the stem (Fig. 1), as was confirmed earlier by histology and histomorphometry analyses on retrieved stems [9]. BONIT-HA is a new generation, electrochemically deposited, biomimetic hydroxyapatite (HA) coating on top of a commercially pure titanium plasma spray (TPS) layer. It is deposited by low-temperature precipitation, is thin (10–20 μm), and has a 3D surface with high porosity (60%) and pore interconnectivity [9, 10, 12, 13]. The coating is fully resorbable and is known to be substituted by bone for about 99% [14]. The anodization surface treatment, DOTIZE, applied on the distal part of the stem, is an electrolytical conversion of the native oxide film on titanium surfaces into a thicker and denser titanium oxide. It shows anti-galling properties and reduces protein adsorption with 19% and bone apposition compared to untreated titanium alloy [9, 10, 15].

Table 1 Baseline demographic data of study cohort

	Centre 1	Centre 2	Total	P value
No. of hips	30	50	80	
Male/female	16/14	29/21	45/35	0.684
Mean (range) age (years)	57.5 (41–71)	56.2 (30–69)	56.7 (30–71)	0.437
Mean (range) BMI (kg/m^2)	27.1 (20–33)	27.0 (18–35)	27.0 (18–35)	0.913
Diagnosis, no. of hips (%)				0.135
Osteoarthritis	27 (90.0%)	41 (82.0%)	68 (85.0%)	
Avascular necrosis	2 (6.7%)	1 (2.0%)	3 (3.8%)	
Posttraumatic arthritis		7 (14.0%)	7 (8.8%)	
Other	1 (3.3%)	1 (2.0%)	2 (2.5%)	

The uncemented HA-coated Trident acetabular cup (Stryker Orthopaedics, Mahwah, NJ, USA) was used in 78 patients (98%) [16], except 2 patients (2.5%) in centre 1 who had cemented SHP ArCom ultra-high molecular weight polyethylene cups (Biomet, Bridgend, UK). Of the 78 uncemented cups, 75 patients (96%) had a ceramic insert (Alumina) and 3 patients (3.8%) had a highly cross-linked polyethylene insert. All patients had a ceramic head (Alumina). Head diameter of 32 mm was used in 52 patients (65%), 28 mm in 14 patients (18%), and 36 mm in 14 patients (18%).

Clinical evaluations

Clinical evaluations were performed preoperatively and postoperatively at 6 months, 1 year, 2 years, 3 years, and 5 years. Evaluated clinical outcome parameters were a hip-specific functional score (Harris Hip Score (HHS)) [17], a patient-centred hip score (Oxford Hip Score (OHS)) [18], and a disease-specific quality-of-life outcome measure (Western Ontario and McMaster Universities Osteoarthritis Index (WOMAC)) [19]. Furthermore, the incidence of thigh pain and overall pain at rest and on weight-bearing was evaluated. The amount of pain was classified as no pain, slight, mild, moderate, marked, or totally disabling [17]. Complications and adverse events were recorded during follow-up, and the resulting survival analysis according to Kaplan-Meier was evaluated at the final follow-up.

Radiographic evaluations

Anteroposterior radiographs of the pelvis and axial radiographs of the operated hips were evaluated immediately postoperative and at follow-up 6 months, 1 year, 2 years, 3 years, and 5 years. Migration was assessed according to the criteria of Malchau et al. [20]. Reactive lines, cancellous condensation ('spotwelds'), cortical hypertrophy, and tip sclerosis were evaluated per Gruen zone [21]. Implant fixation and stability was assessed according to the modified Engh score [22]. Formation of heterotopic bone was evaluated using Brooker's classification [23]. All radiographs were independently assessed by two teams of each two observers (PKA, DK and RtB, PR), consisting of one orthopaedic surgeon of both centres. Both teams of observers were blinded for each other's assessment and the name and details of the patient, as well as for the time of follow-up of the radiographs. Furthermore, both teams evaluated 50 randomly chosen radiographs to determine agreement and to calculate intra-observer and inter-observer reliability. When 95% agreement was established, each team evaluated half of all radiographs of the total patient cohort.

Statistics

SPSS for Windows 17.0.1 (SPSS Inc., Chicago, Illinois, USA) was used for statistical data analysis. Descriptive statistics were used for patient characteristics. Pearson's chi-square test and Student's t test were used to test hypotheses between both study centres for categorical variables and continuous variables respectively. Wilcoxon

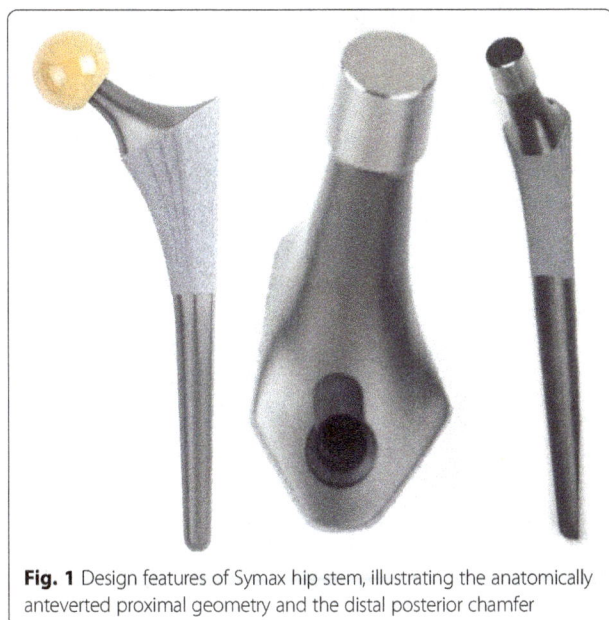

Fig. 1 Design features of Symax hip stem, illustrating the anatomically anteverted proximal geometry and the distal posterior chamfer

signed-rank test was used to analyse whether clinical outcome scores changed statistically significant over time. Statistical significance was set at $p < 0.05$. Results are reported as means, with standard deviation (SD) or range where relevant, or as frequencies. The overall percentage of agreement was used to evaluate observer agreement of radiology results [24]. The Cohen's Kappa was evaluated as a measure of reliability to quantify the agreement between raters, corrected for chance agreement. Kaplan-Meier survival analysis was performed with revision for any reason and with revision of stem for aseptic loosening as the endpoints.

Results

After 5 years of clinical follow-up, 73 patients were evaluated. Follow-up was not completed by one patient because of revision of both stem and cup for recurrent dislocations, one patient had a revision of the insert for squeaking, and five patients were lost to follow-up. One of these patients moved to another geographic area, the remaining four patients discontinued participation for non-hip-related reasons; one patient was from centre 1, and the remaining six patients from centre 2. Retrospective inquiry after a minimum 5-year follow-up learned that there were no hip-related complaints and no revision hip surgery was performed elsewhere.

Clinical evaluations

Mean HHS improved from 58.9 ± 12.0 preoperatively to 98.1 ± 6.1 at 5-year clinical follow-up, mean OHS improved from 38.5 ± 6.0 preoperatively to 16.2 ± 6.4 after 5 years, and mean WOMAC improved from 48.2 ± 13.7 preoperatively to 6.9 ± 9.9 after 5 years of clinical follow-up (Table 2). All clinical outcomes showed statistically significant improvements between preoperative and 6 months postoperative scores ($p < 0.001$), which remained thereafter.

After 5 years, one patient (1.4%) complained of moderate lateral thigh pain at rest and on weight-bearing. No radiographic abnormalities could be detected for this patient. During follow-up, the number of patients with no, or slight, pain at rest improved from 21.3% preoperatively

to 97.3% at 5 years. The number of patients with no, or slight, pain on weight bearing also improved from 2.5% preoperatively to 97.3% at 5 years.

Adverse events

During primary surgery, two patients developed an acetabular fracture for which intraoperative interventions were performed. These patients were not allowed immediate full weight-bearing postoperatively. Four patients had early dislocations, three of them were successfully treated conservatively and the fourth patient underwent revision of both cup and stem for a design with more femoral offset. Conservative treatment of early dislocations in our centres consisted of giving patients more instructions about prohibited movements of deep flexion and internal rotation, and we referred the patients back to their physiotherapists. One patient developed an early deep infection with *Staphylococcus aureus* 1 month after primary surgery. This patient was successfully treated with extensive debridement and with local and systemic antibiotic therapy. The implant could be retained. Finally, one patient complained of squeaking for which revision of the ceramic insert to a highly cross-linked polyethylene insert (X3, Stryker Orthopaedics) was performed.

Survival of the Symax hip stem after 5 years with revision of the stem for any reason as the endpoint is 98.8%, as only 1 patient of the initial 80 patients had a revision of stem and cup for recurrent dislocations (Fig. 2). However, survival of the Symax stem is 100% after 5 years with revision of the stem for loosening as the endpoint.

Radiographic evaluations

The percentage of agreement between both radiology assessment teams for spotweld formation was 94%, with a Cohen's Kappa of 0.380. The percentage of agreement between both radiology assessment teams for other radiological evaluations was 100%, no Cohen's Kappa could be measured for these evaluations. Only distal line formation could not be evaluated with high percentage of agreement, which was calculated at 48%, with a Cohen's Kappa of 0.155.

Table 2 Mean clinical outcome parameters

	Preoperative	6 months	1 year	2 years	3 years	5 years
Mean HHS (± SD)	58.9 (12.0)	94.3 (9.1)	95.2 (10.5)	96.1 (8.7)	97.4 (7.7)	98.1 (6.1)
Wilcoxon (P value)		< 0.001	0.074	0.121	0.015	0.482
Mean OHS (± SD)	38.5 (6.0)	20.0 (9.4)	18.7 (8.1)	17.4 (7.7)	16.0 (7.1)	16.2 (6.4)
Wilcoxon (P value)		< 0.001	0.028	0.072	0.012	0.081
Mean WOMAC (± SD)	48.2 (13.7)	13.0 (14.5)	10.8 (13.7)	9.7 (13.4)	9.0 (13.7)	6.9 (9.9)
Wilcoxon (P value)		< 0.001	0.019	0.673	0.181	0.125

Mean HHS, OHS, and WOMAC with standard deviation (SD) and Wilcoxon ranked sign test evaluating improvement over time between two consecutive follow-up moments

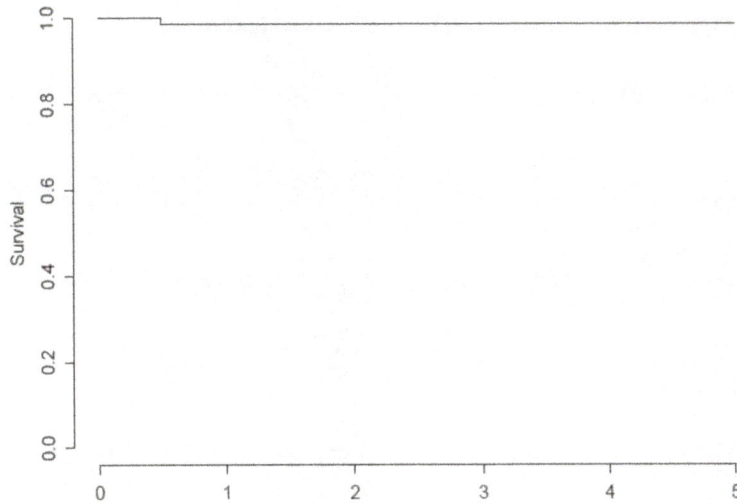

Fig. 2 Kaplan-Meier curve for revision of stem for any reason, in years

Stem position was neutral for all stems. No osteolysis or signs of proximal stress shielding were found during follow-up. One patient (1.3%) showed distal migration of the stem during follow-up. No lines or lucencies were observed around the coated part of the prosthesis at any follow-up time point. The appearance of extensive line formation around the smooth, uncoated, distal part of the stem increased from 10.5% after 6 months to 40% at 5 years. The appearance of distal line formation was most common in Gruen zone 4, 5, and 6 and increased during follow-up (Fig. 3). The appearance of spotwelds increased from 63.2% at 6 months to 90.7% at 5 years, only in the coated proximal Gruen zones 1 and 7 (Fig. 4). Any degree of heterotopic ossifications (Brooker 1 to 4) was seen in 29.7% of patients at 6 months; this number increased to 40.5% at 5 years. Only one patient (1.4%) showed Brooker 4 heterotopic ossification, which was already present at 6 months.

Zone 1	Zone 7
6 months: 0%	6 months: 0%
1 year: 0%	1 year: 0%
2 years: 0%	2 years: 0%
3 years: 0%	3 years: 0%
5 years: 0%	5 years: 0%

Zone 2	Zone 6
6 months: 0%	6 months: 9.2%
1 year: 6.5%	1 year: 15.6%
2 years: 10.4%	2 years: 24.7%
3 years: 15.8%	3 years: 31.6%
5 years: 21.3%	5 years: 38.7%

Zone 3	Zone 5
6 months: 3.9%	6 months: 13.2%
1 year: 11.7%	1 year: 27.3%
2 years: 16.9%	2 years: 32.5%
3 years: 17.1%	3 years: 32.9%
5 years: 24.0%	5 years: 36.0%

Zone 4
6 months: 19.7%
1 year: 52.0%
2 years: 75.3%
3 years: 84.0%
5 years: 86.6%

Fig. 3 Outcomes of radiographic evaluation: reactive line formation

Zone 1		Zone 7
6 months: 51.3%		6 months: 43.4%
1 year: 70.1%		1 year: 59.7%
2 years: 77.9%		2 years: 67.5%
3 years: 82.9%		3 years: 68.4%
5 years: 86.7%		5 years: 77.3%
Zone 2		Zone 6
6 months: 0%		6 months: 0%
1 year: 0%		1 year: 0%
2 years: 0%		2 years: 0%
3 years: 0%		3 years: 0%
5 years: 0%		5 years: 0%
Zone 3		Zone 5
6 months: 0%		6 months: 0%
1 year: 0%		1 year: 0%
2 years: 0%		2 years: 0%
3 years: 0%		3 years: 0%
5 years: 0%		5 years: 0%

Zone 4
6 months: 0%
1 year: 0%
2 years: 0%
3 years: 0%
5 years: 0%

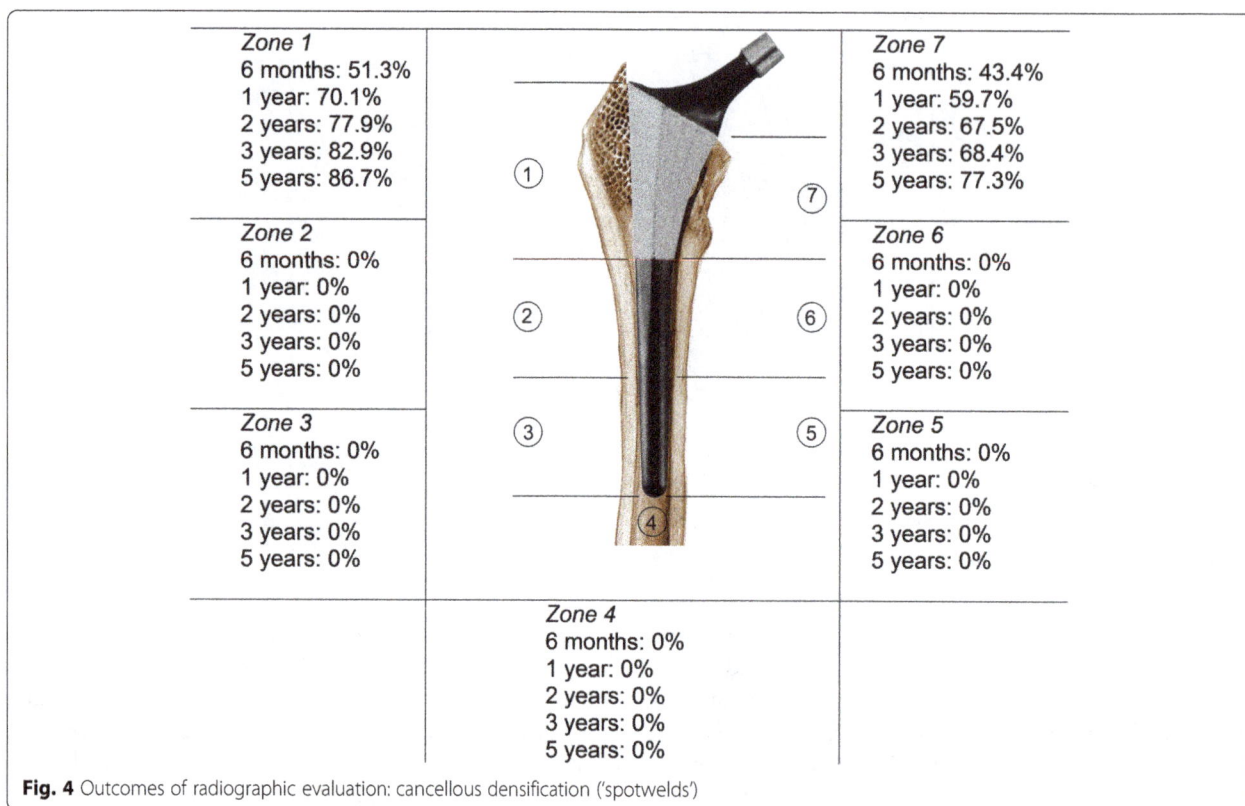

Fig. 4 Outcomes of radiographic evaluation: cancellous densification ('spotwelds')

Discussion

The purpose of this study was to evaluate clinical and radiographic performance of the new uncemented Symax hip stem in a 5-year international study, as part of the 'phased innovation' of a new implant, and to assess whether these outcomes were in line with the design principles and coating properties of the Symax hip stem. Our data showed excellent mid-term clinical and radiographic performances and osseointegration of the Symax hip stem at 5-year clinical follow-up with a Kaplan-Meier survival of 98.8% with revision of the stem for any reason as an endpoint.

The Symax hip stem leads to excellent clinical performance as represented in HHS, OHS, and WOMAC in this 5-year clinical follow-up study. Mean HHS of the Symax hip stem is slightly better compared to the short- and mid-term HHS of the Omnifit hip stem [3, 7, 8, 25, 26]. The Omnifit hip stem is another example of a proximal press fit, HA-coated stem, on which geometry the Symax was optimized. HHS of the Omnifit hip stem during the first 3 years of clinical follow-up was 93 after 6 months, improving to 96 at 3 years [26] and stabilizing to 93 after 6.4 years [27]. The clinical relevance of such small differences in HHS however can be argued as described by Poolman et al., who showed high intra-observer variability for physical examination as part of the HHS [28], and by Wamper et al. who showed limited discriminating power of the HHS because of a ceiling

effect [29]. Nevertheless, the excellent HHS in this study illustrates state of the art performance of the Symax hip stem design.

According to Lieberman et al., we also conducted patient-oriented quality-of-life surveys, like the OHS and WOMAC [30, 31]. The OHS improved over time and led to excellent scores postoperatively [18, 32]. Mean WOMAC score showed the same pattern of improvement over time as OHS [19], confirming high patient satisfaction.

Another interesting observation of this study was that the absence of pain at rest and during weight-bearing. This was seen in 97.3% of the patients after 5 years, while only 1.4% of the patients had moderate lateral thigh pain. Although this result is only slightly better than other contemporary implants based on the same philosophy [8, 26, 27, 33–35], it is clearly superior to older designs that follow different philosophies [36, 37]. This may be related to the distal geometry with posterior chamfer to prevent stem tip impingement. Furthermore, the prevention of distal fixation will also prevent conflicting elasticity issues between the stiffer implant and the more flexible bone.

Longitudinal radiographic evaluations showed signs of enhanced proximal fixation with the consistent appearance of spotwelds in Gruen zones 1 and 7, while on the other hand, no radiolucencies or reactive lines were seen in the coated part of the stem. These signs of proximal fixation combined with increasing line formation around the distal uncoated part of the prosthesis can be explained by the BONIT-HA coating and DOTIZE surface treatment of the Symax hip stem. As illustrated from histomorphometry analyses of retrieval specimens, BONIT-HA coating results in osseointegration over a larger part of the coated stem surface [9, 14]. The highly bioactive biomimetic BONIT-HA coating results in both more extensive bone-implant contact and bone density in periprosthetic regions of interest compared to other currently known hydroxyapatite or porous-coated stems [9, 10]. Enhanced proximal fixation combined with reduced distal bone apposition, caused by the DOTIZE surface treatment, leaves space for relative 'micromotion' between the stiff distal stem and the more elastic bone [25]. This leads to a so-called 'windshield-wiper sign' [33], causing increasing occurrence of distal reactive lines around the Symax hip stem, which proves the theoretical concept of this implant design. With this, distal reactive line formation could be a useful radiographic sign of good proximal fixation. The measure of agreement for distal line formation was only 48% which suggests that this is not a reproducible and useful radiographic sign for evaluation. However, this can be explained by the subjective interpretation of the term 'extensive' distal line formation. A better and uniform definition of the term extensive distal line formation will probably result in a higher measurement of agreement. This makes this radiographic sign more useful for evaluation of proximally fixating uncemented hip stems. The high measure of agreement for spotweld formation and the absence of proximal line formation make them useful and reliable radiographic features for evaluating these kinds of stems radiographically over time. The measure of agreement is more useful to evaluate observer agreement of radiology results compared to Cohen's Kappa, as it is not influenced by the prevalence of the evaluated radiographic signs [24]. So, the absence of proximal line formation in combination with progressive spotweld formation around the coated part and distal line formation should be interpreted as radiographic features of good proximal stem fixation.

Although 5 years of clinical follow-up is too short, a time frame to draw conclusions about final outcome and the survival rates of the Symax hip stem of 98.8%, with revision of the stem for any reason as the end point and with revision of the stem for (a)septic loosening as the end point of 100%, were excellent and meet the 'entry benchmark' criteria for best prostheses following the NICE-criteria [38]. These survival rates correspond to the survival rates of the Symax hip stem in the Danish Hip Arthroplasty Registry (DHR) of 2013 [39]. In the DHR, the Symax hip stem has a survival

rate of 100% after 5 years with revision for aseptic loosening. The survival rate with revision for any reason is 97.7 to 98.1%, depending on the cup used, after 5 years [39]. Based on what is known from other older HA-coated stems, good long-term fixation therefore can be anticipated.

This study had some limitations. Although it was well protocolized regarding surgical technique and postoperative treatment, some minor differences in treatment protocol existed between the two centres that can be interpreted as limitations. Complete excision of the joint capsule during the inclusion period of this study was only predominantly performed in centre 1. Surprisingly, capsulectomy did not seem to influence the occurrence of dislocations in this study, as both centres had two patients with dislocations. There was no difference in the amount of heterotopic bone formation between both study centres, despite the difference in strategies for prevention of it. Some authors have reported a decrease in osseointegration of implants as a result of the use of NSAIDs [40–42], and a nonsignificant increase in implant loosening [43]. However, in line with other reports [44–46], we could not find signs of a difference in bony fixation on conventional radiography between the two centres nor was there more pain reported in one or either centre.

Compared to previous literature of the Symax hip stem, the fact that only one patient showed migration, but no loosening, was in line with the EBRA-FCA study by Buratti et al. [47]. Our results are also in line with the findings of good clinical performance of this implant as was reported in a 1 year prospective study, in which the Symax was compared to the predominantly diaphyseal anchored Hipstar hip stem (Stryker, Duisburg, Germany) and the straight Zweymuller (SL-Plus) hip stem (Plus Orthopedics AG, Rotkreuz, Switzerland) [48]. However, Bergschmidt et al. discontinued using the Symax hip stem because of subsidence of more than 10 mm in two patients and three intraoperative periprosthetic fractures outside the study group. We cannot confirm these complication frequencies in this current study population nor in a multicentre prospective cohort of 300 patients. We therefore do not believe this to be a prosthesis-related problem.

Conclusions

In summary, excellent mid-term clinical and radiographic performance of the Symax hip stem can be reported at 5-year clinical follow-up. This is in line with the design principles and coating properties of this new stem design. Radiographic features of bone remodeling and (proximal) stem fixation around this design show high overall percentage agreement for intra- and inter-observer reliability, making them useful tools for longitudinal follow-up. In view of already available histological and remodeling data, good long-term performance of the Symax hip stem may be anticipated. Further confirmation of long-term result is subject of already initiated follow-up studies of both national and international prospective cohorts.

Abbreviations

BMI: Body mass index; CCD: Centrum-collum-diaphyseal; DEXA: Dual-energy X-ray absorptiometry; GCP: Good Clinical Practice; HA: Hydroxyapatite; HHS: Harris Hip Score; MUMC: Maastricht University Medical Centre; NSAID: Non-steroidal anti-inflammatory drugs; OHS: Oxford Hip Score; RSA: Radiostereometric analysis; SD: Standard deviation; THA: Total hip arthroplasty; TPS: Titanium plasma spray; WOMAC: Western Ontario and McMaster Universities Arthritis Index

Acknowledgements

The authors want to thank Prof. Rudolph Geesink for his contribution to the design of this study. Furthermore, the authors want to thank Liesbeth Jutten for performing study management, data entry, data management and assisting with statistics.

Funding

Research grant was received from Stryker Orthopaedics.

Authors' contributions

DK reorganised clinical database, performed data entry, performed calculations and statistics, wrote and revised the manuscript. PKA co-designed the study, operated, performed clinical evaluations, evaluated radiographs and revised the manuscript. PR operated, performed clinical evaluations, evaluated radiographs and revised the manuscript. JS performed data entry, contributed to data management. CA contributed to study and data management, contributed to writing and revised the manuscript. RtB co-designed the study, operated, performed clinical evaluations, contributed to writing and revised the manuscript. All authors read and approved the final version of this manuscript.

Competing interests

The authors declare that they have no competing interests.

Author details

[1]Department of Orthopaedic Surgery, Research School Caphri, Maastricht University Medical Centre, P. Debyelaan 25, P.O. Box 5800, 6202 AZ Maastricht, the Netherlands. [2]Department of Orthopaedic Surgery, Vejle Hospital, Beriderbakken 4, 7100 Vejle, Denmark.

References

1. Bobyn JD, Glassman AH, Goto H, Krugier JJ, Miller JE, Brooks LE. The effect of stem stiffness on femoral bone resorption after canine porous-coated total hip arthroplasty. Clin Orthop Relat Res. 1990;(261):196–213.

2. Bobyn JD, Mortimer ES, Glassman AH, Engh CA, Miller JE, Brooks LE. Producing and avoiding stress shielding. Laboratory and clinical observations of noncemented total hip arthroplasty. Clin Orthop Relat Res. 1992;274:79–96.

3. Capello WN, D'Antonio JA, Geesink RG, Feinberg JR, Naughton M. Late remodeling around a proximally HA-coated tapered titanium femoral component. Clin Orthop Relat Res. 2009;467:155–65.

4. Engh CA, Bobyn JD. The influence of stem size and extent of porous coating on femoral bone resorption after primary cementless hip arthroplasty. Clin Orthop Relat Res. 1988;231:7–28.

5. Glassman AH, Bobyn JD, Tanzer M. New femoral designs: do they influence stress shielding? Clin Orthop Relat Res. 2006;453:64–74.

6. Huiskes R, Weinans H, Dalstra M. Adaptive bone remodeling and biomechanical design considerations for noncemented total hip arthroplasty. Orthopedics. 1989;12:1255–67.

7. Capello WN, D'Antonio JA, Jaffe WL, Geesink RG, Manley MT, Feinberg JR. Hydroxyapatite-coated femoral components: 15-year minimum followup. Clin Orthop Relat Res. 2006;453:75–80.

8. Hellman EJ, Capello WN, Feinberg JR. Omnifit cementless total hip arthroplasty. A 10-year average followup. Clin Orthop Relat Res. 1999;364:164–74.

9. Broeke ten RHM, Alves A, Baumann A, Arts JJC, Geesink RGT. Bone reaction to a biomimetic third-generation hydroxyapatite coating and new surface treatment for the Symax hip stem. J Bone Joint Surg (Br). 2011;93-B:760–8.

10. Broeke ten RH, Hendrickx RP, Leffers P, Jutten LM, Geesink RG. Randomised trial comparing bone remodelling around two uncemented stems using modified Gruen zones. Hip Int. 2012;22:41–9.

11. Malchau H, Bragdon CR, Muratoglu OK. The stepwise introduction of innovation into orthopedic surgery: The next level of dilemmas. J Arthroplasty. 2011;26:825–31.

12. Barrere F, Layrolle P, Van Blitterswijk CA, De Groot K. Biomimetic coatings on titanium: a crystal growth study of octacalcium phosphate. J Mater Sci Mater Med. 2001;12:529–34.

13. Becker P, Neumann HG, Nebe B, Luthen F, Rychly J. Cellular investigations on electrochemically deposited calcium phosphate composites. J Mater Sci Mater Med. 2004;15:437–40.

14. Szmukler-Moncler S, Perrin D, Ahossi V, Pointaire P. Evaluation of BONIT, a fully resorbable CaP coating obtained by electrochemical deposition, after 6 weeks of healing: a pilot study in the pig maxilla. Key Eng Mater. 2001;192-195:395–8.

15. Becker P, Baumann A, Lüthen F, Rychly J, Kirbs A, Beck U, et al. Spark anodization on titanium and titanium alloys. 10th World Conference on Titanium. Hamburg, Germany 2003;V:3339–3344.

16. D'Antonio JA, Capello WN, Manley MT, Naughton M, Sutton K. A titanium-encased alumina ceramic bearing for total hip arthroplasty: 3- to 5-year results. Clin Orthop Relat Res. 2005;441:151–8.

17. Harris WH. Traumatic arthritis of the hip after dislocation and acetabular fractures: treatment by mold arthroplasty. An end-result study using a new method of result evaluation. J Bone Joint Surg Am. 1969;51:737–55.

18. Dawson J, Fitzpatrick R, Carr A, Murray D. Questionnaire on the perceptions of patients about total hip replacement. J Bone Joint Surg (Br). 1996;78:185–90.

19. Bellamy N, Buchanan WW, Goldsmith CH, Campbell J, Stitt LW. Validation study of WOMAC: a health status instrument for measuring clinically important patient relevant outcomes to antirheumatic drug therapy in patients with osteoarthritis of the hip or knee. J Rheumatol. 1988;15:1833–40.

20. Malchau H, Karrholm J, Wang YX, Herberts P. Accuracy of migration analysis in hip arthroplasty. Digitized and conventional radiography, compared to radiostereometry in 51 patients. Acta Orthop Scand. 1995;66:418–24.

21. Gruen TA, McNeice GM, Amstutz HC. "Modes of failure" of cemented stem-type femoral components: a radiographic analysis of loosening. Clin Orthop Relat Res. 1979;141:17–27.

22. Engh CA, Massin P, Suthers KE. Roentgenographic assessment of the biologic fixation of porous-surfaced femoral components. Clin Orthop Relat Res. 1990; 257:107–28.

23. Brooker AF, Bowerman JW, Robinson RA, Riley LH Jr. Ectopic ossification following total hip replacement. Incidence and a method of classification. J Bone Joint Surg (Am). 1973;55:1629–32.

24. Vet de HC, Mokkink LB, Terwee CB, Hoekstra OS, Knol DL. Clinicians are right not to like Cohen's kappa. BMJ. 2013;346:2125.

25. D'Antonio JA, Capello WN, Crothers OD, Jaffe WL, Manley MT. Early clinical experience with hydroxyapatite-coated femoral implants. J Bone Joint Surg Am. 1992;74:995–1008.

26. D'Antonio JA, Capello WN, Jaffe WL. Hydroxylapatite-coated hip implants. Multicenter three-year clinical and roentgenographic results. Clin Orthop Relat Res. 1992;285:102–15.

27. Capello WN, D'Antonio JA, Feinberg JR, Manley MT. Hydroxyapatite-coated total hip femoral components in patients less than fifty years old. Clinical and radiographic results after five to eight years of follow-up. J Bone Joint Surg Am. 1997;79:1023–9.

28. Poolman RW, Swiontkowski MF, Fairbank JC, Schemitsch EH, Sprague S, Vet de HC. Outcome instruments: rationale for their use. J Bone Joint Surg Am. 2009;91:41–9.

29. Wamper KE, Sierevelt IN, Poolman RW, Bhandari M, Haverkamp D. The Harris hip score: do ceiling effects limit its usefulness in orthopedics? Acta Orthop. 2010;81:703–7.

30. Lieberman JR, Dorey F, Shekelle P, Schumacher L, Kilgus DJ, Thomas BJ, et al. Outcome after total hip arthroplasty. Comparison of a traditional disease-specific and a quality-of-life measurement of outcome. J Arthroplasty. 1997;12:639–45.

31. Lieberman JR, Dorey F, Shekelle P, Schumacher L, Thomas BJ, Kilgus DJ, et al. Differences between patients' and physicians' evaluations of outcome after total hip arthroplasty. J Bone Joint Surg Am. 1996;78:835–8.

32. Ashby E, Grocott MP, Haddad FS. Outcome measures for orthopaedic interventions on the hip. J Bone Joint Surg (Br). 2008;90:545–9.

33. Geesink RG, Hoefnagels NH. Six-year results of hydroxyapatite-coated total hip replacement. J Bone Joint Surg (Br). 1995;77:534–47.

34. Incavo SJ, Havener T, Benson E, McGrory BJ, Coughlin KM, Beynnon BD. Efforts to improve cementless femoral stems in THR: 2- to 5-year follow-up of a high-offset femoral stem with distal stem modification (Secur-Fit Plus). J Arthroplast. 2004;19:61–7.

35. Tonino AJ, Rahmy AI. The hydroxyapatite-ABG hip system: 5- to 7-year results from an international multicentre study. The International ABG Study Group. J Arthroplasty. 2000;15:274–82.

36. Hwang SK, Park JS. Cementless total hip arthroplasty with AML, PCA and HGP prostheses. Int Orthop. 1995;19:77–83.

37. Garcia-Cimbrelo E, Cruz-Pardos A, Madero R, Ortega-Andreu M. Total hip arthroplasty with use of the cementless Zweymuller Alloclassic system. A ten to thirteen-year follow-up study. J Bone Joint Surg (Am). 2003;85:296–303.

38. NHS. Guidance on the Selection of Prostheses for Primary Total Hip Replacement. Technology appraisals guidance, vol. 2. London: National Institute for Health and Clinical Excellence; 2000.

39. Dansk Hoftealloplastik Register. Årsrapport. 2013. http://danskhofteallo plastikregister.dk/wp-content/uploads/2015/11/DHR-årsrapport-2013.pdf. Accessed 4 Apr 2017.

40. Abdul-Hadi O, Parvizi J, Austin MS, Viscusi E, Einhorn T. Nonsteroidal anti-inflammatory drugs in orthopaedics. J Bone Joint Surg Am. 2009;91:2020–7.

41. Dahners LE, Mullis BH. Effects of nonsteroidal anti-inflammatory drugs on bone formation and soft-tissue healing. J Am Acad Orthop Surg. 2004;12:139–43.

42. Trancik T, Mills W, Vinson N. The effect of indomethacin, aspirin, and ibuprofen on bone ingrowth into a porous-coated implant. Clin Orthop Relat Res. 1989;249:113–21.

43. Persson PE, Nilsson OS, Berggren AM. Do non-steroidal anti-inflammatory drugs cause endoprosthetic loosening? A 10-year follow-up of a randomized trial on ibuprofen for prevention of heterotopic ossification after hip arthroplasty. Acta Orthop. 2005;76:735–40.

44. Kjaersgaard-Andersen P, Schmidt SA. Total hip arthroplasty. The role of antiinflammatory medications in the prevention of heterotopic ossification. Clin Orthop Relat Res. 1991;263:78–86.

45. Wurnig C, Schwameis E, Bitzan P, Kainberger F. Six-year results of a cementless stem with prophylaxis against heterotopic bone. Clin Orthop Relat Res. 1999;361:150–8.

46. Heide van der HJ, Hannink G, Buma P, Schreurs BW. No effect of ketoprofen and meloxicam on bone graft ingrowth: a bone chamber study in goats. Acta Orthop. 2008;79:548–54.

47. Buratti CA, D'Arrigo C, Guido G, Lenzi F, Logroscino GD, Magliocchetti G, et al. Assessment of the initial stability of the Symax femoral stem with EBRA-FCA: a multicentric study of 85 cases. Hip Int. 2009;19:24–9.

48. Bergschmidt P, Bader R, Finze S, Gankovych A, Kundt G, Mittelmeier W. Cementless total hip replacement: a prospective clinical study of the early functional and radiological outcomes of three different hip stems. Arch Orthop Trauma Surg. 2010;130:125–33.

11

Cervical lordosis in asymptomatic individuals

Guang-Ming Guo[1†], Jun Li[1†], Qing-Xun Diao[1*], Tai-Hang Zhu[1], Zhong-Xue Song[1], Yang-Yang Guo[1] and Yan-Zheng Gao[2*]

Abstract

Background: Cervical lordosis has important clinical and surgical implications. Cervical spine curvature is reported with considerable variability in individual studies. The aim of this study was to examine the existence and extent of cervical lordosis in asymptomatic individuals and to evaluate its relationship with age and gender.

Methods: A comprehensive literature search was conducted in several electronic databases. Study selection was based on pre-determined eligibility criteria. Random effects meta-analyses were performed to estimate the proportion of asymptomatic individuals with lordosis and the effect size of cervical lordotic curvature in these individuals which followed metaregression analysis to examine the factors affecting cervical lordosis. Data from 21 studies (15,364 asymptomatic individuals, age 42.30 years [95% confidence interval 36.42, 48.18], 54.2% males) were used in the present study.

Results: In this population, 63.99% [95% confidence interval 44.94, 83.03] individuals possessed lordotic curvature. Degree of lordotic curvature differed by method of measurement; 12.71° [6.59, 18.84] with Cobb C2–C7 method and 18.55° [14.48, 22.63] with posterior tangent method. Lordotic curvature was not significantly different between symptomatic and asymptomatic individuals but was significantly higher in males in comparison with females. Age was not significantly associated with lordotic cervical curvature.

Conclusion: Majority of the asymptomatic individuals possesses lordotic cervical curvature which is higher in males than in females but have no relationship with age or symptoms.

Keywords: Cervical spine, Lordosis, Asymptomatic, Age, Gender

Background

Cervical lordosis is important for the efficiency of many processes including mastication, breathing, vocalization, eye movement, and gaze and for the shock absorption during walking and running [1]. Curvature of the cervical spine has important clinical implications [2, 3]. Attainment of moderate cervical lordotic curvature is found to be associated with better surgical outcomes in patients with neurologic deficits [4–6]. Reattainment of cervical lordosis after a surgical intervention is also considered important as compression of nervous tissue may cause injury otherwise [7].

Cervical lordotic curvature starts becoming visible at around 10 weeks of fetal development [8] formed by the posterior wedging when height of vertebrae and discs at anterior side becomes greater than posterior side [1, 9]. Cervical spine in asymptomatic individuals generally attains lordotic alignment but up to 35% of cases exhibit kyphosis [10]. Biomechanically, a lordotic configuration can resist large compressive loads [11] and minimize stress on the vertebral body endplates [12]. Cervical spine distributes the compressive load differently as compared with the rest of the spine; 36% of the compressive load is absorbed by the anterior column and 64% by the posterior facet joints [13, 14].

There are four reliable and predictive line drawing methods for the measurement of cervical lordosis on radiographs: Cobb C2–C7 method, Ishihara's index, Harrison C2–C7 posterior tangent method, and area

* Correspondence: qxdiao_ortho@126.com; gairen513364872@163.com
†Guang-Ming Guo and Jun Li contributed equally to this work.
¹Department of Orthopaedics, Henan Zhoukou Union Orthopaedic Hospital, East Section, Taihao Road, Zhoukou 466000, Henan, China
²Department of Orthopaedics, Henan Province People's Hospital, Zhengzhou 450000, Henan, China

under the curve [15]. Cobb method [16] was proposed for the evaluation of sagittal spinal curvature which was later modified by drawing vertebral endplate lines to construct angles on sagittal radiographs and is frequently used to evaluate cervical lordosis. Ishihara index is another way to measure curvature of the spine which is achieved by summing up the spinal lines connecting the posteroinferior corners of vertebra bodies and to construct additional orthogonal lines [17]. Harrison et al. [18] proposed a geometrical model for the measurement of cervical curvatures in sagittal radiographs which was later modified to an elliptical form to be usable for cervical lordosis as well [19]. There is a wide variation in the cervical lordotic curvature in asymptomatic individuals and patients with related conditions [9, 20, 21]. In asymptomatic individuals, average cervical lordosis is reported variably, e.g., 21.3 by Gore et al. [9], 22.3 by Owens et al. [22], and 34° by Harrison et al. [18], depending also on the method used to measure the curvature.

Increase in lordosis with age is also reported by some studies [9, 23] but not all. Moreover, whereas some studies have found that a non-lordotic sagittal cervical curvature is not related to patient's initial symptoms [9], others have found that non-lordotic cervical curvature correlates with initial panic conditions [20, 21]. These varying observations necessitate having a systematic review of the relevant literature to have reliable estimates of normal lordotic cervical curvature and its affecting factors. The aim of present study was to review the studies which reported cervical curvature in healthy asymptomatic individuals after examining the radiographs with a reliable method, to synthesize the quantitative information pertaining to the cervical lordosis and its relationship with age and gender and morbidity.

Methods

Eligibility criteria

Studies were included if they met following criteria: study (1) included asymptomatic individuals either as sole study population or as controls to symptomatic patients to study normal measures of cervical lordosis, (2) provided values of C2–C7 lordosis angles and/or the proportion of individuals with lordotic curvature, and (3) included adult patients (above 18 years of age). Studies were excluded if (1) reported cervical lordosis measures other than global lordosis (C2–C7 angle), (2) reported segmental lordotic angles but not global lordosis, and (3) reported cervical lordosis measures without mentioning the symptomatic information of individuals/patients.

Search and selection of studies

We searched Embase, Google Scholar, Ovid SP, and PubMed databases for relevant studies by using suitable MeSH and keywords for research papers published before November 2016. The search was not restricted to language or period of publication. The following search terms and strategies were used: (1) cervical-lordosis OR curvature OR lordotic curvature OR alignment; (2) angle OR Cobb angle OR posterior tangent OR theta OR; (3) Radiograph OR X-ray OR Roentgenograph; and (4) various combinations of (1), (2), and (3).

Two reviewers conducted initial database search and independently screened the titles and abstracts identified in the initial search. This followed the observance of the inclusion and exclusion criteria as a result of which full text of articles were identified and later retrieved. If additional data or clarification was necessary, we contacted the study authors. Any disagreement between reviewers was resolved by discussion with other coauthors.

Data and analyses

The following information was collected from each study using a standardized form: study design and location, main inclusion/exclusion criteria, patient demographics, and study outcomes. Data were extracted by two reviewers independently. Cervical curvature measurements were considered if the study utilized either Cobb C2–7 angle (angle between the horizontal line of C2 lower endplate and the horizontal line of C7 lower endplate) or posterior tangent (angle formed by a line projected parallel to the posterior surface of C2 and a line parallel to the posterior surface of C7) method.

Statistical heterogeneity of the required data was tested with a chi-square test, and between-studies inconsistency was quantified by the I^2 index. Meta-analyses were carried out by using Stata software (version 12; Stata Corporation, USA) by pooling the C2–C7 angles reported in individual studies and to generate inverse variance weighted overall effect size as well as effect sizes with regard to method used for the measurement of the lordotic cervical curvature and percentage of asymptomatic individuals with lordotic cervical curvature.

Random effects model was used for the meta-analyses keeping in view significant heterogeneity of the meta-analyzable data. Further analyses were carried out to evaluate the symptomatic and gender differences in cervical lordotic curvature by performing meta-analyses of mean differences using RevMan software (version 5.3; Cochrane collaboration). Meta-regression analyses were also performed to evaluate the effect of age and gender on cervical lordotic curvature using restricted maximum likelihood method in Stata software.

Results

Twenty-one studies [18, 19, 24–42] were selected by following the eligibility criteria (Fig. 1). In these studies, 15,364 asymptomatic or healthy individuals were

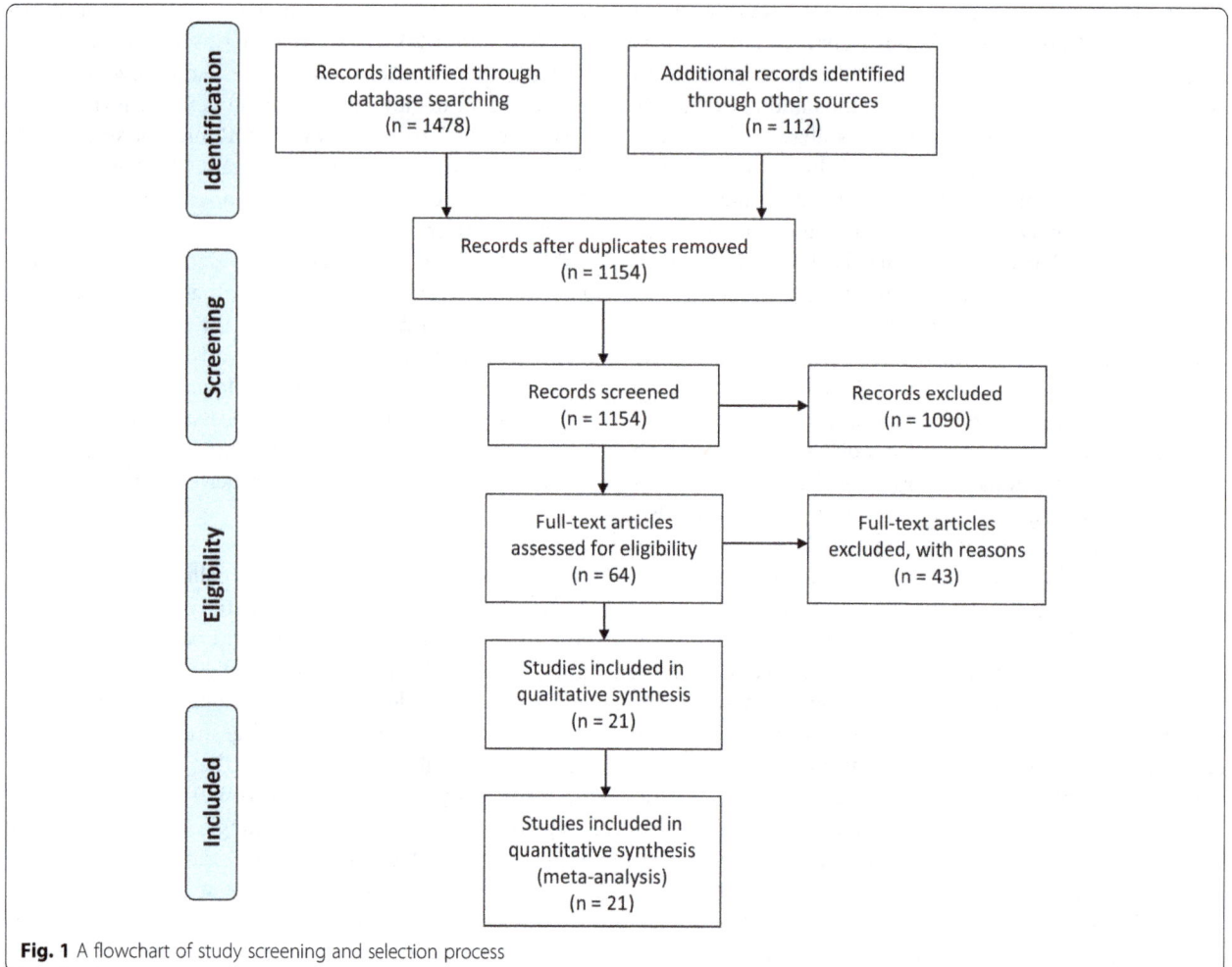

Fig. 1 A flowchart of study screening and selection process

recruited. Age (weighted average) of these individuals was 42.30 years [95% confidence interval 36.42, 48.18], and 54.2% were males. Among the asymptomatic individuals studied, 63.99% [44.94, 83.03] had lordotic curvature while the rest had straight, kyphotic, or sigmoid curvature (dataset, 12455 asymptomatic individuals in 11 studies; Fig. 2).

Eleven of the included studies reported degree of cervical lordotic curvature in 3597 asymptomatic individuals. Overall, cervical lordotic curvature was found to be 16.43° [95% confidence interval 12.69, 20.17]. However, cervical lordotic curvature differed by the method used. In 1046 asymptomatic individuals who underwent measurements with Cobb C2–C7 method, the curvature was found to be 12.71° [6.59, 18.84], whereas in 2551 asymptomatic individuals who underwent measurements with posterior tangent method, the cervical lordotic curvature was 18.55° [14.48, 22.63] (Fig. 3).

Lordotic cervical curvature was not significantly different between symptomatic and asymptomatic individuals (mean difference was 1.79° [– 4.08, 7.67]; $p = 0.55$; Fig. 4). However, lordotic cervical curvature was significantly

higher in males in comparison with that in females (mean difference 4.4° [1.63, 7.17]; $p = 0.002$; Fig. 5).

In the meta-regression analyses, age was not significantly associated with lordotic cervical curvature (coefficient 0.18 [– 0.19, 0.56]; $p = 0.314$) but was significantly associated with the percentage of individuals with lordotic cervical curvature (coefficient 1.43 [0.20, 2.66]; $p = 0.030$; Fig. 6).

Discussion

This meta-analytical review finds that most asymptomatic individuals possess lordotic cervical curvature which averages at about 18° when measured with C2–C7 posterior tangent method. However, Cobb C2–C7 method may underestimate as we have found that use of this method led to an average of about 13° of lordotic cervical angle. We have also observed that there is no significant difference in cervical curvature between symptomatic and asymptomatic individuals but lordotic cervical curvature has been found to be significantly higher in men than in women. However, no significant relationship could be found between lordosis and age,

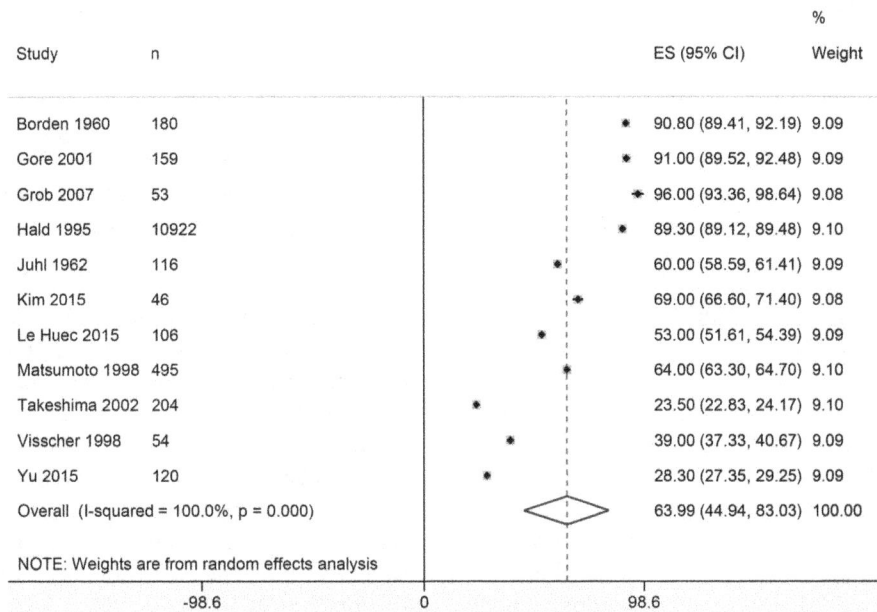

Fig. 2 A forest graph showing the percentage of asymptomatic individuals with lordotic cervical curvature and the overall effect size

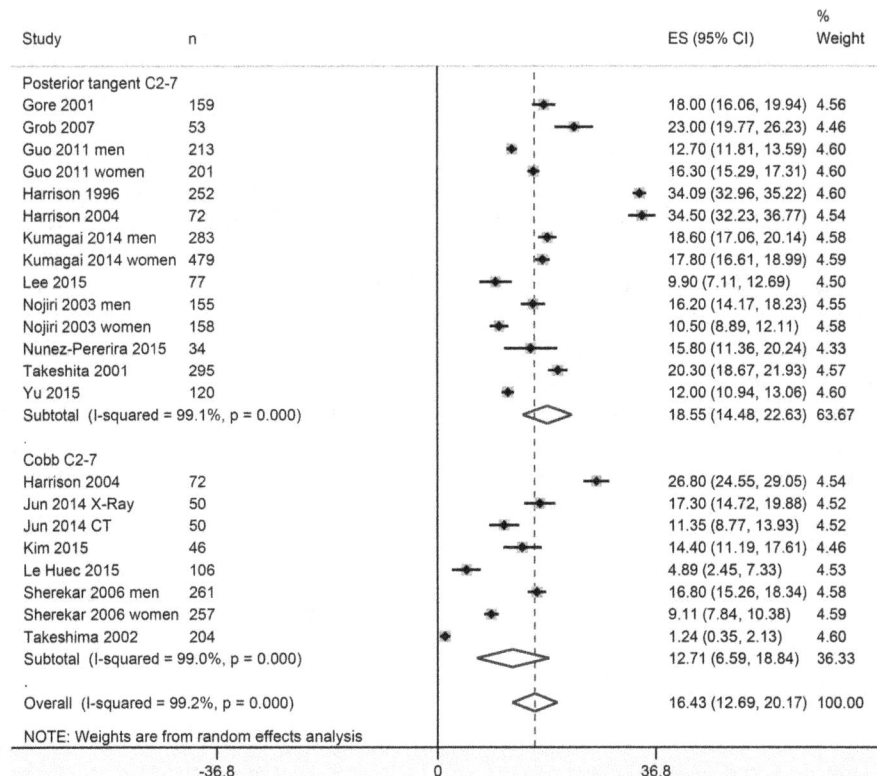

Fig. 3 A forest graph showing the cervical lordotic angles reported by individual studies and the overall effect size as well as the effect sizes of two methods used to measure the cervical curvature

Study or Subgroup	Symptomatic			Asymptomatic			Weight	Mean Difference IV, Random, 95% CI	Mean Difference IV, Random, 95% CI
	Mean	SD	Total	Mean	SD	Total			
Grob 2007	24.3	11.2	54	23	12	53	23.4%	1.30 [-3.10, 5.70]	
Harrison 1996	33.99	9.39	148	34.09	9.16	252	26.2%	-0.10 [-1.99, 1.79]	
Kim 2015	11.1	10.2	95	14.4	11.1	46	24.2%	-3.30 [-7.11, 0.51]	
Yu 2015	20.8	7.8	121	12	5.9	120	26.3%	8.80 [7.05, 10.55]	
Total (95% CI)			418			471	100.0%	1.79 [-4.08, 7.67]	

Heterogeneity: Tau² = 33.40; Chi² = 62.48, df = 3 (P < 0.00001); I² = 95%
Test for overall effect: Z = 0.60 (P = 0.55)

-20 -10 0 10 20
Higher in symptomatic   Higher in asymptomatic

Fig. 4 A forest graph showing no significant difference between symptomatic and asymptomatic individuals in the cervical lordotic angles

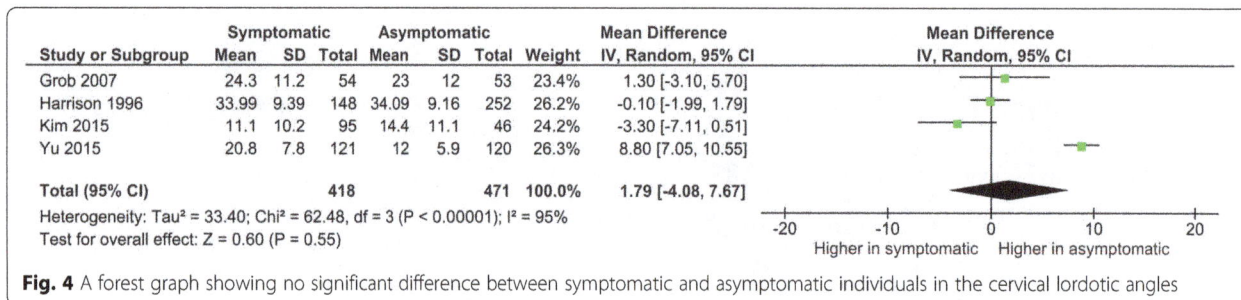

although the percentage of individuals with lordotic cervical curvature increased with age.

In a review study in which the authors analyzed data from studies which evaluated neutral upright sagittal spinal alignment from the occiput to the pelvis in asymptomatic adults, the greatest variation was noted in the cervical spine from C2 to C7 [43]. In this scenario, it becomes difficult to assess the effect of method on cervical curvature, although in a study in which both the methods were used simultaneously, lordotic angle values were found significantly higher with the posterior tangent C2–C7 method than with the Cobb C2–C7 method [19]. A factor that is postulated to affect the level of cervical lordosis is the sagittal shape of odontoid dens [44, 45].

Although meta-regression analysis of the present study could not find a significant association between age and cervical lordotic curvature, increase in lordosis with age is reported by some studies [10, 23]. However, contradictory reports are also available in literature. Milne and Lauder [46], by using an indirect method (surveyor's flexicurve device) in a cross-sectional study of men and women aged 20–90 years, found an increase in kyphosis with age in both older men and women with no lordosis in an increasingly large proportion of both men and women over 60 years of age. Later, Harrison et al. [15] while comparing measurements with flexicurve and radiographic line methods, found that of the 96 flexicurve detected lordotic individuals, only 55 were found to have lordotic curvature on lateral radiographs. In the present study, we have found a positive relationship between the age and the percentage of individuals with lordotic curvature. However, our sample population belonged to rather a middle-aged group.

Lumbar lordosis, sacral inclination, and lumbosacral angulation show a tendency to decrease in individuals aged over 70 years [47]. Using a non-invasive measuring system in 323 asymptomatic individuals, Dreicharf et al. [48] found that total lordosis was significantly reduced by approximately 20% and the range of motion for maximal upper body flexion (RoF) by 12% and extension (RoE) by 31% in the oldest (50–75 years) compared to those in the youngest age cohort (20–29 years). During aging, the lower lumbar spine retains its lordosis and mobility, whereas the middle part flattens and becomes less mobile [48].

Such changes with age may put pressure on cervical spine to change simultaneously causing changes such as increase in lordosis seen by some authors. Whereas in healthy adults (aged 22–50 years), cervical sagittal alignment is found to be associated with thoracic sagittal alignment but not with lumbopelvic alignment [49] and cervical lordosis inversely correlates with thoracic kyphosis [50]; in elderly people, cervical curvature is affected by pelvic sagittal alignment [51]. Lumbar lordosis decreases, and thoracic kyphosis increases with age which results in a compensatory increase in cervical lordosis [10, 17].

Based on a limited data that could be gained under the eligibility criteria of the present study, there was no significant difference between symptomatic and asymptomatic individuals in lordosis angle of the cervical spine. However, this finding is compatible with several related reports. As reviewed by Lippa et al. [52], many studies

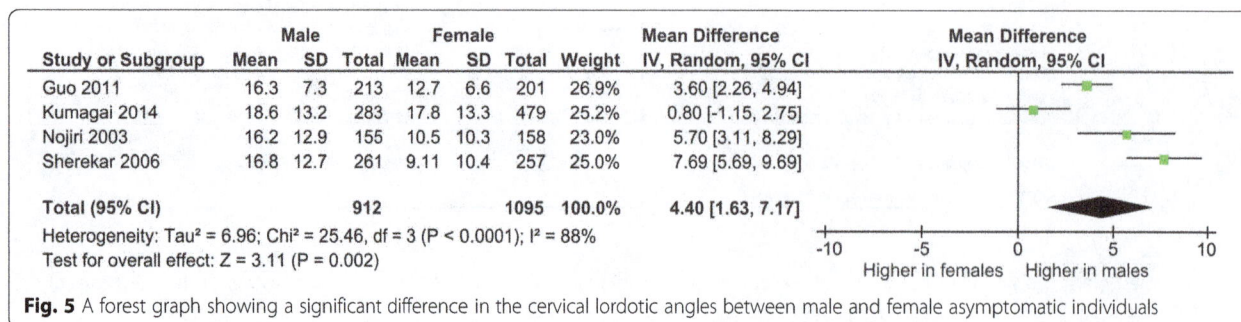

Study or Subgroup	Male			Female			Weight	Mean Difference IV, Random, 95% CI	Mean Difference IV, Random, 95% CI
	Mean	SD	Total	Mean	SD	Total			
Guo 2011	16.3	7.3	213	12.7	6.6	201	26.9%	3.60 [2.26, 4.94]	
Kumagai 2014	18.6	13.2	283	17.8	13.3	479	25.2%	0.80 [-1.15, 2.75]	
Nojiri 2003	16.2	12.9	155	10.5	10.3	158	23.0%	5.70 [3.11, 8.29]	
Sherekar 2006	16.8	12.7	261	9.11	10.4	257	25.0%	7.69 [5.69, 9.69]	
Total (95% CI)			912			1095	100.0%	4.40 [1.63, 7.17]	

Heterogeneity: Tau² = 6.96; Chi² = 25.46, df = 3 (P < 0.0001); I² = 88%
Test for overall effect: Z = 3.11 (P = 0.002)

-10 -5 0 5 10
Higher in females   Higher in males

Fig. 5 A forest graph showing a significant difference in the cervical lordotic angles between male and female asymptomatic individuals

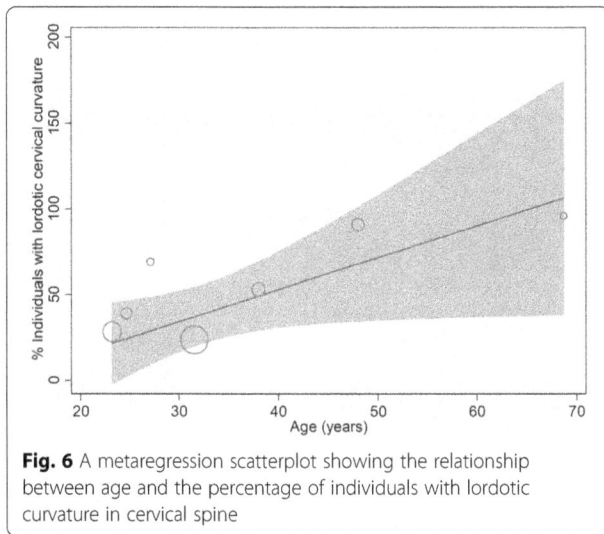

Fig. 6 A metaregression scatterplot showing the relationship between age and the percentage of individuals with lordotic curvature in cervical spine

have found no association between cervical lordotic curvature and symptoms especially the neck pain including whiplash injury in approximately 700 individuals [53–56]. Exceptions can also be found in literature. McAviney et al. [57], after examining 300 cervical X-rays in individuals with and without cervical pain, found a statistically significant association between cervical pain and lordosis of less than 20° (posterior tangent method). However, in the present study, we have found that majority of the included studies which used the posterior tangent method reported less than 20° cervical lordosis in asymptomatic individuals. Therefore, so far, evidence suggests that there exists no association between the degree of cervical lordosis and related symptoms. Even, there is some evidence to suggest that individuals with kyphotic cervical curvature may remain asymptomatic [54]. One of the weaknesses of the present study is that we could not perform subgroup analysis under hyperlordosis and hypolordosis categories. It was due to unavailability of categorical data in reports of the included studies. Only Harrison et al. described this as "The cervical lordosis in both acute and chronic neck pain patients was found to be hypolordotic." We did not try to categorize it because of a wide range of lordosis curvature in asymptomatic individuals and different degrees achieved by the use of two main methods in the included studies. Moreover, in general, we found no association between symptoms and lordosis angle.

Conclusion

Approximately 68% asymptomatic individuals possess lordotic cervical curvature. Average lordotic curvature is estimated at 18° when C2–C7 posterior tangent method was used and 13° with Cobb C2–C7 method. No significant difference in cervical curvature between symptomatic and asymptomatic individuals has been found, but

lordotic cervical curvature was significantly higher in men than in women. No significant relationship was found between lordosis and age, but a positive relationship between the age and the percentage of individuals with lordotic curvature is observed.

Authors' contributions
QXD and GMG were involved in the conception and design; JL and THZ analyzed data; ZXS and YYG contributed in the drafting of the manuscript and revised it critically; YZG approved final version. All authors agreed to be accountable for all aspects of the work. All authors read and approved the manuscript.

Competing interests
All authors declare that they have no competing interests.

References
1. Been E, Shefi S, Soudack M. Cervical lordosis: the effect of age and gender. Spine J. 2017;17(6):880–8.
2. Kawakami M, Tamaki T, Yoshida M, Hayashi N, Ando M, Yamada H. Axial symptoms and cervical alignments after cervical anterior spinal fusion for patients with cervical myelopathy. J Spinal Disord. 1999;12:50–6.
3. Nightingale RW, McElhaney JH, Richardson WJ, Best TM, Myers BS. Experimental impact injury to the cervical spine: relating motion of the head and the mechanism of injury. J Bone Joint Surg Am. 1996;78:412–21.
4. Baba H, Uchida K, Maezawa Y, Furusawa N, Azuchi M, Imura S. Lordotic alignment and posterior migration of the spinal cord following en bloc open-door laminoplasty for cervical myelopathy: a magnetic resonance imaging study. J Neurol. 1996;85:626–32.
5. Swank ML, Sutterlin CE, Bossons CR, Dials BE. Rigid internal fixation with lateral mass plates in multilevel anterior and posterior reconstruction of the cervical spine. Spine. 1997;22:274–82.
6. Stein J. Failure of magnetic resonance imaging to reveal the cause of a progressive cervical myelopathy related to postoperative spinal deformity: a case report. Am J Phys Med Rehabil. 1997;76:73–5.
7. Harrison DE, Cailliet R, Harrison DD, Janik TJ, Holland B. A new 3-point bending traction method for restoring cervical lordosis and cervical manipulation: a nonrandomized clinical controlled trial. Arch Phys Med Rehabil. 2002;83(4):447–53.
8. Bagnall KM, Harris PF, Jones PR. A radiographic study of the human fetal spine. I. The development of the secondary cervical curvature. J Anat. 1977;123:777–82.
9. Broberg KB. On the mechanical behavior of the intervertebral disc. Spine. 1983;8:151–65.
10. Gore D, Sepic S, Gardner G. Roentgenographic findings of the cervical spine in asymptomatic people. Spine. 1986;11:521–4.
11. Miura T, Panjabi MM, Cripton PA. A method to simulate in vivo cervical spine kinematics using in vitro compressive preload. Spine. 2002;27:43–8.
12. Harrison DE, Harrison DD, Janik TJ, Jones EW, Cailliet R, Normand M. Comparison of axial and flexural stresses in lordosis and three buckled configurations of the cervical spine. Clin Biomech. 2001;16:276–84.
13. Albert TJ, Vacarro A. Postlaminectomy kyphosis. Spine (Phila Pa 1976). 1998;23(24):2738–45.
14. Deutsch H, Haid RW, Rodts GE, Mummaneni PV. Postlaminectomy cervical deformity. Neurosurg Focus. 2003;15(3):E5.
15. Harrison DE, Haas JW, Cailliet R, Harrison DD, Holland B, Janik TJ. Concurrent validity of flexicurve instrument measurements: sagittal skin contour of the cervical spine compared with lateral cervical radiographic measurements. J Manip Physiol Ther. 2005;28(8):597–603.
16. Cobb J. Outline for the study of scoliosis. Am Acad Orthop Surg Instr Course Lect. 1948;5:261–75.
17. Ishihara A. Roentgenographic studies on the normal pattern of the cervical curvature. Nippon Seikeigeka Gakkai Zasshi. 1968;42:1033–44.
18. Harrison DD, Janik TJ, Troyanovich SJ, Holland B. Comparisons of lordotic

cervical spine curvatures to a theoretical ideal model of the static sagittal cervical spine. Spine (Phila Pa 1976). 1996;21(6):667–75.

19. Harrison DD, Harrison DE, Janik TJ, Cailliet R, Ferrantelli JR, Haas JW, Holland B. Modeling of the sagittal cervical spine as a method to discriminate hypolordosis: results of elliptical and circular modeling in 72 asymptomatic subjects, 52 acute neck pain subjects, and 70 chronic neck pain subjects. Spine (Phila Pa 1976). 2004;29(22):2485–92.

20. Nagasawa A, Sakakibara T, Takahashi A. Roentgenographic findings of the cervical spine in tension-type headache. Headache. 1993;33:90–5.

21. Kai Y, Oyama M, Kurose S, Inadome T, Oketani Y, Masuda Y. Neurogenic thoracic outlet syndrome in whiplash injury. J Spinal Disord. 2001;14:487–93.

22. Owens E, Hoiris K. Cervical curvature assessment using digitized radiographic analysis. Chiropr Res J. 1990;4:47–62.

23. Kim HJ, Lenke LG, Oshima Y, Chuntarapas T, Mesfin A, Hershman S, et al. Cervical lordosis actually increases with aging and progressive degeneration in spinal deformity patients. Spine Deformity. 2014;2(5):410–4.

24. Borden AG, Rechtman AM, Gershon-Cohen J. The normal cervical lordosis. Radiology. 1960;74:806–9.

25. Gore DR. Roentgenographic findings in the cervical spine in asymptomatic persons: a ten-year follow-up. Spine (Phila Pa 1976). 2001;26(22):2463–6.

26. Grob D, Frauenfelder H, Mannion AF. The association between cervical spine curvature and neck pain. Eur Spine J. 2007;16(5):669–78.

27. Guo Q, Ni B, Yang J, Liu K, Sun Z, Zhou F, Zhang J. Relation between alignments of upper and subaxial cervical spine: a radiological study. Arch Orthop Trauma Surg. 2011;131(6):857–62.

28. Hald HJ, Danz B, Schwab R, Burmeister K, Bahren W. Radiographically demonstrable spinal changes in asymptomatic young men. Rofo. 1995; 163(1):4–8.

29. Juhl JH, Miller SM, Roberts GW. Roentgenographic variations in the normal cervical spine. Radiology. 1962;78:591–7.

30. Jun HS, Chang IB, Song JH, Kim TH, Park MS, Kim SW, Oh JK. Is it possible to evaluate the parameters of cervical sagittal alignment on cervical computed tomographic scans? Spine (Phila Pa 1976). 2014;39(10):E630–6.

31. Kim JH, Kim JH, Kim JH, Kwon TH, Park YK, Moon HJ. The relationship between neck pain and cervical alignment in young female nursing staff. J Korean Neurosurg Soc. 2015;58(3):231–5.

32. Kumagai G, Ono A, Numasawa T, Wada K, Inoue R, Iwasaki H, Iwane K, et al. Association between roentgenographic findings of the cervical spine and neck symptoms in a Japanese community population. J Orthop Sci. 2014; 19(3):390–7.

33. Le Huec JC, Demezon H, Aunoble S. Sagittal parameters of global cervical balance using EOS imaging: normative values from a prospective cohort of asymptomatic volunteers. Eur Spine J. 2015;24(1):63–71.

34. Lee SH, Son ES, Seo EM, Suk KS, Kim KT. Factors determining cervical spine sagittal balance in asymptomatic adults: correlation with spinopelvic balance and thoracic inlet alignment. Spine J. 2015;15(4):705–12.

35. Matsumoto M, Fujimura Y, Suzuki N, Toyama Y, Shiga H. Cervical curvature in acute whiplash injuries: prospective comparative study with asymptomatic subjects. Injury. 1998;29(10):775–8.

36. Nojiri K, Matsumoto M, Chiba K, Maruiwa H, Nakamura M, Nishizawa T, Toyama Y. Relationship between alignment of upper and lower cervical spine in asymptomatic individuals. J Neurosurg. 2003;99(1 Suppl):80–3.

37. Nunez-Pereira S, Hitzl W, Bullmann V, Meier O, Koller H. Sagittal balance of the cervical spine: an analysis of occipitocervical and spinopelvic interdependence, with C-7 slope as a marker of cervical and spinopelvic alignment. J Neurosurg Spine. 2015;23(1):16–23.

38. Sherekar SK, Yadav YR, Basoor AS, Baghel A, Adam N. Clinical implications of alignment of upper and lower cervical spine. Neurol India. 2006;54(3):264–7.

39. Takeshima T, Omokawa S, Takaoka T, Araki M, Ueda Y, Takakura Y. Sagittal alignment of cervical flexion and extension: lateral radiographic analysis. Spine (Phila Pa 1976). 2002;27(15):E348–55.

40. Takeshita K, Murakami M, Kobayashi A, Nakamura C. Relationship between cervical curvature index (Ishihara) and cervical spine angle (C2-7). J Orthop Sci. 2001;6(3):223–6.

41. Visscher CM, de Boer W, Naeije M. The relationship between posture and curvature of the cervical spine. J Manip Physiol Ther. 1998;21(6):388–91.

42. Yu M, Zhao WK, Li M, Wang SB, Sun Y, Jiang L, et al. Analysis of cervical and global spine alignment under Roussouly sagittal classification in Chinese cervical spondylotic patients and asymptomatic subjects. Eur Spine J. 2015; 24(6):1265–73.

43. Kuntz C 4th, Levin LS, Ondra SL, Shaffrey CI, Morgan CJ. Neutral upright sagittal spinal alignment from the occiput to the pelvis in asymptomatic adults: a review and resynthesis of the literature. J Neurosurg Spine. 2007; 6(2):104–12.

44. Koebke J. Morphological and functional studies on the odontoid process of the human axis. Anat Embryol. 1979;155:197–208.

45. Johnson GM. The correlation between surface measurement of the head and neck posture and the anatomic position of the upper cervical vertebrae. Spine. 1998;23:921–7.

46. Milne JS, Lauder IJ. Age effects in kyphosis and lordosis in adults. Ann Hum Biol. 1974;1(3):327–37.

47. Amonoo-Kuofi HS. Changes in the lumbosacral angle, sacral inclination and the curvature of the lumbar spine during aging. Acta Anat (Basel). 1992; 145(4):373–7.

48. Dreischarf M, Albiol L, Rohlmann A, Pries E, Bashkuev M, Zander T, et al. Age-related loss of lumbar spinal lordosis and mobility—a study of 323 asymptomatic volunteers. PLoS One. 2014;9(12):e116186. https://doi.org/10.1371/journal.pone.0116186.

49. Endo K, Suzuki H, Sawaji Y, Nishimura H, Yorifuji M, Murata K, et al. Relationship among cervical, thoracic, and lumbopelvic sagittal alignment in healthy adults. J Orthop Surg (Hong Kong). 2016;24(1):92–6.

50. Hardacker JW, Shuford RF, Capicotto PN, Pryor PW. Radiographic standing cervical segmental alignment in adult volunteers without neck symptoms. Spine (Phila Pa 1976). 1997;22:1472–80.

51. Strine TW, Hootman JM. US national prevalence and correlates of low back and neck pain among adults. Arthritis Rheum. 2007;57:656–65.

52. Lippa L, Lippa L, Cacciola F. Loss of cervical lordosis: what is the prognosis? J Craniovertebr Junction Spine. 2017;8(1):9–14.

53. Matsumoto M, Fujimura Y, Suzuki N, Toyama Y, Shiga H. Cervical curvature in acute whiplash injuries: prospective comparative study with asymptomatic subjects. Injury. 1998;29:775–8.

54. Grob D, Frauenfelder H, Mannion AF. The association between cervical spine curvature and neck pain. Eur Spine J. 2007;16:669–78.

55. Kumagai G, Ono A, Numasawa T, Wada K, Inoue R, Iwasaki H, et al. Association between roentgenographic findings of the cervical spine and neck symptoms in a Japanese community population. J Orthop Sci. 2014;19: 390–7.

56. Shilton M, Branney J, de Vries BP, Breen AC. Does cervical lordosis change after spinal manipulation for non-specific neck pain? A prospective cohort study. Chiropr Man Therap. 2015;23:33.

57. McAviney J, Schulz D, Bock R, Harrison DE, Holland B. Determining the relationship between cervical lordosis and neck complaints. J Manip Physiol Ther. 2005;28:187–93.

12

Combination therapy with low-dose teriparatide and zoledronate contributes to fracture healing on rat femoral fracture model

Yuta Tsubouchi[1], Shinichi Ikeda[2], Masashi Kataoka[3]*[iD] and Hiroshi Tsumura[4]

Abstract

Background: Delay in fracture healing or non-union can be devastating complication. Recent studies have reported that teriparatide (TP) demonstrated effectively on callus formation and mechanical strength and zoledronate (ZA) increased the callus size and resistance at the fracture site in rat fracture model. In this study, the effects of combination therapy with low dose TP and ZA on fracture healing was evaluated.

Methods: From 1 week post-operation, TP (5 times a week administration) and ZA (0.1 mg/kg single administration) were administered by dividing the rats into the following five groups: TP 1 μg group {T(1): TP 1 μg/kg}, ZA group (ZA:0.1 mg/kg), TP1 μg+ZA group {T(1)+ZA: TP 1 μg/kg+ZA}, TP 10 μg+ZA group {T(10)+ZA: TP 10 μg/kg + ZA}, and control group (C: administered saline). Rt femurs were excised 7 weeks after the surgery; bone fusions were evaluated with soft X-ray images on a 4-point scale. And the histopathological examination was performed in demineralized and non-demineralized specimens. Furthermore, the Radiographic Union Scale was conducted in all specimens.

Results: About the bone fusions rates, C, T(1), ZA, T(1)+ZA, and T(10)+ZA groups demonstrated 20.0%, 55.6%, 70.0%, 70.0%, and 80.0%, respectively, and with 4-point scale, each group was 0.50, 1.56, 2.00, 2.60, and 2.80 points, respectively. The callus volume was significantly increased to 16.66 mm^2 and 17.75 mm^2 in the T(1)+ZA and T(10)+ZA groups, respectively, while 10.65 mm^2 ($p < 0.05$) in the C group. Furthermore, the callus area in the T(10)+ZA group was also observed to have significantly increased to 78.78%, compared with 54.63% and 44.11% in the C and T(1)+ZA groups, respectively ($p < 0.01$). Histopathologically, cartilage tissue and immature callus formation were observed at the bone junction in the C group; however, the osseous bridge formation of mature callus was observed in the ZA, T(1)+ZA, and T(10)+ZA groups.

Conclusion: It is suggested that administration of low dose TP and ZA in combination may lead to the treatment of delayed union of fracture. We hope the combination treatment may become one of new therapeutic strategy.

Keywords: Fracture healing, Teriparatide, Zoledronate

* Correspondence: mkataoka@oita-u.ac.jp
[3]Physical Therapy Course of Study, Faculty of Welfare and Health Sciences, Oita University, 700 Dannoharu, Oita 870-1192, Japan
Full list of author information is available at the end of the article

Background

Although improvements in surgical methods for fractures of the femoral shaft have resulted in delayed fracture healing and nonunion in up to 5–10% of patients, subsequent treatment upon the occurrence of nonunion is challenging. Achieving early bone union and returning patients to society under such unfavorable conditions are important issues to address [1].

Teriparatide (TP), which was used in the present study, affects osseous tissue, and its effect varies according to the administration method. While a catabolic effect on the bone is observed during continuous administration, an anabolic effect occurs when it is intermittently administered. Since 2010, TP has been widely used as a therapeutic drug for osteoporosis in Japan; however, it is expected to be clinically applied in the future as a therapeutic agent that promotes fracture healing because of its intense osteogenesis-promoting effect. Coppola et al. reported that TP administration was really effective for the management of non-unions in four cases; however, the efficacy of the TP in delayed or non-unions was not clear [2]. In a rat femoral fracture model, Andreassen et al. administered a post-fracture subcutaneous injection of parathyroid hormone 1–34 (PTH 1–34) for consecutive days at two doses (60 and 200 µg/kg) and reported greater callus formation and strong callus in the group administered 200 µg/kg PTH [3]. However, the continuous administration of 60 or 200 µg/kg PTH is unrealistic and poses pharmacological problems. Considering the administration to humans in clinical practice, examinations should be conducted using a lower dosage. Several studies have investigated the administration of low-dose rhPTH (1–34; 10 µg/kg) in a rat femoral fracture model, in which treatment increased callus bone mineral content (BMC) and bone density, as well as dynamic strength and was thus found to be effective [4, 5].

In contrast, bisphosphonate (BP) has a bone resorption inhibitory action and has been demonstrated to effectively improve bone mineral density (BMD), normalize elevated levels of serum bone metabolism markers, and lower the risk of bone fractures [6, 7]. Furthermore, several reports have studied the effects of BP on the process of bone fracture healing. Most of these reports have demonstrated effectiveness in increasing callus volume (CV) and dynamic strength [8, 9]. In a study conducted to investigate the effects of 0.1-mg/kg zoledronate (ZA) administered in an ovariectomized rat femoral fracture model, it was reported that ZA increased callus strength, bone mass:volume ratio, trabecular width, and trabecular connectivity density during the process of bone fracture healing [10].

Purpose

Although there are not many studies on the effect of combined TP and ZA therapy on the process of bone

fracture healing, the effectiveness of this treatment has been reported; it increases bone mass:volume ratio of the callus as well as bone mass and width [11, 12]. These studies were conducted with the administration of high-dose PTH, which cannot be considered a realistic dose in clinical practice. Therefore, the present study aimed to examine the effect of combined low-dose TP and ZA for bone fracture healing in a refractory rat fracture model using X-ray evaluation and histopathological evaluations of demineralized and non-demineralized specimens.

Methods

Study groups

A total of 50 male Sprague–Dawley rats (12 weeks old; CLEA Japan, Inc., Tokyo, Japan) were divided into five groups. From 1 week post-operation, TP (Forteo, Lilly Japan, Tokyo) (5 times a week administration) and ZA (Novartis Pharma KK Tokyo Japan) (0.1 mg/kg single administration) were administered by dividing the rats into the following 5 groups: TP 1 µg group {T(1): TP 1 µg/kg}, ZA group (ZA:0.1 mg/kg), TP1 µg+ZA group {T(1)+ZA:TP 1 µg/kg+ZA}, TP10 µg+ZA group {T(10)+ZA: TP 10 µg/kg+ZA}, and control group (C: administered saline).

Surgical technique used to construct the femoral fracture model

Approval was obtained from the Oita University animal research committee prior to animal experimentation (Oita University institutional Animal Ethics Committee no.1624003). The Sprague–Dawley rats were anesthetized by an intraperitoneal injection containing 0.3–0.4 ml of 0.15 mg/kg medetomidine + 2 mg/kg midazolam + 2.5 mg/kg butorphanol. The right hind limb was prepared for the operation under standard sterile conditions. With the rat in the lateral position, the right femur was located using the posterolateral approach. The periosteum of the femur was circumferentially incised and elevated and stripped. Then, the femur at osteotomy site was exposed. A transverse osteotomy was performed at the mid-shaft of the femoral bone, the fracture fragments were contacted and stabilized, and the intramedullary was then fixed using a stainless steel wire (diameter, 1.6 mm). The wire was cut on the surface of the intercondylar groove to avoid knee joint motion restriction. The material was applied and wrapped circumferentially around the fracture site. The fascial and skin incisions were closed with a 3–0 nylon suture.

Immediately following surgery and on subsequent days, the rodents received analgesics (buprenorphine subcutaneously and paracetamol). The rodents were housed in separate cages and fed food and water ad libitum, and their conditions were monitored daily. The rats were humanly euthanized 6 weeks after the operation, and the operated right femoral bones were explanted and separated from the stainless steel wire before analysis. We used the left femoral bones, which had not been operated upon, as controls in the biomechanical analysis.

Radiographic analysis

The explanted femoral bones obtained at the 7-week time point were photographed using a Softex X-ray apparatus (Softex CSM-2; Softex, Tokyo, Japan) employing HS Fuji Softex film (Fuji Film, Tokyo, Japan) at 45 cm with 30 kV and 15 mA for 20 s. The fusion was quantified using anteroposterior (A-P) and lateral radiographs. Three blinded independent observers scored the bone formation in each rat using a 4-point scale. Fracture union was judged by visual assessment of the mineralized callus bridging the fracture line in the A-P radiographs (right side: 1 point; left side: 1 point) and lateral radiographs (anterior side: 1 point; posterior side: 1 point). The bone fusion was considered to be more than 2 points with soft X-ray images on a 4-point scale. Furthermore, the Radiographic Union Scale for Tibial fractures in Tibial Fracture (RUST) was conducted in all specimens [13]. The RUST score is based on the presence or absence of callus and of a visible fracture line at the total of four cortices visible on the anteroposterior and lateral radiographs. Its 4-point minimum corresponds to a fracture that is deemed not healed, whereas its 12-point maximum corresponds to a fracture that is deemed healed with all cortices bridged with callus without a fracture line.

Histological analysis

Ten specimens of one group were divided into two kinds of staining. For the HE staining, 4 of 10 specimens were performed, and for the non-demineralized and toluidine blue staining, 6 of 10 specimens were performed in a random manner. After extraction, the femoral bones were dissected, and the specimens were fixed in 70% ethanol. The specimens were then decalcified using a standard 10% decalcifying solution of HCl (Cal-Ex) (Fischer Scientific, Fairlawn, NJ), washed with running tap water, and transferred to 75% ethanol. Serial sagittal sections (5 μm) were carefully cut from the paraffin blocks using a microtome (LS-113; DAIWA-KOKI, Saitama, Japan) at the level of the femoral fracture. The sections were stained with hematoxylin and eosin (HE) and evaluated qualitatively under a light microscope ($n = 4$ per groups).

Furthermore, non-demineralized specimens were obtained from glycolmenthacrylate resin-embedded slices, and the calcification state and cells in the fracture area were observed ($n = 6$ per groups). After staining with toluidine blue, bone morphometry was performed to up to 0.43 mm proximal and distal to the bone fracture area

(Histometry RT CAMERA; System Supply, Tokyo, Japan). Measurement items included callus volume (CV), callus area (CA), and cartilage tissue area (Ca.A).

Statistical methods

One-way ANOVA with Bonferroni post hoc test was used for 4-point test and RUST and the analysis of morphometric results of the treatment groups. All analyses were performed using Statistical Package for the Social Sciences (SPSS V22.0; SPSS, Chicago, IL). Statistical significance was set at < 0.05.

Results

Radiographic analysis

In the C and T(1) group, the fracture line could be clearly identified, and immature callus formation was observed. In particular, callus continuity was not achieved in the C group. Conversely, in the ZA, T(1)+ZA, and T(10)+ZA groups, the fracture line was unclear, the callus was thick, and continuity was confirmed (Fig. 1). On the 4-point scale, the C group scored 0.50 ± 0.85 points, the T(1) group scored 1.56 ± 1.67 points, the ZA group scored 2.00 ± 1.41 points, the T(1)+ZA group scored 2.60 ± 1.90 points, and the T(10)+ZA group scored 2.80 ± 1.69 points, indicating significantly more progress in bone union in the T(1)+ZA and T(10)+ZA groups than in the C group (Table 1). About the bone fusions rates, C, T(1), ZA, T(1)+ZA, and T(10)+ZA groups demonstrated 20.0%, 55.6%, 70.0%, 70.0%, and 80.0%, respectively (Table 1).

The RUST score results, including the evaluation of cortical bone continuity and callus formation, were comparable among the groups, with the C group scoring 5.00 ± 0.82 points, the T(1) group scoring 6.67 ± 2.24 points, the ZA group scoring 7.90 ± 3.10 points, the T(1)+ZA group scoring 9.20 ± 3.65 points, and the T(10)+ZA group scoring 10.2 ± 2.57 points, indicating significantly more progress in bone union in the T(1)+ZA and T(10)+ZA groups than in the C group ($p < 0.01$) (Fig. 2).

Bone histomorphometrical analysis

In the C and T(1) group, verifying the fracture site by HE staining identified the fracture and confirmed extensive chondrogenesis. Furthermore, while several specimens demonstrated thin immature callus formation, callus continuity could not be confirmed in many specimens. Although a few chondrocytes were identified in the T(1)+ZA group, they were enlarged. Compared to the C group, the fracture line was unclear. Furthermore, in the T(10)+ZA group, chondrocytes could not be identified, but mature callus and advanced bone union were confirmed (Fig. 3).

Staining with toluidine blue revealed cartilage tissue and immature callus formation along with the fracture

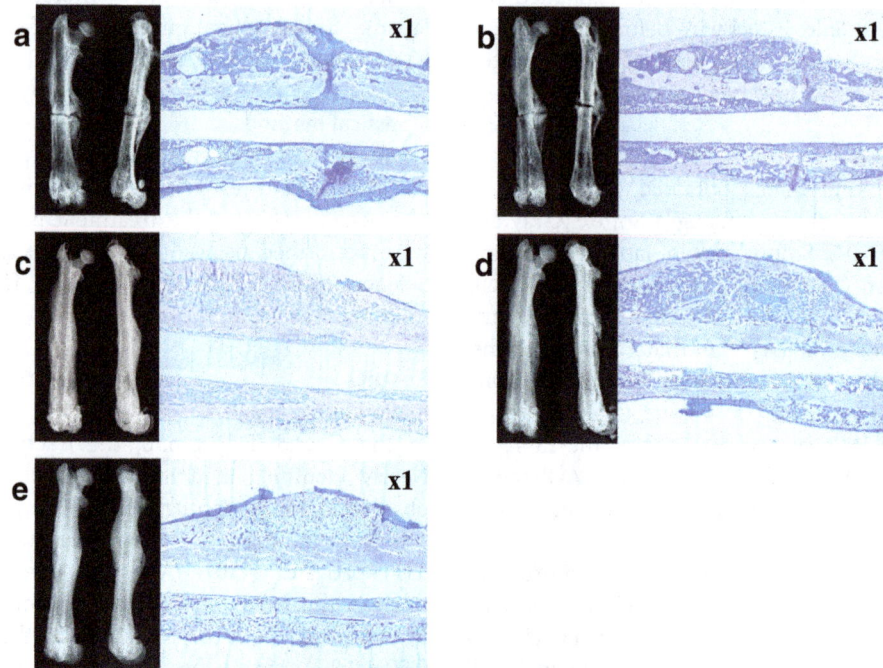

Fig. 1 Bone radiographic and histological findings of rat femur (left: bone radiographic findings, right: histological findings of non-demineralized specimens: toluidine blue staining, × 1). In the C (**a**) and T(1) groups (**b**), a fracture line was observed clearly; however, there were no findings of immature or bridging callus formation. In the ZA (**c**), T(1)+ZA (**d**), and T(10)+ZA group (**e**), the fracture line was unclear and mature bridging callus formation was noted. About bone histological imaging (non-demineralized specimens: toluidine blue staining), in the C (**a**) and T(1) (**b**) groups, immature callus formation and cartilage tissue were observed; however, in the ZA (**c**), T(1)+ZA (**d**), and T(10)+ZA group (**e**), mature bridging callus formation was noted. Furthermore, bone union was seen resulting from endochondral ossification in the ZA (**c**), T(1)+ZA (**d**), and T(10)+ZA group (**e**), and mature bone tissue was identified in the T(10)+ZA group (**e**). Ten specimens of one group were divided into two kinds of staining. For the HE staining, 4 of 10 specimens were performed, and for the non-demineralized and toluidine blue staining, 6 of 10 specimens were performed in a random manner

line in the C and T(1) groups, whereas osseous bridge formation of the mature callus was observed in the ZA, T(1)+ZA, and T(10)+ZA groups. Furthermore, bone union was seen resulting from endochondral ossification in the ZA, T(1)+ZA, and T(10)+ZA groups, and mature bone tissue was identified in the T(10)+ZA group (Fig. 1). Bone histomorphometry revealed CV was 10.65 ± 2.47 mm^2 in the C group, 8.01 ± 1.46 mm^2 in the T(1) group, and 12.79 ± 1.28 mm^2 in the ZA group, but was significantly higher at 16.66 ± 2.35 mm^2 in the T(1)+ZA group and 17.75 ± 2.85 mm^2 in the T(10)+ZA group ($P < 0.01$). Similarly, CA was $54.63\% \pm 5.31\%$ in the C

group, $44.11\% \pm 4.13\%$ in the T(1) group, $62.84 \pm 5.89\%$ in the ZA group, and $62.57\% \pm 2.75\%$ in the T(1)+ZA group, but was significantly higher at $78.78\% \pm 0.85\%$ in the T(10)+ZA group ($P < 0.001$). However, Ca.A was 0.74 ± 0.51 mm^2 in the C group, 0.06 ± 0.11 mm^2 in the T(1) group, 0.01 ± 0.02 mm^2 in the T(1)+ZA group, but it could not be confirmed in the ZA and T(10)+ZA group ($P < 0.05$) (Fig. 4a, b, c).

Discussion

Einhorn et al. reported the molecular mechanism of fracture healing in rodents from a molecular biological

Table 1 Results of bone radiographic statistical analysis of 4-point scale and bone fusion rate

	Control ($n = 10$)	T(1) ($n = 10$)	ZA ($n = 10$)	T(1)+ZA ($n = 10$)	T(10)+ZA ($n = 10$)	ANOVA
Fusion rate (%)	20.0	55.6	70.0	70.0	80.0	
4-point scale	0.50 ± 0.85	1.56 ± 1.67	2.00 ± 1.41	2.60 ± 1.90[a]	2.80 ± 1.69[a]	0.014

All values are mean ± standard deviation

Evaluation of femoral shaft fracture was performed with Softex X-ray apparatus. Fracture union was judged by visual assessment of the mineralized callus bridging the fracture line in the A-P radiographs (right side: 1 point; left side: 1 point) and lateral radiographs (anterior side: 1 point; posterior side: 1 point). The bone fusion was considered to be more than 2 points with soft X-ray images on a 4-point scale. About the bone fusions rates, C, T(1), ZA, T(1)+ZA group, and T(10)+ZA group demonstrated 20.0%, 55.6%, 70.0%, 70.0%, and 80.0% respectively. With the 4-point scale analysis, T(10)+ZA and T(1)+ZA groups were significantly superior to C group in bone union

T(1) teriparatide 1 µg group, *ZA* zoledronate group, *T(1)+ZA* teriparatide 1 µg + zoledronate group, *T(10)+ZA* teriparatide 10 µg + zoledronate group

[a]$p < 0.05$ vs. control group, by post hoc test

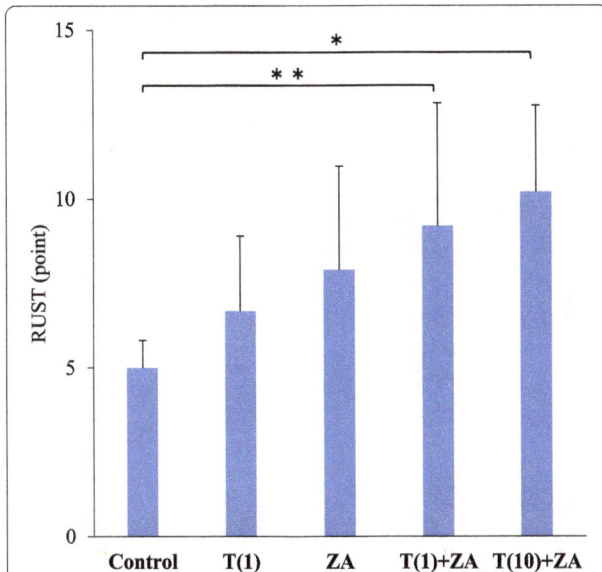

Fig. 2 Results of bone radiographic analysis in RUST. The RUST score is based on the presence or absence of callus and of a visible fracture line at the total of four cortices visible on the anteroposterior and lateral radiographs. Kooistra et al. reported that the reliability and validity of the radiographic union scale in human long bone [13]. In this study, the RUST score was applied to bone union analysis. The RUST score results, including the evaluation of cortical bone continuity and callus formation, were comparable among the groups, with the C group scoring 5.00 ± 0.82 points, the T(1) group scoring 6.67 ± 2.24 points, the ZA group scoring 7.90 ± 3.10 points, the T(1)+ZA group scoring 9.20 ± 3.65 points, and the T(10)+ZA group scoring 10.2 ± 2.57 points, indicating significantly more progress in bone union in the T(1)+ZA and T(10)+ZA groups than in the C group

perspective. Immediately after fracture, hematoma was formed in the fracture gap and transforming growth factor (TGF)-β and platelet-derived growth factor were induced from platelets. Furthermore, interleukin (IL)-2 and IL-6 were derived from inflammatory cells, and TGF-β promoted mesenchymal cell differentiation. Within 24 h after fracture, mesenchymal stem cells secreted bone morphogenetic proteins. In the fracture gap, mesenchymal stem cell differentiation began on day 3 after fracture and cartilage and soft callus began forming. On day 5, at the same site, type II collagen mRNA expression was observed, which peaked on day 9. From around day 14, the soft callus began calcifying, appearing like a primary or secondary spongy bone surrounding the growth plate cartilage. This implies that endochondral ossification occurs after cartilage formation at the site of bone fracture and that membranous ossification occurs near the bone fracture site. The bone that has just been ossified is often fibrous bone, which is remodeled and converted into lamellated bone. It can be said that bone fracture healing is achieved through the combination of all these histological changes [14].

In this study, the periosteum of the femur was circumferentially incised and elevated and stripped, then, the femur at osteotomy site was exposed. A transverse osteotomy was performed at the mid-shaft of the femoral bone; the fracture fragments were contacted and stabilized. We had performed several times of experiments of femoral fracture model, and the average rate of bone union was almost 10–20% of the cases in stripping of periosteum. Cartilage formation is taking place in the cambium layer of the periosteum, and chondrocyte precursor cells also reside in this location. Accordingly, bone union must rely on endochondral ossification. To date, studies have illustrated that TP promotes endochondral ossification from cartilage formation occurring in the fracture gap and promotes membranous ossification near the fracture site. Furthermore, TP promotes callus remodeling and reduces the bridging callus, simultaneously increases the degree of calcification, improves the dynamic quality of callus, and promotes a normal bone fracture healing process.

Nakazawa et al. injected 10 μg/kg of PTH in a rat closed femoral fracture model and analyzed the promotion of bone fracture healing at the molecular level [5]. Compared to the control group, the group administered with PTH radiologically demonstrated remarkable callus formation from the early stage to the late stage in the healing process and exhibited a significantly higher BMC, bone density, and dynamic strength at 4 and 6 weeks after fracture. Several studies have examined bone fracture healing in animals treated with BP. The results of these studies revealed that BP accumulated in the acute fracture site predominantly during the repair phase of bone healing. Furthermore, it was determined that BP not only helped increase callus and bone mass but also increased BMC. Conversely, BP did not affect the start of callus formation.

Regarding the effect of BP on endochondral ossification, it has been suggested that the size and strength of the callus can be controlled by regulating bone remodeling during the healing process. Consequently, the timing and regimen of BP therapy can have a significant impact on the formation and strength of the callus. In our preliminary experiment, we established that 1 week after fracture is the optimal timing of a single intraperitoneal injection of ZA for the rate of bone union, bone formation, and strength testing [15]. Furthermore, Murphy et al. reported that PTH (1–34) increased bone turnover as well as BP turnover [16]. Treatment of combined PTH and BP may be increased effect of BP.

Histopathological findings of the species revealed that ZA treatment not only increases callus formation but also improves trabecular microarchitecture. ZA given systemically as a single dose at the optimal time could reduce catabolic osteoclastic resorption caused by TP.

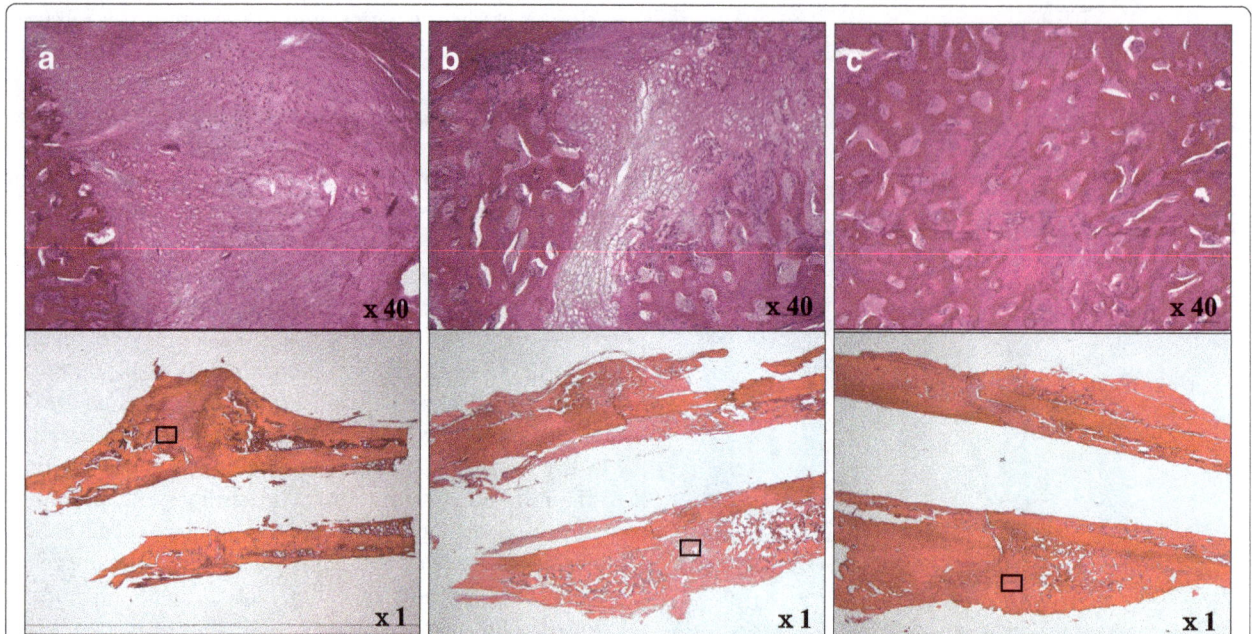

Fig. 3 Bone histological imaging (demineralized specimens: HE staining) (× 1) (× 40). In the C (**a**) and T(1)+ZA groups (**b**), verifying the fracture site by HE staining identified the fracture and confirmed extensive chondrogenesis. Furthermore, while several specimens demonstrated thin immature callus formation, callus continuity could not be confirmed in many specimens. And cartilaginous bone metaplasia was not observed. Although a few chondrocytes, suggesting bone metaplasia, were identified in the T(1)+ZA group (**b**), they were enlarged. Compared to the C group, the fracture line was unclear. Furthermore, in the T(10) + ZA group (**c**), chondrocytes could not be identified, but mature callus and advanced bone union were confirmed (**c**).

However, there were no evidence of ZA-induced suppression of anabolic bone formation caused by TP. The fusion rates in rat femurs administered both ZA and TP were higher than those of rats administered ZA only 6 weeks after surgery.

The present study demonstrated that the synergistic effect of low-dose TP and ZA promoted callus formation, increased callus mass, and helped to promote bone union in a rat refractory fracture model. The synergistic effect of the combination of TP with the anabolic effect and ZA with the anti-catabolic effect was also demonstrated. Because ZA promotes the apoptosis of osteoclasts, remodeling is delayed, which, in turn, can impede the change from fibrous bone to lamellated bone. Hence, detailed

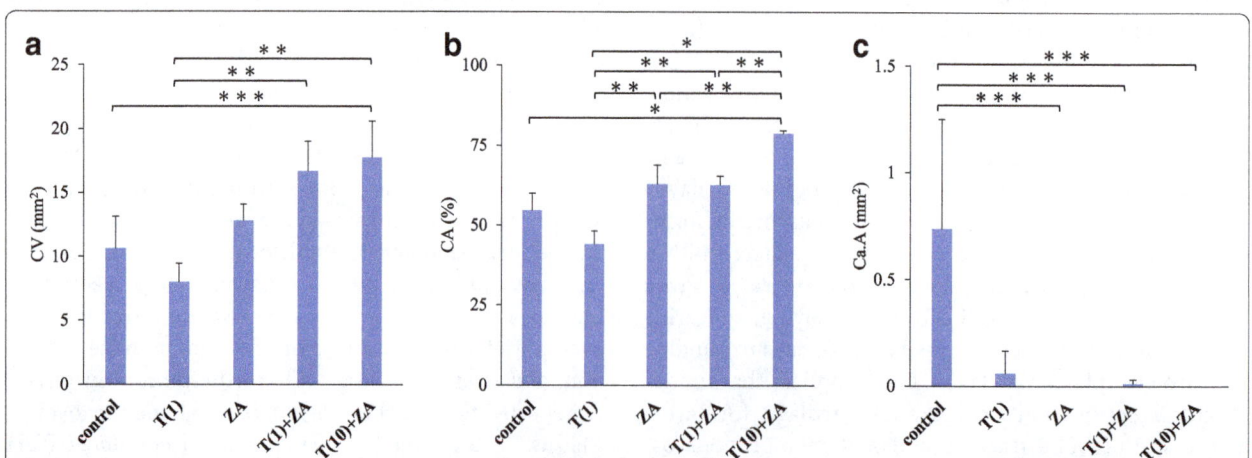

Fig. 4 a, **b**, **c** Results of bone histomorphometry. **a** Callus volume (CV). **b** Callus area(CA). **c** Cartilage tissue area (Ca.A). Bone histomorphometry revealed callus volume (CV); C 10.65 ± 2.47 mm^2, T(1) 8.01 ± 1.46 mm^2, and ZA group 12.79 ± 1.28 mm^2, but was significantly higher at 16.66 ± 2.35 mm^2 in the T(1)+ZA group and 17.75 ± 2.85 mm^2 in the T(10)+ZA group ($P < 0.01$). Similarly, CA was $54.63\% \pm 5.31\%$ in the C group, $44.11\% \pm 4.13\%$ in the T(1) group, $62.84\% \pm 5.89\%$ in the ZA group, and $62.57\% \pm 2.75\%$ in the T(1)+ZA group, but was significantly higher at $78.78\% \pm 0.85\%$ in the T(10)+ZA group ($P < 0.001$). However, Ca.A was 0.74 ± 0.51 mm^2 in the C group, 0.06 ± 0.11 mm^2 in the T(1) group, 0.01 ± 0.02 mm^2 in the T(1)+ZA group, but it could not be confirmed in the ZA and T(10)+ZA group ($P < 0.05$)

investigations of the bone structure through long-term observations are required in the future.

Conclusion

The present experiment shows that administration of low-dose TP and ZA in combination is able to enhance callus formation, increase callus volume, and help to promote bone union in a rat refractory fracture model. We hope the combination treatment may become one of new therapeutic strategy in delay in fracture healing or non-union of patients.

Abbreviations

BMC: Bone mineral content; BMD: Bone mineral density; BP: Bisphosphonate; CA: Callus area; Ca.A: Cartilage tissue area; CV: Callus volume; PTH: Parathyroid hormone; RUST: The Radiographic Union Scale in Tibial Fracture; TP: Teriparatide; ZA: Zoledronate

Acknowledgements

We are grateful to Miss Kaori Abe for excellent technical assistance.

Funding

This work was supported by JSPS KAKENHI Grant Number JP16K12939.

Authors' contributions

YT, SI, and MK carried out the operation. HT conceived of the study design. YT, SI, MK, and HT interpreted the data and drafted the manuscript. All authors read and approved the final manuscript.

Competing interests

The authors declare that they have no competing interests.

Author details

[1]Oita University Hospital Rehabilitation Center, Oita University, 1-1 Idaigaoka, Hasama-machi, Yufu-city, Oita 879-5593, Japan. [2]Department of Rehabilitation Medicine, Faculty of Medicine, Oita University, 1-1 Idaigaoka, Hasama-machi, Yufu-city, Oita 879-5593, Japan. [3]Physical Therapy Course of Study, Faculty of Welfare and Health Sciences, Oita University, 700 Dannoharu, Oita 870-1192, Japan. [4]Department of Orthopaedic Surgery, Faculty of Medicine, Oita University, 1-1 Idaigaoka, Hasama-machi, Yufu-city, Oita 879-5593, Japan.

References

1. Buza JA 3rd, Einhorn T. Bone healing in 2016. Clin Cases Miner Bone Metab. 2016;13(2):101–5.
2. Coppola C, Del Buono A, Maffulli N. Teriparatide in fracture non-unions. Trans Med UniSa. 2015;12(8):47–53.
3. Andreassen TT, Ejersted C, Oxlund H. Intermittent parathyroid hormone (1–34) treatment increases callus formation and mechanical strength of healing rat fractures. J Bone Miner Res. 1999;14(6):960–8.
4. Nakajima A, Shimoji N, Shiomi K, Shimizu S, Moriya H, Einhorn TA, Yamazaki M. Mechanisms for the enhancement of fracture healing in rats treated with intermittent low-dose human parathyroid hormone (1–34). J Bone Miner Res. 2002;17(11):2038–47.
5. Nakazawa T, Nakajima A, Shiomi K, Moriya H, Einhorn TA, Yamazaki M. Effects of low-dose, intermittent treatment with recombinant human parathyroid hormone (1–34) on chondrogenesis in a model of experimental fracture healing. Bone. 2005;37(5):711–9.
6. Chapurlat RD, Palermo L, Ramsay P, Cummings SR. Risk of fracture among women who lose bone density during treatment with alendronate. The fracture intervention trial. Osteoporosis Int. 2005;16(7):842–8.
7. Rebolledo BJ, Unnanuntana A, Lane JM. A comprehensive approach to fragility fractures. J Orthop Trauma. 2011;25(9):566–73.
8. Amanat N, McDonald M, Godfrey C, Bilston L, Little D. Optimal timing of a single dose of zoledronic acid to increase strength in rat fracture repair. J Bone Miner Res. 2007;22(6):867–76.
9. Matos MA, Tannuri U, Guarniero R. The effect of zoledronate during bone healing. J Orthopaed Traumatol. 2010;11(1):7–12.
10. Hao Y, Wang X, Wang L, Lu Y, Mao Z, Ge S, Dai K. Zoledronic acid suppresses callus remodeling but enhances callus strength in an osteoporotic rat model of fracture healing. Bone. 2015;81:702–11.
11. Li YF, Zhou CC, Li JH, Luo E, Zhu SS, Feng G, Hu J. The effects of combined human parathyroid hormone (1-34) and zoledronic acid treatment on fracture healing in osteoporotic rats. Osteoporos Int. 2012;23(4):1463–74.
12. Casanova M, Herelle J, Thomas M, Softley R, Schindeler A, Little D, Schneider P, Müller R. Effect of combined treatment with zoledronic acid and parathyroid hormone on mouse bone callus structure and composition. Bone. 2016;92:70–8.
13. Kooistra BW, Dijkman BG, Busse JW, Sprague S, Schemitsch EH, Bhandari M. The radiographic union scale in tibial fractures: reliability and validity. J Orthop Trauma. 2010;24(Suppl 1):S81–6.
14. Einhorn TA, Gerstenfeld LC. Fracture healing: mechanisms and interventions. Nat Rev Rheumatol. 2015;11(1):45–54.
15. Doi Y, Miyazaki M, Yoshiiwa T, Hara K, Kataoka M, Tsumura H. Manipulation of the anabolic and catabolic responses with BMP-2 and zoledronic acid in a rat femoral fracture model. Bone. 2011;49(4):777–82.
16. Murphy CM, Schindeler A, Cantrill LC, Mikulec K, Peacock L, Little DG. PTH (1-34) treatment increases bisphosphonate turnover in fracture repair in rats. J Bone Miner Res. 2015;30(6):1022–9.

13

New fixation approach for transverse metacarpal neck fracture: a biomechanical study

Yung-Cheng Chiu[1,2], Ming-Tzu Tsai[3], Cheng-En Hsu[4,5], Horng-Chaung Hsu[1,2], Heng-Li Huang[6,7] and Jui-Ting Hsu[6,7*]

Abstract

Background: Fifth metacarpal neck fracture, also known as boxer's fracture, is the most common metacarpal fracture. Percutaneous Kirschner-wire (K-wire) pinning has been shown to produce favorable clinical results. However, the fixation power of K-wires is a major concern. Plate fixation is also a surgical option, but it has the disadvantages of tendon adhesion, requirement of secondary surgery for removal of the implant, and postoperative joint stiffness. A fixation method that causes little soft tissue damage and provides high biomechanical stability is required for patients with fifth metacarpal neck fracture for whom surgical intervention is indicated. The present study proposed fixation using K-wires and a cerclage wire to treat fifth metacarpal neck fracture. The fixation power of this new method was compared with that of K-wires alone and plates.

Methods: We used a saw blade to create transverse metacarpal neck fractures in 16 artificial metacarpal bone specimens, which were then treated with four types of fixation as follows: (1) locking plate with five locking bicortical screws (LP group), (2) regular plate with five bicortical screws (RP group), (3) two K-wires (K group), and (4) two K-wires and a figure-of-eight cerclage wire (KW group). The specimens were tested by using cantilever bending testing on a material testing system. The stiffness of the four fixation types was determined by observing force–displacement curves. Finally, the Kruskal–Wallis test was adopted to process the data, and the Mann–Whitney exact test was performed to conduct paired comparison between the fixation types.

Results: The fixation strength levels of the four fixation approaches for treating fifth metacarpal neck fracture were ranked in a descending order of LP group (24.6 ± 5.1 N/mm, median ± interquartile range) > RP group (22.2 ± 5.8 N/mm) ≅ KW group (20.1 ± 3.2 N/mm) > K group (16.9 ± 3.0 N/mm).

Conclusion: The fixation strength of two K-wires was significantly higher when reinforcement was provided using a figure-of-eight cerclage wire. The strength of the proposed approach is similar to that of a regular plate with five bicortical screws but weaker than that of a locking plate with the same amount of bicortical screws. Cerclage wire-integrated K-wires can be an alternative method that avoids the excessive soft tissue dissection required for plating in open reduction internal fixation for fifth metacarpal neck fracture.

Keywords: Fifth metacarpal neck fracture, Bone plate, K-wire, Cerclage wire

* Correspondence: jthsu@mail.cmu.edu.tw; richard@ms32.url.com.tw
[6]School of Dentistry, College of Dentistry, China Medical University, 91 Hsueh-Shih Road, Taichung 40402, Taiwan
[7]Department of Bioinformatics and Medical Engineering, Asia University, Taichung 413, Taiwan
Full list of author information is available at the end of the article

Background

Metacarpal fractures are common orthopedic injuries [1] that account for 13% of hand fractures and 23% of forearm fractures [2–4]. The fifth metacarpal neck fracture, also known as boxer's fracture, is the most common type of metacarpal fracture, constituting 50% of metacarpal fractures [2]. Because of the activity performed by the intrinsic muscles of the hand, patients with fractures in the fifth metacarpal neck are likely to develop volar angulation deformity. If the fracture is treated nonoperatively, volar malunion with dorsal angulation and joint stiffness is common [5, 6]. Therefore, an increasing number of doctors and patients are opting for surgical treatment instead. The surgical indication of fifth metacarpal fracture is generally considered to be fracture angulation of more than 45° resulting in a considerable decrease in grip strength and range of motion [1, 7].

Of the various fixation methods for metacarpal neck fracture, K-wire fixation is less invasive and has been shown to have outcomes superior to those of plating [1, 3]. Intramedullary pinning has been reported to have better outcomes than crossed and transverse pinning because of its minimal violation of soft tissue [8–10]. Despite causing soft tissue invasion, open reduction and internal fixation (ORIF) still has a role in treating patients with multiple concurrent metacarpal fractures, those who need higher fracture biomechanical stability, those who are unable to protect exposed pins, and those who cannot tolerate a period of immobilization [11]. Plates, available in regular and locking forms, are internal fixation devices commonly used for metacarpal neck fractures. They provide high mechanical strength, but many complications have been reported, including metacarpal head avascular necrosis, nonunion, severe tendon irritation, and high rate of stiffness due to excessive soft tissue damage [1, 7, 12–14]. For the minimization of soft tissue damage and reduction of implant profiles in ORIF, we propose a novel fixation method that integrates K-wires with a cerclage wire. This new method may provide higher mechanical stability and avoid the complications that arise from the use of plates.

The purpose of our study was to investigate the degree of strength that a cerclage wire can add to K-wires and to compare the biomechanical stability of this new fixation method with that achieved using two commonly used plate methods.

Methods

Specimen preparation

Obtaining an adequate number of real human specimens with identical bone quality and size is difficult, so we used artificial metacarpal bone (3B Scientific GmbH, Hamburg, Germany) in our experiments. A total of 16 artificial metacarpal bone specimens were employed. A metacarpal neck fracture was generated in the specimens using a 0.4-mm saw blade. The fracture distance was 13 mm from the distal articular surface.

Fixation approaches and stability test

The specimens were assigned to four fixation technique groups, and all fixations were performed by a single senior hand surgeon (Yung-Cheng Chiu).

- Group 1—Locking plate with five locking bicortical screws (LP group). The specimens were fixed using a six-hole Y-shaped locking plate and 2.3-mm-diameter locking screws (Stryker, Germany). The locking plate was fixed at the dorsum of the metacarpal using three bicortical proximal locking screws and two bicortical distal locking screws (Fig. 1a).
- Group 2—Regular plate, nonlocking, with five bicortical screws (RP group). The specimens were fixed using a six-hole Y-shaped nonlocking plate and 2.3-mm-diameter compression screws (Stryker, Germany). The nonlocking plate was fixed at the dorsum of the metacarpal with three bicortical proximal compression screws and two bicortical distal compression screws (Fig. 1b).
- Group 3—Two K-wires (K group). The specimens were stabilized using two 1.5-mm-diameter K-wires inserted from the dorsal medial and lateral sides of the metacarpal head, penetrated the fracture site, and fed out from the proximal volar cortex; fracture reduction was maintained with manual axial compression during the surgery (Fig. 1c).
- Group 4—Two K-wires with figure-of-eight cerclage wire (KW group). The specimens were stabilized using two 1.5-mm-diameter K-wires inserted from the dorsal medial and lateral sides of the metacarpal head, penetrated through the fracture site, and fed out from the proximal volar cortex; fracture reduction was maintained with manual axial compression during the surgery. Subsequently, an 18-gauge needle was mounted on an electric drill to serve as the wire guide. Two wire guides were drilled transversely into the distal and proximal parts of the fractured metacarpal parallel at approximately 0.5 cm from the fracture site. A 25-gauge stainless steel wire was used to pass the two wire guides to shape the wire into a figure of eight at the dorsum of the metacarpal after the two needles were withdrawn (Fig. 1d and Fig. 2).

Before mechanical testing, the proximal end of each specimen was held in a custom fixture using molded epoxy clamps. Cantilever bending tests were conducted using a material testing system (JSV-H1000, Japan Instrumentation System, Nara, Japan) (Fig. 3). Following preloading to 5 N, a perpendicular load was applied to

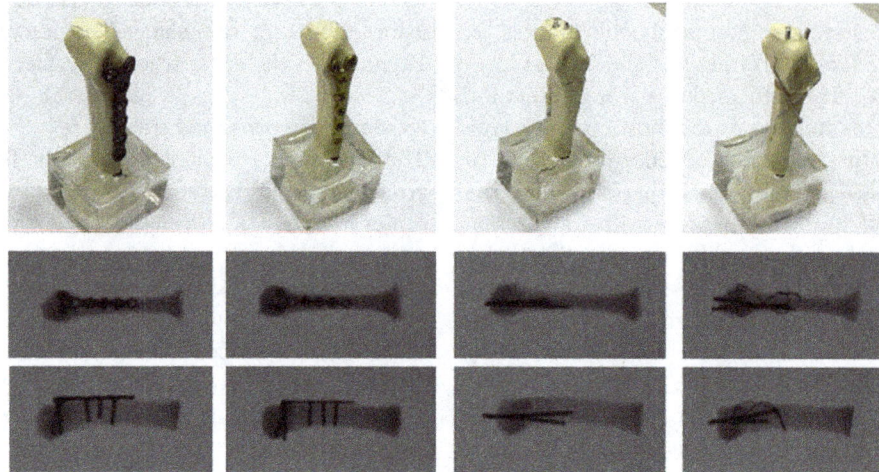

Fig. 1 Artificial metacarpal bones and four fixation types of the metacarpal neck fracture. **a** Locking plate with five locking bicortical screws (LP group). **b** Regular plate with five bicortical screws (RP group). **c** Two K-wires (K group). **d** Two K-wires and a figure-of-eight cerclage wire (KW group). Radiographs of the four fixation types in superior and lateral views are also shown

the dorsal side of the specimen at a distance of 53 mm from the fixture until failure. The crosshead speed was 10 mm/min. The experimental setup was similar to that used in other studies [12, 15]. Force–displacement data were recorded, and the bending stiffness of each specimen was determined.

Statistical analysis

The stiffness of the specimens with metacarpal neck fracture and four fixation types are summarized as the median value (interquartile range [IQR]). The Kruskal–Wallis test was used to compare the differences between the four fixation types. Post hoc pairwise comparisons were conducted using the Mann–Whitney test. Statistical significance was set at $P < 0.05$. All statistical analyses were performed using SPSS Version 19 (IBM Corporation, Armonk, NY, USA).

Results

The experimental results are presented in Table 1 and Fig. 4. The highest median stiffness was obtained for the LP group specimens and was equal to 24.6 ± 5.1 N/mm. The median of the RP group (22.2 ± 5.8 N/mm) was slightly higher than that of the KW group (20.1 ± 3.2 N/mm), but the difference was nonsignificant. The most unstable fixation type was that in the K group, for which the median stiffness was only 16.9 ± 3.0 N/mm, 15.9 and 23.9% lower than that for the KW and RP groups, respectively. The fixation stiffness of the four types of fixation in fifth metacarpal neck fracture thus followed the order LP group > RP group ≅ KW group > K group.

Discussion

Fifth metacarpal neck fracture is a common hand fracture. K-wires and plates are the commonly used internal

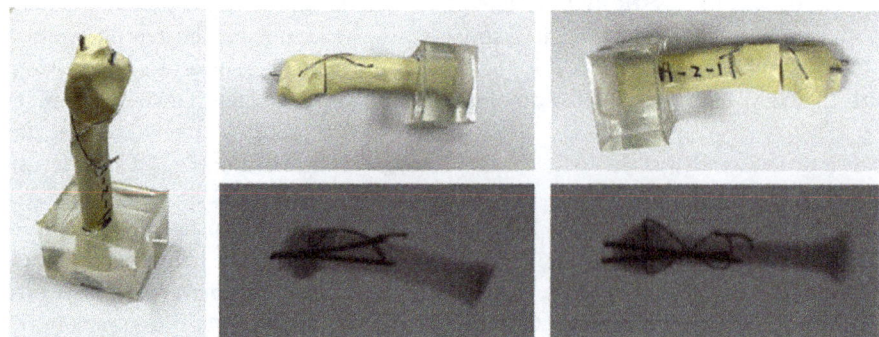

Fig. 2 Details of the fixation approach employing two K-wires and a figure-of-eight cerclage wire (KW group)

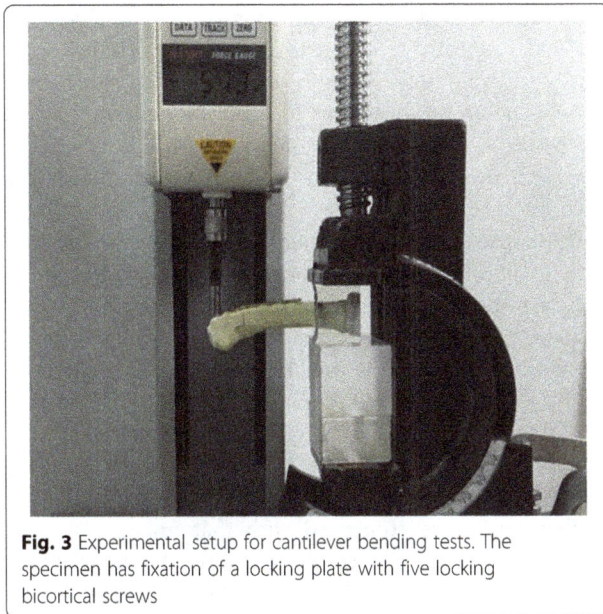

Fig. 3 Experimental setup for cantilever bending tests. The specimen has fixation of a locking plate with five locking bicortical screws

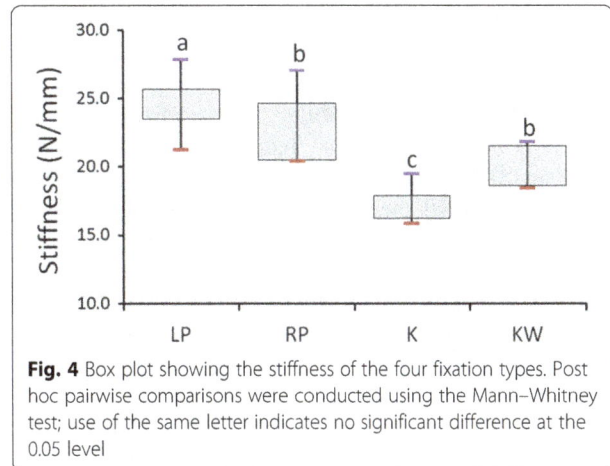

Fig. 4 Box plot showing the stiffness of the four fixation types. Post hoc pairwise comparisons were conducted using the Mann–Whitney test; use of the same letter indicates no significant difference at the 0.05 level

fixation devices; however, numerous complications and high rates of postoperative joint stiffness are reported due to the excessive soft tissue damage that these devices cause [1, 7, 12–14]. Herein, we proposed a mixed fixation of K-wires and a cerclage wire. This fixation approach requires less soft tissue dissection than plate insertion, has mechanical strength comparable to that of a nonlocking plate, and may avoid the complications caused by plate fixation. Additionally, the cost of the proposed approach is considerably lower than that of plate fixation.

In this study, we used artificial metacarpal bones to conduct experiments because of difficulty with acquiring bones from corpses with consistent qualities. Fifth metacarpal neck fracture is often experienced by young people, but obtaining metacarpal bones from the corpses of young people is particularly difficult. Consequently, studies have tended to conduct experiments using porcine or artificial metacarpal bones [12, 16–18]. This study compared the strength of different osteosynthesis techniques for fixation and therefore entailed selecting specimens with almost identical geometrics and material properties. Accordingly, artificial bones were employed because of their uniformity and consistency [19].

Table 1 Stiffness (unit: N/mm) of the four fixation types used to fix metacarpal neck fracture

Group	Median	IQR	Max	Min	P
LP	24.6	5.1	27.9	21.3	0.001
RP	22.2	5.8	27.1	20.4	
K	16.9	3.0	19.5	15.9	
KW	20.1	3.2	21.8	18.5	

According to the American Society for Testing and Materials (ASTM) F-1839-08, "Standard Specification for Rigid Polyurethane Foam for Use as a Standard Material for Testing Orthopaedic Devices and Instruments" states that "the uniformity and consistent properties of rigid polyurethane foam make it an ideal material for comparative testing of bone screws and other medical devices and instruments" [20].

We conducted cantilever bending tests, which differ slightly from the physiological loading tests commonly used in a clinical setting. However, no existent in vitro biomechanical test is able to reflect actual amounts of physiological loading. In addition to the cantilever bending test, previous studies have adopted tests including the three-point bending test [17], modified three-point bending test [13, 21, 22], four-point bending test [16, 18], and torsional test [12, 23]. We employed the cantilever bending test instead of a bending test mainly because the aim of the study was to explore fixation approaches for metacarpal neck fracture not metacarpal shaft fracture. Previously, the maximum fracture force and stiffness were common indexes for scholars to determine fixation strength [12, 14, 16, 17, 21, 23]. In this study, however, the strength was assessed by evaluating the stiffness alone. We assumed that during fracture healing, no matter what fixation is used, refracture of the fifth metacarpal neck as a result of an extremely strong active or passive force does not and should never occur. By contrast, stiffness indicates the structure stiffness of a fixation. Thus, measuring stiffness is more meaningful than measuring the maximum fracture force in clinical practice.

Research has identified that bone plate fixation is the strongest fixation [16, 24–27]. Similarly, the present study determined that the stiffness of the fixation using two K-wires was lower than that using a locking plate and regular plate. Malasitt et al. [13] compared the strength of K-wire and locking plate fixation by conducting experiments on porcine second metacarpals and revealed that the K-wire fixation exhibited higher initial stiffness. The experiments of the present study verified that the stiffness of locking plate fixation (24.61 + 5.12 N/mm) was higher than that of regular plate fixation (22.17 + 5.12 N/mm). Likewise, Ochman et al. [14] implemented modified three-point bending tests to examine pig metacarpal specimens with various types of fixation. The results indicated that when monocortical bone fixation was employed, the stiffness of the fixation using a locking plate (83 + 35 N/mm) was higher than that using a regular plate (46 + 12 N/mm). Doht et al. [21] also conducted modified three-point bending tests on pig metacarpal bones. Despite the mean stiffness of the locking plate group exceeding that of the regular plate group, the difference was nonsignificant.

The stiffness of the KW group was lower than that of the LP group, but no significant difference was discovered between that of the KW and RP groups. Additionally, KW fixation exhibited much greater stiffness than K-wire fixation, indicating that using two K-wires and one figure-of-eight cerclage wire to treat fifth metacarpal neck fracture is reliable.

An increasing amount of evidence is demonstrating that some innovative procedures and modern, fashionable, expensive locking plates do not always achieve superior outcomes to nonsurgical treatment or use of a simple fixation device (e.g., K-wires) [28–30]. Orthopedic and trauma surgeons should consider the possibility of nonsurgical treatment before resorting to an operation. Maffulli indicated that if surgical intervention is inevitable, fixation using devices with a low profile should be prioritized [31]. Pinning fractured bones using K-wires is a reliable approach in treating boxer's fracture. Compared with plate fixation, K-wire fixation requires less soft tissue dissection [9] and thus results in a lower rate of postoperative extensor tendon adhesion. Nonetheless, K-wire fixation does have some disadvantages, including exposed hardware, a longer period of immobilization, and lower resistance to angulation and rotational deformity force wire migration, and these disadvantages make this method inappropriate for some patients [32, 33]. Requiring much less soft tissue dissection than what is needed in plate fixation, K-wire and figure-of-eight cerclage wire fixation prevents K-wires from migrating, avoids hardware exposure, and has similar strength to plate fixation, resisting deformity forces and thus potentially reducing the postoperative immobilization period. The proposed surgical treatment modality (two K-wires and one figure-of-eight cerclage wire) had lower profile than plates, which may reduce complications caused by using a plate, including tendon irritation, joint stiffness, and metacarpal head ischemia necrosis. Regarding the cost-effectiveness, the costs of locking plate and regular

plate fixation at our institution are US$1500 and US$200, respectively, whereas that of KW fixation using two K-wires and one figure-of-eight cerclage wire is only US$5. Therefore, given our aforementioned results and the present discussion, we conclude that KW fixation is a feasible alternative fixation for treating fifth metacarpal neck fracture.

The approach of integrating a figure-of-eight cerclage wire to two K-wires and adopted in the present study was inspired by the use of tension band wiring (TBW) fixation [34] in a previous study to treat patella transverse fracture. TBW is widely employed to treat limb fractures, including distal clavicle fracture [35], olecranon fracture [36], and medial malleolar fracture [37]. The advantages of TBW are (1) higher antirotation force [3] compared with that in K-wire fixation, (2) higher antibending force compared with that in wire fixation, and (3) lower profile compared with the bone plate, which reduces tendon irritation. Therefore, bones heal more effectively when TBW is applied at the tension side of a fracture [38, 39]. In our proposed method, TBW is inserted in the dorsal side of the fractured fifth metacarpal neck because this fixation is mechanically advantageous. Usually, the fractured fifth metacarpal neck is tilted toward the palm because of the traction power of intrinsic muscle, meaning that the dorsal side is the tension side. By using the fixation of two K-wires and one figure-of-eight cerclage wire, the dorsal tension side became the compression side, enabling the dorsal volar cortex (fractured bones) to heal faster.

This study was subject to several limitations. First, to ensure that the specimens used had the same geometry and material properties, we used artificial bones to conduct experiments. Although artificial bones have been used previously [12, 40], they are not able to simulate the actual properties of human bones such as inhomogeneity and anisotropy and do not have the actual structure of trabecular bones. Second, as was the case in most previous in vitro biomechanical experiments, the fracture pattern created was a simple fracture [12, 16–18]. Third, we conducted cantilever bending tests to assess the fixation strength of the distinct fixation types, and such testing does not reflect all actual physiological conditions; in fact, no mechanical testing is able to reflect all actual physiological conditions. Fourth, as previous studies have indicated [18, 19], artificial and animal bones do not contain soft tissues such as muscles, ligaments, and tendons. Although the absolute values measured in this study will hence be different from those under actual conditions, we held that this difference would not influence the ranking of the four fixation types regarding their fixation strength. In the future, we will collect clinical results to evaluate the effect of soft tissue when the two K-wires and a figure-of-eight cerclage wire fixation approach is employed.

Conclusion

In this study, we proposed a new fixation approach with two K-wires and one figure-of-eight cerclage wire for treating fifth metacarpal neck fracture in patients for whom open reduction internal fixation is indicated. On the basis of the experimental design and limitations, we conclude that the figure-of-eight cerclage wire significantly increases the biomechanical stability of the two K-wires. The fixation strength of the proposed fixation is similar to that of a regular plate with five bicortical screws but weaker than that of a locking plate with five bicortical screws. Integrating a figure-of-eight cerclage wire with K-wires is an alternative fixation method that avoids the excessive soft tissue dissection that occurs in open reduction internal fixation for fifth metacarpal neck fracture.

Abbreviations
K group: Two K-wire group; KW group: Two K-wires and a figure-of-eight cerclage wire group; LP group: Locking plate with five locking bicortical screw group; RP group: Regular plate with five bicortical screw group; TBW: Tension band wiring

Funding
This work was supported by grants from the Ministry of Health and Welfare, Taiwan (MOHW107-TDU-B-212-123004). In addition, this study was partially supported by the Ministry of Science and Technology, Taiwan (MOST 106-2221-E-039-002).

Authors' contributions
YC, HCH, and JH participated in the design of the study. YC, CH, HLH, and JH carried out the measurement. YC, MT, CH, and JH carried out the statistical analysis. YC, MT, and JH conceived of the study, participated in its design and coordination, and drafted the manuscript. All authors read and approved the final manuscript.

Competing interests
No authors of this study have any financial and personal relationships with other people or organizations, which could result in an inappropriate influence of this study. The authors declare that they have no competing interests.

Author details
[1]School of Medicine, China Medical University, Taichung 404, Taiwan.
[2]Department of Orthopedic Surgery, China Medical University Hospital, Taichung 404, Taiwan, Republic of China. [3]Department of Biomedical Engineering, Hungkuang University, Taichung 433, Taiwan. [4]Department of Orthopaedics, Taichung Veterans General Hospital, Taichung 407, Taiwan.
[5]Sports Recreation and Health Management Continuing Studies-Bachelor's Degree Completion Program, Tunghai University, Taichung 407, Taiwan.
[6]School of Dentistry, College of Dentistry, China Medical University, 91 Hsueh-Shih Road, Taichung 40402, Taiwan. [7]Department of Bioinformatics and Medical Engineering, Asia University, Taichung 413, Taiwan.

References
1. Padegimas EM, Warrender WJ, Jones CM, Ilyas AM. Metacarpal neck fractures: a review of surgical indications and techniques. Arch Trauma Res. 2016;5(3):e32933.
2. Boussakri H, Elidrissi M, Azarkane M, Bensaad S, Bachiri M, Shimi M, Elibrahimi A, Elmrini A. Fractures of the neck of the fifth metacarpal bone, treated by percutaneous intramedullary nailing: surgical technique, radiological and clinical results study (28 cases). Pan Afr Med J. 2014;18:187.
3. Facca S, Ramdhian R, Pelissier A, Diaconu M, Liverneaux P. Fifth metacarpal neck fracture fixation: locking plate versus K-wire? Orthop Traumatol Surg Res. 2010;96(5):506–12.
4. Potenza V, Caterini R, De Maio F, Bisicchia S, Farsetti P. Fractures of the neck of the fifth metacarpal bone. Medium-term results in 28 cases treated by percutaneous transverse pinning. Injury. 2012;43(2):242–5.
5. Harris AR, Beckenbaugh RD, Nettrour JF, Rizzo M. Metacarpal neck fractures: results of treatment with traction reduction and cast immobilization. Hand (N Y). 2009;4(2):161–4.
6. Wong KP, Hay RA, Tay SC. Surgical outcomes of fifth metacarpal neck fractures—a comparative analysis of dorsal plating versus tension band wiring. Hand Surg. 2015;20(1):99–105.
7. Kollitz KM, Hammert WC, Vedder NB, Huang JI. Metacarpal fractures: treatment and complications. Hand (N Y). 2014;9(1):16–23.
8. Wong TC, Ip FK, Yeung SH. Comparison between percutaneous transverse fixation and intramedullary K-wires in treating closed fractures of the metacarpal neck of the little finger. J Hand Surg. 2006;31(1):61–5.
9. Schädel-Höpfner M, Wild M, Windolf J, Linhart W. Antegrade intramedullary splinting or percutaneous retrograde crossed pinning for displaced neck fractures of the fifth metacarpal? Arch Orthop Trauma Surg. 2007;127(6):435–40.
10. Winter M, Balaguer T, Bessiere C, Carles M, Lebreton E. Surgical treatment of the boxer's fracture: transverse pinning versus intramedullary pinning. J Hand Surg Eur Vol. 2007;32(6):709–13.
11. Leinberry C, Ukomadu U, Ilyas A, Metacarpal fractures and carpometacarpal fracture-dislocations. 1st ed New Delhi: Jaypee Brothers Medical Publishers Ltd;. 2013;
12. Barr C, Behn AW, Yao J. Plating of metacarpal fractures with locked or nonlocked screws, a biomechanical study: how many cortices are really necessary? Hand (N Y). 2013;8(4):454–9.
13. Malasitt P, Owen JR, Tremblay M-A, Wayne JS, Isaacs JE. Fixation for metacarpal neck fracture: a biomechanical study. Hand. 2015;10(3):438–43.
14. Ochman S, Vordemvenne T, Paletta J, Raschke MJ, Meffert RH, Doht S. Experimental fracture model versus osteotomy model in metacarpal bone plate fixation. TheScientificWorldJOURNAL. 2011;11:1692–8.
15. Nicklin S, Ingram S, Gianoutsos MP, Walsh WR. In vitro comparison of lagged and nonlagged screw fixation of metacarpal fractures in cadavers. J Hand Surg. 2008;33(10):1732–6.
16. Bozic KJ, Perez LE, Wilson DR, Fitzgibbons PG, Jupiter JB. Mechanical testing of bioresorbable implants for use in metacarpal fracture fixation. J Hand Surg. 2001;26(4):755–61.
17. Curtis BD, Fajolu O, Ruff ME, Litsky AS. Fixation of metacarpal shaft fractures: biomechanical comparison of intramedullary nail crossed K-wires and plate-screw constructs. Orthop Surg. 2015;7(3):256–60.
18. Liodaki E, Wendlandt R, Waizner K, Schopp BE, Mailander P, Stang F. A biomechanical analysis of plate fixation using unicortical and bicortical screws in transverse metacarpal fracture models subjected to 4-point bending and dynamical bending test. Medicine. 2017;96(27):e6926.
19. Elfar J, Stanbury S, Menorca RMG, Reed JD. Composite bone models in orthopaedic surgery research and education. J Am Acad Orthop Surg. 2014;22(2):111.
20. American Society for Testing and Materials A. ASTM F1839 - 08 Standard specification for rigid polyurethane foam for use as a standard material for testing orthopedic devices and instruments.

21. Doht S, Meffert RH, Raschke MJ, Blunk T, Ochman S. Biomechanical analysis of the efficacy of locking plates during cyclic loading in metacarpal fractures. TheScientificWorldJOURNAL. 2014;2014:648787.

22. Ochman S, Doht S, Paletta J, Langer M, Raschke MJ, Meffert RH. Comparison between locking and non-locking plates for fixation of metacarpal fractures in an animal model. J Hand Surg. 2010;35(4):597–603.

23. Eu-Jin Cheah A, Behn AW, Comer G, Yao J. A biomechanical analysis of 2 constructs for metacarpal spiral fracture fixation in a cadaver model: 2 large screws versus 3 small screws. J Hand Surg. 2017;42(12):1033 e1–6.

24. Black D, Mann R, Constine R, Daniels A. Comparison of internal fixation techniques in metacarpal fractures. J Hand Surg. 1985;10(4):466–72.

25. Firoozbakhsh KK, Moneim MS, Doherty W, Naraghi FF. Internal fixation of oblique metacarpal fractures. A biomechanical evaluation by impact loading. Clinical Orthopaedics and Related Research. 1996;325:296–301.

26. Mann R, Black D, Constine R, Daniels A. A quantitative comparison of metacarpal fracture stability with five different methods of internal fixation. J Hand Surg. 1985;10(6):1024–8.

27. Meunier MJ, Hentzen E, Ryan M, Shin AY, Lieber RL. Predicted effects of metacarpal shortening on interosseous muscle function. J Hand Surg. 2004;29(4):689–93.

28. Handoll H, Brealey S, Rangan A, Torgerson D, Dennis L, Armstrong A, Chuang L-H, Cross B, Dumville J, Gardner S. Protocol for the ProFHER (PROximal Fracture of the Humerus: Evaluation by Randomisation) trial: a pragmatic multi-centre randomised controlled trial of surgical versus non-surgical treatment for proximal fracture of the humerus in adults. BMC Musculoskelet Disord. 2009;10(1):140.

29. Handoll H, Keding A, Corbacho B, Brealey S, Hewitt C, Rangan A. Five-year follow-up results of the PROFHER trial comparing operative and non-operative treatment of adults with a displaced fracture of the proximal humerus. The Bone & Joint Journal. 2017;99(3):383–92.

30. Rangan A, Handoll H, Brealey S, Jefferson L, Keding A, Martin BC, Goodchild L, Chuang L-H, Hewitt C, Torgerson D. Surgical vs nonsurgical treatment of adults with displaced fractures of the proximal humerus: the PROFHER randomized clinical trial. JAMA. 2015;313(10):1037–47.

31. Maffulli N. We are operating too much. J Orthop Traumatol. 2017;18(4):289–92.

32. Sharma H, Taylor GR, Clarke NM. A review of K-wire related complications in the emergency management of paediatric upper extremity trauma. Ann R Coll Surg Engl. 2007;89(3):252–8.

33. Wong KY, Mole R, Gillespie P. Kirschner wire breakage during removal requiring retrieval. Case reports in surgery. 2016;2016:7515760.

34. Osteotomies MM, Müller ME, Allgöwer M, Schneider R, et al., editors. Manual of internal fixation: techniques recommended by the AO-ASIF Group. Berlin Heidelberg New York: Springer-Verlag; 1979.

35. Kao F-C, Chao E-K, Chen C-H, Yu S-W, Chen C-Y, Yen C-Y. Treatment of distal clavicle fracture using Kirschner wires and tension-band wires. J Trauma Acute Care Surg. 2001;51(3):522–5.

36. Claessen F, van den Bekerom MPJ, van Dijk CN, Carel Goslings J, Kerkhoffs G, Doornberg JN. Tension band wiring for simple olecranon fractures: evaluation of surgical technique. J Orthop Traumatol : official journal of the Italian Society of Orthopaedics and Traumatology. 2017;18(3):275–81.

37. Ostrum RF, Litsky AS. Tension band fixation of medial malleolus fractures. J Orthop Trauma. 1992;6(4):464–8.

38. Ali M, Kuiper J, John J. Biomechanical analysis of tension band wiring (TBW) of transverse fractures of patella. Chin J Traumatol. 2016;19(5):255–8.

39. Zens M, Goldschmidtboeing F, Wagner F, Reising K, Sudkamp NP, Woias P. Polydimethylsiloxane pressure sensors for force analysis in tension band wiring of the olecranon. Technol Health Care : official journal of the European Society for Engineering and Medicine. 2016;24(6):909–17.

40. Hiatt SV, Begonia MT, Thiagarajan G, Hutchison RL. Biomechanical comparison of 2 methods of intramedullary K-wire fixation of transverse metacarpal shaft fractures. J Hand Surg. 2015;40(8):1586–90.

14

Roles and mechanisms of leptin in osteogenic stimulation in cervical ossification of the posterior longitudinal ligament

Bin Feng[†], Shiliang Cao[†], Jiliang Zhai, Yi Ren, Jianhua Hu, Ye Tian[*] and Xisheng Weng[*] (iD)

Abstract

Background: Hyperleptinemia is a common feature of obese people, and leptin, an adipocyte-derived cytokine, is believed to be an important factor in the pathogenesis of cervical ossification of the posterior longitudinal ligament(C-OPLL). So this research was to identify the relation between the serum leptin and bone metabolic markers and how the leptin induced osteogenic effect in C-OPLL.

Methods: Sixty-four samples were selected to determine the concentration of leptin, insulin, and alkaline phosphatase. And the association of leptin with these factors was also examined. We also evaluate the effect of leptin on the development of C-OPLL and further explored the possible underlying mechanism in vitro.

Results: We found that serum leptin concentrations were higher in females than in males. Serum leptin and ALP concentrations were increased significantly in C-OPLL females compared to non-OPLL females. In OPLL subjects, the serum leptin concentration corrected for body mass index correlated negatively with the ALP concentrations. In C-OPLL cells, leptin treatment led to a significant increase in mRNA expressions of ALP and OCN and formation of mineralized nodule. Our experiments reported here that osteogenic effect of leptin in C-OPLL cells could be mediated via ERK1/2, p38 MAPK, and/or JNK signaling pathways.

Conclusions: From this research, we got that leptin treatment led to a significant increase in mRNA expressions of ALP and OCN and formation of mineralized nodule. And the osteogenic effect of leptin in C-OPLL cells could be mediated via ERK1/2, p38 MAPK, and/or JNK signaling pathways.

Keywords: Leptin, Ossification of the posterior longitudinal ligament (OPLL), Gender, Bone metabolic markers, Signaling pathway

Background

Ossification of the posterior longitudinal ligament (OPLL) is a common musculoskeletal disease, characterized by ectopic bone formation of the spinal ligament preferentially at the cervical spine [1, 2]. As OPLL commonly involved in cervical spine resulting in myelopathy or radiculopathy, in this condition, we said it cervical OPLL(C-OPLL). Enlarged ossified ligament compresses

the spinal cord and nerve roots, eventually leads to the neurological deficit [3, 4]. Its prevalence is higher among Asian populations, and in Chinese populations, the average prevalence is reported to be 3.08% [5–8].

Although the exact pathogenesis of C-OPLL remains unclear, leptin is supposed to be an important factor in the pathogenesis of C-OPLL. Leptin, a product of the ob gene which is expressed by adipocyte tissue and released into circulation, is a prominent regulator of body weight and fat [9, 10]. Investigations have indicated that leptin can stimulate the proliferation and osteogenic differentiation of embryonic cells, bone marrow stromal cells (BMSCs), and osteoblastic cells [11–13]. Leptin has been found to have

* Correspondence: TianYe@pumch.cn; DoctorWXS@126.com
[†]Bin Feng and Shiliang Cao contributed equally to this work.
Department of Orthopedics Surgery, Peking Union Medical College Hospital, Chinese Academy of Medical Sciences & Peking Union Medical College, Beijing 100730, China

both positive and negative effects on bone mass [14]. Leptin positively regulates bone formation through direct actions on bone, when administrated peripherally [10, 15], and suppresses bone formation and increases resorption through a hypothalamic relay, when infused centrally [16]. Previous study indicates that serum leptin may be associated with the development of heterotopic ossification of the spinal ligament [17]. However, the association between leptin and OPLL is still controversial and needs to be clarified further. And the mechanism of leptin in the development of OPLL has seldom been studied.

In this study, to clarify the association between leptin and C-OPLL, we measured serum leptin concentrations in C-OPLL patients and non-OPLL controls and corrected these levels using individual body mass index (BMI). Then, we analyzed the possible mechanism of leptin in the development of OPLL in vitro.

Methods

Patients

Totally, 64 samples were used for the research, including 35 cervical OPLL (24 males and 11 females) patients who underwent anterior cervical decompression surgery and 29 non-OPLL (15 males and 14 females) controls; the majority of who had cervical degenerative disorders were enrolled into this study. The diagnosis of cervical OPLL was confirmed by computer tomography (CT), X-ray photographs, and magnetic resonance imaging (MRI) of the cervical spine. This study was approved by the Ethics Committee of Peking Union Medical College Hospital, and informed consents were obtained from all patients.

Previous data indicated that there are important gender-based differences in the regulation and action of leptin in humans, and leptin levels are higher in women than in men. We subdivided the OPLL and non-OPLL groups according to gender. The mean age of OPLL males, non-OPLL males, OPLL females, and non-OPLL females was 59.04 ± 9.32, 57.40 ± 11.04, 57.25 ± 8.68, and 61.95 ± 10.93 years, respectively. The mean BMI (weight in kilograms divided by the square of height in meters) of the four groups was 26.47 ± 3.46, 25.26 ± 4.46, 25.49 ± 3.05, and 24.1 ± 3.37 kg/m^2, respectively.

Blood samples

Blood samples were collected from all patients between 8:00 and 10:00 after overnight fasting and the serum immediately frozen at -80 °C until analysis. Serum leptin and insulin concentrations were measured using a commercially available enzyme-linked immunosorbent assay (ELISA) kit (Elabscience). The serum concentrations of bone formation markers, alkaline phosphatase (ALP), were measured using BCIP/NBT ALP Color Development Kit (Beyotime Biotechnology). The

concentration of glycosylated serum protein (GSP), which can effectively reflect the average glucose concentration of the patients in the past 2~3 weeks, was also detected using GSP test kit (Solarbio life sciences).

Spinal ligament samples

During the anterior cervical decompression surgery, posterior longitudinal ligament specimens were aseptically harvested from OPLL patients and rinsed with phosphate-buffered saline. Surrounding tissue was carefully removed under a dissecting microscope.

Cell cultures

The collected ligaments were mincing into approximately 0.5 mm^3 pieces and washed twice with phosphate-buffered saline (PBS). Then, the ligament fragments were plated into 6 cm culture dishes and maintained in low-glucose Dulbecco's modified Eagle's media (DMEM) (supplemented with 10% FBS, 1% L-glutamine, 100 units/ml of penicillin G sodium, 10 mM-glycerophosphate, and 100 µg/ml of streptomycin sulfate) in a humidified atmosphere of 95% air and 5% CO_2 at 37 °C. The cells derived from the explants were removed from the dishes with 0.02% EDTA, 0.05% trypsin for further passage. The first to third passage cells were used in the following study.

CCK8 assay

Cell proliferation was measured by CCK8 dye reduction assay. Briefly, 5×10^3 cells were seeded into 96-well plates overnight and exposed to the leptin at distinct concentrations (0, 50, 100, 200, 400 ng/ml) for different times (4 and 7 days). Then, the cells were incubated with 10 µl of CCK8 for 1 h at 37 °C. The absorbance was measured at 450 nm using a microplate reader.

Real-time PCR

3×10^6 cells in logarithmic phase were plated into 6-well dishes for 24 h, then the cells were exposed to the leptin at different concentrations (0, 50, 100, 200 ng/ml). After 96 h, total RNA was extracted from the cells using Trizol reagents (Invitrogen), and the RNA concentration was detected. Two micrograms of total RNA were reverse-transcribed using Reverse Transcription Kit (Invitrogen) for real time-PCR (RT-PCR). Primers used for amplification were as follows: ALP, 5′-TCCCAGTTG AGGAGGAGAA-3′ (forward), 5′-CCAGGAAGATGAT GAGGTTC-3′ (reverse); osteocalcin (OCN), 5′-AGCG AGGTAGTGAAGAGAC-3′ (forward), 5′-CCTGAAAGC CGATGTGGT-3′ (reverse); β-actin, 5′-ATCATGTTTGA GACCTTCAACA-3′(forward), 5′-CATCTCTTGCTCGA AGTCCA3′ (reverse). Polymerase chain reaction amplification was carried out in a volume of 25 µl containing 12.5 µl 2× PCR mix, 10.5 µl nuclease-free water, 1 µl cDNA, and 1 μl primer. The melting curves were also prepared during the amplifications. All products were normalized to β-actin mRNA levels. Each specimen was repeated three times.

Mineralization assay

1×10^4 cells were plated into 12-well dishes and maintained in DMEM with 10% FBS. On confluence, designated day 0, cells were exposed to leptin medium containing DMEM supplemented with 10% FBS, 1% L-glutamine, 100 units/ml of penicillin G sodium and 100 μg/ml of streptomycin sulfate, 10 mM-glycerophosphate, and 100 ng/ml leptin. Alizarin red assay (Sigma) was performed at 72 and 96 h to determine the mineralization. Briefly, cells were washed with D-hank's and fixed with 4% paraformaldehyde for 20–30 min at room temperature. Fixed cultures were incubated with 1% alizarin red for 20–30 min at 37 °C and washed with distilled water for three times to remove the excessive dye. Extracellular matrix mineral-bound stains were visualized and photographed under a microscope.

ALP activity assay

ALP activity was evaluated using commercially available kits. Cells were cultured in 6-well plates for 3–5 h and exposed to the leptin at different concentrations (0, 50, 100, 200 ng/ml). After 96 h, cells were washed with PBS and fixed in 4% polyoxymethylene for 10 min, and stained with BCIP/NBT ALP Color Development Kit (Beyotime Biotechnology) according to the manufacturer's instructions.

Western blotting

Cells were harvested, and equal amounts of protein were loaded onto 10% sodium dodecyl sulfate polyacrylamide gel electrophoresis (SDS–PAGE) gels for 2 h at 100 V and subsequently transferred onto polyvinylidene difluoride (PVDF) membranes (Millipore). The membrane was blocked with 5% skim milk for 1 h at room temperature. After washing three times with Tris-buffered saline (TBS) containing 0.1% Tween 20 (TBST), the membranes were incubated with appropriately diluted Phospho-p44/42 MAPK, p44/42 MAPK, Phospho-JNK/SAPK, JNK/SAPK, Phospho-p38 MAPK, and p38 MAPK (Beyotime, Shanghai, China) antibodies at 4 °C overnight. Then, the membranes were washed as before and incubated with horseradish peroxidase-conjugated secondary antibodies (anti-mouse or anti-rabbit) for 1 h at room temperature. After that, these membranes were washed thoroughly, to eliminate the unspecific antibody. At last, proteins were detected using enhanced chemiluminescence (ECL) blotting reagents according to the manufacturer's instruction.

Statistical analysis

Data was analyzed using mean ± SD. Student's t test was used to compare the data between OPLL and non-OPLL groups. Tukey's multiple comparison test was used to analyze the variance of the data and to estimate the level of significance. $p < 0.05$ was considered significant.

Results

Serum leptin concentrations and leptin/BMI ratios in OPLL and non-OPLL patients

As shown in Table 1, compared with the male subjects, both non-OPLL and OPLL groups had significantly higher serum leptin concentration in females. In females, serum leptin/BMI ratio in the OPLL group was 1.6-fold higher than that in the non-OPLL group ($p < 0.05$); meanwhile, serum concentrations of bone metabolism biomarkers ALP also increased significantly ($p < 0.05$). However, in male subjects, there was no obvious difference in serum leptin concentration between the OPLL and non-OPLL groups, and ALP concentrations showed no difference either. The serum insulin concentrations were higher in OPLL groups than that in non-OPLL groups in both female and male subjects. However, the difference was not statistically significant.

Table 1 Clinical characteristics of female and male OPLL and serum concentration of leptin, insulin, and ALP

Female OPLL versus non-OPLL			
	Non-OPLL ($n = 14$)	OPLL ($n = 11$)	p (Student's t)
Age (year)	61.95 ± 10.93	57.25 ± 8.68	N.S.
Height (cm)	1.61 ± 0.05	1.62 ± 0.05	N.S.
Weight (kg)	62.79 ± 9.86	66.83 ± 10.55	N.S.
BMI (kg/m)	24.10 ± 3.37	25.49 ± 3.05	N.S.
Serum leptin (ng/ml)	22.30 ± 9.21	37.68 ± 25.22	< 0.05
Leptin/BMI	0.93 ± 0.33	1.50 ± 0.97	< 0.05
Serum insulin (μU/ml)	19.00 ± 8.60	22.90 ± 13.20	N.S.
Serum ALP	7.17 ± 1.11	8.05 ± 0.73	< 0.05
Male OPLL versus non-OPLL			
	Non-OPLL ($n = 15$)	OPLL ($n = 24$)	p (Student's t)
Age (year)	57.4 ± 11.04	59.04 ± 9.32	N.S.
Height (cm)	170 ± 4.20	170 ± 7.07	N.S.
Weight (kg)	73.53 ± 13.68	76.61 ± 12.99	N.S.
BMI (kg/m)	25.26 ± 4.46	26.47 ± 3.46	N.S.
Serum leptin (ng/ml)	13.45 ± 6.32	16.69 ± 6.90	N.S.
leptin/BMI	0.52 ± 0.19	0.65 ± 0.25	N.S.
Serum insulin (μU/ml)	22.10 ± 11.00	29.20 ± 30.00	N.S.
Serum ALP	7.25 ± 1.57	7.97 ± 1.63	N.S.

Correlation of leptin/BMI with serum insulin and biochemical maker, ALP

To determine the factors associated with the leptin/BMI ratio in OPLL subjects, we examined the correlation between leptin/BMI ratios and serum insulin, ALP level (Fig. 1). There was only a relatively weak, non-significant positive correlation between the leptin/BMI ratio and serum insulin in females. In contrast, in male groups, the serum insulin concentration showed a weak, non-significant negative correlation with the leptin/BMI ratio. ALP concentrations were correlated negatively with the leptin/BMI ratio both in OPLL male groups and female groups, whereas male OPLL groups showed a significant correlation ($r = -0.473$, $p < 0.05$). There was no significant correlation between the leptin/BMI ratios and serum insulin, ALP level, in non-OPLL subjects (data not shown).

Effect of leptin on the proliferation of OPLL cells

To investigate the molecular mechanism underlying leptin-stimulated OPLL, the effect of leptin on cell proliferation of OPLL cells was evaluated by CCK8 method. As shown in Fig. 2, the leptin had no significant effect on the proliferation of OPLL cells with various leptin concentration (0, 50, 100, 200 ng/ml) at different periods of time (4 and 9 days).

Effect of leptin on the osteogenic differentiation of OPLL cells

We then examined the osteogenic differentiation of OPLL cells by RT-PCR and ALP activity assay. RT-PCR analysis showed that leptin treatment resulted in a significant increase in mRNA expression of ALP and osteocalcin (OCN) in OPLL cells, and the effect was most obvious at 50 ng/ml leptin concentration (Fig. 3a, b). ALP activity assay demonstrated that the activity of ALP was significantly elevated in response to leptin stimulation in OPLL cells, and the effect was dose-dependent (Fig. 3c).

Apart from makers of osteogenic differentiation, we further examined the formation of mineralized nodules by alizarin red staining. Mineralization assays showed that under 100 ng/ml leptin stimulation, the cell matrix began to mineralize, and crystals appeared at 72 h. The mineralized nodules increased significantly at 96 h (Fig. 4a, b indicated by red arrows), compared with the absence of leptin treatment OPLL cells. There was no mineralization observed in the negative control (NC) group.

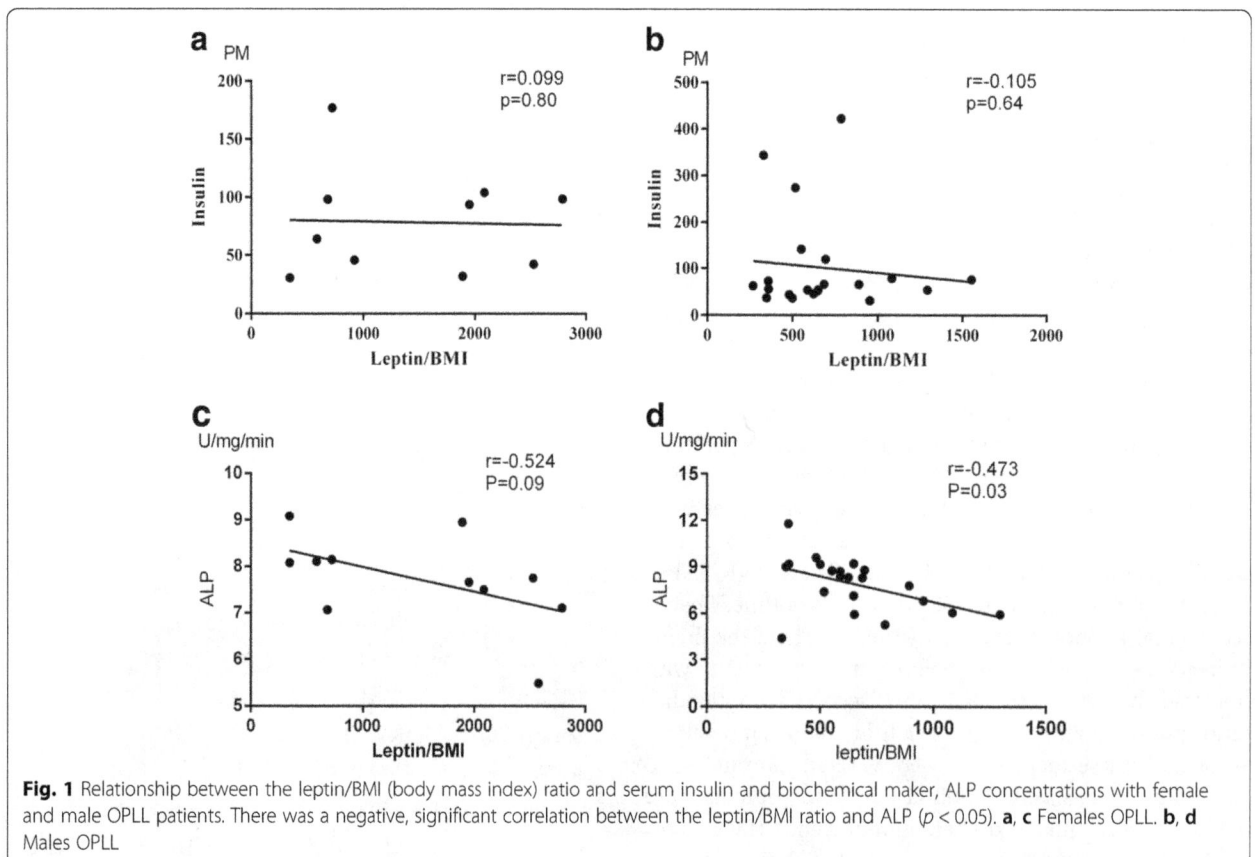

Fig. 1 Relationship between the leptin/BMI (body mass index) ratio and serum insulin and biochemical maker, ALP concentrations with female and male OPLL patients. There was a negative, significant correlation between the leptin/BMI ratio and ALP ($p < 0.05$). **a, c** Females OPLL. **b, d** Males OPLL

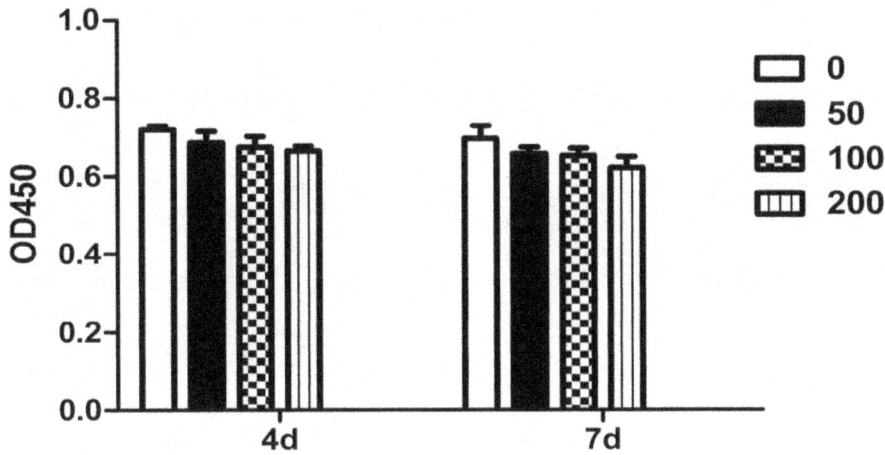

Fig. 2 Effect of leptin on the proliferation of OPLL cells

Pathways involved in the leptin-stimulated osteogenic differentiation of OPLL cells

To learn more about the mechanism underlying the osteogenic effect of leptin, we further examined the status of ERK, JNK, and p38 phosphorylation in response to leptin treatment in OPLL cells. Proteins were extracted from OPLL cells at different time after 100 ng/ml leptin treatment. The immunoblot results showed that leptin stimulated the phosphorylation of ERK1/2, p38 MAPK, and JNK in a time-dependent manner and the effect was most obvious at 1 h, while the total expression levels of ERK1/2, p38 MAPK, and JNK were unchanged over the time of leptin treatment (Fig. 5).

Discussion

Many investigations have indicated that leptin is involved in many bone diseases [18–21]. OPLL is a common bone disease caused by heterotopic bone formation

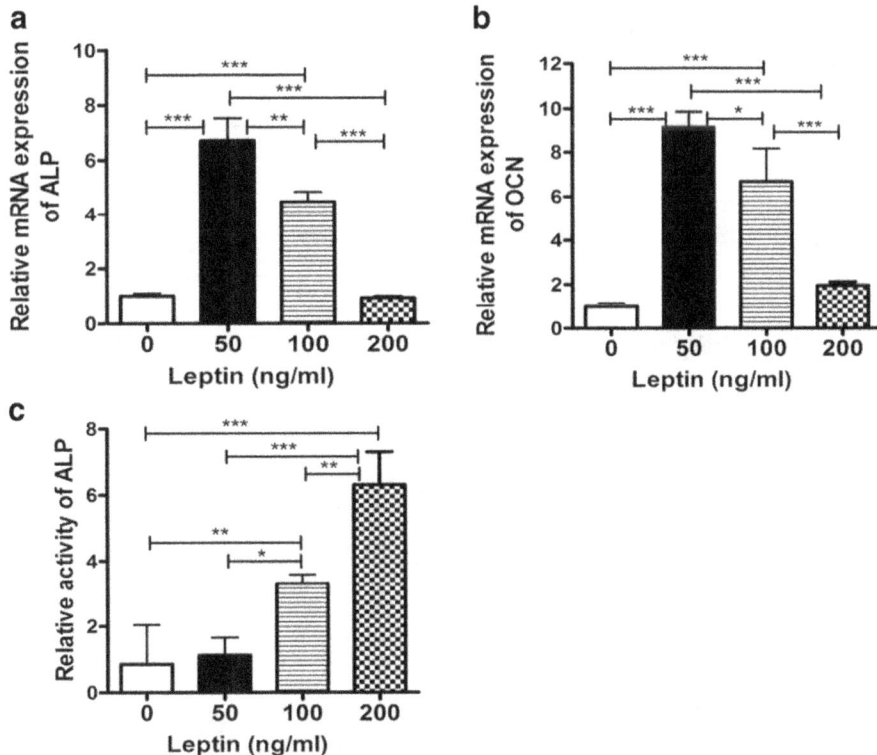

Fig. 3 Effects of leptin on osteocalcin and ALP mRNA expressions and activity in OPLL cells. **a** ALP mRNA expression. **b** OCN mRNA expression. **c** ALP activity measurement. $*p < 0.05$; $**p < 0.001$; $***p < 0.0001$

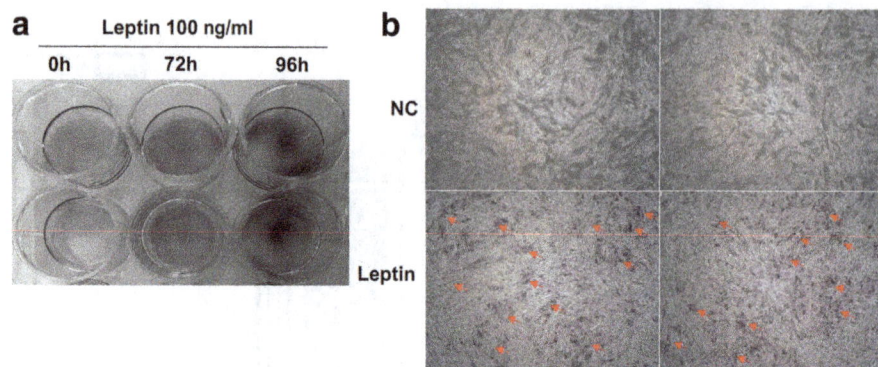

Fig. 4 Effects of leptin on the formation of mineralized nodules in OPLL cells. **a** Different time points of leptin stimulation. **b** Leptin (100 ng/ml) stimulated for 96 h. Mineralized nodules are indicated by red arrows in the figure. NC, negative control

of the posterior longitudinal ligament. Obesity is considered to be the major risk factor of OPLL [5, 22]. Recent studies showed that hyperleptinemia, a common feature of obese people, was closely correlated with OPLL [18]. These studies suggest that leptin, an adipocyte-derived cytokine, plays a critical role in connecting at molecular levels the phenotypical manifestation of obesity and the pathological development of OPLL.

In this study, we firstly determined the association between serum leptin concentration and bone metabolic markers in patients with OPLL. Our results demonstrated that female subjects had significantly higher serum leptin concentration compared with male subjects, in both

OPLL and non-OPLL groups. Serum leptin/BMI ratio in the OPLL groups was higher than that in the non-OPLL groups ($p < 0.05$) in female subjects. However, there was no obvious difference in the male subjects. Further analysis indicated that the leptin/BMI ratio correlated negatively with the ALP concentrations in both OPLL male and female groups, whereas male groups showed a significant correlation ($r = -0.473$, $p < 0.05$). Nevertheless, there were only 11 subjects, and the individual difference was great, which resulted in no statistically significant difference. This result suggests that leptin can inhibit bone formation in vivo, which was in accordance with the report of Elefteriou et al. [23], which demonstrated in

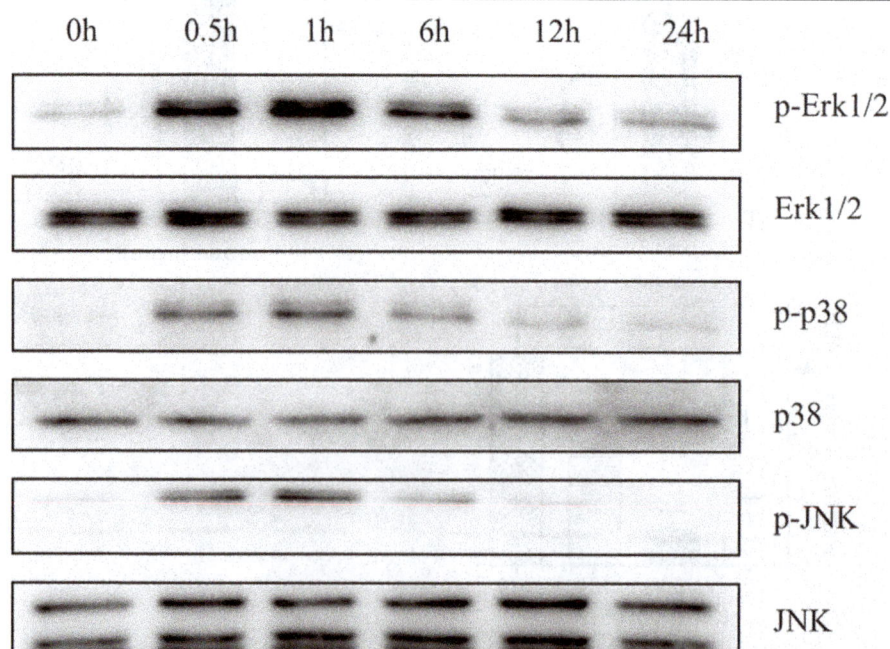

Fig. 5 Activation of ERK1/2, p38MAPK, and JNK signaling pathway in OPLL cells after 100 ng/ml leptin treatment

animal experiments that leptin was a determinant of bone formation and leptin anti-osteogenic function was conserved in vertebrates. We also found that in the female group, the leptin/BMI ratio was weakly correlated positively with serum insulin levels in female OPLL, whereas the negative correlation was observed in male OPLL group, which was consistent with the previous studies [17, 24, 25].

To further validate the role of leptin in OPLL, we performed OPLL cell differentiation experiments in vitro. And the cell experiments were derived from multiple individuals. We found that leptin treatment can lead to a significant increase in mRNA expressions of ALP and OCN in OPLL cells; the effect was most significant at 50 ng/ml leptin concentration. ALP activity assay demonstrated that the activity of ALP was significantly elevated in response to leptin stimulation in a dose-dependent manner in OPLL cells. Furthermore, leptin can induce the cell matrix mineralization, nodules, and crystals in OPLL cells, whereas it had no appreciable effect on the proliferation of OPLL cells. Our findings prove that leptin plays an important role in osteogenic differentiation and mineralization of OPLL cells, which is consistent with the previous reports [26–28] that peripheral leptin was essential for normal bone resorption and enhancement of bone formation.

At the same time, in this study, we try to confirm the molecular mechanism involved in leptin-stimulated osteogenesis in OPLL cells. It is believed that leptin exerted its biological function through binding to its receptors, which in turn transduced the signal through the activation of specific pathways. Previous studies indicated that leptin can activate many signaling pathways involving the JK/signal transducer and activator of transcription (JAK/STAT), as well as PI3-K and MAPK, to regulate chondrocyte differentiation [29–33]. However, the involvement in leptin induction of osteogenic differentiation has not been studied. In our study, we found that leptin increased the expressions of ALP and OCN in a dose-dependent manner and the formation of mineralized nodule. At the same time, the phosphorylation of ERK1/2, JNK, and p38MAPK was activated by leptin. In summary, these results indicated that ERK1/2, JNK, and p38MAPK might be the signaling pathways mediating leptin-stimulated osteogenic differentiation in OPLL cells. This was helpful for the further studies on investigating the molecular mechanism underlying osteogenic commitment of OPLL cells.

The main limitation in this study was that the sample size was small, especially in the OPLL female group, which resulted in no statistically significant difference of the serum insulin concentrations between OPLL and non-OPLL females, as well as no significant correlations between leptin and both insulin and ALP. Nevertheless, even with the limitation of the sample size, in this study, our results were consistent with the results of preceding studies.

In conclusion, we found that leptin may negatively regulate bone formation in vivo, through a central hypothalamic relay, whereas positively promoted the osteogenic differentiation in vitro through the peripheral pathway as previous studies report [23, 28, 34]. Furthermore, activated ERK1/2, JNK, and p38MAPK signaling pathways might mediate leptin-stimulated osteogenic differentiation in OPLL cells. The results of our research may have significant enlightenment in understanding the mechanisms of spinal ligament growth. And further studies are needed to confirm our findings and to evaluate other possible mechanisms involved.

Conclusions

From this research, we found that serum leptin concentration was higher in female subjects compared with male subjects in both C-OPLL and non-OPLL groups. Serum leptin and ALP concentrations increased significantly in C-OPLL female compared to non-OPLL female. In both male and female with OPLL, the serum leptin concentration corrected for BMI correlated negatively with the ALP concentrations. In C-OPLL cells, leptin treatment led to a significant increase in mRNA expressions of ALP and OCN and the formation of mineralized nodule. The osteogenic effect of leptin in C-OPLL cells might be mediated via ERK1/2, p38 MAPK, and/or JNK signaling pathways.

Abbreviation
ALP: Alkaline phosphatase activity; CCK-8: Cell Counting Kit-8; C-OPLL: Cervical OPLL; DMEM: Dulbecco's modified Eagle's medium; ERK: Extracellular signal-regulated kinase; FBS: Fetal bovine serum; GSP: Glycosylated serum protein; JNK: c-Jun NH2-terminal kinase; MAPK: Mitogen-activated protein kinase; OCN: Osteocalcin; OPLL: Ossification of the posterior longitudinal ligament

Acknowledgements
We acknowledge the assistance of Peking Union Medical College Central Laboratory with the technical guidance.

Funding
This study was supported by a grant from the National Natural Science Foundation of Youth in China (No. 81401758).

Authors' contributions
SLC and YR performed the experiments. JLZ and JHH analyzed and interpreted the data. BF, XSW, and YT devised the experiments and wrote the manuscript, with input from all co-authors. All authors read and approved the final manuscript.

Competing interests

The authors declare that they have no competing interests.

References

1. Chen Y, Wang X, Yang H, et al. Upregulated expression of PERK in spinal ligament fibroblasts from the patients with ossification of the posterior longitudinal ligament. Eur Spine J. 2014;23:447–54.
2. Shi L, Cai G, Shi J, et al. Ossification of the posterior ligament is mediated by osterix via inhibition of the beta-catenin signaling pathway. Exp Cell Res. 2016;349:53–9.
3. Matsunaga S, Kukita M, Hayashi K, et al. Pathogenesis of myelopathy in patients with ossification of the posterior longitudinal ligament. J Neurosurg. 2002;96:168–72.
4. Kawaguchi Y, Nakano M, Yasuda T, et al. Serum biomarkers in patients with ossification of the posterior longitudinal ligament (OPLL): inflammation in OPLL. PLoS One. 2017;12:e0174881.
5. Nakajima M, Takahashi A, Tsuji T, et al. A genome-wide association study identifies susceptibility loci for ossification of the posterior longitudinal ligament of the spine. Nat Genet. 2014;46:1012–6.
6. Nakajima M, Kou I, Ohashi H, et al. Identification and functional characterization of RSPO2 as a susceptibility gene for ossification of the posterior longitudinal ligament of the spine. Am J Hum Genet. 2016;99:202–7.
7. Tanaka T, Ikari K, Furushima K, et al. Genomewide linkage and linkage disequilibrium analyses identify COL6A1, on chromosome 21, as the locus for ossification of the posterior longitudinal ligament of the spine. Am J Hum Genet. 2003;73:812–22.
8. Tsuyama N. Ossification of the posterior longitudinal ligament of the spine. Clin Orthop Relat Res. 1984;(184):71–84.
9. Jiang H, Chen Y, Chen G, et al. Leptin accelerates the pathogenesis of heterotopic ossification in rat tendon tissues via mTORC1 signaling. J Cell Physiol. 2018;233(2):1017–28.
10. Philbrick KA, Wong CP, Branscum AJ, et al. Leptin stimulates bone formation in ob/ob mice at doses having minimal impact on energy metabolism. J Endocrinol. 2017;232:461–74.
11. Fan D, Chen Z, Chen Y, et al. Mechanistic roles of leptin in osteogenic stimulation in thoracic ligament flavum cells. J Biol Chem. 2007;282:29958–66.
12. Zheng B, Jiang J, Luo K, et al. Increased osteogenesis in osteoporotic bone marrow stromal cells by overexpression of leptin. Cell Tissue Res. 2015;361:845–56.
13. Lamghari M, Tavares L, Camboa N, et al. Leptin effect on RANKL and OPG expression in MC3T3-E1 osteoblasts. J Cell Biochem. 2006;98:1123–9.
14. Motyl KJ, Rosen CJ. Understanding leptin-dependent regulation of skeletal homeostasis. Biochimie. 2012;94:2089–96.
15. Steppan CM, Crawford DT, Chidsey-Frink KL, et al. Leptin is a potent stimulator of bone growth in ob/ob mice. Regul Pept. 2000;92:73–8.
16. Ducy P, Amling M, Takeda S, et al. Leptin inhibits bone formation through a hypothalamic relay: a central control of bone mass. Cell. 2000;100:197–207.
17. Ikeda Y, Nakajima A, Aiba A, et al. Association between serum leptin and bone metabolic markers, and the development of heterotopic ossification of the spinal ligament in female patients with ossification of the posterior longitudinal ligament. Eur Spine J. 2011;20:1450–8.

18. Shirakura Y, Sugiyama T, Tanaka H, et al. Hyperleptinemia in female patients with ossification of spinal ligaments. Biochem Biophys Res Commun. 2000;267:752–5.
19. Scotece M, Mobasheri A. Leptin in osteoarthritis: focus on articular cartilage and chondrocytes. Life Sci. 2015;140:75–8.
20. Upadhyay J, Farr OM, Mantzoros CS. The role of leptin in regulating bone metabolism. Metabolism. 2015;64:105–13.
21. Vuolteenaho K, Koskinen A, Moilanen E. Leptin—a link between obesity and osteoarthritis. Applications for prevention and treatment. Basic Clin Pharmacol Toxicol. 2014;114:103–8.
22. Shingyouchi Y, Nagahama A, Niida M. Ligamentous ossification of the cervical spine in the late middle-aged Japanese men. Its relation to body mass index and glucose metabolism. Spine. 1996;21:2474–8.
23. Elefteriou F, Takeda S, Ebihara K, et al. Serum leptin level is a regulator of bone mass. Proc Natl Acad Sci U S A. 2004;101:3258–63.
24. Akune T, Ogata N, Seichi A, et al. Insulin secretory response is positively associated with the extent of ossification of the posterior longitudinal ligament of the spine. J Bone Joint Surg. 2001;83a:1537–44.
25. Dagogo-Jack S, Fanelli C, Paramore D, et al. Plasma leptin and insulin relationships in obese and nonobese humans. Diabetes. 1996;45:695–8.
26. Cornish J, Callon K, Bava U, et al. Leptin directly regulates bone cell function in vitro and reduces bone fragility in vivo. J Endocrinol. 2002;175:405–15.
27. Zheng B, Jiang J, Chen Y, et al. Leptin overexpression in bone marrow stromal cells promotes periodontal regeneration in a rat model of osteoporosis. J Periodontol. 2017;88:808–18.
28. Turner RT, Kalra SP, Wong CP, et al. Peripheral leptin regulates bone formation. J Bone Miner Res Off J Am Soc Bone Miner Res. 2013;28:22–34.
29. Ben-Eliezer M, Phillip M, Gat-Yablonski G. Leptin regulates chondrogenic differentiation in ATDC5 cell-line through JAK/STAT and MAPK pathways. Endocrine. 2007;32:235–44.
30. Nepal M, Li L, Cho HK, et al. Kaempferol induces chondrogenesis in ATDC5 cells through activation of ERK/BMP-2 signaling pathway. Food Chem Toxicol. 2013;62:238–45.
31. Oh HK, Choi YS, Yang YI, et al. Leptin receptor is induced in endometriosis and leptin stimulates the growth of endometriotic epithelial cells through the JAK2/STAT3 and ERK pathways. Mol Hum Reprod. 2013;19:160–8.
32. Ohba S, Lanigan TM, Roessler BJ. Leptin receptor JAK2/STAT3 signaling modulates expression of Frizzled receptors in articular chondrocytes. Osteoarthr Cartil. 2010;18:1620–9.
33. Otero M, Lago R, Gómez R, et al. Phosphatidylinositol 3-kinase, MEK-1 and p38 mediate leptin/interferon-gamma synergistic NOS type II induction in chondrocytes. Life Sci. 2007;81:1452–60.
34. Chen XX, Yang T. Roles of leptin in bone metabolism and bone diseases. J Bone Miner Metab. 2015;33:474–85.

15

Calcar screws and adequate reduction reduced the risk of fixation failure in proximal humeral fractures treated with a locking plate: 190 patients followed for a mean of 3 years

Sjur Oppebøen[1]* ⓘ, Annette K. B. Wikerøy[1], Hendrik F. S. Fuglesang[1,2], Filip C. Dolatowski[1,2] and Per-Henrik Randsborg[1]

Abstract

Background: Fixation of proximal humeral fractures (PHF) with locking plates has gained popularity over conservative treatment, but surgery may be complicated with infection, non-union, avascular necrosis (AVN) of the humeral head and fixation failure. Failure to achieve structural support of the medial column has been suggested to be an important risk factor for fixation failure. The aims of this study were to examine the effect of calcar screws and fracture reduction on the risk of fixation failure and to assess long-term shoulder pain and function.

Methods: This was a single-centre retrospective study of 190 adult PHF patients treated with a locking plate between 2011 and 2014. Reoperations due to fixation failure were the primary outcome. Risk factors for fixation failure were assessed using the Cox regression analysis. Postoperative shoulder pain and function were assessed by the Oxford Shoulder Score (OSS).

Results: Thirty-one of 190 (16%) patients underwent a reoperation: 14 (7%) due to fixation failure, 10 (5%) due to deep infection and 2 (1%) due to AVN. The absence of calcar screws and fixation with residual varus malalignment (head-shaft angle < 120°) both increased the risk of fixation failure with an adjusted hazard ratio (95% CI) of 8.6 (1.9–39.3; $p = 0.005$) and 4.9 (1.3–17.9; $p = 0.02$), respectively. The median (interquartile range) OSS was 40 (27–46).

Conclusion: The use of calcar screws, as well as the absence of postoperative varus malalignment, significantly reduced the risk of fixation failure. We, therefore, recommend the use of calcar screws and to avoid residual varus malalignment to improve the medial support of proximal humeral fractures treated with a locking plate.

Keywords: Proximal humeral fracture, Locking plate fixation, Fixation failure, Calcar screws, Reoperation, Long-term shoulder function

* Correspondence: sjur_oppeboen@hotmail.com
[1]Department of Orthopaedic Surgery, Akershus University Hospital, Lørenskog, Norway
Full list of author information is available at the end of the article

Background

Proximal humeral fractures (PHFs) represent the third most frequent fragility fracture [1]. The incidence of surgical treatment has increased, and fracture fixation with locking plates has become a popular treatment [2]. Cochrane reviews do not support this trend [3]. Patients treated surgically probably need more subsequent surgery than conservatively treated patients [4]. Reoperation rates after primary fixation of PHFs may reach 30% [5] due to mechanical fixation failure, surgical site infection, screw perforation or avascular necrosis (AVN) of the humeral head. Failure to achieve structural support of the medial column has been suggested to be an important risk factor for fixation failure [6–9].

We, therefore, studied the effect of calcar screws and postoperative varus malalignment on the risk of fixation failure in adult patients with a PHF treated with a locking plate. A secondary aim was to assess long-term shoulder pain and function reported by these patients.

Methods

The patients were retrospectively identified by a digital search for locking plate fixations of PHF performed at Akershus University Hospital, Norway, between January 2011 and December 2014. We identified 229 eligible adult patients (18 years and above). As explained in Table 1, 39 (17%) patients were not included, and we did not send the OSS questionnaire to 43 patients.

For the final analyses, 190 patients were included. The patients' medical records were reviewed for patient, fracture and procedural characteristics. Furthermore, we recorded clinical and radiological results including surgically related complications and reoperations. Patients were retrospectively observed until whichever of the following events first occurred: re-operation, end of study period or death. The individual times to events were used in the Cox regression analyses, and the end of the study period was July 30, 2016, for all patients.

Two of the authors (SO and AKBW), blinded for the clinical outcome, assessed pre- and post-operative anteroposterior (AP) and trans-scapular shoulder radiographs stored in the hospital's digital image database. Patients were categorised in two groups by the presence

or absence of calcar screws as seen in postoperative radiographs (Fig. 1). Calcar screws were defined as obliquely placed 3.5 mm screws locked to the plate and with purchase in the inferomedial quadrant of the humeral head [10]. Pre and postoperative fracture malalignment was evaluated by measuring the head-shaft angle (HSA) using the method described by Agel [11] (Fig. 1). Consistent with previously published data, postoperative varus malalignment was defined as an HSA < 120° [12] and an HSA of 135° defined the physiological reference value [13]. Fractures were categorised according to the number of fragments as two, three or four part fractures, corresponding to the Arbeitsgemeinschaft für osteosynthesefragen/Orthopaedic Trauma Association's (AO/OTA) classification A, B or C type fractures, respectively [14].

Patient-reported shoulder pain and function were assessed by a validated Norwegian version of the Oxford Shoulder Score (OSS), consisting of 12 questions with scores ranging from 0 (worst possible result) to 4 (best possible result) [15]. OSS was graded as poor (< 36 points), good (36–41 points) and excellent (> 41 points) [16]. The OSS questionnaire was mailed to 147 of 190 (77%) patients during June and July, 2016, and 43 patients (23%) were not eligible to complete the questionnaire (Table 1).

During the study period, our centre considered patients with the following fracture characteristics for open reduction and locking plate fixation: an HSA < 105° (varus displacement), an HSA > 180° (valgus displacement) and displacement of the tuberosities more than 5 mm and/or less than 50% contact between the shaft and the head fragments. Patients who were offered locking plate fixation, received general anaesthesia, an inter-scalene brachial plexus block, or both, and were positioned in a beach chair position. Open reduction was performed through either a classic deltopectoral approach or by the less invasive deltoid split approach, depending on fracture characteristics and surgeon's preference. The surgeon reduced the fracture under fluoroscopic guidance by the aid of non-absorbable sutures placed in the rotator cuff and temporary fixation with Kirschner wires. A 5-hole locking plate (PHILOS,

Table 1 Reasons for patient exclusion. 190 patients were included for final analysis

Excluded from all outcomes (39 patients)	Not invited to complete OSS (43 patients)
• Primary treatment delayed more than 3 weeks (15 patients)	• Deceased (23 patients)
• Surgery performed due to non-union following conservative treatment (8 patients)	• Considered non-compliant (dementia/alcoholism/drug abuse) (11 patients)
• Isolated fracture of the greater tuberosity (5 patients)	• A concomitant fracture in the same upper extremity (4 patients)
• Neurovascular injury at presentation (2 patients)	• Patients with pre-existing shoulder complaints (3 patients)
• Open fracture (2 patients)	• Did not speak Norwegian (2 patients)
• Other reasons (7 patients)	

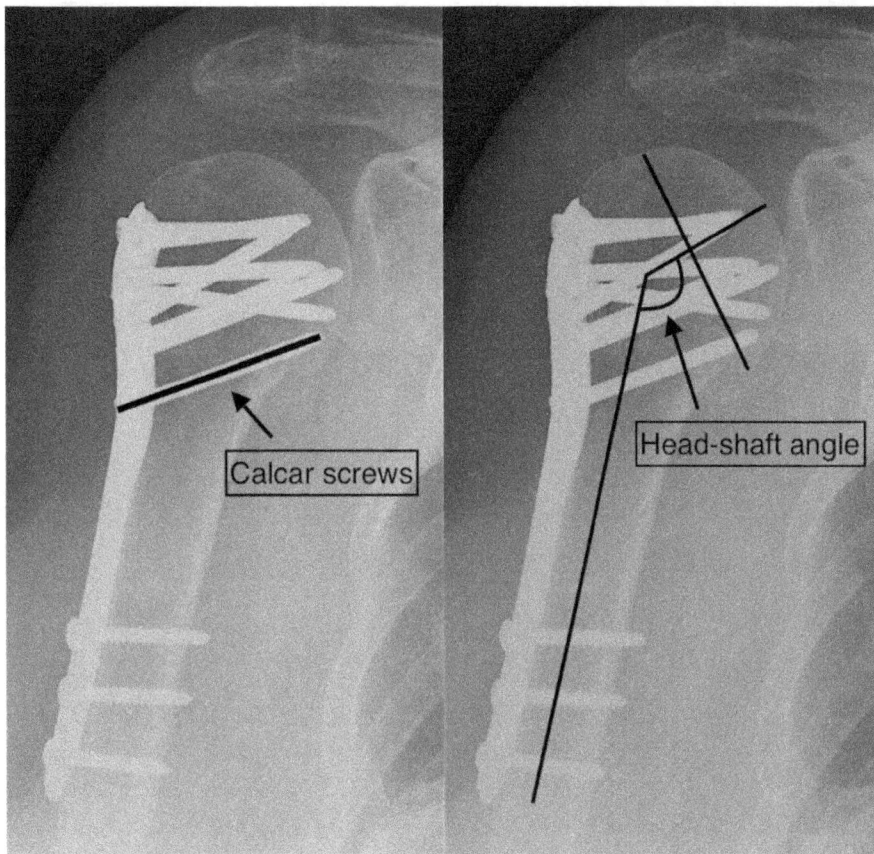

Fig. 1 Correct positioning of the calcar screws with purchase in the inferiomedial quadrant of the humeral head (left). Measurement of the head-shaft angle (HSA). The HSA is the angle created between a line perpendicular to the anatomical neck plane and the axis of the humerus shaft (right)

DePuy Synthes, West Chester, Pennsylvania, USA) was temporarily fixed to the reduced fracture fragments using Kirschner wires and the cuff sutures and approximated to the humeral shaft using a 3.5 mm cortical screw. If a deltoid split approach was used, the shaft screws were placed percutaneously or through a mini-open approach. Finally, 3.5 mm locking screws were inserted into the humeral head after subtracting 5 mm screw length from the joint line contour to minimise the risk of subsequent perforation. No patients received medial buttress plate or allograft reinforcement during the study period. Bone substitute (HydroSet, Stryker, or STRUCSURE CP, Smith & Nephew) was used in valgus impacted fractures at the surgeon's discretion. All patients received three doses of perioperative antibiotic prophylaxis (cloxacillin 2 g + 1 g + 1 g, or clindamycin 600 mg + 300 mg + 300 mg in case of penicillin allergy).

Physiotherapists instructed all patients orally and in writing in post-operative rehabilitation exercises as per local guidelines. Patients were routinely scheduled for follow-up after 6–8 weeks (Fig. 2). Patients with prolonged pain, radiologically evident loss of reduction, fixation failure, non-union or AVN were scheduled for additional follow-ups. These patients were followed every 6–8 weeks with radiographs until union, or until they were scheduled for revision surgery with re-fixation or arthroplasty.

Statistics

The Shapiro–Wilk test was used to assess continuous variables for normal distribution. Normally distributed variables were described by means and standard deviations (SDs) and non-normally distributed variables by medians and interquartile ranges (IQRs). The corresponding statistical tests used to compare differences between the two groups were independent two-sample t test and the Mann–Whitney U test. Categorical variables were described as numbers and percentages, and differences between groups were compared using z-statistics. Inter-rater reliability (IRR) for radiological measurements was assessed using the intraclass correlation coefficient (ICC). The Cox proportional hazards regression analysis was used to assess risk factors for fixation failure. The assumption of proportional hazards was tested by inspection of log-minus-log plots. In the multivariable Cox regression, the variables were adjusted for age and

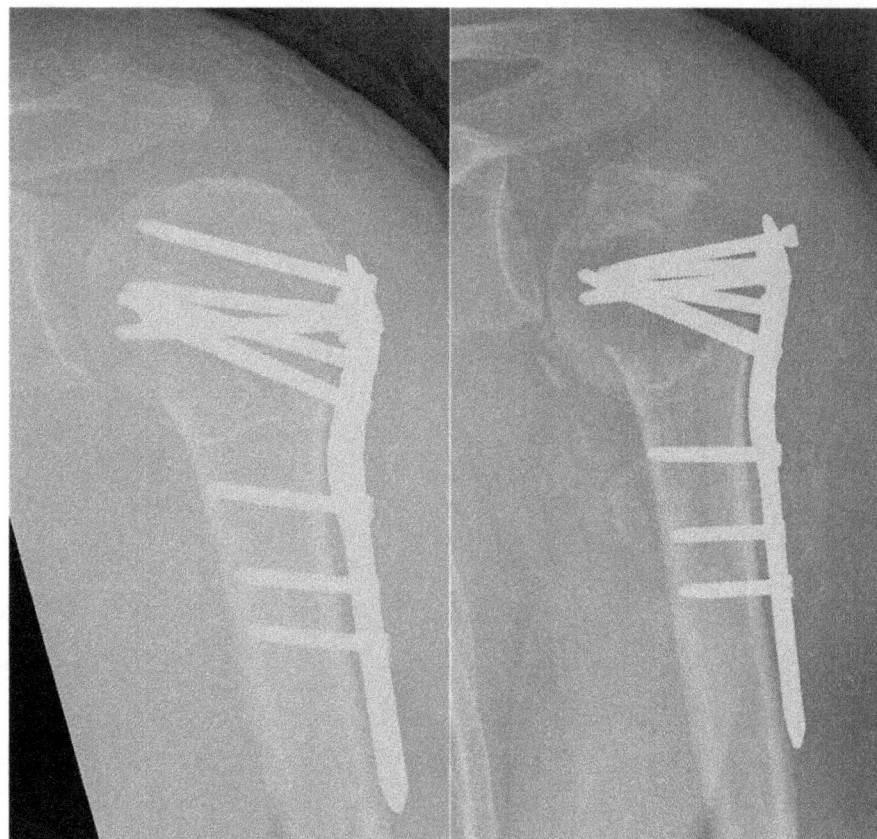

Fig. 2 A proximal humeral fracture in a 68-year-old female treated with a locking plate without calcar screws (left). Failure of fixation with varus collapse 6 weeks after primary surgery (right)

Table 2 Patient, fracture and procedural characteristics in 190 patients with a proximal humeral fracture

	No calcar screws (n = 93)	Calcar screws (n = 97)	Mean difference or relative risk (95% CI)	p value
Age (years), mean (SD)	65 (15)	69 (13)	4.7 (0.7–8.7)	0.02 [b]
median (IQR)	68 (17)	70 (20)	–	0.06 [c]
Women	64 (69)	68 (70)	1.0 (0.8–1.2)	0.8 [d]
Smokers	21 (23)	27 (28)	0.8 (0.5–1.3)	0.4 [d]
Diabetes	13 (14)	8 (8)	1.7 (0.7–3.9)	0.2 [d]
Non-compliance	9 (10)	7 (7)	1.3 (0.5–3.5)	0.5 [d]
ASA III or IV	31 (33)	23 (24)	1.4 (0.9–2.2)	0.1 [d]
3 or 4 part fracture type	68 (73)	74 (76)	1.0 (0.8–1.1)	0.6 [d]
Fracture dislocation	7 (8)	6 (6)	1.2 (0.4–3.5)	0.7 [d]
Preoperative varus < 105°	22 (24)	21 (22)	1.1 (0.6–1.8)	0.7 [d]
Preoperative valgus > 180°	16 (17)	19 (20)	0.9 (0.5–1.6)	0.7 [d]
Medial comminution	54 (58)	75 (77)	0.8 (0.6–0.9)	0.006 [d]
Surgical approach: deltoid split	69 (74)	40 (41)	1.8 (1.4–2.3)	< 0.001 [d]
Residual varus malalignment < 120° [a]	6 (7)	5 (5)	1.3 (0.4–4.0)	0.7 [d]

Percentages in parenthesis unless stated otherwise
CI confidence interval, SD standard deviation, IQR Interquartile range, ASA American Society of Anaesthesiologists
[a]n = 88 and 93, [b]Independent two-sample t test, [c] Mann–Whitney test, [d]z statistics

sex. Statistical analyses were performed using the IBM SPSS version 24 for Mac.

Ethics

The regional ethical committee of south east Norway reviewed and delegated the approval of this study (reference no. 2015/1435) to the Data Protection Official at Akershus University Hospital who granted the ethics approval (reference no. 15–128).

Results

Ninety-three of 190 (49%) patients were operated without calcar screws and 97 of 190 (51%) with calcar screws. The median follow-up time was 35 (range 0.3–65) months, and the median time for the last radiological examination was 3, 4 (range 0,03–53) months.

Patient demographics, fracture characteristics and perioperative circumstances, categorised by application of calcar screws are presented in Table 2.

Patients operated without calcar screws were nearly 5 years younger than those operated with calcar screws (mean difference = 4.7 (95% CI: 0.7–8.7); p = 0.02). Patients with an intact medial column of the proximal humerus were more often operated without calcar screws, and these fractures were more often approached by deltoid split. Patients with preoperative varus (HSA < 105°) were more often fixated in residual varus malalignment (HSA < 120°) compared to those who presented with a preoperative HSA > 105° (8 of 11 (73%) versus 33 of 170 (19%); p < 0.001). Thirty-one of 190 (16%) patients with PHF treated with a locking plate required a reoperation: 14 (7%) due to fixation failure, 10 (5%) due to deep surgical site infection and 2 (1%) due to avascular necrosis of the humeral head. In addition, 5 (3%) patients underwent hardware removal due to presumably implant-related local shoulder pain. Patients operated without calcar screws more often required a reoperation than those who received calcar screws (12 of 93 (13%) versus 2 of 97 (2%); p = 0.005) (Table 3).

Patients operated without calcar screws had a 6-fold increased risk of a reoperation due to fixation failure compared to those who received calcar screws (hazard ratio (HR) = 6.5 (95% CI 1.5–28.9; p = 0.02) (Table 4).

Adjusting for age and gender, the risk of fixation failure without the use of calcar screws was even greater (HR = 8.6 (95% CI 1.9–39.3; p = 0.005) (Table 5).

Fixation of the humeral head with a residual varus malalignment (HSA < 120°) also increased the risk of reoperations due to fixation failure (HR = 5.2 (95% CI 1.5–18.7; p = 0.01), and adjusting for age and gender, HR = 4.9 (95% CI 1.3–17.9; p = 0.02). The interrater agreement for measurements of the postoperative HSA was excellent (ICC (95% CI) = 0.91 (0.88–0.93) [17].

There were 132 of 148 (89%) patients who completed the OSS questionnaire. The median long-term shoulder function was 40 (IQR 27–46). OSS was available for 19 of 31 (61%) patients who needed a reoperation and for 113 of 117 (97%) patients who did not undergo secondary surgery. Patients who did not require secondary surgery had a significantly better shoulder score than those who underwent a reoperation (median OSS (IQR) = 41 (33–46) versus 25 (13–32); p < 0.001).

Discussion

We found that the use of calcar screws and adequate reduction of the fracture, to achieve medial support, significantly reduced the risk of a reoperation due to fixation failure in patients with a PHF treated with a locking plate.

Medial support can be restored by anatomical reduction in fractures without medial comminution to reduce the risk of fixation failure. In fractures with medial comminution, calcar screws, medialization and impaction of the humeral shaft onto the humeral head or both, may restore a medial support [10]. Alternatively, some authors advocate the use of an additional medial buttress plate [18], allograft reinforcement [19, 20], bone substitution [9, 21] or intramedullary nailing [22–24].

Although we were aware of the possible importance of calcar screws during the study period, calcar screws were only used in half of the patients. One possible explanation was that the less invasive deltoid split approach was introduced during the study period, and that calcar screws were initially avoided using this approach to prevent iatrogenic axillary nerve injury. However, with increased experience with the deltoid split approach, calcar screws could be placed safely [25]. A cadaveric

Table 3 Reoperations in 190 patients with a proximal humeral fracture treated with a locking plate

Indication	No calcar screws (n = 93)	Calcar screws (n = 97)	Relative risk (95% CI)	p value
Fixation failure	12 (13)	2 (2)	6.3 (1.4–27.2)	0.01 [a]
Deep infection	4 (4)	6 (6)	0.7 (0.2–2.4)	0.6 [a]
Avascular necrosis	1 (1)	1 (1)	1.0 (0.06–16.4)	1.0 [a]
Local pain	3 (3)	2 (2)	1.6 (0.3–9.2)	0.6 [a]

Percentages in parenthesis
CI confidence interval
[a] z statistics

Table 4 Risk factors for fixation failure. Univariate Cox regression analysis with time to fixation failure as outcome

Covariate	n	Hazard ratio	95% CI	p value
Age, increase of 1 year	69 [b]	1.05	(1.0 to 1.1)	0.04
Sex				
Women	133	1 [a]		
Men	57	0.59	(0.2 to 2.1)	0.4
Smoker				
No	142	1 [a]		
Yes	48	0.80	(0.2 to 2.9)	0.7
Diabetes				
No	169	1 [a]		
Yes	21	0.61	(0.1 to 4.7	0.6
Non-compliant				
No	173	1 [a]		
Yes	17	5.35	(1.7 to 17.1)	0.005
ASA classification				
ASA I-II	136	1 [a]		
ASA III-IV	54	2.7	(1.0 to 7.7)	0.06
Fracture classification				
2 part	48	1 [a]		
3 or 4 part	142	2.1	(0.5 to 9.5)	0.3
Fracture dislocation				
No	177	1 [a]		
Yes	13	2.3	(0.5 to 10.3)	0.3
Preoperative varus < 105°				
No	147	1 [a]		
Yes	43	2.8	(1.0 to 8.0)	0.06
Preoperative valgus > 180°				
No	155	1 [a]		
Yes	35	1.8	(0.6 to 5.7)	0.3
Medial comminution				
No	60	1 [a]		
Yes	130	1.9	(0.5 to 6.6)	0.3
Surgical approach				
Deltopectoral	82	1 [a]		
Deltoid split	108	0.5	(0.2 to 1.5)	0.3
Calcar screws				
Yes	97	1 [a]		
No	93	6.5	(1.5 to 28.9)	0.02
Adequate reduction > 120°				
Yes	179	1 [a]		
No (varus)	11	5.2	(1.5 to 18.7)	0.01

CI Confidence Interval, *ASA* American Society of Anaesthesiologists
[a]Reference category, [b]median age

Table 5 Multivariate Cox proportional hazards analyses with time to fixation failure as outcome

Covariate	n	Hazard ratio	95% CI	p value
Calcar screws				
Yes	97	1 [a]		
No	93	8.6	(1.9 to 39.3)	0.005
Adequate reduction > 120°				
Yes	179	1 [a]		
No (residual varus)	11	4.9	(1.3 to 17.9)	0.02

[a] Reference category

study has shown improved stability in the fracture with calcar screws, both in fractures with medial comminution and in fractures with intact medial column, suggesting the use of calcar screws in all PHFs in an osteoporotic bone [26]. On the other side, calcar screws may not be sufficient to prevent fixation failure if the fracture is fixed in varus and may not be essential when there is good medial support [27].

In keeping with a previous study, we found that postoperative varus malalignment significantly increased the risk of a reoperation due to fixation failure [12]. Interestingly we did not find that preoperative varus was an independent risk factor for fixation failure, which contradicts the findings presented by Jung et al. [28]. However, both pre and postoperative varus malalignment have been associated with an increased risk of fixation failure [29]. Residual postoperative varus was more often found in patients who presented with a preoperative varus malalignment, and surgeons should be aware that such PHF subtypes may be especially at risk for fixation failure.

In the present retrospective cohort study, the number of reoperations (16%) was in the lower range of previously published data in two systematic review articles, ranging from 13 to 30% [5, 30]. Patients who underwent a reoperation reported poor long-term shoulder function, compared to good shoulder function reported by those who did not undergo a secondary surgery. The poorer outcomes following revision surgery are in line with other studies [31, 32], which points out the importance of a successful first intervention. The overall long-term shoulder function in our cohort was good, which is consistent with a multicentre randomised controlled trial that compared surgical treatment to conservative treatment in adult patients with PHF [33]. The authors of that study did not find any advantage of surgical over conservative management in terms of shoulder pain and function after 2 years. However, critics have questioned the recruitment process, as 1000 of 1250 (80%) eligible patients were not included, counting 87 patients with a "clear indication for surgery" [34].

Primary reverse total shoulder arthroplasty (RTSA) has been advocated to avoid revision surgery following inadequate reduction and unstable fixation [35]. RTSA has gained popularity and showed promising results, especially in elderly patients [36], also when compared to locking plate fixation [37]. However, RTSA complications are potentially adverse and include prosthetic joint infection, instability, neurological injury, scapular notching and periprosthetic fractures [38]. Still, RTSA may be a relevant choice for the primary surgical treatment of displaced PHFs among patients aged 65 years and above with poor rotator cuff status and high risk of healing complications [9, 39]. However, there are few level I trials, and two ongoing randomised controlled multicentre trials compare treatment of PHFs with locking plate versus RTSA [18] and locking plate versus RTSA or versus conservative treatment [40]. Hopefully, these trials will prove high-level evidence and guide the surgical treatment of proximal humeral fractures accordingly.

The main limitations of the current study were the retrospective design, possibly missing complications treated at other hospitals, and the lack of a matched control group to assess shoulder function in conservatively treated patients. Furthermore, we did not have radiographs of the contralateral uninjured shoulder, possibly introducing classification bias when evaluating the postoperative malalignment. The main strengths of our study were the number of patients and the high response rate for OSS questionnaires (89%).

Conclusion

Medial support seems to be important to enhance stability and to avoid fixation failure in proximal humeral fractures and, hence, revision surgeries. In the present retrospective cohort study of 190 patients with a proximal humeral fracture treated with a locking plate, the use of calcar screws and the absence of postoperative varus malalignment (head-shaft angle > 120°), significantly reduced the risk of fixation failure. We, therefore, recommend the use of calcar screws and to avoid residual varus malalignment to improve the medial support of proximal humeral fractures treated with a locking plate.

Abbreviations
AVN: Avascular necrosis; HSA: Head-shaft angle; ICC: Intraclass correlation coefficient; IRR: Inter-rater reliability; OSS: Oxford Shoulder Score; PHF: Proximal humeral fractures; RTSA: Reverse total shoulder arthroplasty

Authors' contributions
SO designed the study,, collected and analysed the data and wrote the manuscript. AKBW, HFSF, FCD and PHR designed the study, analysed the data and revised the manuscript. All authors read and approved the final manuscript.

Competing interests
All authors declare that they have not received any financial payments or other benefits from any commercial entity related to the subject of this article. The authors declare that they have no competing interests.

Author details
[1]Department of Orthopaedic Surgery, Akershus University Hospital, Lørenskog, Norway. [2]Faculty of Medicine, University of Oslo, Oslo, Norway.

References
1. Lauritzen JB, Schwarz P, Lund B, McNair P, Transbol I. Changing incidence and residual lifetime risk of common osteoporosis-related fractures. Osteoporos Int. 1993;3(3):127–32.
2. Sumrein BO, Huttunen TT, Launonen AP, Berg HE, Fellander-Tsai L, Mattila VM. Proximal humeral fractures in Sweden-a registry-based study. Osteoporos Int. 2017;28(3):901–7.
3. Handoll HH, Brorson S. Interventions for treating proximal humeral fractures in adults. Cochrane Database Syst Rev. 2015;11:CD000434.
4. Bell JE, Leung BC, Spratt KF, Koval KJ, Weinstein JD, Goodman DC, Tosteson AN. Trends and variation in incidence, surgical treatment, and repeat surgery of proximal humeral fractures in the elderly. J Bone Joint Surg Am. 2011;93(2):121–31.
5. Launonen AP, Lepola V, Flinkkila T, Laitinen M, Paavola M, Malmivaara A. Treatment of proximal humerus fractures in the elderly: a systemic review of 409 patients. Acta Orthop. 2015;86(3):280–5.
6. Kralinger F, Unger S, Wambacher M, Smekal V, Schmoelz W. The medial periosteal hinge, a key structure in fractures of the proximal humerus: a biomechanical cadaver study of its mechanical properties. J Bone Joint Surg Br. 2009;91(7):973–6.
7. Osterhoff G, Ossendorf C, Wanner GA, Simmen HP, Werner CM. The calcar screw in angular stable plate fixation of proximal humeral fractures--a case study. J Orthop Surg Res. 2011;6:50.
8. Yang P, Zhang Y, Liu J, Xiao J, Ma LM, Zhu CR. Biomechanical effect of medial cortical support and medial screw support on locking plate fixation in proximal humeral fractures with a medial gap: a finite element analysis. Acta Orthop Traumatol Turc. 2015;49(2):203–9.
9. Laux CJ, Grubhofer F, Werner CML, Simmen HP, Osterhoff G. Current concepts in locking plate fixation of proximal humerus fractures. J Orthop Surg Res. 2017;12(1):137.
10. Gardner MJ, Weil Y, Barker JU, Kelly BT, Helfet DL, Lorich DG. The importance of medial support in locked plating of proximal humerus fractures. J Orthop Trauma. 2007;21(3):185–91.
11. Agel J, Jones CB, Sanzone AG, Camuso M, Henley MB. Treatment of proximal humeral fractures with Polarus nail fixation. J Shoulder Elb Surg. 2004;13(2):191–5.
12. Agudelo J, Schurmann M, Stahel P, Helwig P, Morgan SJ, Zechel W, Bahrs C, Parekh A, Ziran B, Williams A, et al. Analysis of efficacy and failure in proximal humerus fractures treated with locking plates. J Orthop Trauma. 2007;21(10):676–81.
13. Jeong J, Bryan J, Iannotti JP. Effect of a variable prosthetic neck-shaft angle and the surgical technique on replication of normal humeral anatomy. J Bone Joint Surg Am. 2009;91(8):1932–41.
14. Marsh JL, Slongo TF, Agel J, Broderick JS, Creevey W, DeCoster TA, Prokuski L, Sirkin MS, Ziran B, Henley B, et al. Fracture and dislocation classification compendium - 2007: orthopaedic trauma association classification, database and outcomes committee. J Orthop Trauma. 2007;21(10 Suppl):S1–133.
15. Ekeberg OM, Bautz-Holter E, Tveita EK, Keller A, Juel NG, Brox JI. Agreement, reliability and validity in 3 shoulder questionnaires in patients with rotator cuff disease. BMC Musculoskelet Disord. 2008;9:68.
16. Randsborg PH, Fuglesang HF, Rotterud JH, Hammer OL, Sivertsen EA. Long-term patient-reported outcome after fractures of the clavicle in patients aged 10 to 18 years. J Pediatr Orthop. 2014;34(4):393–9.
17. Cicchetti DV. Guidelines, criteria, and rules of thumb for evaluating normed and standardized assessment instruments in psychology. Psychol Assess. 1994;6(4):284–90.
18. Fjalestad T, Iversen P, Hole MO, Smedsrud M, Madsen JE. Clinical investigation for displaced proximal humeral fractures in the elderly: a randomized study of two surgical treatments: reverse total prosthetic

replacement versus angular stable plate Philos (the DELPHI-trial). BMC Musculoskelet Disord. 2014;15:323.

19. Katthagen JC, Schwarze M, Meyer-Kobbe J, Voigt C, Hurschler C, Lill H. Biomechanical effects of calcar screws and bone block augmentation on medial support in locked plating of proximal humeral fractures. Clin Biomech (Bristol, Avon). 2014;29(7):735–41.

20. Hinds RM, Garner MR, Tran WH, Lazaro LE, Dines JS, Lorich DG. Geriatric proximal humeral fracture patients show similar clinical outcomes to non-geriatric patients after osteosynthesis with endosteal fibular strut allograft augmentation. J Shoulder Elb Surg. 2015;24(6):889–96.

21. Schliemann B, Wahnert D, Theisen C, Herbort M, Kosters C, Raschke MJ, Weimann A. How to enhance the stability of locking plate fixation of proximal humerus fractures? An overview of current biomechanical and clinical data. Injury. 2015;46(7):1207–14.

22. Gadea F, Favard L, Boileau P, Cuny C, d'Ollone T, Saragaglia D, Sirveaux F. Sofcot: fixation of 4-part fractures of the proximal humerus: can we identify radiological criteria that support locking plates or IM nailing? Comparative, retrospective study of 107 cases. Orthop Traumatol Surg Res. 2016;102(8): 963–70.

23. Kloub M, Holub K, Polakova S. Nailing of three- and four-part fractures of the humeral head -- long-term results. Injury. 2014;45(Suppl 1):S29–37.

24. Dilisio MF, Nowinski RJ, Hatzidakis AM, Fehringer EV. Intramedullary nailing of the proximal humerus: evolution, technique, and results. J Shoulder Elb Surg. 2016;25(5):e130–8.

25. Gardner MJ, Boraiah S, Helfet DL, Lorich DG. The anterolateral acromial approach for fractures of the proximal humerus. J Orthop Trauma. 2008; 22(2):132–7.

26. Ponce BA, Thompson KJ, Raghava P, Eberhardt AW, Tate JP, Volgas DA, Stannard JP. The role of medial comminution and calcar restoration in varus collapse of proximal humeral fractures treated with locking plates. J Bone Joint Surg Am. 2013;95(16):e113–(111–117).

27. Bai L, Fu Z, An S, Zhang P, Zhang D, Jiang B. Effect of calcar screw use in surgical neck fractures of the proximal humerus with unstable medial support: a biomechanical study. J Orthop Trauma. 2014;28(8):452–7.

28. Jung SW, Shim SB, Kim HM, Lee JH, Lim HS. Factors that influence reduction loss in proximal humerus fracture surgery. J Orthop Trauma. 2015;29(6):276–82.

29. Hardeman F, Bollars P, Donnelly M, Bellemans J, Nijs S. Predictive factors for functional outcome and failure in angular stable osteosynthesis of the proximal humerus. Injury. 2012;43(2):153–8.

30. Gupta AK, Harris JD, Erickson BJ, Abrams GD, Bruce B, McCormick F, Nicholson GP, Romeo AA. Surgical management of complex proximal humerus fractures—a systematic review of 92 studies including 4500 patients. J Orthop Trauma. 2015;29(1):54–9.

31. Jost B, Spross C, Grehn H, Gerber C. Locking plate fixation of fractures of the proximal humerus: analysis of complications, revision strategies and outcome. J Shoulder Elb Surg. 2013;22(4):542–9.

32. Kristensen MR, Rasmussen JV, Elmengaard B, Jensen SL, Olsen BS, Brorson S. High risk for revision after shoulder arthroplasty for failed osteosynthesis of proximal humeral fractures. Acta Orthop. 2018;89(3):345–50.

33. Rangan A, Handoll H, Brealey S, Jefferson L, Keding A, Martin BC, Goodchild L, Chuang LH, Hewitt C, Torgerson D, et al. Surgical vs nonsurgical treatment of adults with displaced fractures of the proximal humerus: the PROFHER randomized clinical trial. JAMA. 2015;313(10):1037–47.

34. Dean BJ, Jones LD, Palmer AJ, Macnair RD, Brewer PE, Jayadev C, Wheelton AN, Ball DE, Nandra RS, Aujla RS, et al. A review of current surgical practice in the operative treatment of proximal humeral fractures: does the PROFHER trial demonstrate a need for change? Bone Joint Res. 2016;5(5): 178–84.

35. Cazeneuve JF, Cristofari DJ. Grammont reversed prosthesis for acute complex fracture of the proximal humerus in an elderly population with 5 to 12 years follow-up. Rev Chir Orthop Reparatrice Appar Mot. 2006;92(6): 543–8.

36. Iacobellis C, Berizzi A, Biz C, Camporese A. Treatment of proximal humeral fractures with reverse shoulder arthroplasty in elderly patients. Musculoskelet Surg. 2015;99(1):39–44.

37. Giardella A, Ascione F, Mocchi M, Berlusconi M, Romano AM, Oliva F, Maradei L. Reverse total shoulder versus angular stable plate treatment for proximal humeral fractures in over 65 years old patients. Muscles Ligaments Tendons J. 2017;7(2):271–8.

38. Cheung E, Willis M, Walker M, Clark R, Frankle MA. Complications in reverse total shoulder arthroplasty. J Am Acad Orthop Surg. 2011;19(7):439–49.

39. Kancherla VK, Singh A, Anakwenze OA. Management of acute proximal humeral fractures. J Am Acad Orthop Surg. 2017;25(1):42–52.

40. Launonen AP, Lepola V, Flinkkila T, Strandberg N, Ojanpera J, Rissanen P, Malmivaara A, Mattila VM, Elo P, Viljakka T, et al. Conservative treatment, plate fixation, or prosthesis for proximal humeral fracture. A prospective randomized study. BMC Musculoskelet Disord. 2012;13:167.

16

Training with Hybrid Assistive Limb for walking function after total knee arthroplasty

Kenichi Yoshikawa[1], Hirotaka Mutsuzaki[2*], Ayumu Sano[1], Kazunori Koseki[1], Takashi Fukaya[3], Masafumi Mizukami[4] and Masashi Yamazaki[5]

Abstract

Background: The Hybrid Assistive Limb (HAL, CYBERDYNE) is a wearable robot that provides assistance to patients while walking, standing, and performing leg movements based on the intended movement of the wearer. We aimed to assess the effect of HAL training on the walking ability, range of motion (ROM), and muscle strength of patients after total knee arthroplasty (TKA) for osteoarthritis and rheumatoid arthritis, and to compare the functional status after HAL training to the conventional training methods after surgery.

Methods: Nine patients (10 knees) underwent HAL training (mean age 74.1 ± 5.7 years; height 150.4 ± 6.5 cm; weight 61.2 ± 8.9 kg), whereas 10 patients (11 knees) underwent conventional rehabilitation (mean age 78.4 ± 8.0 years; height 150.5 ± 10.0 cm; weight 59.1 ± 9.8 kg). Patients underwent HAL training during 10 to 12 (average 14.4 min a session) sessions over a 4-week period, 1 week after TKA. There was no significant difference in the total physical therapy time including HAL training between the HAL and control groups. Gait speed, step length, ROM, and muscle strength were evaluated.

Results: The nine patients completed the HAL training sessions without adverse events. The walking speed and step length in the self-selected walking speed condition, and the walking speed in the maximum walking speed condition were greater in the HAL group than in the control group at 4 and 8 weeks ($P < 0.05$). The step length in the maximum walking speed condition was greater in the HAL group than in the control group at 2, 4, and 8 weeks ($P < 0.05$). The extension lag and knee pain were lower in the HAL group than in the control group at 2 weeks ($P < 0.05$). The muscle strength of knee extension in the HAL group was greater than that in the control group at 8 weeks ($P < 0.05$).

Conclusion: HAL training after TKA can improve the walking ability, ROM, and muscle strength compared to conventional physical therapy for up to 8 weeks after TKA. Since the recovery of walking ability was earlier in the HAL group than in the control group and adverse events were not observed in this pilot study, HAL training after TKA can be considered a safe and effective rehabilitation intervention.

Keywords: Total knee arthroplasty, Osteoarthritis, Rheumatoid arthritis, Robot assisted training, Hybrid assistive limb

* Correspondence: mutsuzaki@ipu.ac.jp
[2]Department of Orthopaedic Surgery, Ibaraki Prefectural University of Health Sciences, 4669-2 Ami, Ami-machi, Inashiki-gun, Ibaraki 300-0394, Japan
Full list of author information is available at the end of the article

Background

Total knee arthroplasty (TKA) is one of the most common surgeries for severe osteoarthritis (OA) and rheumatoid arthritis (RA) [1, 2]. Although it is possible to eventually obtain higher physical function and quality of life (QOL) through rehabilitation [3], physical function decreases immediately after TKA [4–6]. Moreover, studies suggest that walking speed and walking ability require about 1 year of recovery after TKA [6, 7]. In addition, knee extension lag occurs early after surgery, and restriction on range of active extension is observed [8–10]. Therefore, gaining improved walking function efficiently is particularly important for patients after TKA.

Robot-assisted training (RAT) has been developed since the early 2000s. There are several reports demonstrating improvements in walking ability through the application of RAT in patients with central nervous system diseases, such as stroke [11], spinal cord injury [12], and cerebral palsy [13]. However, there are few reports that confirm the effect of RAT in postoperative rehabilitation after TKA [14].

The Hybrid Assistive Limb (HAL, Cyberdyne Corporation, Tsukuba, Japan) is an assisted training device. HAL is a wearable robot that interactively provides motion according to the wearer's voluntary drive [15]. Details of the HAL system have been reported in preliminary studies [16, 17]. Both single leg and two leg versions of the HAL are available, and the choice depends on the wearer's requirements. The HAL detects the bioelectrical signals generated by the wearer's muscle activity or the floor-reaction-force signals caused by the wearer's weight shifts, or both. HAL enables lower limb exercise and gait training with voluntary drive, and has the advantages of both voluntary drive and ambulatory performance. Most other exoskeleton devices use autonomously generated predefined motion. In contrast, HAL provides motion in response to the wearer's voluntary drive. The wearer operates HAL by adjusting his or her own muscle activity. Clinical trials of training using HAL have been already conducted for patients with stroke [18, 19], spinal cord injury [20], cerebral palsy [21], and neuromuscular diseases [22], and its clinical safety has been confirmed.

The study by Tanaka et al. [23] has been the only randomized controlled trial that compared the lower limb function between groups of patients who underwent training with HAL and conventional therapy after TKA. Although actual measured values were not described in the article, an immediate improvement within 1 week was observed with the use of HAL. This study was a short-term evaluation and was conducted for up to 3 weeks after surgery, and did not examine the improvement in range of motion (ROM). Moreover, the two-legged HAL was used in this study. Furthermore, the patients in this study had OA only, and RA was not included. The authors suggested that the single leg HAL may be better for functional recovery after TKA owing to its lighter weight and because it allows freedom of movements in the unaffected leg. Yoshioka et al. [24] showed an improvement of postoperative extension lag using a single joint type HAL (HAL-SJ), which is equipped with only one actuator to the knee joint motion for TKA patients, and Fukaya et al. [25] reported an improvement of postoperative walking ability in a case report of a single leg version of HAL. We hypothesized that the assistive benefit of HAL also reduces knee extension lag and improves walking ability and pre-operative function of TKA patients not only with OA but also with RA compared with conventional physical therapy.

Therefore, the purpose of this study was to evaluate the effect of training using the single leg version of HAL on walking ability, knee ROM, muscle strength, pain, and physical function, and to compare the functional status after HAL training with the conventional therapy alone and with the pre-operative functional status for up to 8 weeks after TKA for OA and RA.

Methods

Subjects

All subjects were admitted to our hospital between February 2015 and January 2018. Patients diagnosed with severe OA and RA via varus deformation of the knee by X-ray examination and who underwent primary TKA by a senior surgeon (H.M.) were included in the study. During this period, a total of 21 consecutive patients (23 knees) underwent primary TKA. The patients were categorized into two groups before undergoing surgery (HAL and control groups). The patients who agreed to receive HAL training and their physique allowed for HAL device were in the HAL group, because the size of a single leg HAL was in size medium only at that time. The other patients were in the control group. The patients in the HAL group underwent HAL training (average 14.4 ± 5.9 min a session) and conventional physical therapy (60 to 80 min a day) during the HAL intervention period. The HAL training started 1 to 5 weeks after TKA (HAL intervention period). The total number of HAL interventions ranged from 10 to 12 during the 4-week period. The patients in the control group underwent only conventional physical therapy (60 to 120 min a day) after TKA during the HAL intervention period of the HAL group. There was no significant difference in the total physical therapy time including HAL training between both groups during the HAL intervention period. 5 weeks after TKA, the patients in the both groups underwent same physical therapy. The physical therapy details in the both groups are summarized in Table 1. Eleven patients (12 knees) were included in the

Table 1 Details of physical therapy and HAL training protocol

	HAL group	Control group	P value
HAL training	Single leg version HAL (size M)	None	
	1 week to 5 weeks after TKA (4 weeks)		
	Number of sessions: 11.6 ± 0.8		
	Average duration of session: 14.4 ± 5.9 min		
	●Knee ROM exercises (less than 20 min)		
	●Gait training (less than 20 min)		
Conventional PT	1 day after TKA to hospital discharge		
	5 or more days a week		
	60 to 80 min a day (during the HAL intervention period)	60 to 120 min a day (during the HAL intervention period)	
	●CPM: from 3 days after TKA		
	●FWB: from 1 week after TKA		
	●Gait training (flat ground, outdoor, irregular terrain)		
	●Stair climbing training		
	●Joint ROM training		
	●Muscle strengthening		
	●Balancing training (sitting and standing positions)		
	●ADL training (toilet, bathing, bedside tasks, etc.)		
	●Bicycle ergometer training		
	●Various physical exercises for returning to work		
	●Self-exercise education		
Total PT time including HAL training during HAL intervention period	26.5 ± 4.2 (h)	28.2 ± 5.2 (h)	0.434

Values are expressed as numbers or as mean ± SD
Abbreviation: *TKA*, total knee arthroplasty; *ROM*, range of motion; *PT*, physical therapy; *CPM*, continuous passive movement; *FWB*, full weight-bearing; *ADL*, activities of daily living

HAL group, whereas 10 patients (11 knees) were in the control group. Among the 11 patients allocated to the HAL group, 2 patients withdrew consent. One of the two patients could not continue the study because of worsening of depression (6 times HAL sessions were done). Another patient withdrew, because it was troublesome to continue the study (6 times HAL sessions were done). Therefore, 9 patients (10 knees) underwent HAL training. Before this study, 4 and 2 patients in the HAL and control groups, respectively, had already undergone TKA on the contralateral side. The pre-operative characteristics and baseline values did not differ significantly between the two groups (Table 2).

The ethics committee of Ibaraki Prefectural University of Health Sciences approved the study (no. e155). We explained the purpose of the study to the patients in verbal and written forms, and written consent was obtained from all patients. The protocol of this study was registered in the University Hospital Medical Information Network Clinical Trials Registry (UMIN000017623).

Surgical procedure

The surgical procedure was similar to that described in our previous report [26]. Under general anesthesia, a midline skin incision was made, and a medial parapatellar approach was used. The patella was not replaced, and the posterior cruciate ligament was retained. The implants used were the NexGen® or Persona® (Zimmer, Warsaw, IN, USA) for the femoral component and the NexGen CR Stem Tibia or NexGen Trabecular Metal Monoblock Tibia (Zimmer, Warsaw, IN, USA) for the tibial component.

HAL training

The single leg version of the HAL (size medium) (Table 1) was placed on the operative side, and the Cybernic Voluntary Control (CVC) mode was used. The gain in assistive torque at each joint in response to the bioelectrical signals was controlled by a therapist so that the patient could move the knee joint sufficiently and easily within the ROM without aggravating pain or presence of pain and extension lag, and the walk pattern was as normal and symmetrical as possible. First, repetitive

Table 2 Preoperative baseline characteristics of subjects

Characteristics		HAL group 9 patients (10 knees)	Control group 10 patients (11 knees)	P value
Age		74.1 ± 5.7	78.4 ± 8.0	0.180
Sex	Male/female	1/8	2 / 8	1.000
Weight (kg)		61.2 ± 8.9	59.1 ± 9.8	0.612
Height (m)		150.4 ± 6.5	150.5 ± 10.0	0.985
BMI (kg/m^2)		27.1 ± 3.9	26.3 ± 5.3	0.719
Disease	OA/RA	8/2	10/1	0.587
TKA operated side	right/left	6/4	5/6	0.670
Contralateral side TKA		4	2	0.350

Values are expressed as numbers or as mean ± SD
Abbreviation: *BMI*, body mass index; *OA*, osteoarthritis; *RA*, rheumatoid arthritis; *TKA*, total knee arthroplasty

knee flexion/extension exercises within the range where pain was not aggravated or was absent were performed for less than 20 min with the patient in the sitting position. Second, gait training with HAL was conducted on a level ground at a speed that the subject was comfortable with while still maintaining good gait posture, as judged by a physical therapist, for less than 20 min. To prevent falls, a wheeled walker was used during gait training with HAL (Fig. 1).

Outcome measures

Indicators related to walking ability were as follows: self-selected walking speed (SWS) [27]; maximum walking speed (MWS) [27]; mean step length at SWS (SL-SWS) and MWS (SL-MWS); and cadence at SWS and MWS. SWS and MWS were measured according to the time taken to cover the intermediate 10 m of a total distance. Measurement was performed as many times as possible, up to a maximum of three times, and the fastest time was used. To calculate SL and cadence, the number of steps in the 10-m measurement section of the MWS or SWS test was counted. These were evaluated before the surgery and at weeks 2, 4, and 8.

The assessments related to knee function were as follows: ROM of knee flexion and extension motion on passive and active movements on the operated side; torque of knee extension and knee flexion as muscle strength of quadriceps and hamstrings; and Western Ontario and McMaster Universities Osteoarthritis Index (WOMAC) [28]. WOMAC validated for the Japanese patients who had TKA surgery was divided into subscales of pain (WOMAC-p) and physical function (WOMAC-f) [29]. ROM was measured by using a medical goniometer in 5 ° increments with the patients in the sitting position or the supine position. Torques of knee were measured with an isometric mode using Biodex System 4 (Biodex Medical Systems, NY, USA). The knee joint was fixed in 60 ° of knee flexion, and the maximum knee joint flexion and extension torque were measured. Both torques were measured in 3 sets every 5 s, and peak torque values were used. The value obtained by dividing the peak torque value by each body weight was used for analysis. ROM, both torques, and both WOMAC subscale scores were measured before the surgery and at weeks 2, 4, and 8. Four kinds of ROM were measured before the surgery and at weeks 1, 2, 3, 4, and 8.

Statistical analysis

Differences in pre-operative subject characteristics were analyzed using a Student's *t* test or the Wilcoxon's rank

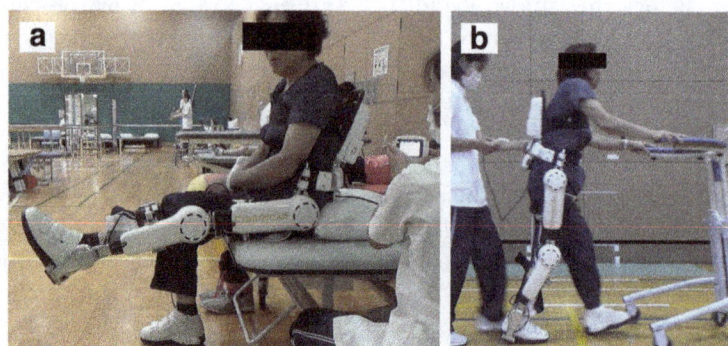

Fig. 1 Hybrid Assistive Limb (HAL) training. Knee extension and flexion exercise while sitting, with HAL on the sagittal plane (**a**). Gait training, with HAL on the sagittal plane (**b**)

sum test, as appropriate, for continuous variables, and Fisher's exact test for categorical variables. For all outcome measures, two-way mixed analysis of variance (ANOVA) with repeated measures factor (from before surgery to week 8) and between-subjects factor (HAL group or control group) were performed for assessing 2 factor's main effects and interaction between the 2 factors. If main effects of the repeated measures factor (time effect) or interactions satisfied significant level ($P < 0.05$) or significant large effect size ($\eta_p^2 > 0.14$), Tukey's honestly significant difference was used for within-group comparisons of the outcomes at the various assessment time points [30]. If main effects of the between-subjects factor (intervention effect) or interactions satisfied a significant level ($P < 0.05$) or significant large effect size ($\eta_p^2 > 0.14$), Student's t test was used for comparison between groups at the various assessment time points [30]. All analyses were performed with IBM SPSS Statistics version 24.0 (International Business Machines Corporation, Chicago, USA). Level of significance was set at $P < 0.05$.

Results

The 9 patients completed the HAL training sessions without adverse events. All 9 patients (10 knees) in the HAL group and 10 patients (11 knees) in the control group were evaluated until week 4. At weeks 8, 4, and 5 patients were discharged from the hospital in the HAL and control groups, respectively (Fig. 2).

The results of walking ability are summarized in Table 3. At weeks 4 and 8, the SWS in the HAL group were greater than in the control group ($P = 0.030$ and $P = 0.022$, respectively). The SWS in the HAL group exceeded the pre-operative value as early as week 4, and only the HAL group showed significantly greater SWS at week 8 than in the pre-operative period ($P = 0.045$) (two-way ANOVA; intervention effect $P = 0.121$ and $\eta_p^2 = 0.223$; time effect $P < 0.001$ and $\eta_p^2 = 0.544$; and interactions $P = 0.304$ and $\eta_p^2 = 0.112$).

At weeks 4 and 8, the MWS in the HAL group was greater than that in the control group ($P = 0.006$ and $P = 0.027$, respectively) (two-way ANOVA; intervention effect $P = 0.021$ and $\eta_p^2 = 0.430$; time effect $P = 0.001$ and $\eta_p^2 = 0.532$; and interactions $P = 0.111$ and $\eta_p^2 = 0.198$).

The SL at SWS in the HAL group was greater than that in the control group at weeks 4 ($P = 0.002$) and 8 ($P = 0.011$). In the within-group comparison, only the HAL group was found to have significantly greater SL at SWS at weeks 4 and 8 than those at week 2 ($P = 0.026$ and $P = 0.003$, respectively) (two-way ANOVA; intervention effect $P = 0.048$ and $\eta_p^2 = 0.337$; time effect $P = 0.017$ and $\eta_p^2 = 0.341$; and interactions $P = 0.271$, $\eta_p^2 = 0.123$).

The SL at MWS in the HAL group was also greater than that in the control groups at weeks 2 ($P = 0.016$), 4 ($P = 0.001$), and 8 ($P = 0.003$). In the within-group comparison, only the HAL group was found to have significantly greater SL at MWS at week 4 than at week 2 ($P = 0.010$) (two-way ANOVA; intervention effect $P = 0.003$ and $\eta_p^2 = 0.594$; time

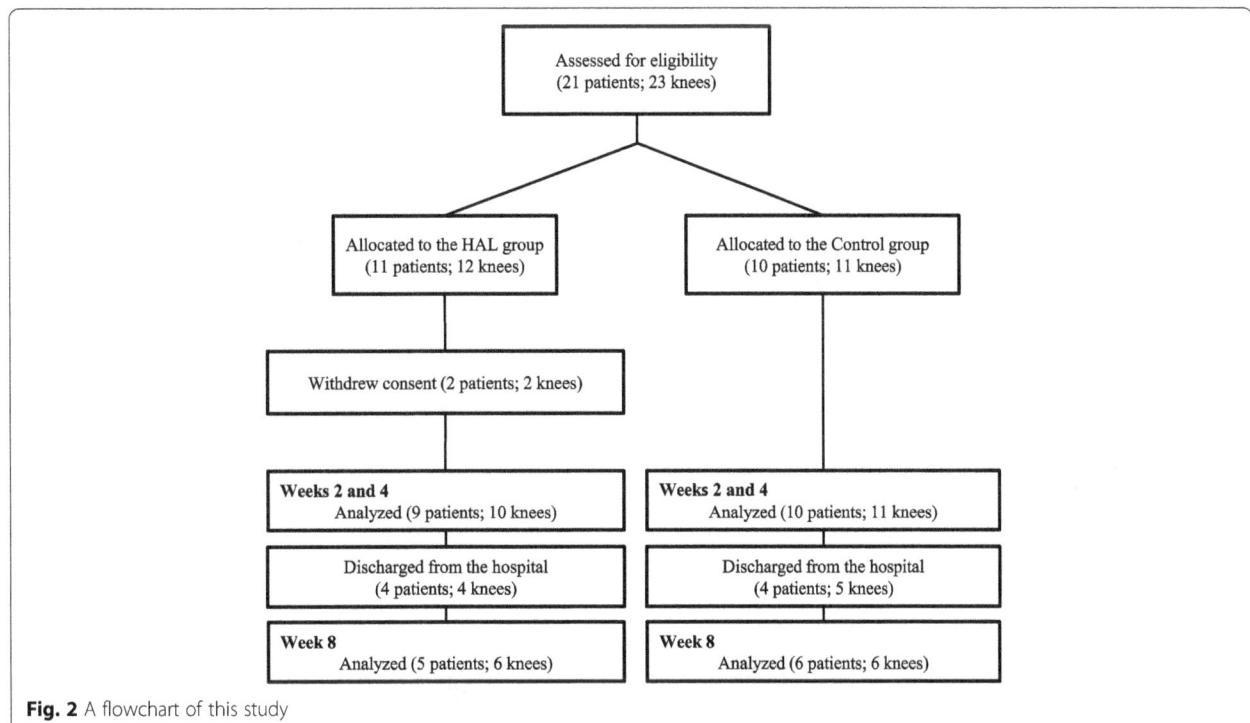

Fig. 2 A flowchart of this study

Table 3 Walking ability in the HAL and control groups

Response	Visit	HAL group Mean ± SD		Control group Mean ± SD		P value	
SWS (m/s)	Pre	1.08 ± 0.29	(n = 10)	1.04 ± 0.26	(n = 11)	0.794	
	Week 2	0.87 ± 0.19	(n = 10)	0.77 ± 0.27	(n = 11)	0.366	
	Week 4	1.20 ± 0.09	(n = 10)	0.99 ± 0.26	(n = 11)	0.030	*
	Week 8	1.34 ± 0.11	(n = 6)	1.05 ± 0.23	(n = 6)	0.022	*
MWS (m/s)	Pre	1.41 ± 0.33	(n = 10)	1.35 ± 0.21	(n = 11)	0.588	
	Week 2	1.25 ± 0.38	(n = 10)	1.01 ± 0.34	(n = 11)	0.137	
	Week 4	1.61 ± 0.32	(n = 10)	1.24 ± 0.23	(n = 11)	0.006	**
	Week 8	1.63 ± 0.09	(n = 6)	1.35 ± 0.24	(n = 6)	0.027	*
SL at SWS (m)	Pre	0.59 ± 0.11	(n = 10)	0.57 ± 0.11	(n = 11)	0.656	
	Week 2	0.54 ± 0.05	(n = 10)	0.50 ± 0.09	(n = 11)	0.215	
	Week 4	0.63 ± 0.03	(n = 10)	0.53 ± 0.07	(n = 11)	0.002	**
	Week 8	0.67 ± 0.03	(n = 6)	0.56 ± 0.08	(n = 6)	0.011	*
SL at MWS (m)	Pre	0.67 ± 0.10	(n = 10)	0.62 ± 0.09	(n = 11)	0.274	
	Week 2	0.62 ± 0.06	(n = 10)	0.52 ± 0.10	(n = 11)	0.016	*
	Week 4	0.70 ± 0.05	(n = 10)	0.58 ± 0.07	(n = 11)	0.001	**
	Week 8	0.73 ± 0.03	(n = 6)	0.61 ± 0.07	(n = 6)	0.003	**
Cadence at SWS (m)	Pre	108.1 ± 13.7	(n = 10)	109.9 ± 11.1	(n = 11)		
	Week 2	96.2 ± 13.7	(n = 10)	91.5 ± 22.9	(n = 11)		
	Week 4	115.1 ± 6.9	(n = 10)	111.3 ± 20.7	(n = 11)		
	Week 8	119.9 ± 5.3	(n = 6)	113.1 ± 13.4	(n = 6)		
Cadence at MWS (m)	Pre	125.4 ± 14.9	(n = 10)	130.7 ± 11.2	(n = 11)		
	Week 2	120.0 ± 25.3	(n = 10)	114.0 ± 28.4	(n = 11)		
	Week 4	137.7 ± 21.2	(n = 10)	127.8 ± 18.1	(n = 11)		
	Week 8	133.9 ± 10.0	(n = 6)	133.4 ± 20.6	(n = 6)		

Abbreviations: SWS, self-selected walking speed; MWS, maximum walking speed; SL, step length
*$P < 0.05$; **$P < 0.01$

effect $P < 0.001$ and $\eta_p^2 = 0.586$; and interactions $P = 0.063$ and $\eta_p^2 = 0.212$).

The results of changes in the ROM are summarized in Table 4. At weeks 2 and 4, the passive knee extension ROM was significantly greater in the HAL group than in the control group ($P = 0.034$ and $P = 0.006$, respectively) (two-way ANOVA; intervention effect $P = 0.135$ and $\eta_p^2 = 0.209$; time effect $P = 0.071$ and $\eta_p^2 = 0.238$; and interactions $P = 0.419$ and $\eta_p^2 = 0.082$). At weeks 2 and 3, the active knee extension ROM was significantly greater in the HAL group than in the control group ($P = 0.005$ and $P = 0.048$, respectively) (two-way ANOVA; intervention effect $P = 0.120$ and $\eta_p^2 = 0.225$; time effect $P = 0.082$ and $\eta_p^2 = 0.204$; and interactions $P = 0.262$ and $\eta_p^2 = 0.124$).

The results of muscle strength are summarized in Table 5. The knee extension torque was significantly higher in the HAL group than in the control group at week 8 ($P = 0.014$) (two-way ANOVA; intervention effect $P = 0.233$ and $\eta_p^2 = 0.173$; time effect $P = 0.009$ and $\eta_p^2 = 0.530$; and interactions $P = 0.422$ and $\eta_p^2 = 0.092$).

The results of WOMAC are summarized in Table 6. The WOMAC-P in the HAL group at week 2 was greater than that in the control group ($P = 0.021$), and the lowering of pain was recognized early in the HAL group (two-way ANOVA; intervention effect $P = 0.336$ and $\eta_p^2 = 0.103$; time effect $P = 0.002$ and $\eta_p^2 = 0.427$; and interactions $P = 0.023$ and $\eta_p^2 = 0.293$ in the WOMAC-P, and intervention effect $P = 0.073$ and $\eta_p^2 = 0.313$; time effect $P = 0.019$ and $\eta_p^2 = 0.304$; and interactions $P = 0.109$ and $\eta_p^2 = 0.198$ in the WOMAC-F, respectively).

The results of two-way ANOVA in the cadence at SWS and MWS, the passive and active knee flexion ROM and the torque of knee flexion showed a significant effect only in the time effect.

Discussion

The walking speed in the HAL group was better than that in the control group at weeks 4 and 8. In addition, the SWS of the HAL group exceeded the pre-operative

Table 4 Range of motion in the HAL and control groups

Response	Visit	HAL group Mean ± SD		Control group Mean ± SD		P value	
Knee ROM (degree)							
Passive extension	Pre	− 4.0 ± 8.4	(n = 10)	− 6.4 ± 5.0	(n = 11)	0.440	
	Week 1	− 5.0 ± 3.3	(n = 10)	− 8.6 ± 6.4	(n = 11)	0.117	
	Week 2	− 3.0 ± 4.2	(n = 10)	− 7.7 ± 5.2	(n = 11)	0.034	*
	Week 3	− 2.0 ± 3.5	(n = 10)	− 5.9 ± 4.9	(n = 11)	0.051	
	Week 4	− 0.5 ± 1.6	(n = 10)	-5.5 ± 4.7	(n = 11)	0.006	**
	Week 8	− 0.8 ± 2.0	(n = 6)	-4.2 ± 3.8	(n = 6)	0.086	
Active extension	Pre	− 7.0 ± 5.4	(n = 10)	− 6.8 ± 5.6	(n = 11)	0.940	
	Week 1	− 10.5 ± 7.6	(n = 10)	− 13.2 ± 7.2	(n = 11)	0.416	
	Week 2	−5.0 ± 5.3	(n = 10)	− 12.3 ± 5.2	(n = 11)	0.005	**
	Week 3	− 4.0 ± 3.9	(n = 10)	− 7.7 ± 4.1	(n = 11)	0.048	*
	Week 4	− 3.5 ± 4.1	(n = 10)	-6.4 ± 6.0	(n = 11)	0.220	
	Week 8	− 2.5 ± 2.7	(n = 6)	-5.8 ± 3.8	(n = 6)	0.110	
Passive flexion	Pre	126.0 ± 20.2	(n = 10)	119.1 ± 18.4	(n = 11)		
	Week 1	95.3 ± 16.9	(n = 10)	95.5 ± 7.6	(n = 11)		
	Week 2	103.5 ± 11.1	(n = 10)	102.7 ± 8.8	(n = 11)		
	Week 3	109.5 ± 9.8	(n = 10)	108.2 ± 9.3	(n = 11)		
	Week 4	115.8 ± 9.2	(n = 10)	110.9 ± 10.9	(n = 11)		
	Week 8	122.5 ± 11.7	(n = 6)	117.8 ± 11.4	(n = 6)		
Active flexion	Pre	123.0 ± 22.4	(n = 10)	115.0 ± 17.0	(n = 11)		
	Week 1	85.5 ± 25.1	(n = 10)	85.0 ± 12.2	(n = 11)		
	Week 2	96.0 ± 14.3	(n = 10)	94.1 ± 10.9	(n = 11)		
	Week 3	100.0 ± 21.6	(n = 10)	99.5 ± 13.5	(n = 11)		
	Week 4	108.0 ± 15.1	(n = 10)	104.1 ± 13.0	(n = 11)		
	Week 8	115.8 ± 13.6	(n = 6)	109.2 ± 11.6	(n = 6)		

*$P < 0.05$; **$P < 0.01$

SWS by as early as 4 weeks, and only the HAL group showed significantly better SWS at week 8 than in the pre-operative period. This difference exceeded the minimum clinically meaningful change in walking speed suggested for people with knee pain [31, 32]; thus, clinically meaningful changes were obtained early in the HAL group. Early recovery beyond the pre-operative period allows early discharge and early social reversion. In past studies, the post-operative walking speed did not recover to the pre-operative speed at 4 or 8 weeks

Table 5 Muscle strength in the HAL and control groups

Response	Visit	HAL group Mean ± SD		Control group Mean ± SD		P value	
Knee extension torque (Nm/kg)	Pre	1.10 ± 0.64	(n = 10)	0.91 ± 0.31	(n = 11)	0.373	
	Week 2	0.68 ± 0.43	(n = 10)	0.67 ± 0.23	(n = 10)	0.924	
	Week 4	0.93 ± 0.32	(n = 10)	0.85 ± 0.23	(n = 11)	0.541	
	Week 8	1.15 ± 0.12	(n = 6)	0.88 ± 0.17	(n = 5)	0.014	*
Knee flex torque (Nm/kg)	Pre	0.56 ± 0.22	(n = 10)	0.51 ± 0.22	(n = 11)		
	Week 2	0.36 ± 0.15	(n = 10)	0.41 ± 0.15	(n = 10)		
	Week 4	0.45 ± 0.16	(n = 10)	0.41 ± 0.15	(n = 11)		
	Week 8	0.51 ± 0.12	(n = 6)	0.50 ± 0.15	(n = 5)		

*$P < 0.05$

Table 6 Knee pain and functionality in the HAL and control groups

Response	Visit	HAL group Mean ± SD		Control group Mean ± SD		P value	
WOMAC-P	Pre	72.0 ± 13.4	(n = 10)	60.0 ± 23.2	(n = 11)	0.169	
	Week 2	78.0 ± 15.7	(n = 10)	59.1 ± 18.4	(n = 11)	0.021	*
	Week 4	79.0 ± 12.4	(n = 10)	80.0 ± 13.6	(n = 11)	0.863	
	Week 8	88.0 ± 5.7	(n = 5)	79.2 ± 14.6	(n = 6)	0.218	
WOMAC-F	Pre	82.2 ± 16.9	(n = 10)	74.6 ± 15.0	(n = 11)	0.287	
	Week 2	82.8 ± 14.5	(n = 9)	69.6 ± 19.0	(n = 10)	0.110	
	Week 4	86.5 ± 10.6	(n = 10)	83.3 ± 11.3	(n = 11)	0.515	
	Week 8	92.6 ± 6.6	(n = 5)	85.3 ± 5.7	(n = 6)	0.077	

Abbreviations: Western Ontario and McMaster Universities Osteoarthritis Index *WOMAC-P*, Subscale of pain in WOMAC; *WOMAC-F*, Subscale of function in WOMAC
*$P < 0.05$

postoperatively [33, 34], but was found to recover by 12 weeks [4, 5, 7, 31]. Owing to the early recovery in walking speed, it can be stated that HAL training can be an effective rehabilitation intervention for patients after TKA.

At weeks 2 and 3, the active knee extension ROM in the HAL group was better than that in the control group. Extension lag has been reported to be associated with muscle strain reduction in the quadriceps muscles [9]. Improvement in extension lag at week 2 implies recovery of knee extension, possibly through a potential neuromuscular mechanism [8, 35], and might have led to an improvement in the knee extension torque in the HAL group than in the control group, which was observed at weeks 8. In a case report where a HAL-SJ was applied after TKA [26], the authors suggested that improvement in the extension lag was brought about by the HAL-SJ-mediated promotion of muscle and nerve function in the quadriceps muscle. Due to the assistance during knee motion, the extension lag during walking decreased, and it was believed that the increase in step length led to an improvement in walking speed. Similarly, in our previous study on HAL training in stroke patients, improvements in walking speed accompanied by improvements in gait symmetry and increase in step length were observed [36]. The torque assistance provided by the HAL allows the therapist to gradually adjust the magnitude of the myoelectric potential emitted by the patient in real time, and it allows the adjustment of the degree of effort required by the patient to walk almost normally. The involvement of repetitive movements and voluntary activities is an important factor for motor learning [37, 38]. HAL training for post-TKA patients seems to be a voluntary iterative exercise of sensory feedback of normal joint movement and walking pattern.

The WOMAC-P score was significantly greater in the HAL group than in the control group, indicating that postoperative pain was relieved by early as week 2.

Knee pain is associated with abnormal muscle activity [39], co-contraction [40], and weakness [41], and it is known to affect extension lag [10] and walking ability [42]. By using HAL, gradual assistance is provided to patients so that pain is not experienced or aggravated, and exercises are conducted so as not to cause co-contraction of the flexion and extension muscles at an early stage. These may have contributed to the improvement in walking ability and the reduction in extension lag.

In the HAL group, the patients could participate in all sessions without experiencing adverse events. HAL training after TKA can therefore be considered safe. In fact, the time of HAL training is unexpectedly less than the set time limit, and it seems that the cost effectiveness and wearing time of HAL training should be evaluated in future trials.

Limitations

Although there is no difference between the two groups in terms of patients' background, this study was non-randomized and non-blinded with a small number of patients. Since the size of single leg HAL was medium only at that time, only the patients who agreed to receive HAL training and their physique allowed for HAL device underwent HAL training. Moreover, there is no data over 8 weeks. Therefore, in the future, a randomized controlled trial with a larger number of patients and longer follow-up is necessary to consider as potential bias risks. However, the intervention procedure and evaluation items in this study are reasonable, and this pilot study can be helpful in planning the future randomized controlled trial. Although there is no significant difference between the two groups in the number of cases that already undergone TKA on the contralateral side and the total physical therapy time including HAL training, it is necessary to align these precisely in the future study.

Conclusion

HAL training after TKA can improve walking speed, step length, early active knee extension ROM, and muscle strength without severe pain better than conventional rehabilitation for up to 8 weeks after TKA. Since the recovery of walking ability was earlier in the HAL group than in the control group and no adverse events were noted, HAL training can be considered a safe and effective rehabilitation intervention for patients who have undergone TKA. Since this study was a preliminary study, a randomized controlled trial with a larger number of patients and loner follow-up is necessary in the future.

Abbreviations

ADL: Activities of daily living; ANOVA: Analysis of variance; CVC: Cybernic Voluntary Control; HAL: Hybrid Assistive Limb; MWS: Maximum walking speed; OA: Osteoarthritis; QOL: Quality of life; RA: Rheumatoid arthritis; RAT: Robot-assisted training; ROM: Range of motion; SL-MWS: Step length at maximum walking speed; SL-SWS: Step length at self-selected walking speed; SWS: Self-selected walking speed; TKA: Total knee arthroplasty; WOMAC: Western Ontario and McMaster Universities Osteoarthritis Index; WOMAC-f: Subscale of function in WOMAC; WOMAC-p: Subscale of pain in WOMAC

Acknowledgements

We are grateful to the physical therapists at Ibaraki Prefectural University of Health Sciences Hospital who helped in the intervention and assessment.

Funding

This work was supported by Grant-in-Aid for Project Research (1655) from Ibaraki Prefectural University of Health Sciences.

Authors' contributions

KY participated in the design of the study, performed the data collection, analysis, and interpretation, and drafted and revised the manuscript. HM participated in the design of the study and analysis, collected patient's informed consent, performed TKAs, and drafted and revised the manuscript. AS and KK performed the HAL training and assessments. TF performed the assessments. MM and MY participated in the coordination and design of the study and in finalizing the manuscript. All authors read and approved the final manuscript.

Competing interests

The authors declare that they have no competing interests.

Author details

[1]Department of Physical Therapy, Ibaraki Prefectural University of Health Sciences Hospital, 4773 Ami, Ami-machi, Inashiki-gun, Ibaraki 300-0331, Japan. [2]Department of Orthopaedic Surgery, Ibaraki Prefectural University of Health Sciences, 4669-2 Ami, Ami-machi, Inashiki-gun, Ibaraki 300-0394, Japan. [3]Department of Physical Therapy, Faculty of Health Sciences, Tsukuba International University, 6-8-33 Manabe, Tsuchiura, Ibaraki 300-0051, Japan. [4]Department of Physical Therapy, Ibaraki Prefectural University of Health Sciences, 4669-2 Ami, Ami-machi, Inashiki-gun, Ibaraki 300-0394, Japan. [5]Department of Orthopaedic Surgery, Faculty of Medicine, University of Tsukuba, 1-1-1 Tennodai, Tsukuba, Ibaraki 305-8575, Japan.

References

1. Sanna M, Sanna C, Caputo F, Piu G, Salvi M. Surgical approaches in total knee arthroplasty. Joints. 2013;1:34.
2. Gøthesen Ø, Espehaug B, Havelin L, Petursson G, Lygre S, Ellison P, et al. Survival rates and causes of revision in cemented primary total knee replacement: a report from the Norwegian arthroplasty register 1994–2009. Bone Joint J. 2013;95:636–42.
3. Ethgen O, Bruyere O, Richy F, Dardennes C, Reginster J-Y. Health-related quality of life in total hip and total knee arthroplasty: a qualitative and systematic review of the literature. JBJS. 2004;86:963–74.
4. Mizner RL, Petterson SC, Snyder-Mackler L. Quadriceps strength and the time course of functional recovery after total knee arthroplasty. J Orthop Sports Phys Ther. 2005;35:424–36.
5. Turcot K, Sagawa Y Jr, Fritschy D, Hoffmeyer P, Suva D, Armand S. How gait and clinical outcomes contribute to patients' satisfaction three months following a total knee arthroplasty. J Arthroplast. 2013;28:1297–300.
6. Pua YH, Seah FJ, Clark RA, Lian-Li Poon C, Tan JW, Chong HC. Factors associated with gait speed recovery after total knee arthroplasty: a longitudinal study. Semin Arthritis Rheum. 2017;46:544–51.
7. Yoshida Y, Mizner RL, Ramsey DK, Snyder-Mackler L. Examining outcomes from total knee arthroplasty and the relationship between quadriceps strength and knee function over time. Clin Biomech. 2008;23:320–8.
8. Sakamoto R, Takemasa S, Nakagawa N. Extensor lag after the total knee arthroplasty for the knee oseteoarthritis. Bulletin of Kobe University Graduate School of Health Sciences. 2009;24:29-39.
9. Sprague RB. Factors related to extension lag at the knee joint. J Orthop Sports Phys Ther. 1982;3:178–82.
10. Gotlin RS, Hershkowitz S, Juris PM, Gonzalez EG, Scott WN, Insall JN. Electrical stimulation effect on extensor lag and length of hospital stay after total knee arthroplasty. Arch Phys Med Rehabil. 1994;75:957–9.
11. Mehrholz J, Elsner B, Werner C, Kugler J, Pohl M. Electromechanical-assisted training for walking after stroke updated evidence. Stroke. 2013;44:e127-e8.
12. Cheung EYY, Ng TKW, Yu KKK, Kwan RLC, Cheing GLY. Robot-assisted training for people with spinal cord injury: a meta-analysis. Arch Phys Med Rehabil. 2017;98:2320–31.
13. Carvalho I, Pinto SM, das Virgens Chagas D, dos Santos JLP, de Sousa Oliveira T, Batista LA. Robotic gait training for individuals with cerebral palsy: a systematic review and meta-analysis. Arch Phys Med Rehabil. 2017;98:2332–44.
14. Henderson KG, Wallis JA, Snowdon DA. Active physiotherapy interventions following total knee arthroplasty in the hospital and inpatient rehabilitation settings: a systematic review and meta-analysis. Physiotherapy. 2018;104:25–35.
15. Kawamoto H, Kamibayashi K, Nakata Y, Yamawaki K, Ariyasu R, Sankai Y, et al. Pilot study of locomotion improvement using hybrid assistive limb in chronic stroke patients. BMC Neurol. 2013;13:141.
16. Kawamoto H, Taal S, Niniss H, Hayashi T, Kamibayashi K, Eguchi K, et al., editors. Voluntary motion support control of robot suit HAL triggered by bioelectrical signal for hemiplegia. Conf Proc IEEE Eng Med Biol Soc. 2010; 2010:462-6.
17. Suzuki K, Mito G, Kawamoto H, Hasegawa Y, Sankai Y. Intention-based walking support for paraplegia patients with robot suit HAL. Adv Robot. 2007;21:1441–69.
18. Nilsson A, Vreede KS, Haglund V, Kawamoto H, Sankai Y, Borg J. Gait training early after stroke with a new exoskeleton–the hybrid assistive limb: a study of safety and feasibility. J Neuroeng Rehabil. 2014;11:92.
19. Watanabe H, Tanaka N, Inuta T, Saitou H, Yanagi H. Locomotion improvement using a hybrid assistive limb in recovery phase stroke patients: a randomized controlled pilot study. Arch Phys Med Rehabil. 2014;95:2006–12.
20. Sczesny-Kaiser M, Höffken O, Aach M, Cruciger O, Grasmücke D, Meindl R, et al. HAL® exoskeleton training improves walking parameters and normalizes cortical excitability in primary somatosensory cortex in spinal cord injury patients. J Neuroeng Rehabil. 2015;12:1.

21. Matsuda M, Mataki Y, Mutsuzaki H, Yoshikawa K, Takahashi K, Enomoto K, et al. Immediate effects of a single session of robot-assisted gait training using Hybrid Assistive Limb (HAL) for cerebral palsy. J Phys Ther Sci. 2018;30:207–12.

22. Sugimura Y, Takahashi T, Iijima Y, Nakajima H, Fujiya Y, Shimosegawa Y, et al. The efficacy of treatment using hybrid assistive limb for patients with neuromuscular disease. J Neurol Sci. 2017;381:836.

23. Tanaka Y, Oka H, Nakayama S, Ueno T, Matsudaira K, Miura T, et al. Improvement of walking ability during postoperative rehabilitation with the hybrid assistive limb after total knee arthroplasty: a randomized controlled study. SAGE Open Med. 2017;5:2050312117712888.

24. Yoshioka T, Sugaya H, Kubota S, Onishi M, Kanamori A, Sankai Y, et al. Knee-extension training with a single-joint hybrid assistive limb during the early postoperative period after total knee arthroplasty in a patient with osteoarthritis. Case Rep Orthop. 2016;2016:9610745.

25. Fukaya T, Mutsuzaki H, Yoshikawa K, Sano A, Mizukami M, Yamazaki M. The training effect of early intervention with a hybrid assistive limb after total knee arthroplasty. Case Rep Orthop. 2017;2017:1.

26. Mutsuzaki H, Takeuchi R, Mataki Y, Wadano Y. Target range of motion for rehabilitation after total knee arthroplasty. J Rural Med. 2017;12:33–7.

27. Bohannon RW. Comfortable and maximum walking speed of adults aged 20—79 years: reference values and determinants. Age Ageing. 1997;26:15–9.

28. Bellamy N, Buchanan WW, Goldsmith CH, Campbell J, Stitt LW. Validation study of WOMAC: a health status instrument for measuring clinically important patient relevant outcomes to antirheumatic drug therapy in patients with osteoarthritis of the hip or knee. Rheumatol. 1988;15:1833–40.

29. Hashimoto H, Hanyu T, Sledge CB, Lingard EA. Validation of a Japanese patient-derived outcome scale for assessingtotal knee arthroplasty: comparison with Western Ontario and McMaster Universities osteoarthritis index (WOMAC). J Orthop Sci. 2003;8:288–93.

30. Huck SW. Reading statistics and research sixth edition. 6th ed. Boston: Pearson; 2012.

31. Abbasi-Bafghi H, Fallah-Yakhdani HR, Meijer OG, de Vet HC, Bruijn SM, Yang L-Y, et al. The effects of knee arthroplasty on walking speed: a meta-analysis. BMC Musculoskelet Disord. 2012;13:66.

32. White DK, Felson DT, Niu J, Nevitt MC, Lewis CE, Torner JC, et al. Reasons for functional decline despite reductions in knee pain: the multicenter osteoarthritis study. Phys Ther. 2011;91:1849–56.

33. Fusi S, Campailla E, Causero A, di Prampero P. The locomotory index: a new proposal for evaluating walking impairments. Int J Sports Med. 2002;23:105–11.

34. Parent E, Moffet H. Comparative responsiveness of locomotor tests and questionnaires used to follow early recovery after total knee arthroplasty. Arch Phys Med Rehabil. 2002;83:70–80.

35. Kennedy JC, Alexander IJ, Hayes KC. Nerve supply of the human knee and its functional importance. Am J Sports Med. 1982;10:329–35.

36. Yoshikawa K, Mizukami M, Kawamoto H, Sano A, Koseki K, Sano K, et al. Gait training with Hybrid Assistive Limb enhances the gait functions in subacute stroke patients: a pilot study. NeuroRehabilitation. 2017;40:87–97.

37. Pennycott A, Wyss D, Vallery H, Klamroth-Marganska V, Riener R. Towards more effective robotic gait training for stroke rehabilitation: a review. J Neuroeng Rehabil. 2012;9:65.

38. Lotze M, Braun C, Birbaumer N, Anders S, Cohen LG. Motor learning elicited by voluntary drive. Brain. 2003;126:866–72.

39. Rice DA, McNair PJ. Quadriceps arthrogenic muscle inhibition: neural mechanisms and treatment perspectives. Semin Arthritis Rheum. 2010;40:250–66.

40. Preece SJ, Jones RK, Brown CA, Cacciatore TW, Jones AK. Reductions in co-contraction following neuromuscular re-education in people with knee osteoarthritis. BMC Musculoskelet Disord. 2016;17:372.

41. Perry J, Davids JR. Gait analysis: normal and pathological function. NJ: Slack; 1992. p. 815.

42. Lee I-h, S-y P. A comparison of gait characteristics in the elderly people, people with knee pain, and people who are walker dependent people. J Phys Ther Sci. 2013;25:973–6.

17

Effects of bisphosphonates in preventing periprosthetic bone loss following total hip arthroplasty

Jialing Shi[1†], Guang Liang[2†], Rongzhi Huang[1], Liang Liao[2*] and Danlu Qin[3*]

Abstract

Background: Periprosthetic bone loss following total hip arthroplasty (THA) was a well-known phenomenon. This systematic review was to assess the effectiveness of bisphosphonates (BPs) for decreasing periprosthetic bone resorption.

Methods: The MEDLINE, EMBASE, and Cochrane Library databases were searched up to March 2018. Randomized controlled trials compared the effects between administrating BPs and placebo or no medication were eligible; the target participants were patients who underwent THA. Mean differences (MD) and 95% confidence interval (95% CI) were calculated by using the random-effects models. Statistical analyses were performed by RevMan 5.3 software.

Results: Fourteen trials involving 620 patients underwent THA were retrieved. BPs significantly prevented the loss of periprosthetic bone mineral density at 1 year (MD, 0.06 [95% CI, 0.03 to 0.08], $p < 0.001$), between 2 and 4 years (MD, 0.04 [95% CI, 0.01 to 0.07], $p = 0.02$), and more than 5 years after THA (MD, 0.08 [95% CI, 0.06 to 0.11], $p < 0.001$). Both serum bone alkaline phosphatase (MD, -7.28 [95% CI, -9.81 to -4.75], $p < 0.001$) and urinary N-telopeptide of type I collagen (MD, -24.37 [95% CI, -36.37 to -12.37], $p < 0.001$) in BP group were significantly lower. Subgroup analyses showed that the third-generation BPs were more effective in decreasing periprosthetic bone loss than the first and second generation within 1 year after THA ($p = 0.001$).

Conclusion: BPs were beneficial to decreasing periprosthetic bone loss. The third-generation BPs showed significantly efficacy for patients in short-term observation.

Keywords: Bisphosphonates, Total hip arthroplasty, Bone resorption, Meta-analysis

Background

Total hip arthroplasty (THA) has become the most effective therapy for severe osteoarthritis [1–3]. It was estimated that approximately 572,000 patients will demand primary THA in the USA by the year 2030 [4]. Periprosthetic bone resorption following THA was a well-known phenomenon [5]. It may increase late-occurring periprosthetic fractures [6]. Moreover, bone resorption may decrease the primary stability of the implant and lead to progressive implant loosening [7], which was considered as the most common reason for revision [8]. Compared with primary THA, the risk of local and systemic complications increased and favorable benefits decreased in revision surgeries [9]. Therefore, strategies for inhibiting periprosthetic bone resorption and maintaining bone stock were essential.

Bisphosphonates (BPs), a family of drugs with a strong anti-osteoclast activity, were widely used for the first-line treatment of osteoporosis [10]. Mass data had showed that BPs inhibited bone resorption, increased bone mineral density, and reduced the risk of fractures [11]. Nevertheless, there was still controversy about the

* Correspondence: 237586233@qq.com; 53595883@qq.com
[†]Jialing Shi and Guang Liang contributed equally to this work.
[2]The first affiliated Hospital of Guangxi Medical University, The First Clinical Medical College, No. 6, Shuang Yong Road, Nanning 530021, Guangxi Zhuang Autonomous Region, China
[3]Department of the Second Endocrinology Ward, Jiangbin Hospital of Guangxi Zhuang Autonomous Region, Nanning 530021, Guangxi Zhuang Autonomous Region, China
Full list of author information is available at the end of the article

effect and mechanism of BPs on inhibiting periprosthetic bone loss after THA. Some studies indicated that BPs had no significant effect on suppressing bone loss after THA [12, 13]. In contrast, previous meta-analyses suggested BPs could inhibit early bone resorption around the implant [14–17]. However, these studies only included randomized controlled trials (RCTs) published before 2011. And target participants were not only THA but also total knee arthroplasty (TKA) and hemiarthroplasty in some studies. Compared with previous articles, this meta-analysis complemented the latest RCTs and had a larger sample size (620 patients). Moreover, it applied more rigorous eligibility of criteria and excluded trials involving TKA or hemiarthroplasty to reduce heterogeneity.

It was essential to perform a meta-analysis based on the latest evidence. This systematic review was to assess the effectiveness of BPs for decreasing periprosthetic bone resorption.

Methods
Literature search
The electronic literature search lasted up to 10 March 2018. Without language restrictions, reviewers searched PubMed (1966 to present), EMBASE (1980 to present), Ovid (1860 to present), and the Cochrane Library (Issue 1, 2017) by using the following items: "total hip arthroplasty," "bisphosphonates," "bone resorption," and their associated words. Reference lists of all the selected studies were hand-searched for any additional trials. Two reviewers independently assessed trials for inclusion and resolved disagreements by discussion.

Inclusion and exclusion criteria
Studies were eligible for inclusion: (1) target participants were patients who underwent THA, (2) compared the effects between administrating BPs and placebo or no medication, and (3) randomized controlled trials. We excluded studies if (1) participants had a history of metabolic bone diseases, bone tumor, or renal failure; (2) the same randomized controlled trial was reanalyzed with a shorter follow-up.

Outcome measure
The primary outcome was periprosthetic bone mineral density (BMD) because this data is the most intuitive index to reflect the extent of periprosthetic bone loss. In order to analyze the bone turnover activity, researchers also collected the data of biochemical bone turnover (serum bone alkaline phosphates (BAP, U/L) and urinary N-telopeptide of type I collagen (NTX-I, nmol/mmol Cr)) as the second outcome.

Quality assessment
Two reviewers independently assessed quality. Quality assessment consisted of random sequence generation, allocation concealment, blinding, incomplete outcome data, selective reporting, and other potential bias.

Data extraction
The data was extracted in table that included the first author, year of publication, original country, primary disease, type of THA, type of BPs, control group, the number of participants, treatment duration, time of following, and the number of loss to follow-up. If the data was not reported in the text or the table in the article, it was extrapolated from the accompanying graphs. Reviewers asked the corresponding author of the eligible study for additional information when necessary.

Statistical analysis
Statistical analysis was performed using Review Manager 5.3. Mean differences (MD) and 95% confidence interval (95% CI) were calculated for continuous outcomes. Meta-analysis was done according to a random-effects model. $P < 0.05$ was considered statistically significant. Heterogeneity was tested by using chi-square test with significance being set at $p > 0.1$ and I-square (I^2) was used to estimate total variation across studies due to heterogeneity in percentage. I^2 greater than 50% was considered as denoting substantial heterogeneity.

Result
Study identification
The search identified 1625 potentially relevant references. Four hundred forty trials were excluded for duplicates. And 1185 trials were eliminated all based on titles and abstracts but 22 trials. After requiring full-text review, 14 trials met the inclusion criteria. Eight trials were excluded for several reasons: participants underwent hemiarthroplasty (two trials), shorter follow-up and reanalyzed data (three trials), and shared groups of participants because participants, authors, and designs were similar (three trials). The rest of 14 trials were included in qualitative synthesis. Finally, these 14 trials published from 2004 to 2017 were included in our systematic review [18–31] (Fig. 1).

Characteristic of the studies
The included 14 studies were published from 2004 to 2017, with 318 participants receiving BPs and 302 receiving placebo or no medication. Table 1 provided more detailed information on these studies. Types of BPs were consisted of alendronate (six trials), etidronate (two trials), risedronate (three trials), pamidronate (one trial), zoledronate (one trial), and clodronate (one trial). G 1–2 BPs (etidronate, clodronate, and pamidronate) have simple R2 side

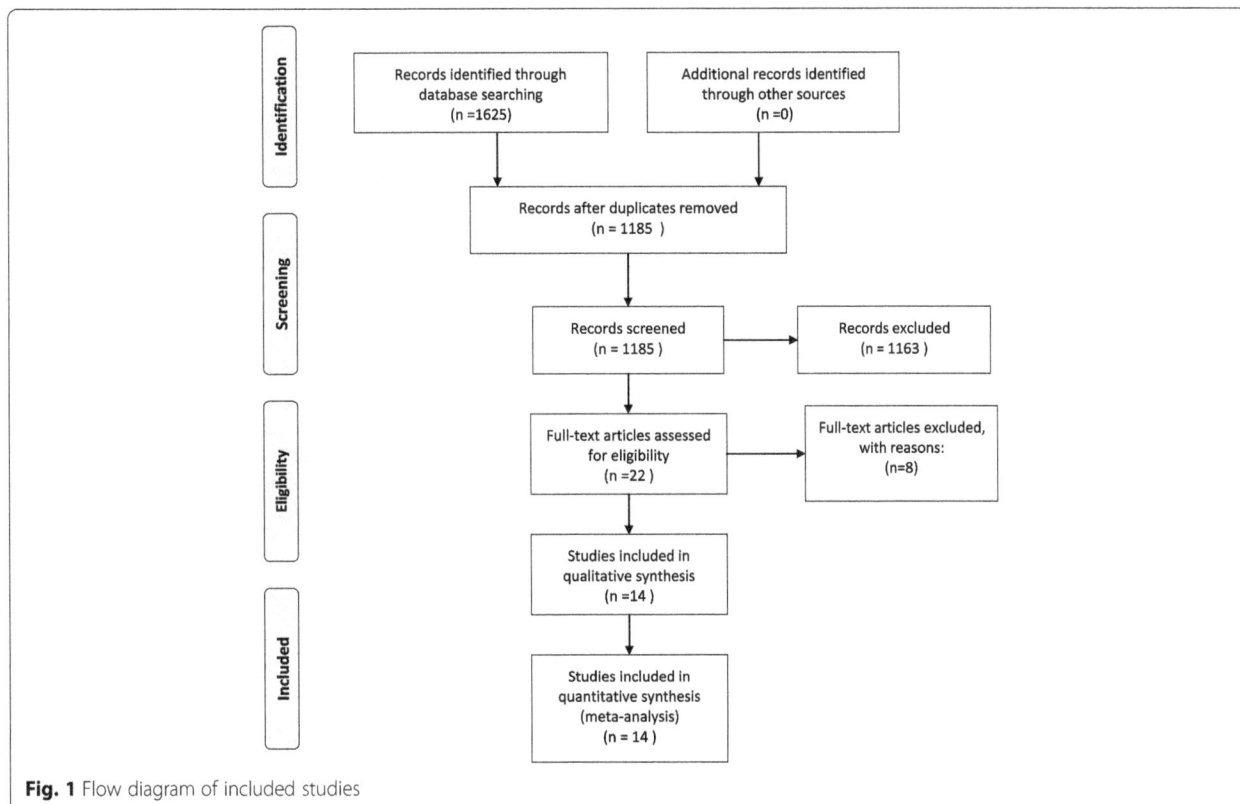

Fig. 1 Flow diagram of included studies

chains. And G 3 BPs (alendronate, risedronate, and zole-dronate) were developed by modifying the R2 side chain to include an amino group and heterocyclic structures. The dose and the duration of BP administration were different among the studies. The sample size ranged from 16 to 91 patients. Eleven trials reported BMD at different time points after THA surgery (ranged from 24 weeks to more than 9 years), and four trials reported biochemical markers of postoperativebone turnover markers. Table 2 provided outcomes of the 14 including articles.

Publication bias

The quality of included trials was assessed by the Cochrane collaboration's tool for assessing risk of bias (Fig. 2). All included trials were randomized controlled trials, most of which were low risk of bias and documented randomization, allocation concealment, blinding, and complete outcomes.

Periprosthetic bone mineral density (BMD)

BMD at 1 year after THA

Eleven trials including 465 participants compared BPs with placebo or no medication at 1 year after THA. As showed in Fig. 3, periprosthetic bone resorption in the BP group was significantly less than that in the control group (MD, 0.06 [95% CI, 0.03 to 0.08], $p < 0.001$). Both G 3 BPs and G 1–2 BPs observably inhibit bone

resorption, respectively [(MD, 0.03 [95% CI, 0.01 to 0.06], $p = 0.01$); (MD, 0.09 [95% CI, 0.07 to 0.11], $p < 0.001$)]. The difference in BMD between G 3 BP group and the control group was greater than that in between G 1–2 BP group and the control group ($p = 0.001$).

In subgroup analysis, the efficacy of BPs for BMD was significant in the uncemented THA subgroup (MD, 0.05 [95% CI, 0.02 to 0.09], $p = 0.002$), but no significant difference in cemented THA subgroup (MD, 0.06 [95% CI, 0.00 to 0.13], $p = 0.05$). These two subgroup difference was not significant ($p = 0.76$). The duration of BP administration more than 6 months dramatically inhibit bone resorption (MD, 0.07 [95% CI, 0.04 to 0.09], $p < 0.001$). And it seemly obtained more benefit for BMD than the duration less than 6 months, but no difference was showed between the subgroup analysis ($p = 0.45$) (Table 3).

BMD between 2 to 4 years after THA

Six trials including 250 participants compared BPs with placebo or no medication between 2 to 4 years after THA. As showed in Fig. 4, periprosthetic bone resorption in the BP group was significantly less than that in the control group (MD, 0.04 [95% CI, 0.01 to 0.07], $p = 0.02$). G 3 BPs observably inhibit bone resorption (MD, 0.05 [95% CI, 0.01 to 0.10], $p = 0.03$), but not in G 1–2 BP subgroup (MD, 0.01 [95% CI, – 0.04 to 0.06], $p = 0.69$).

Table 1 Characteristics of the 14 including articles

Study (author/year)	Country	Primary disease	Type of THA	Type of BPs	Control group	Men BPs	Men control	Women BPs	Women control	Treatment duration BPs	Treatment duration control	Time of following BPs	Time of following control	Loss to follow-up BPs	Loss to follow-up control
Tapaninen TS/2010 [18]	Finland	Primary hip osteoarthritis	Uncemented	Alendronate (G$_3$)	Calcium	2	5	5	4	0.5 year	0.5 year	5 years	5 years	0	0
Trevisan C/2010 [19]	Italy	NA	Uncemented	Clodronate (G$_2$)	No medication	26	27	16	22	1 year	No medication	1 year	1 year	4	8
Arabmotlagh M/2009 [20]	Germany	Degenerative osteoarthritis	Uncemented	Alendronate (G$_3$)	No medication	16	9	13	11	5/10 weeks	No medication	6 years	6 years	2	1
Yamasaki S/2007 [21]	Japan	Osteoarthritis secondary to acetabular dysplasia	Uncemented	Risedronate (G$_3$)	Placebo	2	2	17	19	0.5 year	0.5 year	0.5 year	0.5 year	3	0
Fokter SK/2006 [22]	Slovenia	Primary or secondary osteoarthritis	Cemented	Etidronate (G$_1$)	Placebo	6	3	12	10	1 year	1 year	1 year	1 year	2	1
Arabmotlagh M/2006 [23]	Germany	Degenerative primary osteoarthritis	Uncemented	Alendronate (G$_3$)	Placebo	14	12	13	12	0.5 year	0.5 year	52 weeks	52 weeks	0	0
Yamaguchi K/2004 [24]	Japan	Osteoarthritis secondary to hip dysplasia	Uncemented	Etidronate (G$_1$)	No medication	5	2	26	22	1 year	No medication	30 months	30 months	2	0
Iwamoto N/2011 [25]	Japan	Osteoarthritis	Uncemented	Alendronate (G$_3$)	No medication	4	5	16	17	48 weeks	no medication	48 weeks	48 weeks	2	0
Kinov P/2006 [26]	Bulgaria	Osteoarthritis, osteonecrosis, or hip fracture	Cemented or hybrid	Risedronate (G$_3$)	Placebo	4	5	8	7	0.5 year	0.5 year	0.5 year	0.5 year	0	0
Shetty N/2006 [27]	England	Primary or secondary osteoarthritis	Hybrid	Pamidronate (G$_2$)	Placebo	12	10	6	9	50 days	50 days	5 years	5 years	1	1
Scott DF/2013 [28]	America	NA	Uncemented	Zoledronate (G$_3$)	Placebo + calcium	12	11	15	13	Twice administration	Twice administration	2 years	2 years	0	0
Yukizawa Y/2017 [29]	Japan	Osteoarthritis	Uncemented	Alendronate (G$_3$)	No medication	4	7	14	9	≥ 2 years	no medication	≥ 9 years	≥ 9 years	0	0
Muren O/2015 [30]	Sweden	Osteoarthritis	Uncemented	Risedronate (G$_3$)	Placebo + calcium	20	18	10	13	0.5 year	0.5 year	4 years	4 years	0	0
Nehme A/2003 [31]	Lebanon	Degenerative hip disease	Cemented	Alendronate (G$_3$)	Placebo + calcium	NA	NA	NA	NA	2 years	2 years	2 years	2 years	0	0

THA total hip arthroplasty, BPs bisphosphonates, NA not applicable

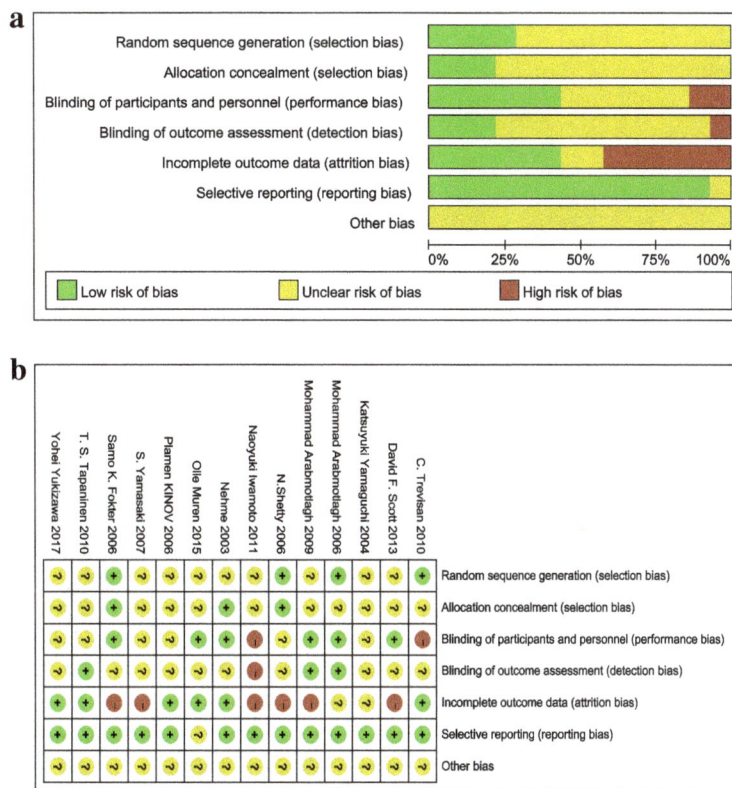

Fig. 2 Quality assessment. **a** Risk of bias graph: the author's judgments about each risk of bias item presented as percentages across all included studies. **b** Risk of bias summary: the author's judgments about each risk of bias item for all included studies

In subgroup analysis, the efficacy of BPs for BMD was significant in the cemented THA subgroup (MD, 0.07 [95% CI, 0.03 to 0.11], $p = 0.0003$). But no significant difference was observed comparing uncemented THA group with cemented THA group ($p = 0.46$). The duration of BP administration more than 6 months dramatically inhibit bone resorption (MD, 0.06 [95% CI, 0.03 to 0.10], $p = 0.0003$). However, subgroup difference was not significant on the treatment duration ($p = 0.32$) (Table 3).

BMD at more than 5 years after THA

Four trials including 136 participants compared BPs with placebo or no medication at more than 5 years after THA. As showed in Fig. 5, periprosthetic bone resorption in the BP group was significantly less than that in the control group (MD, 0.08 [95% CI, 0.06 to 0.11], $p < 0.001$). G 3 BPs observably inhibit bone resorption (MD, 0.09 [95% CI, 0.07 to 0.11], $p < 0.001$). No difference was showed in G 1–2 BP subgroup (MD, 0.01 [95% CI, – 0.09 to 0.11], $p = 0.85$).

In subgroup analysis, the duration of BP administration more than 6 months dramatically inhibit bone resorption (MD, 0.09 [95% CI, 0.07 to 0.11], $p < 0.001$). However, subgroup difference was not significant on the treatment duration ($p = 0.12$) (Table 3).

Serum bone alkaline phosphatase (BAP)

Four trials including 179 participants compared BPs with placebo or no medication on serum bone alkaline phosphatase. BAP in the control group were significantly higher than that in the BP group (MD, – 7.28 [95% CI, – 9.81 to – 4.75], $p < 0.001$) (Fig. 6). Reviewers did not performed subgroup analyses for BAP as the eligible trials were not enough.

Urinary N-telopeptide of type I collagen (NTX-I)

Two trials including 104 participants compared BPs with placebo or no medication on NTX-I. NTX-I in the BP group were significantly lower than that in the control group (MD, – 24.37 [95% CI, – 36.3 to – 12.37], $p < 0.001$) (Fig. 7). Reviewers did not perform subgroup analyses for BAP as the eligible trials were not enough.

Discussion

This systematic review indicated that BPs could significantly decrease periprosthetic bone resorption at short-, medium-, and long-term observation. The third-generation BPs (G 3 BPs) showed significant efficacy for patients. In addition, this review found that both BAP and NTX-I in the BP group were significantly lower than that in the control group. In subgroup analysis, administration of BPs

Table 2 Outcomes of the 14 including articles

Study (author/year)	BMD (mean ± SD) (g/cm²)			BAP (mean ± SD) (U/L) (BPs vs. control)	NTX-I (mean ± SD) (nmol/mmol Cr) (BPs vs. control)
	1 year (BPs vs. control)	2–4 years (BPs vs. control)	≥ 5 years (BPs vs. control)		
Tapaninen TS/2010 [18]	−0.04 ± 0.09 vs. − 0.12 ± 0.10	−0.05 ± 0.12 vs. − 0.18 ± 0.21	−0.06 ± 0.12 vs. − 0.16 ± 0.24	NA	NA
Trevisan C/2010 [19]	−0.04 ± 0.07 vs. − 0.07 ± 0.08	NA	NA	NA	NA
Arabmotlagh M/2009 [20]	−0.02 ± 0.16 vs. − 0.04 ± 0.09	NA	−0.02 ± 0.17 vs. − 0.06 ± 0.20	NA	NA
Yamasaki S/2007 [21]	NA	NA	NA	21.5 ± 7.7 vs. 31.2 ± 9.6	39.2 ± 15.9 vs.70.3 ± 27.7
Fokter SK/2006 [22]	−0.06 ± 0.07 vs. − 0.06 ± 0.23	NA	NA	NA	NA
Arabmotlagh M/2006 [23]	0 ± 0.16 vs. − 0.07 ± 0.22	NA	NA	17.9 ± 6 vs. 27.1 ± 8.9	NA
Yamaguchi K/2004 [24]	−0.06 ± 0.12 vs. − 0.12 ± 0.14	−0.09 ± 0.13 vs. − 0.13 ± 0.13	NA	25.2 ± 6.6 vs. 29.6 ± 8.7	52.5 ± 29.2 vs. 71.3 ± 17.8
Iwamoto N/2011 [25]	0 ± 0.12 vs. − 0.08 ± 0.14	NA	NA	NA	NA
Kinov P/2006 [26]	NA	NA	NA	19.93 ± 6.6 vs. 26.9 ± 5.9	NA
Shetty N/2006 [27]	−0.01 ± 0.07 vs. − 0.02 ± 0.14	−0.02 ± 0.05 vs. − 0.01 ± 0.16	−0.02 ± 0.01 vs. − 0.03 ± 0.2	NA	NA
Scott DF/2013 [28]	0.80 ± 10.4 vs. − 6.03 ± 13.2	−0.16 ± 14.0 vs. − 7.13 ± 12.7	NA	NA	NA
Yukizawa Y/2017 [29]	−0.04 ± 0.02 vs. − 0.13 ± 0.02	NA	−0.12 ± 0.03 vs. − 0.21 ± 0.02	NA	NA
Muren O/2015 [30]	NA	−0.19 ± 0.02 vs. − 0.22 ± 0.03	NA	NA	NA
Nehme A/2003 [31]	−0.24 ± 0.07 vs. − 0.32 ± 0.07	−0.09 ± 0.06 vs. − 0.16 ± 0.06	NA	NA	NA

BPs bisphosphonates, *BMD* bone mineral density, *BAP* serum bone alkaline phosphates, *NTX-I* urinary N-telopeptide of type I collagen, *NA* not applicable

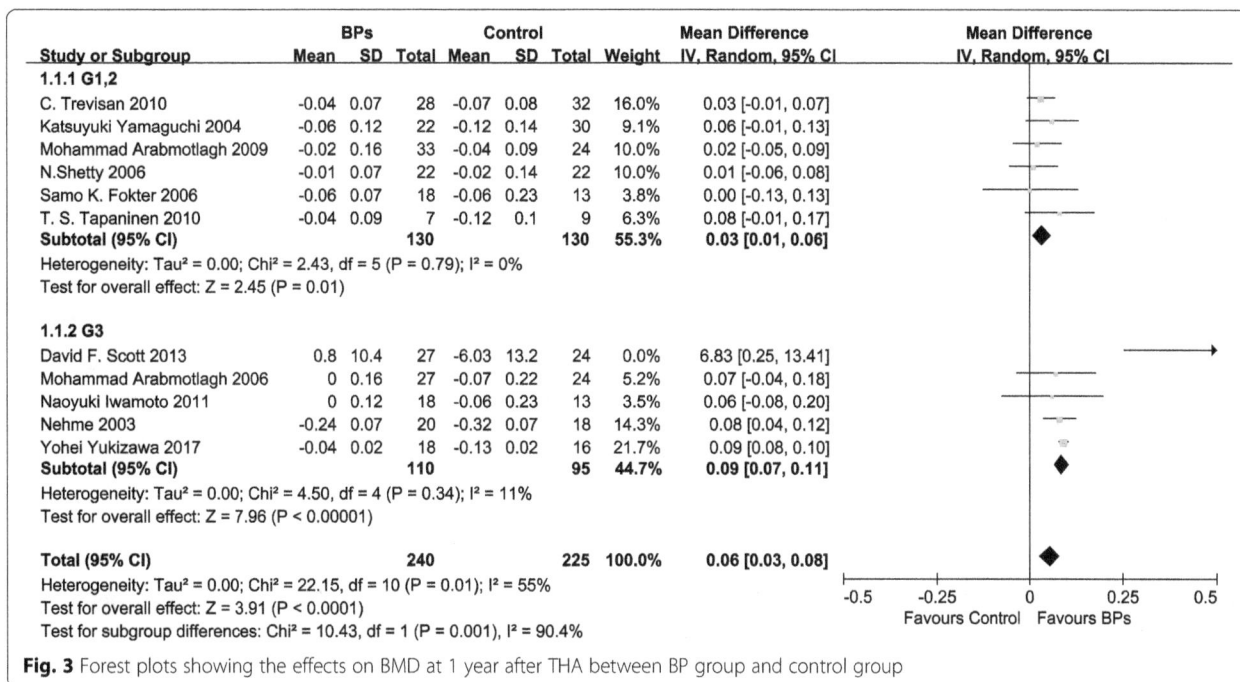

Study or Subgroup	BPs Mean	SD	Total	Control Mean	SD	Total	Weight	Mean Difference IV, Random, 95% CI
1.1.1 G1,2								
C. Trevisan 2010	-0.04	0.07	28	-0.07	0.08	32	16.0%	0.03 [-0.01, 0.07]
Katsuyuki Yamaguchi 2004	-0.06	0.12	22	-0.12	0.14	30	9.1%	0.06 [-0.01, 0.13]
Mohammad Arabmotlagh 2009	-0.02	0.16	33	-0.04	0.09	24	10.0%	0.02 [-0.05, 0.09]
N.Shetty 2006	-0.01	0.07	22	-0.02	0.14	22	10.0%	0.01 [-0.06, 0.08]
Samo K. Fokter 2006	-0.06	0.07	18	-0.06	0.23	13	3.8%	0.00 [-0.13, 0.13]
T. S. Tapaninen 2010	-0.04	0.09	7	-0.12	0.1	9	6.3%	0.08 [-0.01, 0.17]
Subtotal (95% CI)			**130**			**130**	**55.3%**	**0.03 [0.01, 0.06]**
Heterogeneity: Tau² = 0.00; Chi² = 2.43, df = 5 (P = 0.79); I² = 0%								
Test for overall effect: Z = 2.45 (P = 0.01)								
1.1.2 G3								
David F. Scott 2013	0.8	10.4	27	-6.03	13.2	24	0.0%	6.83 [0.25, 13.41]
Mohammad Arabmotlagh 2006	0	0.16	27	-0.07	0.22	24	5.2%	0.07 [-0.04, 0.18]
Naoyuki Iwamoto 2011	0	0.12	18	-0.06	0.23	13	3.5%	0.06 [-0.08, 0.20]
Nehme 2003	-0.24	0.07	20	-0.32	0.07	18	14.3%	0.08 [0.04, 0.12]
Yohei Yukizawa 2017	-0.04	0.02	18	-0.13	0.02	16	21.7%	0.09 [0.08, 0.10]
Subtotal (95% CI)			**110**			**95**	**44.7%**	**0.09 [0.07, 0.11]**
Heterogeneity: Tau² = 0.00; Chi² = 4.50, df = 4 (P = 0.34); I² = 11%								
Test for overall effect: Z = 7.96 (P < 0.00001)								
Total (95% CI)			**240**			**225**	**100.0%**	**0.06 [0.03, 0.08]**
Heterogeneity: Tau² = 0.00; Chi² = 22.15, df = 10 (P = 0.01); I² = 55%								
Test for overall effect: Z = 3.91 (P < 0.0001)								
Test for subgroup differences: Chi² = 10.43, df = 1 (P = 0.001), I² = 90.4%								

Fig. 3 Forest plots showing the effects on BMD at 1 year after THA between BP group and control group

Table 3 Subgroup analysis of association between BPs and BMD for each variable

Variable	No. of trials	No. of participants BPs	Control	MD	95% CI	p value
1 year after THA						
Type of THA						
Cemented	2	38	31	0.06	0.00–0.13	0.76
Uncemented	9	202	194	0.05	0.02–0.09	
Treatment duration of BPs						
≤ 6 months	5	96	88	0.04	− 0.01–0.10	0.32
> 6 months	6	124	122	0.07	0.04–0.09	
2–4 year after THA						
Type of THA						
Cemented	1	20	18	0.05	0.02–0.09	0.46
Uncemented	4	80	88	0.07	0.03–0.11	
Treatment duration of BPs						
≤ 6 months	4	86	86	0.03	− 0.03–0.09	0.32
> 6 months	2	36	42	0.06	0.03–0.10	
≥ 5 year after THA						
Type of THA						
Cemented	0	0	0	Not estimable	Not estimable	NA
Uncemented	3	54	45	0.09	0.07–0.11	
Treatment duration of BPs						
≤ 6 months	3	54	48	0.03	− 0.03–0.10	0.12
> 6 months	1	18	16	0.09	0.07–0.11	

THA total hip arthroplasty, BPs bisphosphonates, MD mean differences, CI confidence interval, NA not applicable

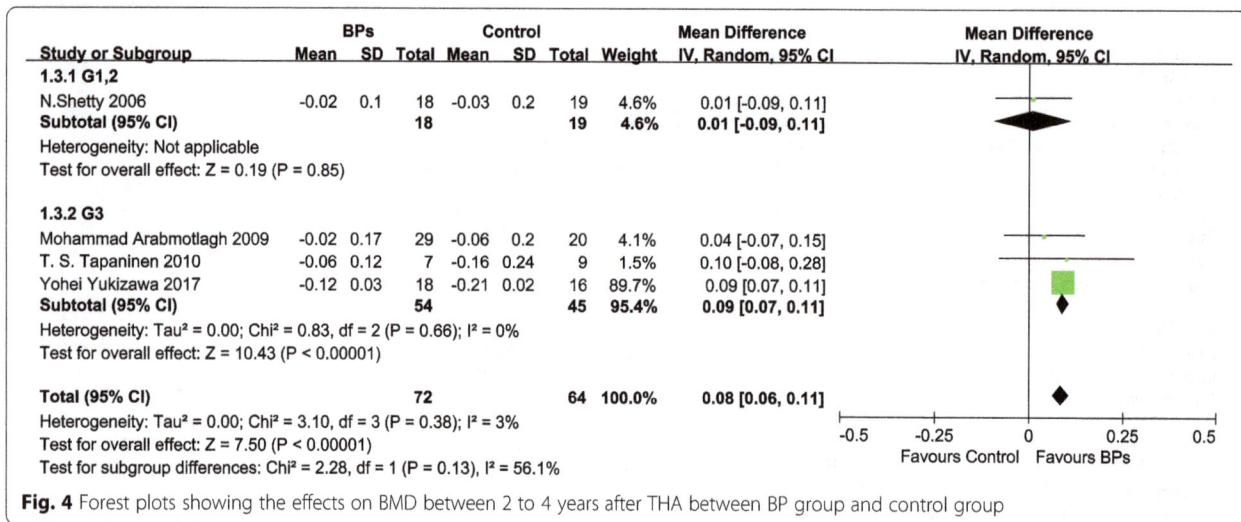

Study or Subgroup	BPs Mean	SD	Total	Control Mean	SD	Total	Weight	Mean Difference IV, Random, 95% CI
1.3.1 G1,2								
N.Shetty 2006	-0.02	0.1	18	-0.03	0.2	19	4.6%	0.01 [-0.09, 0.11]
Subtotal (95% CI)			**18**			**19**	**4.6%**	**0.01 [-0.09, 0.11]**
Heterogeneity: Not applicable								
Test for overall effect: Z = 0.19 (P = 0.85)								
1.3.2 G3								
Mohammad Arabmotlagh 2009	-0.02	0.17	29	-0.06	0.2	20	4.1%	0.04 [-0.07, 0.15]
T. S. Tapaninen 2010	-0.06	0.12	7	-0.16	0.24	9	1.5%	0.10 [-0.08, 0.28]
Yohei Yukizawa 2017	-0.12	0.03	18	-0.21	0.02	16	89.7%	0.09 [0.07, 0.11]
Subtotal (95% CI)			**54**			**45**	**95.4%**	**0.09 [0.07, 0.11]**
Heterogeneity: Tau² = 0.00; Chi² = 0.83, df = 2 (P = 0.66); I² = 0%								
Test for overall effect: Z = 10.43 (P < 0.00001)								
Total (95% CI)			**72**			**64**	**100.0%**	**0.08 [0.06, 0.11]**
Heterogeneity: Tau² = 0.00; Chi² = 3.10, df = 3 (P = 0.38); I² = 3%								
Test for overall effect: Z = 7.50 (P < 0.00001)								
Test for subgroup differences: Chi² = 2.28, df = 1 (P = 0.13), I² = 56.1%								

Fig. 4 Forest plots showing the effects on BMD between 2 to 4 years after THA between BP group and control group

more than 6 months seemly obtained more benefit for BMD than the duration less than 6 months at long-term observation.

Compared with placebo or no medication, patient in BP group obtained more benefit for BMD especially in the G 3 BP group. Previous studies indicated that aseptic loosening was associated with poor bone quality [32]. The surrounding bone stock provided primary stability of the prosthesis and osseointegration, sealed the bone-implant interfaces, and reduced the implant migration. It was a key factor to avoid aseptic loosening [33]. In the current analysis, BPs could effectively decrease short, medium, and long phase of periprosthetic bone resorption. Besides, low-bone mineral density was a major risk factor for osteoporotic fracture [34]. Meanwhile, the rate of bone loss was an important risk factor for osteoporotic fracture [35]. In our eligible trials, the most of participants were

over 50 years old and some of them are postmenopausal women who underwent osteoporosis. Thus, the risk of fracture was high in these participants and it may threaten the longevity of the implant. So BPs may be beneficial for reducing the risk of periprosthetic fracture. In support of us, Alhambra et al. [36] suggested that the use of BPs decreased the fracture risk among THA patients who received BPs as primary prevention (hazard ratio 0.56, 95% CI 0.38 to 0.82) and also among THA patients who had experienced a previous osteoporotic fracture (HR 0.48, 95% CI 0.23 to 0.99).

Base on the present evidence, this study suggested that G 3 BPs were more effective in decreasing periprosthetic bone loss than G 1–2 BPs. Variations in the structure of the side chains determine the strength with which the biphosphonate binds to bone, the distribution through bone, and the amount of time, and it remains in the bone

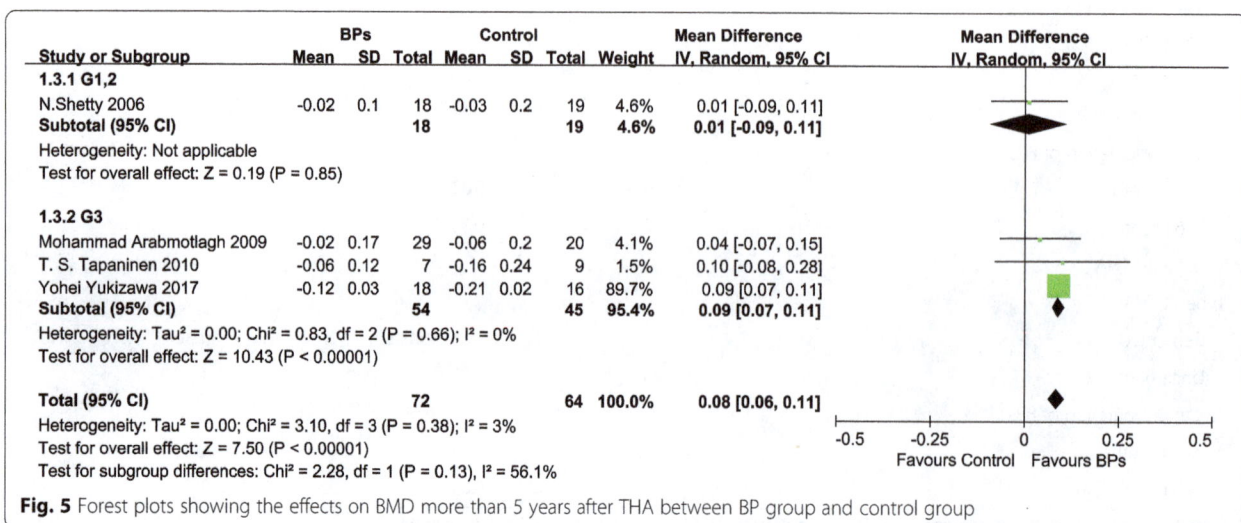

Study or Subgroup	BPs Mean	SD	Total	Control Mean	SD	Total	Weight	Mean Difference IV, Random, 95% CI
1.3.1 G1,2								
N.Shetty 2006	-0.02	0.1	18	-0.03	0.2	19	4.6%	0.01 [-0.09, 0.11]
Subtotal (95% CI)			**18**			**19**	**4.6%**	**0.01 [-0.09, 0.11]**
Heterogeneity: Not applicable								
Test for overall effect: Z = 0.19 (P = 0.85)								
1.3.2 G3								
Mohammad Arabmotlagh 2009	-0.02	0.17	29	-0.06	0.2	20	4.1%	0.04 [-0.07, 0.15]
T. S. Tapaninen 2010	-0.06	0.12	7	-0.16	0.24	9	1.5%	0.10 [-0.08, 0.28]
Yohei Yukizawa 2017	-0.12	0.03	18	-0.21	0.02	16	89.7%	0.09 [0.07, 0.11]
Subtotal (95% CI)			**54**			**45**	**95.4%**	**0.09 [0.07, 0.11]**
Heterogeneity: Tau² = 0.00; Chi² = 0.83, df = 2 (P = 0.66); I² = 0%								
Test for overall effect: Z = 10.43 (P < 0.00001)								
Total (95% CI)			**72**			**64**	**100.0%**	**0.08 [0.06, 0.11]**
Heterogeneity: Tau² = 0.00; Chi² = 3.10, df = 3 (P = 0.38); I² = 3%								
Test for overall effect: Z = 7.50 (P < 0.00001)								
Test for subgroup differences: Chi² = 2.28, df = 1 (P = 0.13), I² = 56.1%								

Fig. 5 Forest plots showing the effects on BMD more than 5 years after THA between BP group and control group

Study or Subgroup	BPs Mean	SD	Total	Control Mean	SD	Total	Weight	Mean Difference IV, Random, 95% CI	Mean Difference IV, Random, 95% CI
Katsuyuki Yamaguchi 2004	25.2	6.6	34	29.6	8.7	30	32.3%	-4.40 [-8.22, -0.58]	
Mohammad Arabmotlagh 2006	17.9	6	27	27.1	8.9	24	27.8%	-9.20 [-13.42, -4.98]	
Plamen KINOV 2006	19.9	6.6	12	26.9	5.9	12	21.1%	-7.00 [-12.01, -1.99]	
S. Yamasaki 2007	21.5	7.7	19	31.2	9.6	21	18.8%	-9.70 [-15.07, -4.33]	
Total (95% CI)			92			87	100.0%	-7.28 [-9.81, -4.75]	

Heterogeneity: Tau² = 1.36; Chi² = 3.76, df = 3 (P = 0.29); I² = 20%
Test for overall effect: Z = 5.64 (P < 0.00001)

Scale: -20, -10, 0, 10, 20 — Favours Control / Favours BPs

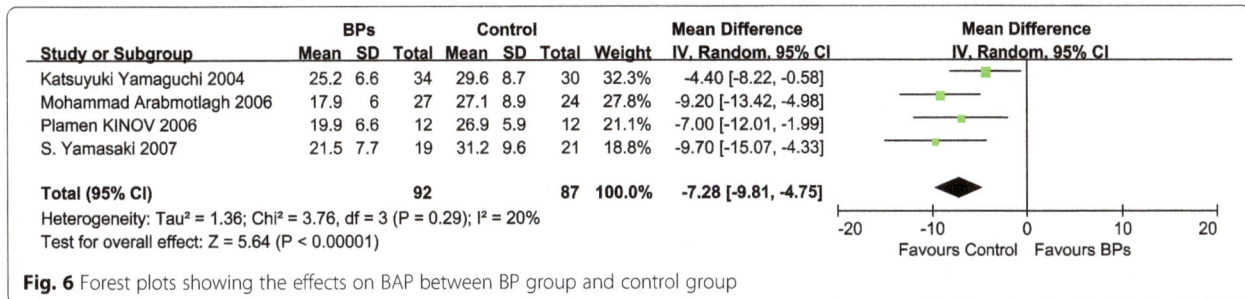

Fig. 6 Forest plots showing the effects on BAP between BP group and control group

after treatment is discontinued [37]. G 1–2 BPs (etidronate, clodronate, pamidronate, and olpadronate) have simple R2 side chains [38]. Differently, G 3 BPs (alendronate, neridronate, olpadronate, risedronate, ibandronate, and zoledronate) were developed by modifying the R2 side chain to include an amino group and heterocyclic structures, which were found to be up to 1000 times more potent with respect to antiresorptive activity [10]. What is more, G 3 BPs selectively inhibited the cholesterol pathway and subsequently disrupted the osteoclast cytoskeleton with associated osteoclast inactivation [39]. Therefore, G 3 BPs had less effect on osteoblasts and bone formation compared with G 1 BPs [40]. Black and bone also demonstrated the safety of 10 years' treatment with alendronate for osteoporosis in postmenopausal women [41, 42]. Our result was consistent with it, which also can be applied to inhibit periprosthetic bone resorption.

The significantly lower BAP value in BP group suggested that an influence of BPs may play a role on osteoblast function. Previous studies had found that G 3 BPs had inhibitory effects on terminal differentiation of osteoblasts for bone remodeling, consequently leading to a delay in bone healing [43]. Besides, the unusual mid-shaft long bone fractures were observed in some patients receiving BPs for osteoporosis [44, 45]. Lately, Park et al. demonstrated treatment with BPs more than 5 years was associated with an increased risk of subtrochanteric or femoral shaft fractures [46]. So further investigations were necessary to clarify the duration of BPs or to monitor the bone markers to avoid oversuppression of bone turnover.

With regard to NTX-I, the current analysis suggested that BPs has a strong effect on anti-osteoclast activity. Bone resorption also occurred in the later period, that

was focal bone resorption at the prosthesis-bone interface, as a part of the host response to wear debris generated from the prosthesis materials [47, 48]. The wear debris stimulated the release of pro-inflammatory cytokines at the prosthesis-bone interface membrane, the differentiation and activation of osteoclasts, then gave rise to periprosthetic osteolyticlesions [49]. This wear-related osteolysis could also lead to aseptic loosening, which accounting for over 60% of revision surgeries [50]. BPs have been shown promising in reducing osteoclast activity in animal models of particle-induced osteolysis. Shanbhag et al. advocated it for the first time that oral alendronate treatment (5 mg/day for 6 months) could reduce periprosthetic osteolysis in a cementless THA canine model of wear particle-induced osteolysis [51]. Then, Wise et al. further demonstrated that high-dose intravenous zoledronate therapy (10 µg/kg/week) decreased periprosthetic cortical bone porosity and enhanced its mechanical strength in a similar model [52]. In clinical trials, Nishii et al. suggested that alendronate treatment could prevent and restore periprosthetic osteolysis, which was generally thought to require surgical intervention [53].

Bhandari M et al. indicated that BPs presented more efficacies for the cemented group than the uncemented group [16]. However, the report has only included six RCTs of THA and did not conduct any subgroup analysis according to the follow-up time. In the current review, the efficacy of BPs for BMD was significant in the uncemented subgroup at short-term observation, but significant in the cemented subgroup at medium-term observation. Many uncemented implants are larger than cemented implants; thus, stiff stems of uncemented THA may produce more stress shielding and result in greater

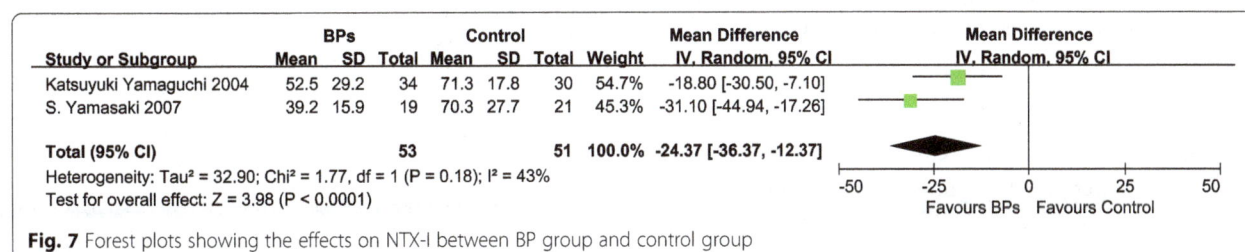

Study or Subgroup	BPs Mean	SD	Total	Control Mean	SD	Total	Weight	Mean Difference IV, Random, 95% CI	Mean Difference IV, Random, 95% CI
Katsuyuki Yamaguchi 2004	52.5	29.2	34	71.3	17.8	30	54.7%	-18.80 [-30.50, -7.10]	
S. Yamasaki 2007	39.2	15.9	19	70.3	27.7	21	45.3%	-31.10 [-44.94, -17.26]	
Total (95% CI)			53			51	100.0%	-24.37 [-36.37, -12.37]	

Heterogeneity: Tau² = 32.90; Chi² = 1.77, df = 1 (P = 0.18); I² = 43%
Test for overall effect: Z = 3.98 (P < 0.0001)

Scale: -50, -25, 0, 25, 50 — Favours BPs / Favours Control

Fig. 7 Forest plots showing the effects on NTX-I between BP group and control group

bone loss at short-term observation [54]. At long-term observation, cemented particles can induce osteoclast differentiation and lead to greater bone resorption compared with uncemented particles [55]. Therefore, the effects of BPs may be magnified by this difference. It may explain BPs worked differently on cemented and uncemented THA. However, only three RCTs were involved in cemented subgroup, which may be difficult to avoid publication bias. To explore the potential efficacies of BPs in different types of THA, more high-quality RCTs were needed.

Administration of BPs more than 6 months seemly obtained more benefit for BMD than the duration less than 6 months. In this subgroup analysis, BMD in more than 6-month group were higher than that in less than 6-month group at all terms of observation. However, the subgroup difference was not significant. These results suggested a significant association of BPs' long treatment duration with inhibited periprosthetic bone resorption, but the current analysis may lack statistical power to show this association. It was consistent with the previous meta-analysis [17].

Four studies that explored the potential efficacies of BPs have been published [14–17]. However, they had the following limitations: (1) most of them ignored the difference between generation of BPs and did not describe it separately. (2) Target participants in some studies included not only THA but also TKA and hemiarthroplasty. In contrast to previous meta-analyses, this analysis applied more rigorous eligibility criteria and excluded trials involving TKA or hemiarthroplasty to reduce heterogeneity. Furthermore, this analysis not only focused on the efficacies between different generations of BPs, but also discussed effects on treatment duration and types of THA.

Meanwhile, some limitations of this current meta-analysis should be taken into account. First, BMD and biochemical bone turnover outcomes were used to extrapolate the risk of implant revision in this study. However, revision rate in the later follow-up was more objective and ideal. Second, the limited numbers of studies and participants in long-term observation could decrease the strength of our results. Therefore, further RCTs were needed to determine whether a maximum benefit obtainable by BPs, whether benefits increase with increasing duration of administration, whether benefits persist after administration stop, and whether BAP or NTX-I is still suppressed in the later follow-up.

Conclusion

In conclusion, this study indicated that BPs were beneficial to decreasing periprosthetic bone loss following THA. In short-term observation, G 3 BPs showed greater efficacy for patients.

Abbreviations
95% CI: 95% confidence interval; BAP: Bone alkaline phosphates; BMD: Bone mineral density; BPs: Bisphosphonates; I²: I-square; MD: Mean differences; NTX-I: Urinary N-telopeptide of type I collage; THA: Total hip arthroplasty

Acknowledgements
We are grateful to all colleagues in our department for their generous support.

Funding
This study was supported by the fund of the Natural Science Foundation of Guangxi Province (2016JB140086). The funders had no role in study design, data collection and analysis, decision to publish, or preparation of the manuscript.

Authors' contributions
JS drafted the article and prepared all figures. GL acquired the data and prepared all tables. RH performed the statistical analysis. LL and DQ designed this study. All authors read and approved the final manuscript.

Competing interests
The authors declare that they have no competing interests.

Author details
¹Guangxi Medical University, No. 22, Shuang Yong Road, Nanning 530021, Guangxi Zhuang Autonomous Region, China. ²The first affiliated Hospital of Guangxi Medical University, The First Clinical Medical College, No. 6, Shuang Yong Road, Nanning 530021, Guangxi Zhuang Autonomous Region, China. ³Department of the Second Endocrinology Ward, Jiangbin Hospital of Guangxi Zhuang Autonomous Region, Nanning 530021, Guangxi Zhuang Autonomous Region, China.

References
1. Harris WH, Sledge CB. Total hip and total knee replacement. N Engl J Med. 1990;323(11):7.
2. Engh CA, Culpepper WJ, Engh CA, Virginia A. Long-term results of use of the anatomic medullary locking prosthesis in total hip arthroplasty. J Bone Joint Surg. 1997;79(2):8.
3. Xenos JS, Callaghan JJ, Heekin RD, Hopkinson WJ, Savory CG, Moore MS. The porous-coated anatomic total hip prosthesis, inserted without cement. A prospective study with a minimum of ten years of follow-up. J Bone Joint Surg. 1999;81(1):9.
4. Kurtz S, Ong K, Lau E, Mowat F, Halpern M. Projections of primary and revision hip and knee arthroplasty in the United States from 2005 to 2030. J Bone Joint Surg Am. 2007;89(4):780–5. https://doi.org/10.2106/JBJS.F.00222.
5. Venesmaa PK, Kpoger HPJ, Miettinen HJA, Jurvelin JS, Suomalainen OT, Alhava EM. Monitoring of periprosthetic BMD after uncemented total hip arthroplasty with dual-energy X-ray absorptiometry—a 3-year follow-up study. J Bone Miner Res. 2001;16(6):6.
6. Lindahl H. Epidemiology of periprosthetic femur fracture around a total hip arthroplasty. Injury. 2007;38(6):651–4. https://doi.org/10.1016/j.injury.2007.02.048.
7. Kobayashi S, Saito N, Horiuchi H, Iorio R, Takaoka K. Poor bone quality or hip structure as risk factors affecting survival of total-hip arthroplasty. Lancet. 2000;355(9214):1499–504. https://doi.org/10.1016/s0140-6736(00)02164-4.

8. Havelin LI, Engesæter LB, Espehaug B, Furnes O, Lie SA, Vollset SE. The Norwegian arthroplasty register 11 years and 73,000 arthroplasties. Acta Orthop Scand. 2000;71(4):17.

9. de Steiger RN, Miller LN, Prosser GH, Graves SE, Davidson DC, Stanford TE. Poor outcome of revised resurfacing hip arthroplasty. Acta Orthop. 2010; 81(1):72–6. https://doi.org/10.3109/17453671003667176.

10. Morris CD, Einhorn TA. Current concepts review—bisphosphonates in orthopaedic surgery. J Bone Joint Surg. 2005;87-A:10.

11. Woolf AD, Åkesson K. Preventing fractures in elderly people. Br Med J. 2003;327:7.

12. Wells VM, Hearn TC, McCaul KA, Anderton SM, Wigg AER, Graves SE. Changing incidence of primary total hip arthroplasty and total knee arthroplasty for primary osteoarthritis. J Arthroplast. 2002;17(3):267–73. https://doi.org/10.1054/arth.2002.30414.

13. Sibanda N, Copley LP, Lewsey JD, Borroff M, Gregg P, MacGregor AJ, et al. Revision rates after primary hip and knee replacement in England between 2003 and 2006. PLoS Med. 2008;5(9):11. https://doi.org/10.1371/journal. pmed.0050179.

14. Zhao X, Hu D, Qin J, Mohanan R, Chen L. Effect of bisphosphonates in preventing femoral periprosthetic bone resorption after primary cementless total hip arthroplasty: a meta-analysis. J Orthop Surg Res. 2015;10:65. https:// doi.org/10.1186/s13018-015-0206-8.

15. Knusten AR, Ebramzadeh E, Longjohn DB, Sangiorgio SN. Systematic analysis of bisphosphonate intervention on periprosthetic BMD as a function of stem design. J Arthroplast. 2014;29(6):1292–7. https://doi.org/10.1016/j.arth. 2014.01.015.

16. Bhandari M, Bajammal S, Guyatt GH, Griffith L, Busse JW, Schunemann H, et al. Effect of bisphosphonates on periprosthetic bone mineral density after total joint arthroplasty. A meta-analysis. J Bone Joint Surg. 2005;87-A:10.

17. Lin T, Yan SG, Cai XZ, Ying ZM. Bisphosphonates for periprosthetic bone loss after joint arthroplasty: a meta-analysis of 14 randomized controlled trials. Osteoporos Int. 2012;23(6):1823–34. https://doi.org/10.1007/s00198-011-1797-5.

18. Tapaninen TS, Venesmaa PK, Jurvelin JS, Miettinen HJA, Kröger HPJ. Alendronate reduces periprosthetic bone loss after uncemented primary total hip arthroplasty—a 5-year follow-up of 16 patients. Scand J Surg. 2010;99:6.

19. Trevisan C, Ortolani S, Romano P, Isaia G, Agnese L, Dallari D, et al. Decreased periprosthetic bone loss in patients treated with clodronate: a 1-year randomized controlled study. Calcif Tissue Int. 2010;86(6):436–46. https://doi.org/10.1007/s00223-010-9356-1.

20. Arabmotlagh M, Pilz M, Warzecha J, Rauschmann M. Changes of femoral periprosthetic bone mineral density 6 years after treatment with alendronate following total hip arthroplasty. J Orthop Res. 2009;27(2):183–8. https://doi.org/10.1002/jor.20748.

21. Yamasaki S, Masuhara K, Yamaguchi K, Nakai T, Fuji T, Seino Y. Risedronate reduces postoperative bone resorption after cementless total hip arthroplasty. Osteoporos Int. 2007;18(7):1009–15. https://doi.org/10.1007/s00198-007-0339-7.

22. Fokter SK, Komadina R, Repse-Fokter A. Effect of etidronate in preventing periprosthetic bone loss following cemented hip arthroplasty: a randomized, double blind, controlled trial. Wien Klin Wochenschr. 2006; 118(Suppl 2):23–8. https://doi.org/10.1007/s00508-006-0556-7.

23. Arabmotlagh M, Rittmeister M, Hennigs T. Alendronate prevents femoral periprosthetic bone loss following total hip arthroplasty: prospective randomized double-blind study. J Orthop Res. 2006;24(7):1336–41. https:// doi.org/10.1002/jor.20162.

24. Yamaguchi K, Masuhara K, Yamasaki S, Fuji T, Seino Y. Effects of discontinuation as well as intervention of cyclic therapy with etidronate on bone remodeling after cementless total hip arthroplasty. Bone. 2004;35(1): 217–23. https://doi.org/10.1016/j.bone.2004.03.017.

25. Iwamoto N, Inaba Y, Kobayashi N, Ishida T, Yukizawa Y, Saito T. A comparison of the effects of alendronate and alfacalcidol on bone mineral density around the femoral implant and in the lumbar spine after total hip arthroplasty. J Bone Joint Surg Am. 2011;93(13):1203–9. https://doi.org/10. 2106/JBJS.I.01714.

26. Kinov P, Tivchev P, Doukova P, Leithner A. Effect of risedronate on bone metabolism after total hip arthroplasty a prospective randomised study. Acta Orthop Belg. 2006;72(1):7.

27. Shetty N, Hamer AJ, Stockley I, Eastell R, Wilkinson JM. Clinical and radiological outcome of total hip replacement five years after pamidronate therapy: a trial extension. J Bone Joint Surg. 2006;88-B:7. https://doi.org/10. 1302/0301-620x.88b10.

28. Scott DF, Woltz JN, Smith RR. Effect of zoledronic acid on reducing femoral bone mineral density loss following total hip arthroplasty: preliminary results of a prospective randomized trial. J Arthroplasty. 2013;28(4):671–5. https://doi.org/10.1016/j.arth.2012.08.007.

29. Yukizawa Y, Inaba Y, Kobayashi N, Choe H, Kubota S, Saito T. Efficacy of alendronate for the prevention of bone loss in calcar region following total hip arthroplasty. J Arthroplast. 2017;32(7):2176–80. https://doi.org/10.1016/j. arth.2017.02.036.

30. Muren O, Akbarian E, Salemyr M, Boden H, Eisler T, Stark A, et al. No effect of risedronate on femoral periprosthetic bone loss following total hip arthroplasty. A 4-year follow-up of 61 patients in a double-blind, randomized placebo-controlled trial. Acta Orthop. 2015;86(5):569–74. https:// doi.org/10.3109/17453674.2015.1041846.

31. Nehme A, Maalouf G, Tricoire JL, Giordano G, Chiron P, Puget J. Effect of alendronate on periprosthetic bone loss after cemented primary total hip arthroplasty: a prospective randomized study. Rev Chir Orthop Reparatrice Appar Mot. 2003;6:593–8.

32. Nixon M, Taylor G, Sheldon P, Iqbal SJ, Harper W. Does bone quality predict loosening of cemented total hip replacements. J Bone Joint Surg. 2007;89-B: 6. https://doi.org/10.1302/0301-620X.89B10.

33. Sundfeldt M, Carlsson LV, Johansson CB, Thomsen P, Gretzer C. Aseptic loosening, not only a question of wear: a review of different theories. Acta Orthop. 2006;77(2):21. https://doi.org/10.1080/17453670610045902.

34. Marshall D, OlofJohnell, Wedel H. Meta-analysis of how well measures of bone mineral density predict occurrence of osteoporotic fractures. Br Med J. 1996;312:6.

35. Riis BJ, Hansen MA, Jensen AM, Overgaard K, Christiansen C. Low bone mass and fast rate of bone loss at menopause equal risk factors for future fracture: a 15-year follow-up study. Bone. 1996;19:4.

36. Prieto-Alhambra D, Javaid MK, Judge A, Maskell J, Kiran A, Fd V, et al. Fracture risk before and after total hip replacement in patients with osteoarthritis potential benefits of bisphosphonate use. Arthritis Rheum. 2011;64:10. https://doi.org/10.1002/art.30214.

37. Russell RG, Watts NB, Ebetino FH, Rogers MJ. Mechanisms of action of bisphosphonates: similarities and differences and their potential influence on clinical efficacy. Osteoporos Int. 2008;19:27.

38. MR M. Bisphosphonates. Endocrinol Metab Clin North Am. 2003;32:19.

39. Fisher JE, Rodan GA, Reszka AA. In vivo effects of bisphosphonates on the osteoclast mevalonate pathway. Endocrinology. 2000;141:4.

40. Russell RGG, Rogers MJ, Frith JC, Luckman SP, Coxon FP, Benford HL, et al. The pharmacology of bisphosphonates and new insights into their mechanisms of action. J Bone Miner Res. 1999;14:13.

41. Black DM, Schwartz AV, Ensrud KE, Cauley JA, Levis S, Quandt SA, et al. Effects of continuing or stopping alendronate after 5 years of treatment: the Fracture Intervention Trial Long-term Extension (FLEX) a randomized trial. J Am Med Assoc. 2006;296:12.

42. Bone HG, Hosking D, Devogelaer J-P, Tucci JR, Emkey RD, Tonino RP, et al. Ten years' experience with alendronate for osteoporosis in postmenopausal women. N Engl J Med. 2004;350(12):11.

43. Nagashima M, Sakai A, Uchida S, Tanaka S, Tanaka M, Nakamura T. Bisphosphonate (YM529) delays the repair of cortical bone defect after drill-hole injury by reducing terminal differentiation of osteoblasts in the mouse femur. Bone. 2005;36:10. https://doi.org/10.1016/j.bone.2004. 11.013.

44. Lenart BA, Lorich DG, Lane JM. Atypical fractures of the femoral diaphysis in postmenopausal women taking alendronate. N Engl J Med. 2008;358(12):3.

45. Neviaser AS, Lane JM, Lenart BA, Edobor-Osula F, Lorich DG. Low-energy femoral shaft fractures associated with alendronate use. J Orthop Trauma. 2008;22:5.

46. Park-Wyllie LY, Mamdani MM, Juurlink DN, Hawker GA, Gunraj N, Austin PC, et al. Bisphosphonate use and the risk of subtrochanteric or femoral shaft fractures in older women. JAm Med Assoc. 2011;305:7.

47. Goldring SR, Jasty M, Roelke MS, Rourke CM, Bringhurst FR, Harris WH. Formation of a synovial-like membrane at the bone-cement interface. Its role in bone resorption and implant loosening after total hip replacement. Arthritis Rheum. 1986;29:7.

48. Wilkinson JM, Little DG. Bisphosphonates in orthopedic applications. Bone. 2011;49:8. https://doi.org/10.1016/j.bone.2011.01.009.

49. Tuan RS, Lee FY-I, Konttinen Y, Wilkinson, Smith RL. What are the local and systemic biological reactions and mediators to wear debris and what host factors determine or modulate the biological response to wear particles? J Am Acad Orthop Surg. 2008;16:10.

50. Herberts P, Malchau H. Long-term registration has improved the quality of hip replacement a review of the Swedish THR register comparing 160,000 cases. Acta Orthop Scand. 2000;71(2):11.

51. Shanbhag AS, Hasselman CT, Rubash HE. The John Charnley award. Inhibition of wear debris mediated osteolysis in a canine total hip arthroplasty model. Clin Orthop Relat Res. 1997;344:11.

52. Wise LM, Waldman SD, Kasra M, Cheung R, Binnington A, Kandel RA, et al. Effect of zoledronate on bone quality in the treatment of aseptic loosening of hip arthroplasty in the dog. Calcif Tissue Int. 2005;77:9. https://doi.org/10.1007/s00223-005-0062-3.

53. Nishii, Takashi, Sugano, Nobuhiko, Miki, Hidenobu. Restoration of periprosthetic osteolysis by systemic alendronate treatment. J Bone Joint Surg Br. 2008;90:5.

54. Huiskes R, Stolk J. Biomechanics and preclinical testing of artifical joints: the hip. In: Basic orthopaedic biomechanics and mechanobiology; 2005. p. 72.

55. Sabokbar A, Fujikawa Y, Brett J. Increased osteoclastic differentiation by PMMA particle-associated macrophages: inhibitory effect by interleukin 4 and leukemia inhibitory factor. Acta Orthop Scand. 1996;67:593–8.

18

Evaluation of bone marrow-derived mesenchymal stem cell quality from patients with congenital pseudoarthrosis of the tibia

Ismail Hadisoebroto Dilogo[1,2,3*] (iD), Fajar Mujadid[1], Retno Wahyu Nurhayati[2,4] and Aryadi Kurniawan[3]

Abstract

Background: The treatment of congenital pseudoarthrosis of the tibia (CPT) remains challenging in pediatric orthopedics due to the difficulties in bone union, continuous angulation, joint stiffness, and severe limb length discrepancy. Mesenchymal stem cells (MSCs) therapy offers a complementary approach to improve the conventional surgical treatments. Although the autologous MSC treatment shows a promising strategy to promote bone healing in CPT patients, the quality of MSCs from CPT patients has not been well studied. The purpose of this study is to investigate the quality of MSCs isolated from patients with CPT.

Methods: The bone marrow-derived MSCs from the fracture site and iliac crest of six CPT patients were isolated and compared. The cumulative population doubling level (cPDL), phenotype characteristics, and trilineage differentiation potency were observed to assess the quality of both MSCs.

Results: There were no significant differences of the MSCs derived from the fracture site and the MSCs from the iliac crest of the subjects, in terms of cPDL, phenotype characteristics, and trilineage differentiation potency (all $p > 0.05$). However, MSCs from the fracture site had a higher senescence tendency than those from the iliac crest.

Conclusion: MSC quality is not the main reason for delayed bone regeneration in those with CPT. Thus, autologous MSC is a promising source for treating CPT patients

Keywords: Pseudoarthrosis, Mesenchymal stem cells, Osteocytes, Cell differentiation

Backgrounds

Congenital pseudoarthrosis of the tibia (CPT) is a rare disorder indicated by non-union or false joint, tibial bowing, reduced growth in distal tibial epiphysis, and shortening of the tibia [1], affecting at least 1 in 250,000 people [2]. The clinical manifestations of this condition often appear within the first year of life; however, in some cases, the symptoms develop after reaching the adolescence [3]. The main cause of CPT remains unclear; however, about 40–80% of incidence is related to genetic mutation of *NF1*

gene, resulting in dysregulation of a multifunctional protein termed as neurofibromin [4–6].

The treatment of CPT remains challenging in pediatric orthopedics due to the difficulties in bone union, continuous angulation, joint stiffness, and severe limb length discrepancy [7]. Amputation often becomes the only choice when repeated surgeries resulted in failure or worst condition in CPT patients. Mesenchymal stem cell (MSC) therapy offers a complementary approach to improve the conventional surgical treatments [8, 9]. Although the autologous MSC treatment shows a promising strategy to promote bone healing in CPT patients, the quality of MSCs from CPT patients has not been well studied.

Although various protocols for isolating human MSCs from different sources exist, minimal criteria have been concluded to be a standard consensus to identify cells as MSCs [10]. The Mesenchymal and Tissue Stem Cell Committee of the International Society for Cellular

* Correspondence: ismailortho@gmail.com; ismailorthofkui@yahoo.co.id
[1]Integrated Service Unit of Stem Cell Medical Technology, Dr. Cipto Mangunkusumo General Hospital (RSCM), Jl. Diponegoro No 71, Salemba, Cental Jakarta 10430, Indonesia
[2]Stem Cell and Tissue Engineering Cluster, Indonesian Medical Education and Research Institute (IMERI), Faculty of Medicine, Universitas Indonesia, Jl. Salemba Raya No 6, Salemba, Cental Jakarta 10430, Indonesia
Full list of author information is available at the end of the article

Therapy proposes that at least three characteristics are required to define human MSCs, first: become plastic-adherent when cultured in standard conditions; second: express CD105, CD73, and CD90, and lack expression of CD45, CD34, CD14, or CD11b, CD79a, or CD19 and HLA-DR surface proteins; and third: can differentiate into osteogenic, adipogenic and chondrogenic lineages (trilineage differentiation) [11].

In the current study, we evaluated and compared the characteristics of MSCs isolated from the iliac crest and fracture site of the tibia from six CPT patients. The phenotypic characteristics and the cumulative population doubling time (cPDL) from both sources were analyzed to assess the trilineage differentiation and proliferation capacities of MSCs from the CPT patients. Finally, proliferation of MSCs from the CPT patients was compared with MSCs from healthy donors for clarifying if MSC quality is the reason for delayed bone regeneration in the CPT patients.

Methods
Subjects
Six patients involved in this study were diagnosed with CPT. The patients have been tested for HIV types 1 and 2, HBV, HCV, syphilis, and TORCH prior to the study. Ages of the patients were 15 years or younger. The bone marrow was aspirated from the iliac crest and the fracture site of the tibia from these CPT patients. For healthy (non-CPT) subjects, six participants (age 20–50 years old) were medically examined and showed no symptoms of CPT. MSCs from these healthy subjects were collected from bone marrow of iliac crest.

Isolation of bone marrow-derived MSCs [12]
Ten milliliters of bone marrow aspirates were diluted by 10 ml complete medium containing α-MEM (Life Technologies, USA) with 10% of platelet lysate (Indonesian Red Cross, Indonesia), 10 IU/ml of heparin sodium (Pratapa Nirmala, Indonesia), 2 mM of GlutaMAX, 100 units/ml of penicillin G sodium, 100 μg/ml of streptomycin sulfate, and 2.5 μg/ml of amphotericin (Life Technologies). Samples were centrifuged at 400×g for 10 min. The supernatant was discarded, and the pellet was diluted by an equal volume of complete medium. Fifteen milliliters of diluted cells were transferred into 75-cm^2 T-Flask and incubated at 37 °C in normoxia condition. Cells were harvested after 80–90% confluent and then sub-cultured until fifth passage. Viability and the number of cells were analyzed by a dye-excluding method with trypan blue [13–15]. The cPDL was calculated based on the following formula:

$$cPDL = 3.32 \ (\log N - \ \log N_0) + X$$

where N = final cell number (cells/mL), N_0 = initial cell number (cells/mL), and X = initial population doubling level.

MSC phenotypic characterization
MSCs were harvested after the fifth passage. Cells were treated with trypsin for 5 min at 37 °C to detach the adherent cells. After being washed with phosphate-buffered saline, the cells (2×10^5) were stained with human MSC analysis kit (BD Biosciences, USA) according to the company instruction. Fluorescence antibody cocktails contained positive markers (CD73, CD90, and CD105) and negative markers/NEG (CD34, CD11b, CD19, CD45, and HLA-DR). The stained cells were subsequently loaded into a flow cytometer (FACSCalibur; BD Biosciences)

Senescence assay
A cellular senescence test was performed by a Senescence Cells Histochemical Staining Kit from Sigma-Aldrich (USA) at the fifth passage according to the manufacturer's protocol. Percentage of senescent cell was observed under an inverted microscope with ×100 magnification in five fields of view and analyzed by ImageJ 1.50i software (National Institute of Health, USA) [16].

Differentiation assay
Differentiation assay was conducted to confirm the MSC plasticity. At the fifth passage, cultured cells were harvested and transferred to specific inducing media for chondrogenic, osteogenic, and adipogenic differentiations. The cells were cultured in complete medium to induce spontaneous chondrogenic differentiation. Osteogenic and adipogenic potencies were evaluated by culturing the cells in StemPro Osteogenesis and Adipocyte Differentiation Kits (ThermoFisher Scientific, USA), respectively. All cultures were incubated at 37 °C under a normoxia condition. The induced cells were analyzed after 7, 14, and 21 days of culturing.

For the differentiation assays, the cells were stained with 1% of alcian blue, 2% of alizarin red, and 1.4% oil red O for evaluating their capacity to undergo chondrogenesis, osteogenesis, and adipogenesis, respectively. Percentage of staining area was observed in five fields of view with 100-fold magnification. Differentiation potential was measured as percentage of stained area by ImageJ 1.50i software [17, 18].

Statistics
SPSS 15.0 software was used to analyze the significant difference between MSCs from the iliac crest bone marrow and fracture site bone marrow, in terms of cPDL, percentage of senescent cells, phenotype characteristics, and differentiation potencies. Numerical data was analyzed using independent t test or Mann-Whitney test.

Results
Bone marrow-derived cells gradually attached in plastic surface when cultured in the presence of serum. The

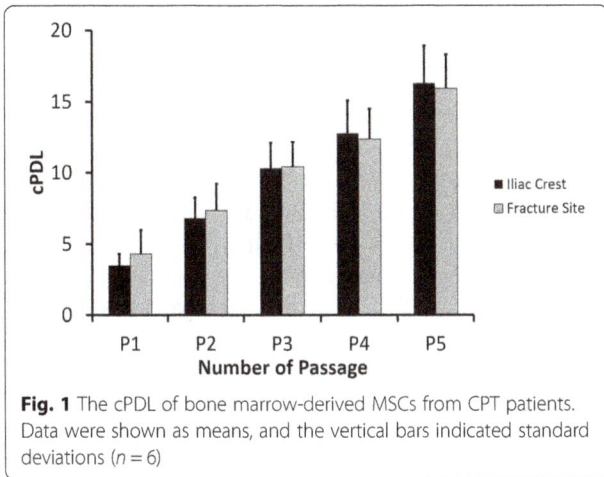

Fig. 1 The cPDL of bone marrow-derived MSCs from CPT patients. Data were shown as means, and the vertical bars indicated standard deviations (n = 6)

adherent cells were subsequently used for further analyses in this study. Afterwards, the cPDL was evaluated to compare the proliferation capacity of bone marrow-derived MSCs from the fracture site and iliac crest of CPT patients. The cPDL from both sources increased from the first passage (P1) to the fifth passage (P5) (Fig. 1), indicating that the MSCs were actively proliferating. In the same passage number, there was no significant difference ($p > 0.05$) of cPDL from MSCs isolated from the iliac crest and fracture site of those with CPT.

After the fifth passage, we evaluated the purity of cultured cells by flow cytometry analysis. More than 99% cultured cells were positive for CD73/CD90, and over 85% were CD105 positive (Fig. 2). Non-MSCs including cells marked positive with CD34/CD11b/CD19/CD45/HLA-DR were less than 0.5%. These results suggested that

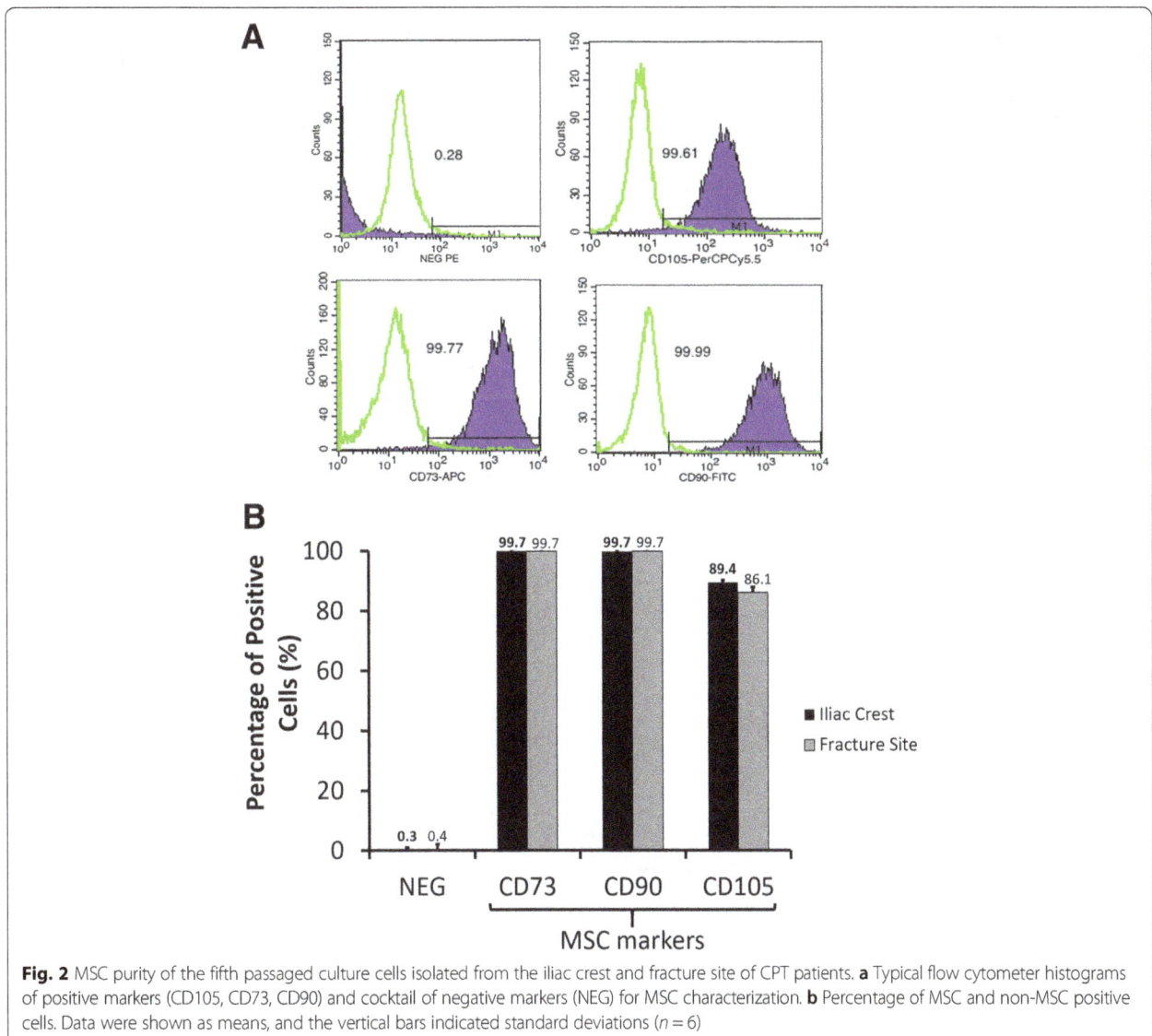

Fig. 2 MSC purity of the fifth passaged culture cells isolated from the iliac crest and fracture site of CPT patients. **a** Typical flow cytometer histograms of positive markers (CD105, CD73, CD90) and cocktail of negative markers (NEG) for MSC characterization. **b** Percentage of MSC and non-MSC positive cells. Data were shown as means, and the vertical bars indicated standard deviations (n = 6)

up to the fifth passage, the iliac crest- and fracture site-derived cells maintained the MSC phenotypes.

Figure 3 showed the positive result of chondrogenic differentiation assay as the blue-stained area. Chondrocyte population appeared on day 14 after incubation. Both of bone marrow-derived cells showed an increased chondrocyte population by incubation periods. There was no significant different ($p > 0.05$) of chondrogenic potency between cells isolated from the iliac crest and fracture site of CPT patients.

The data tendency from the osteogenic differentiation assay was similar with that from the chondrogenic differentiation assay. Osteocyte population gradually formed after 7 days of incubation. There is no significantly difference ($p > 0.05$) of osteogenic potency between the cells isolated from the iliac crest and fracture site (Fig. 4).

Red-stained oil droplets represented the positive result of adipogenic differentiation assay (Fig. 5a). Both of the MSCs were able to differentiate into adipogenic lineage after 7 days of incubation. Moreover, the percentage of adipocyte population became higher after 14 and 21 days of incubation (Fig. 5b). Nevertheless, there was no significant difference ($p > 0.05$) in adipogenic differentiation potency of MSCs from the iliac crest and fracture site of CPT patients.

Primary cells have a finite proliferation capacity and undergo senescence state after repeated proliferation. On the fifth passage, the percentage of senescence cells of MSCs isolated from the iliac crest and fracture site was assessed. As shown in Fig. 6, there was a tendency for MSCs from the fracture site to have a higher percentage of senescent cells than MSCs from the iliac crest.

Figure 7 summarized the cPDL of iliac crest-isolated MSCs from healthy (non-CPT) and CPT patients. The cPDL of CPT patients were slightly higher than those of non-CPT subjects. These result suggested that MSC proliferation from CPT patients were comparable with MSC from healthy subjects.

Discussion

Treatment for CPT is challenging because patients experience the disorder at a very young age, and success rate of the treatment varies. Surgical treatments for CPT patients frequently involve internal or external fixation with or without bone grafting to improve bone consolidation [19]. Repeated surgical treatments are often needed; however, inevitable outcomes can still occur, i.e., more severe condition or in a worst case lead to amputation [20].

Currently, stem cell therapy offers a regenerative approach to improve the outcome of conventional surgical treatments. MSC therapy has attracted attention due to the potency to improve the surgical methods of CPT treatment by promoting bone and surrounding tissue

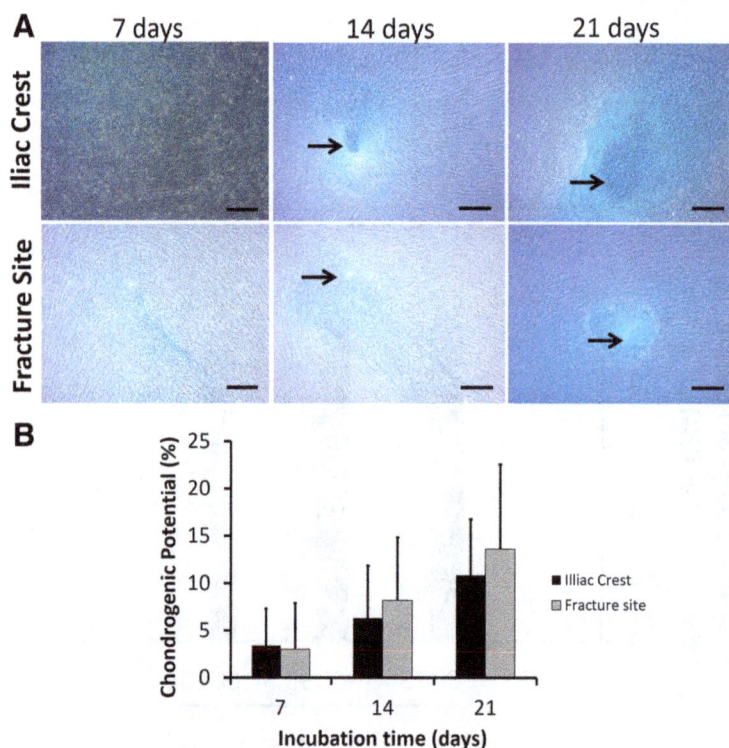

Fig. 3 Chondrogenic differentiation of MSCs isolated from the iliac crest and fracture site of the tibia from CPT patients. **a** Representative microscopic images of chondrogenic assays. Bars and black arrows indicate 100 μm and chondrocytes population, respectively. **b** Percentage of chondrogenic differentiation potential. Data were shown as means, and the vertical bars indicated standard deviations ($n = 6$)

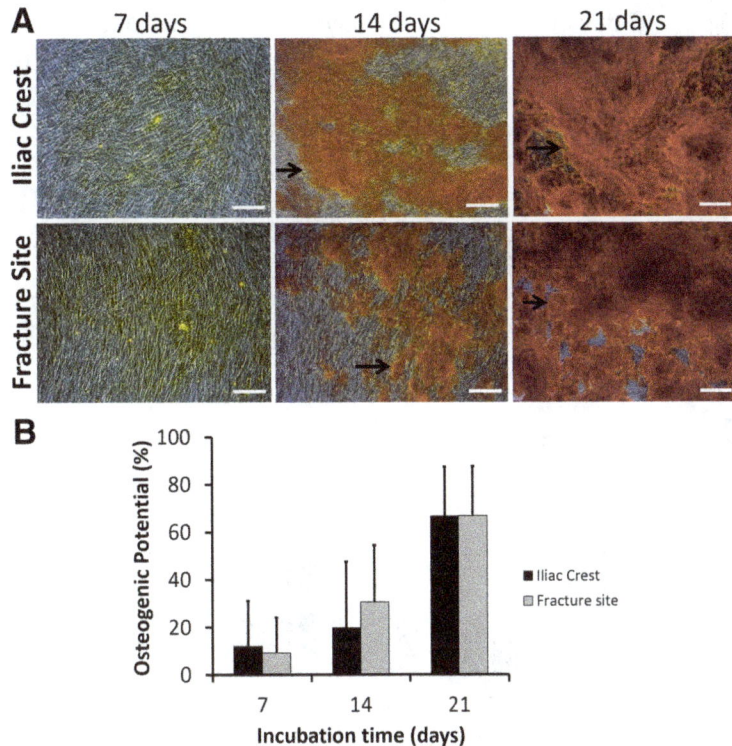

Fig. 4 Osteogenic differentiation of MSCs isolated from the iliac crest and fracture site of the tibia from CPT patients. **a** Representative microscopic images of osteogenic assays. Bars and black arrows indicate 100 μm and osteocytes population, respectively. **b** Percentage of osteogenic differentiation potential. Data were shown as means, and the vertical bars indicated standard deviations ($n = 6$)

regeneration. It is likely that autologous MSCs (from a patient's own body) are more popular than allogeneic MSCs (from a donor). Nevertheless, the studies about MSC quality from CPT patients are still limited.

Bone marrow of the iliac crest is the common source for MSC isolation [21] while a few studies reported a success on isolating MSCs from the bone marrow of the tibia [22]. The number of MSCs in the tibia is typically much lower than that in the iliac crest [22]. In the current study, we evaluated the quality of MSCs from six patients with CPT. MSCs were isolated from the bone marrow of the fracture site of the tibia and iliac crest. The isolated MSCs were cultured on standard culture media with 10% human serum, and passaging was conducted after the cells reached confluence. Experimental data showed that the cPDL increased from the first passage to the fifth passage, suggesting that the cells were actively proliferating. There was no significant difference ($p > 0.05$) in terms of cPDL between MSCs isolated from the iliac crest and those from the fracture site of the tibia in CPT patients.

The MSC specific markers, including CD73, CD90, and CD105 antibodies, were analyzed after the fifth passage. It was clarified that more than 99% of cultured cells were able to express CD73 and CD90 proteins. The CD105$^+$ cells were 89% and 86% for MSCs from the iliac crest and fracture site of tibia, respectively. Ng et al. [23] reported

the percentage of CD105 cells of human MSCs was around 86% in late passage (sixth passage). The expression of CD105 in human MSCs reduced significantly when human MSCs were cultured in serum-free media; however, the cells could maintain the trilineage potencies [24]. Although CD105 expression is often associated with chondrogenic potential, a recent study clearly stated that enriched CD105 MSCs did not show superior chondrogenic potential [25]. Thus, as long as expressing double-positive CD73/CD90 markers, the cells are potentially classified as MSC. Cells expressing negative markers for MSCs (CD34, CD11b, CD19, CD45, and HLA-DR) in our study were less than 0.5% even after fifth passage.

Surprisingly, percentage of senescent cells from fracture site-derived MSCs was significantly higher than iliac crest-derived MSCs. A study from Bajada et al. [26] investigated the growth potential of MSCs isolated from the fibrocartilaginous tissue at atrophic non-union site. They reported that, in standard culture condition, the proportion of senescent MSCs from this site was higher that MSCs from bone marrow of iliac crest. Their report showed a corresponding agreement with our finding, even though the patient conditions or tissue site were different.

Trilineage potencies of MSCs isolated from CPT patients were evaluated by culturing the cells in specific inducing media. Spontaneous chondrogenic differentiation

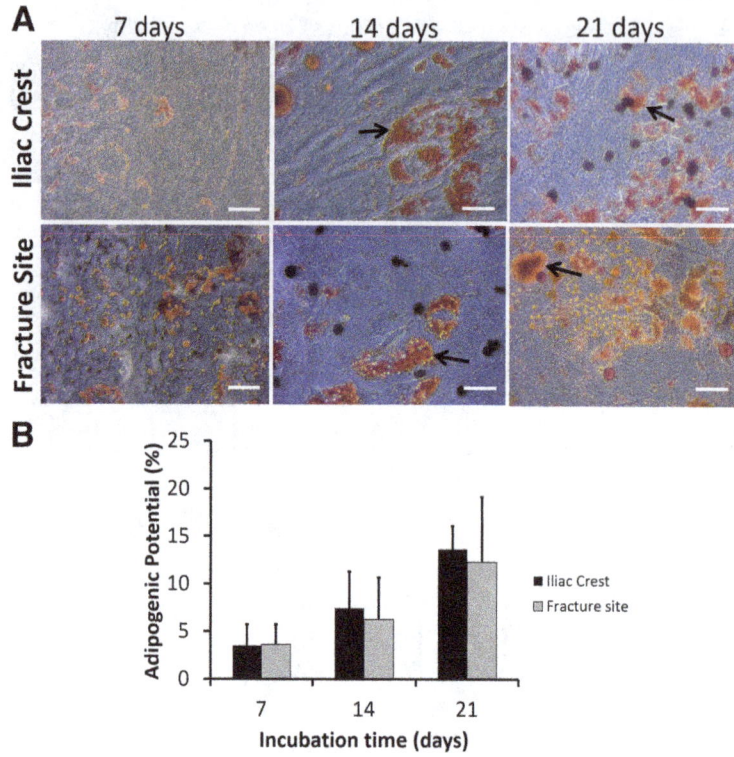

Fig. 5 Adipogenic differentiation of MSCs isolated from the iliac crest and fracture site of the tibia from CPT patients. **a** Representative microscopic images of adipogenic assays. Bars and black arrows indicate 100 μm and adipocytes population, respectively. **b** Percentage of adipogenic differentiation potential. Data were shown as means and the vertical bars indicated standard deviations ($n = 6$)

was detected after culturing the cells over 2 weeks. Similarly, adipogenic differentiation was visually noticed after 2 weeks in adipogenic-stimulating media. In case of osteogenic differentiation, about 10% showed osteogenic potency after a week of induction. The trilineage differentiation potencies increased after longer incubation time. There was no significant difference of trilineage potencies from MSCs isolated from the iliac crest or

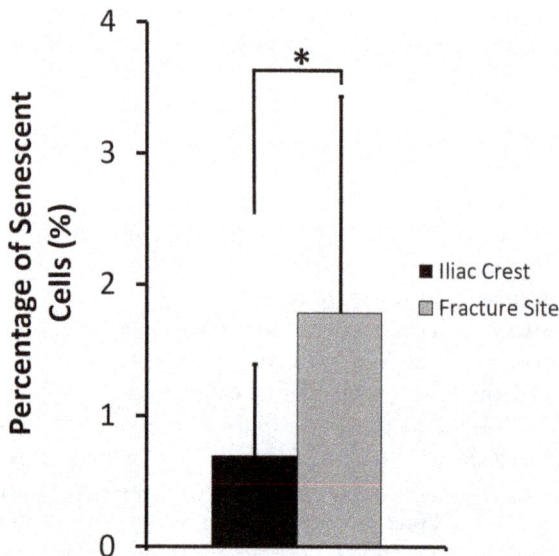

Fig. 6 Percentage of senescent cells from the fifth passaged MSCs isolated from CPT patients. Data were shown as means, and the vertical bars indicated standard deviations ($n = 6$). The value of $p < 0.05$ (*) was indicated based on a paired t test

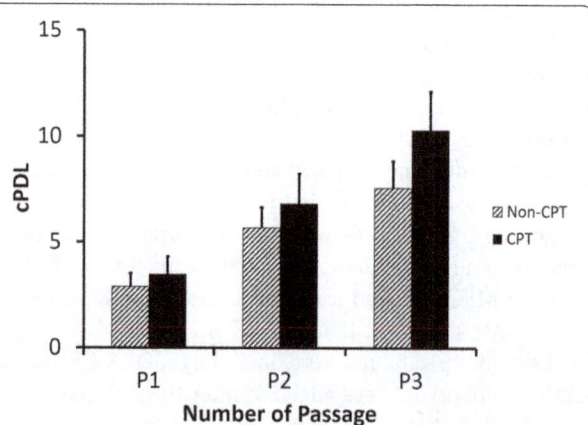

Fig. 7 The cPDL of iliac crest-derived MSCs from healthy (non-CPT) and CPT patients. Data were shown as means and the vertical bars indicated standard deviations ($n = 6$)

Evaluation of bone marrow-derived mesenchymal stem cell quality from patients with congenital...

161

fracture site of tibia from CPT patients. A case report [27] in a 2-year-old CPT patient suggested that MSCs from his fibrous tissue were able to differentiate into osteogenic, chondrogenic, and adipogenic cells, showing a similar tendency with our finding; the difference was our study used bone marrow-derived MSCs and involved more number of CPT patients.

The cPDL of MSCs from CPT patients was then compared with MSCs from healthy subjects. It was hypothesized that low MSC proliferation might affect the slow bone healing in CPT patients. Surprisingly, the MSC's cPDL from CPT patients were higher than that of healthy subjects, indicating that CPT-derived MSCs were proliferating in a comparable level with healthy MSCs. In this study, it was difficult to recruit a healthy bone marrow donor with a similar age range with CPT patients. We expected that higher cPDL in CPT patients than in healthy donors was merely caused by age difference.

Conclusion

The MSC characteristics from the fracture site of the tibia and the iliac crest of CPT patients were similar, in terms of proliferation capacity and trilineage differentiation. It was noticed that the proliferation capacity of iliac crest-derived MSCs from CPT patients was comparable with those from healthy persons. The findings in this study are expected to promote the use of autologous MSC therapy for CPT patients.

Abbreviations
cPDL: Cumulative population doubling time; CPT: Congenital pseudoarthrosis of the tibia; HBV: Hepatitis B virus; HCV: Hepatitis C virus; HIV: Human immunodeficiency virus; MSC: Mesenchymal stem cell; TORCH: Toxoplasma gondii, other viruses (HIV, measles, and so on), rubella (German measles), cytomegalovirus, and herpes simplex

Acknowledgements
we acknowledge to Dr. Zarkasyi Ari Mukti and Dr Anissa Feby Caningtika for helping during the study especially in sample and data collecting.

Funding
This work was supported by a Penelitian Unggulan Perguruan Tinggi (PUPT) Universitas Indonesia Research Grant from the Ministry of Research, Technology and Higher Education, Republic of Indonesia (Grant Number: 1709/UN2.R12/HKP.05.00/2016).

Authors' contributions
IHD is responsible for designing the studies, isolating the bone marrow from the patients/subjects, and creating the idea. FM performed the experiments, conducted the data analysis, and wrote the manuscript. RWN conducted the data analysis and wrote the manuscript. AK took part in isolating the bone marrow from the subjects. All authors read and approved the final manuscript.

Competing interests
The authors declare that they have no competing interests.

Author details
[1]Integrated Service Unit of Stem Cell Medical Technology, Dr. Cipto Mangunkusumo General Hospital (RSCM), Jl. Diponegoro No 71, Salemba, Cental Jakarta 10430, Indonesia. [2]Stem Cell and Tissue Engineering Cluster, Indonesian Medical Education and Research Institute (IMERI), Faculty of Medicine, Universitas Indonesia, Jl. Salemba Raya No 6, Salemba, Cental Jakarta 10430, Indonesia. [3]Department of Orthopaedic and Traumatology, Faculty of Medicine, Universitas Indonesia - Dr. Cipto Mangunkusumo General Hospital, Jl. Diponegoro No 71, Salemba, Cental Jakarta 10430, Indonesia. [4]Department of Biochemistry and Molecular Biology, Faculty of Medicine, Universitas Indonesia, Jl. Salemba Raya No. 6, Central Jakarta 10430, Indonesia.

References
1. Hardinge K. Congenital anterior bowing of the tibia. The significance of the different types in relation to pseudarthrosis. Ann R Coll Surg Engl. 1972; 51(1):17–30.
2. Hefti F, Bollini G, Dungl P, Fixsen J, Grill F, Ippolito E, Romanus B, Tudisco C, Wientroub S. Congenital pseudarthrosis of the tibia: history, etiology, classification, and epidemiologic data. J Pediatr Orthop B. 2000;9:11–5.
3. Andersen KS. Radiological classification of congenital pseudarthrosis of the tibia. Acta Orthop Scand. 1973;44(6):719–27.
4. DeClue JE, Cohen BD, Lowy DR. Identification and characterization of the neurofibromatosis type 1 protein product. P Natl Acad Sci USA. 1991;88:9914–8.
5. Abramowicz A, Gos M. Neurofibromin in neurofibromatosis type 1 mutations in NF1 gene as a cause of disease. Dev Period Med. 2014;18(3):297–306.
6. Crawford AH, Schorry EK. Neurofibromatosis update. J Pediatr Orthop. 2006; 26:413–23.
7. Pannier S. Congenital pseudarthrosis of the tibia. Orthop Traumatol-Sur. 2011;97:750–61.
8. Magnani M, Racano C, Abati C, Granchi D, Vescovi V, Stilli S. Use of MSC in the treatment of the congenital pseudoarthrosis in children. Surg Sci. 2014;5:555–61.
9. Tikkanen J, Leskelä HV, Lehtonen ST, Vähäsarja V, Melkko J, Ahvenjärvi L, Pääkkö E, Väänänen K, Lehenkari P. Attempt to treat congenital pseudarthrosis of the tibia with mesenchymal stromal cell transplantation. Cytotherapy. 2010;12(5):593–604.
10. Secunda R, Vennila R, Mohanashankar AM, Rajasundari M, Jeswanth S, Surendran R. Isolation, expansion and characterisation of mesenchymal stem cells from human bone marrow, adipose tissue, umbilical cord blood and matrix: a comparative study. Cytotechnology. 2015;67(5):793–807.
11. Dominici M, Le Blanc K, Mueller I, Slaper-Cortenbach I, Marini F, Krause D, Deans R, Keating A, Dj P, Horwitz E. Minimal criteria for defining multipotent mesenchymal stromal cells. Cytotherapy. 2006;8(4):315–7.
12. Pawitan JA, Feroniasanti L, Kispa T, Dilogo IH, Fasha I, Kurniawati T, Liem IK. Simple method to isolate mesenchymal stem cells from bone marrow using xeno-free material: a preliminary study. Int J PharmTech Res. 2015;7(2):354–9.
13. Ng CP, Sharif ARM, Health DE, Chow JW, Zhang CBY, Chan-Park MB, Hammond PT, Chan JKY, Griffith LG. Enhanced ex vivo expansion of adult mesenchymal stem cells by mesenchymal stem cell ECM. Biomaterials. 2014;35:4046–57.
14. Nobuhiro I, Lin LR, Reddy VN. Effect of growth factors on proliferation and differentiation in human lens epithelial cells in early subculture. Invest Opthal Vis Sci. 1995;36:2304–12.
15. Shebaby W, Abdalla EK, Saad F, Faour WH. Data on isolating mesenchymal stromal cells from human adipose tissue using a collagenase-free method. Data Brief. 2016;6:974–9.
16. Schneider CA, Rasband WS, Eliceiri KW. NIH image to ImageJ: 25 years of image analysis. Nat Methods. 2012;9(7):671–5.
17. Birmingham E, Niebur GL, McHugh PE, Shaw G, Barry FP, McNamara LM. Osteogenic differentiation of mesenchymal stem cells is regulated by osteocyte and osteoblast cells in a simplified bone niche. Eur Cell Mater. 2012;2012(23):13–27.

18. Nora CCV, Camassola M, Bellagamba B, Ikuta N, Cristoff AP, Meirelles LS, Ayres R, Margis R, Nardi NB. Molecular analysis of the differentiation potential of murine mesenchymal stem cells from tissues of endodermal or mesodermal origin. Stem Cells Dev. 2012;21:1761–8.

19. Granchi D, Devescovi V, Baglio SR, Magnani M, Donzelli O, Baldini N. A regenerative approach for bone repair in congenital pseudarthrosis of the tibia associated or not associated with type 1 neurofibromatosis: correlation between laboratory findings and clinical outcome. Cytotherapy. 2012;14(3):306–14.

20. Shah H, Rousset M, Canavese F. Congenital pseudoarthrosis of the tibia: management and complications. Indian J Orthop. 2012;46(6):616–26.

21. Ullah I, Subbarao RB, Rho GJ. Human mesenchymal stem cells - current trends and future prospective. Biosci Rep. 2015;35(2).

22. Narbona-Carceles J, Vaquero J, Suárez-Sancho S, Forriol F, Fernández-Santos ME. Bone marrow mesenchymal stem cell aspirates from alternative sources: is the knee as good as the iliac crest? Injury. 2014;45(Suppl 4):S42–7.

23. Ng CP, Sharif AR, Heath DE, Chow JW, Zhang CB, Chan-Park MB, Hammond PT, Chan JK, Griffith LG. Enhanced ex vivo expansion of adult mesenchymal stem cells by fetal mesenchymal stem cell ECM. Biomaterials. 2014;35(13): 4046–57.

24. Mark P, Kleinsorge M, Gaebel R, Lux CA, Toelk A, Pittermann E, David R, Steinhoff G, Ma N. Human mesenchymal stem cells display reduced expression of CD105 after culture in serum-free medium. Stem Cells Int. 2013;2013:698076.

25. Cleary MA, Narcisi R, Focke K, van der Linden R, Brama PA, van Osch GJ. Expression of CD105 on expanded mesenchymal stem cells does not predict their chondrogenic potential. Osteoarthr Cartilage. 2016;24(5):868–72.

26. Bajada S, Marshall MJ, Wright KT, Richardson JB, Johnson WE. Decreased osteogenesis, increased cell senescence and elevated Dickkopf-1 secretion in human fracture non union stromal cells. Bone. 2009;45:726–35.

27. Diaz-Solano D, Wittig O, Motta JD, Cardier JE. Isolation and characterization of multipotential mesenchymal stromal cells from congenital pseudoarthrosis of the tibia: case report. Anat Rec. 2015;298:1804–14.

19

Comparative effectiveness and safety of tranexamic acid plus diluted epinephrine to control blood loss during total hip arthroplasty

Zhao Wang[1] and Hao-jie Zhang[2*]

Abstract

Background: The standard protocol to achieve haemostasis during total hip arthroplasty (THA) is uncertain. Tranexamic acid plus diluted epinephrine (DEP) and tranexamic acid (TXA) alone are the two most common alternatives. The purpose of this study was to compare the efficacy and safety of TXA plus DEP to treat blood loss in THA patients.

Methods: Published randomized controlled trials (RCTs) were identified from the following electronic databases: PubMed, Embase, Web of Science, Cochrane Library and Google from inception to July 10, 2018. Studies comparing TXA plus DEP with TXA alone to treat blood loss were included. Either a random-effects model or a fixed-effects model was used for meta-analysis depending on the heterogeneity. We used the need for transfusion as the primary outcome. Stata 12.0 was used for meta-analysis.

Results: Six studies involving 703 patients were included in the present meta-analysis. The pooled results demonstrated that TXA plus DEP was associated with a lower transfusion rate than TXA alone (RR = 0.57, 95% CI 0.38–0.86, $P = 0.006$). Furthermore, TXA plus DEP was associated with less total blood loss and hidden blood loss by approximately 209.79 ml and 297.74 ml, respectively, than TXA alone. There was no significant difference in terms of intraoperative blood loss or the occurrence of deep venous thrombosis or haematoma between the TXA plus DEP and TXA alone groups ($P > 0.05$).

Conclusions: Our meta-analysis suggested that TXA plus DEP significantly decreased the need for transfusion, total blood loss and hidden blood loss among THA patients. Furthermore, TXA plus DEP did not increase the occurrence of DVT or haemostasis. Additional long-term follow-up RCTs are needed to identify the optimal doses of TXA and DEP.

Keywords: Tranexamic acid, Blood loss, Total hip arthroplasty, Meta-analysis

Introduction

Total hip arthroplasty (THA) is an effective treatment for end-stage hip osteoarthritis (OA) [1]. By 2030, the demand for primary THA is estimated to increase to 572,000 [2]. THA is associated with a large amount of intraoperative blood loss and hidden blood loss [3]. Extensive blood loss results in cardiovascular complications and the need for a blood transfusion [4, 5]. Blood transfusion carries the risk of hepatitis virus transmission and immunomodulation, increasing economic costs and prolonging the length of hospital stay [6]. Therefore, there is an urgent need to identify a safe, effective method of reducing blood loss and blood transfusions after THA.

Several alternatives are available for minimizing blood loss after THA. These include topical fibrin sealants, topical or intravenous tranexamic acid (TXA) [7, 8], aminocaproic acid [3, 9] or diluted epinephrine (DEP) [10]. Recently, administration TXA plus DEP has become popular for THA patients [11]. DEP enhances coagulation by several mechanisms [12]. Nevertheless, whether TXA plus DEP is superior to TXA alone remains unclear. To

* Correspondence: 2046293417@qq.com
[2]Department of Orthopaedics, The 82rn Hospital of People's Liberation Army of China, No. 100, Jiankangdong Road, Huai'an, Jiangsu, China
Full list of author information is available at the end of the article

further explore these issues and to identify the best haemostatic techniques for THA, we performed a meta-analysis of all the available randomized controlled trials (RCTs) of patients with THA.

Methods

This review was conducted according to the Preferred Reporting Items for Systematic Reviews and Meta-Analysis Statement issued in 2011 [13]. Ethical approval was not necessary for this study, as only de-identified pooled data from individual studies were analysed.

Search strategies

We searched PubMed, Embase and Cochrane CENTRAL for relevant studies from the time of inception of these databases to July 10, 2018. The following groups of keywords and medical terms were used for the literature search: "tranexamic acid" AND "epinephrine" (OR "total hip arthroplasty" OR "total hip replacement" OR arthroplasty OR "THA" "THR") AND (random* OR prospective* OR trial*). The language was not restricted to English. We also conducted an additional search by screening the references of eligible studies.

Study eligibility

We evaluated each identified RCT against the following predetermined selection criteria:

i. Study population: adults with hip OA eligible for primary THA.
ii. Interventions: the review focused on topical or intravenous TXA plus topical DEP, which are commonly used in the management of blood loss after THA, as commonly reported in the literature.
iii. Comparator: direct comparisons among any of the four core therapeutic interventions (i.e. DEP alone, topical or intravenous TXA alone and a control group).
iv. Outcome measures: the primary outcomes for this review were the need for transfusion, total blood loss, blood loss in drainage and the occurrence of deep venous thrombosis (DVT).

Data extraction

Two authors independently extracted the general characteristics and outcomes from the included studies. The following data were extracted from each study: first author, publication year, location, age and number of patients in the intervention and control groups, doses of TXA and DEP, outcomes, transfusion threshold and

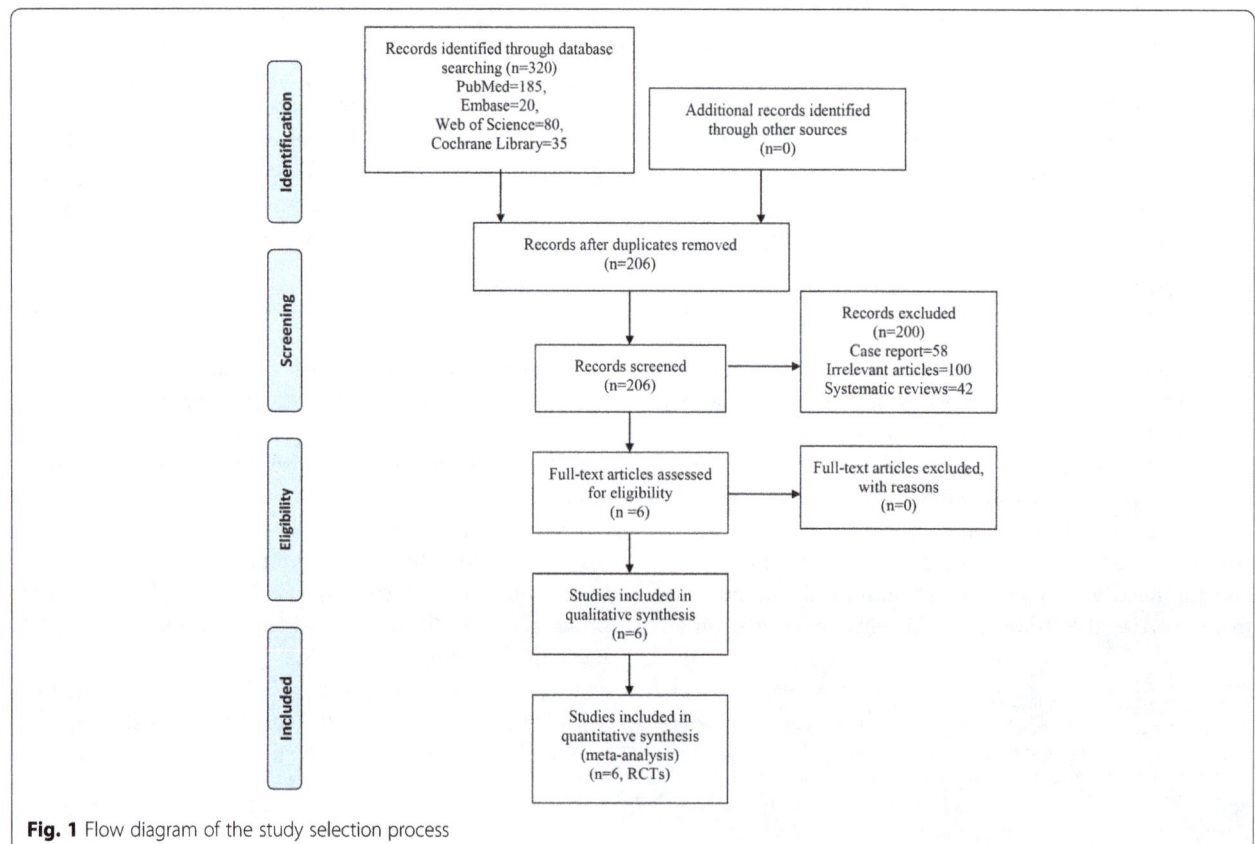

Fig. 1 Flow diagram of the study selection process

Table 1 General characteristic of the included studies. 1, need for transfusion; 2, total blood loss; 3, hidden blood loss; 4, intraoperative blood loss; 5, the occurrence of DVT; 6, the occurrence of hematoma

Author	Country	Age (years, I/C)	No. of patients (n)	Interventions	Dose of intervention	Outcomes	Transfusion threshold	Follow-up
Gao F 2015	China	58.6 vs 61.7	53 vs 54	Topical TXA + topical DEP vs topical TXA	TXA (3 g), DEP (0.25 mg, 1:200000)	1, 2, 3, 4, 5, 6	Hb < 70 g/l	3 months
Jans O 2016	Denmark	67 vs 69	50 vs 50	Intravenous TXA + intravenous DEP vs intravenous TXA	TXA (1 g), DEP (0.05 μg kg^{-1} min^{-1})	2,3,	Hb < 80 g/l	At discharge
Liu JL 2018	China	50.0 vs 50.2 vs 51.8	65 vs 65 vs 65	Intravenous TXA + DEP vs intravenous TXA + topical DEP vs intravenous TXA	IV DEP (1 mg), IV TXA (10 mg/kg), topical DEP (0.25 mg, 1:200000)	1, 2, 3, 4, 5, 6	Hb < 70 g/l	2 weeks
Wang JW 2017	China	67 vs 69	45 vs 45	Topical TXA + topical DEP vs topical TXA	TXA (3 g), DEP (0.25 mg, 1:200000)	1, 2, 3, 4, 5, 6	Hb < 80 g/l	2 months
Zhang JK 2017	China	62.5 vs 63.1	21 vs 34	Topical TXA + topical DEP vs topical TXA	TXA (3 g), DEP (0.25 mg, 1:200000)	1, 2, 3, 4, 5, 6	Hb < 80 g/l	6 months
Zhang JZ 2017	China	59.8 vs 60.3 vs 58.6	52 vs 52 vs 52	Topical 1 g TXA + topical low dose DEP vs topical 1 g TXA + topical high dose DEP vs topical TXA	TXA (1 g), DEP (0.125 mg, 0.25 mg, 1:200000)	1, 2, 3, 4, 5	Hb < 70 g/l	3 months

follow-up. The differences in the extracted data were discussed by a panel of all the reviewers. When there were no clear data or missing data from the included studies, we tried to contact the corresponding author to obtain the relevant data.

Quality assessment

Two reviewers independently evaluated the risk of bias using the Cochrane risk-of-bias tool. Seven major domains of bias (selection bias (random sequence generation), selection bias (allocation concealment), performance bias, detection bias, attrition bias, reporting bias and other bias) in each trial were reviewed. Disagreements between the reviewers were resolved by discussion.

Statistically analysis

The risk ratios (RRs) with 95% confidence intervals (CIs) were calculated for the need for transfusion and the occurrence of DVT. The weighted mean difference (WMD) and corresponding CIs were calculated for continuous data (total blood loss, blood loss in drainage). Heterogeneity was explored for all the meta-analyses and quantified using I^2 statistics. When I^2 value was > 50%, this was considered substantial heterogeneity

	Random sequence generation (selection bias)	Allocation concealment (selection bias)	Blinding of participants and personnel (performance bias)	Blinding of outcome assessment (detection bias)	Incomplete outcome data (attrition bias)	Selective reporting (reporting bias)	Other bias
Gao F 2015	+	+	+	+	+	+	+
Jans O 2016	+	+	+	+	+	+	+
Liu JL 2018	?	?	+	+	+	+	+
Wang JW 2017	?	?	+	+	+	+	+
Zhang JK 2017	+	?	?	?	+	+	+
Zhang JZ 2017	+	+	+	+	+	+	+

Fig. 2 Risk of bias summary for the included RCTs. +, low risk of bias; –, high risk of bias; ?, unclear risk of bias

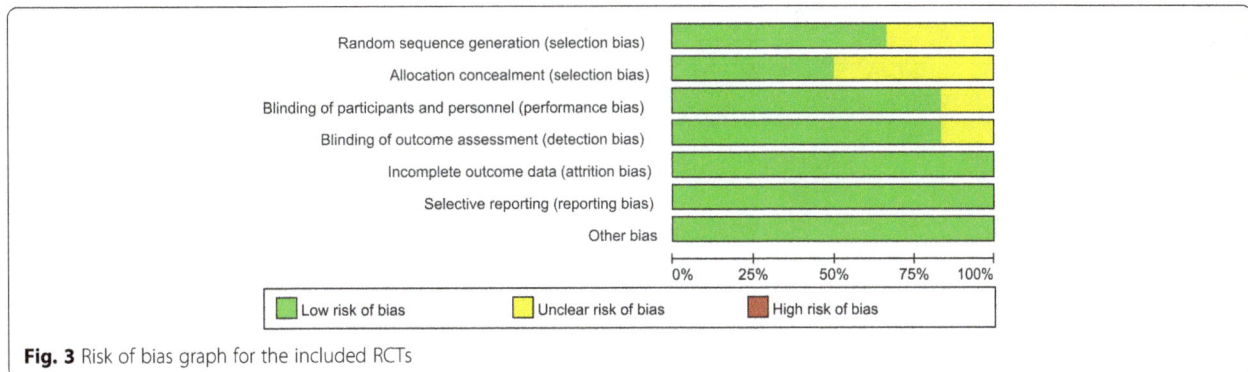

Fig. 3 Risk of bias graph for the included RCTs

between studies. If there was a large clinical heterogeneity, a random-effects model was applied to pool the outcome data. A P value < 0.05 was considered statistically significant. All statistical analyses were performed using Stata 12.0 (Stata Corp., College Station, TX). Subgroup analysis was further performed according to the following variables: risk of bias (low or unclear/high), IV TXA dose (≥ 2 g or < 2 g), topical dose (≥ 2 g or < 2 g) and transfusion protocol (strict or loose). We categorized the TXA dose of 30 mg/kg into the subgroup of ≥ 2 g. Sensitivity analysis was also performed by omitting each of the studies in turn.

Quality of evidence assessment

We used the Grading of Recommendations Assessment, Development and Evaluation (GRADE) methodology to assess the quality of evidence. The assessment includes five items: risk of bias, inconsistency, indirectness, imprecision and publication bias. Each outcome was rated as high, moderate, low or very low. Summary tables were

constructed using GRADE Pro version 3.6 (GRADE Working Group).

Results

Search results

A flowchart of study search and selection is presented in Fig. 1. We identified 320 references (PubMed = 185, Embase = 20, Web of Science = 80, Cochrane Library = 35) in our initial literature search. There were no additional records identified through other sources. After removing duplicates using Endnote X7 software, there were 206 studies remaining. Subsequently, 200 studies were excluded according to the inclusion criteria. Finally, 6 trials with 703 patients met our inclusion criteria and were included in the meta-analysis [14–19]. The general characteristics of the included studies can be seen in Table 1. All trials were published after the year 2015. Five studies were performed in China, and one was performed in Denmark. The mean age of the patients

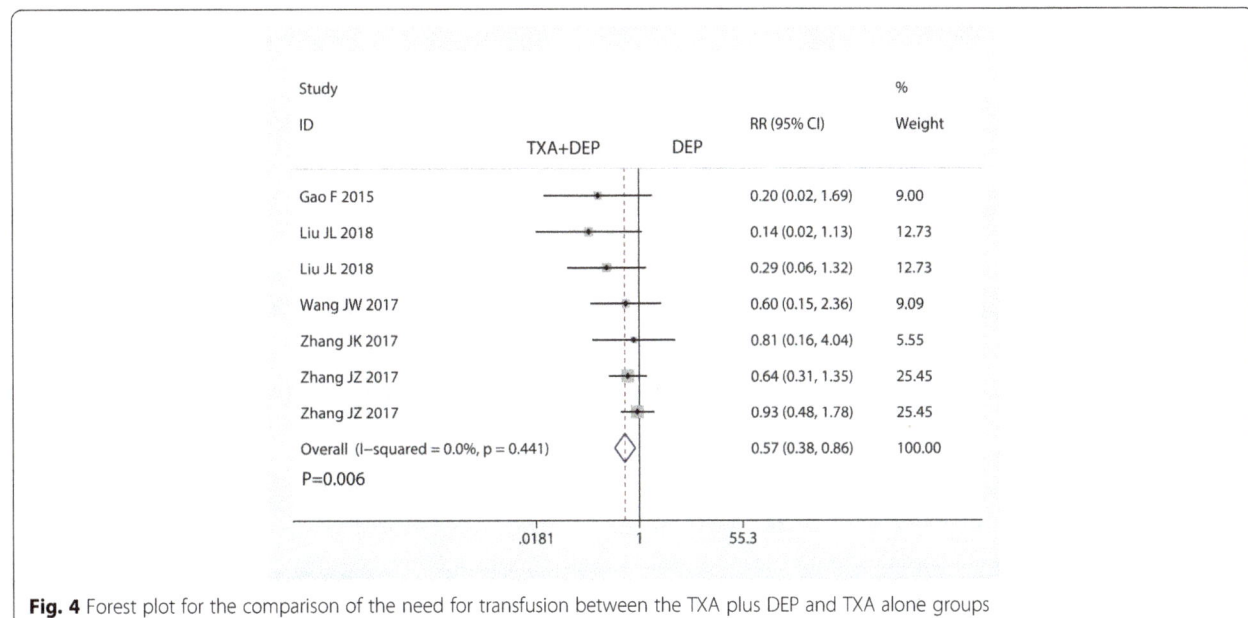

Fig. 4 Forest plot for the comparison of the need for transfusion between the TXA plus DEP and TXA alone groups

Table 2 Subgroup analysis for the need for transfusion

Subgroup	No. trials	RR (95% CI)	P value	I^2 (%)	Test of interaction, P
Risk of bias					
Low	4	0.60 (0.38, 0.95)	0.028	35.5	0.047
Unclear/high	3	0.50 (0.21, 1.16)	0.105	0	
Dose of TXA					
Low	4	0.60 (0.38, 0.93)	0.014	34.1	0.125
High	3	0.50 (0.16, 0.84)	0.023	0	
Transfusion protocol					
Strict	3	0.43 (0.18, 1.05)	0.064	0	0.043
Loose	4	0.63 (0.40, 0.98)	0.041	14.5	

ranged from 50.0 to 69 years. Patients' ages ranged from 21 to 65 years, and all were less than 100 years old.

Quality assessment

Data regarding the risk of bias summary and risk of bias graphs for each study are presented in Figs. 2 and 3, respectively. Three studies had a low risk of bias. The other studies were considered to have an unclear risk of bias.

Quality of evidence assessment

The GRADE evidence profiles are presented in Additional file 1. The GRADE level of evidence was low for total blood loss, hidden blood loss and intra-operative blood loss; it was moderate for the need for transfusion and the occurrence of DVT and haematoma.

Results of the meta-analysis
Need for transfusion

Five studies were available with information regarding transfusion rate. The pooled results demonstrated that TXA plus DEP was associated with a lower transfusion rate than TXA alone (RR = 0.57, 95% CI 0.38–0.86, P = 0.006, Fig. 4). No heterogeneity was detected (I^2 = 0%, P = 0.441), and thus, a fixed-effects model was used. The results of the subgroup analysis are shown in Table 2. The findings of a decreased need for transfusion were consistent for different doses of TXA except for the risk of bias and transfusion protocol.

Total blood loss

Five studies were available for analysis of total blood loss. TXA plus DEP led to significantly less total blood

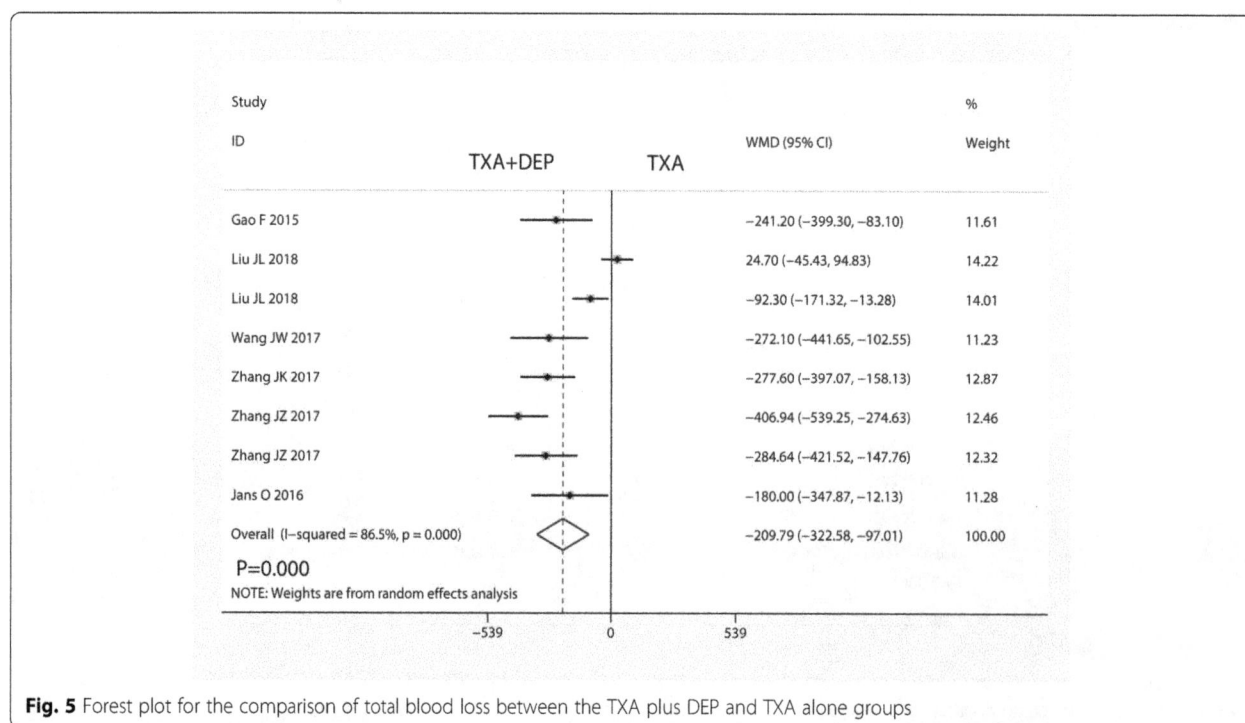

Fig. 5 Forest plot for the comparison of total blood loss between the TXA plus DEP and TXA alone groups

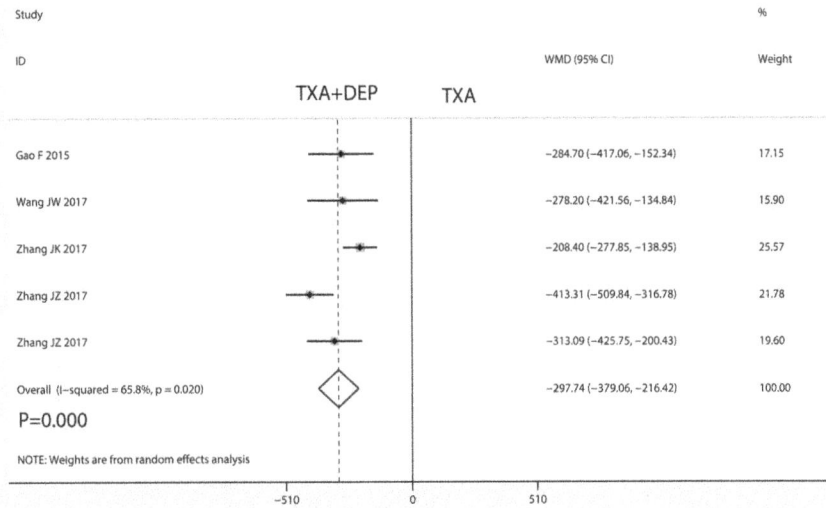

Fig. 6 Forest plot for the comparison of hidden blood loss between the TXA plus DEP and TXA alone groups

loss than TXA alone (WMD = – 209.79, 95% CI – 322.58 to – 97.02, $P = 0.000$; $I^2 = 86.5\%$, $P = 0.000$, Fig. 5). Thus, we used a random-effects model to pool the relevant data.

Hidden blood loss
Five studies were available for analysing hidden blood loss. TXA plus DEP led to significantly less hidden blood loss

than TXA alone (WMD = – 297.74, 95% CI – 379.06 to – 216.42, $P = 0.000$; $I^2 = 65.8\%$, $P = 0.020$, Fig. 6). Thus, we used a random-effects model to pool the relevant data.

Intraoperative blood loss
Four studies were available for analysis of intraoperative blood loss. TXA plus DEP led to significantly less hidden blood loss than TXA alone (WMD = – 74.35, 95% CI –

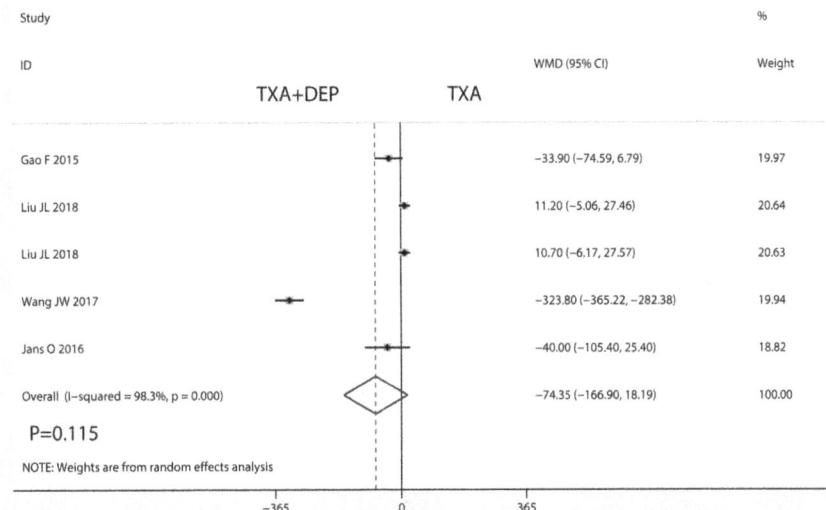

Fig. 7 Forest plot for the comparison of intraoperative blood loss between the TXA plus DEP and TXA alone groups

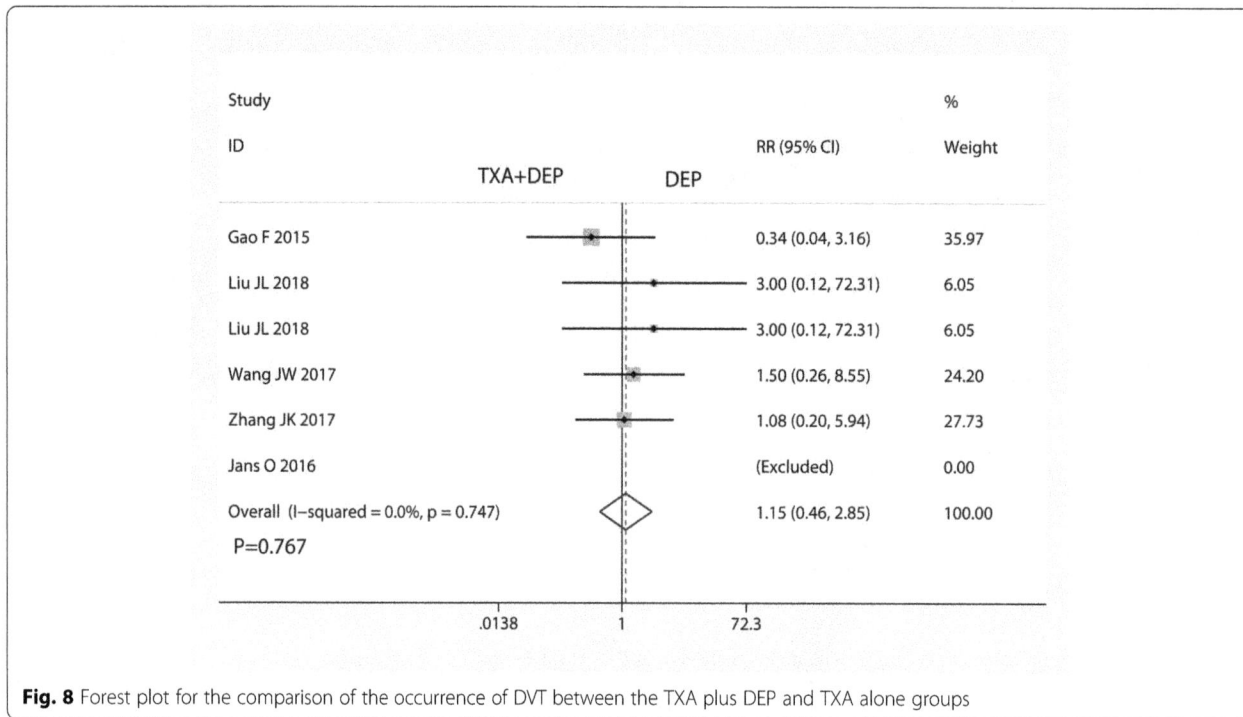

Fig. 8 Forest plot for the comparison of the occurrence of DVT between the TXA plus DEP and TXA alone groups

166.90 to 18.19, $P = 0.115$; $I^2 = 98.3\%$, $P = 0.000$, Fig. 7). Thus, we used a random-effects model to pool the relevant data.

The occurrence of DVT and haematoma

Five studies reported the occurrence of DVT. There was no significant difference in the occurrence of DVT between the TXA plus DEP and TXA alone groups (RR = 1.15, 95% CI 0.46–2.85, $P = 0.767$, Fig. 8). No heterogeneity was detected ($I^2 = 0\%$, $P = 0.747$); thus, a fixed-effects model was used. Four studies reported the occurrence of haematoma. There was no significant difference in the occurrence of DVT between the TXA plus DEP and the TXA alone groups in terms of the

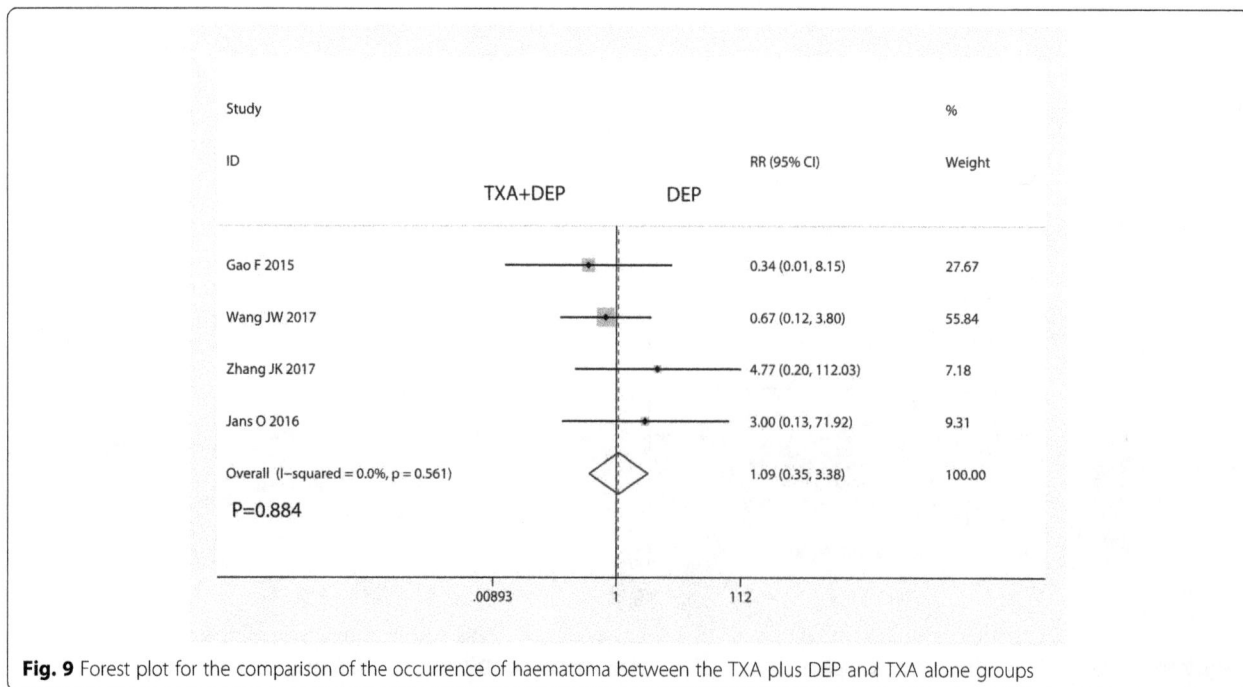

Fig. 9 Forest plot for the comparison of the occurrence of haematoma between the TXA plus DEP and TXA alone groups

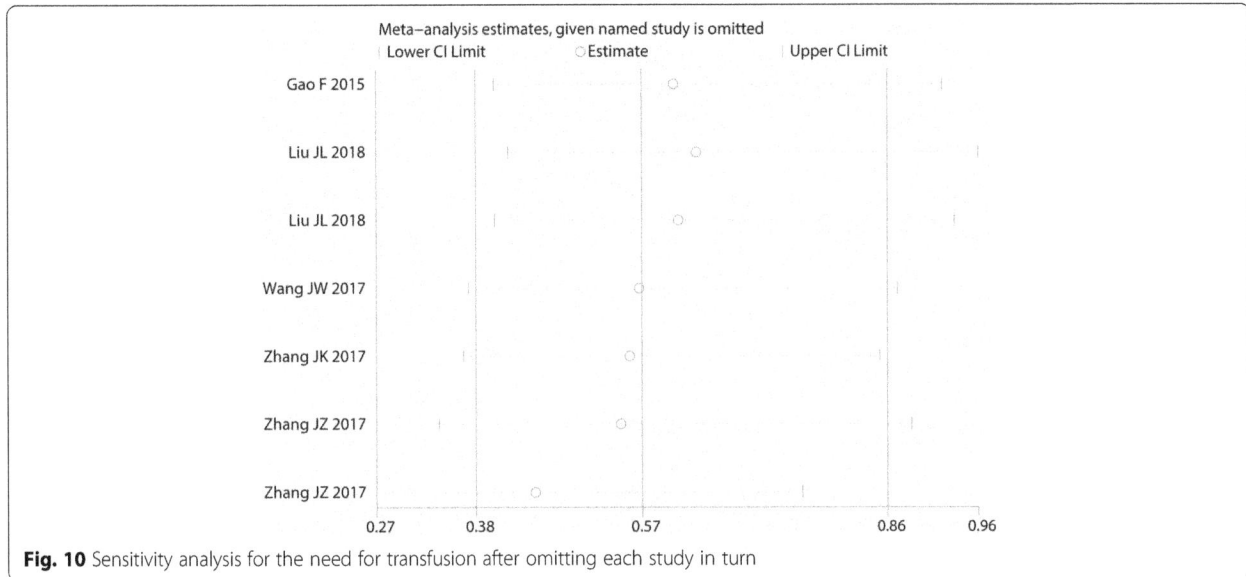

Meta–analysis estimates, given named study is omitted

| Lower CI Limit | Estimate | Upper CI Limit |

Fig. 10 Sensitivity analysis for the need for transfusion after omitting each study in turn

occurrence of haematoma (RR = 1.09, 95% CI 0.35–3.38, $P = 0.884$, Fig. 9). No heterogeneity was detected ($I^2 = 0\%$, $P = 0.561$); thus, a fixed-effects model was sued.

Sensitivity analysis, publication bias

We performed a sensitivity analysis for the need for transfusion (Fig. 10. The results showed that after omitting the included studies, in turn, the overall effects did not change. The funnel plots were visually assessed and revealed no asymmetry (Fig. 11); no evidence of publication bias was determined by the Egger linear regression test for the need for transfusion ($P = 0.72$, Fig. 12),

Discussion

In the current meta-analysis, we evaluated the efficacy and safety of TXA plus DEP for patients with THA. On the basis of the pooled estimates, TXA plus DEP was associated with significantly less total blood loss and subsequent need for transfusion than TXA alone. The use of tanezumab was not associated with a significantly increased risk of DVT or haematoma.

This was not the first meta-analysis. Yu et al. [20] conducted a meta-analysis comparing TXA plus DEP for blood loss after total joint arthroplasty (THA and total knee arthroplasty). Thus, we could not determine whether TXA plus DEP was certain to have a significant

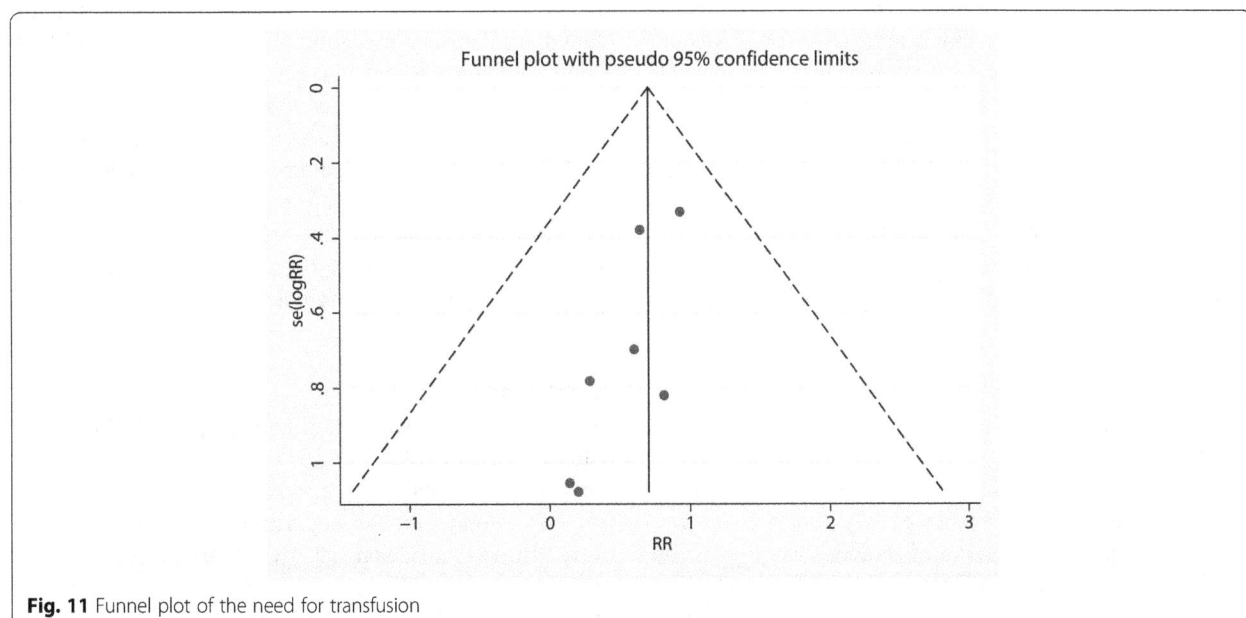

Funnel plot with pseudo 95% confidence limits

Fig. 11 Funnel plot of the need for transfusion

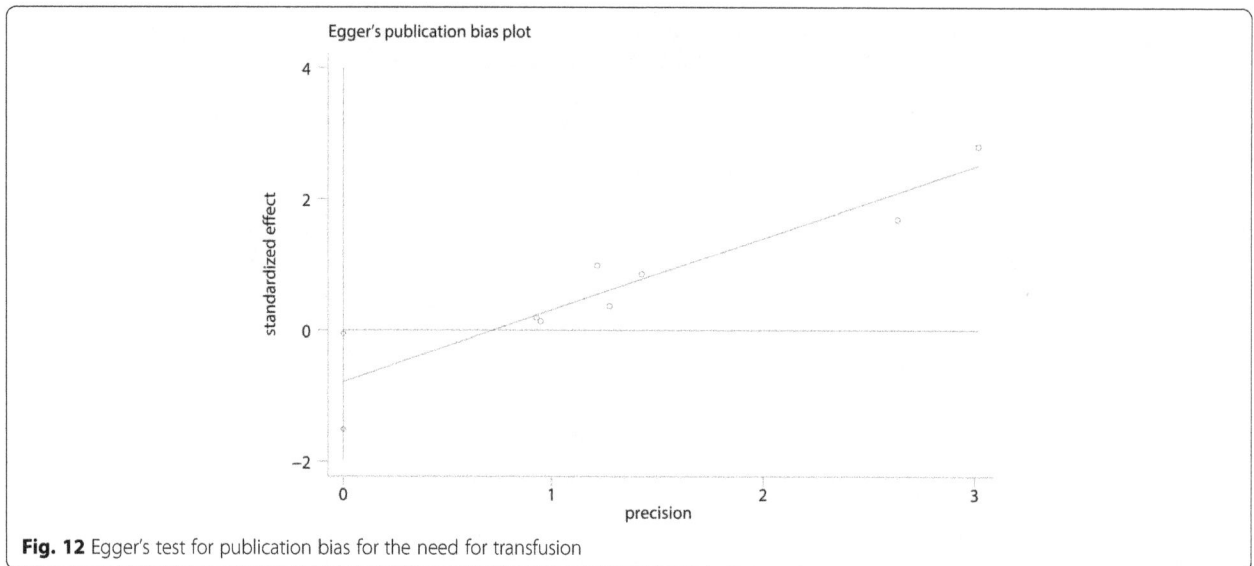

Fig. 12 Egger's test for publication bias for the need for transfusion

influence on controlling blood loss among patients undergoing THA alone. Moreover, Yu et al. [20] only included two studies that focused on THA. In this meta-analysis, we ultimately included six studies totalling 703 patients, adding the statistical power of at least 535 cases. Our meta-analysis was the latest and the most comprehensive one, and it generally concurs and further reinforces the results of the previous meta-analysis. Finally, we performed a subgroup-analysis and evaluated the quality of evidence using GRADE to help healthcare professionals make clinical decisions.

The current meta-analysis demonstrated that TXA plus DEP has a beneficial effect on total blood loss. TXA plus DEP was associated with less total blood loss by 209.79 ml than TXA alone. Several meta-analyses have found that TXA has a beneficial role in reducing blood loss in THA patients without increasing DVT occurrence [21, 22]. TXA can be administered by several routes including topical [23], intravenous [24] and oral [25]. Studies have shown that there was no significant difference among these routes in terms of the total blood loss. Concerning DEP, Jans O et al. [15] strongly suggested that intravenous DEP could be beneficial for reducing blood loss after THA. The administration of low-dose DEP could act as a procoagulant by increasing platelet aggregation, resulting in an instant 20–30% increase in platelet count [26]. Furthermore, DEP could activate α-adrenergic and β-adrenergic receptors; therefore, DEP could stimulate the release of several coagulation factors [27].

We measured hidden blood loss between the TXA plus DEP and TXA alone groups. We found that TXA plus DEP significantly reduced hidden blood loss by 297.74 ml compared with TXA alone. In THA patients, significant blood loss can occur after wound closure, and

the proportion of this blood loss is called hidden blood loss. Hidden blood loss accounts for as much as 60% of the total perioperative blood loss [28]. With the administration of DEP, the procoagulant effects could last for 1–2 h; therefore, oozing could be decreased.

Regarding complications, we measured the occurrences of DVT and haematoma formation. We found that there was no significant difference between the occurrences of DVT and haematoma formation. Regarding the administration of TXA, DVT was the major concern. Several meta-analyses have identified that administration with TXA does not increase the occurrence of DVT [29]. Due to the incidence rate being relatively small, there is a need for studies to further clarify the risk [30].

There were several limitations in this meta-analysis: (1) the doses of TXA and DEP varied among the included studies, and the optimal doses of TXA and DEP require further exploration; (2) heterogeneity was large in terms of total blood loss and hidden blood loss, and these two outcomes should be interpreted cautiously; (3) the follow-up period varied among the included studies; thus, complications of TXA plus DEP may have been underestimated; and (4) the sample size was relatively small in the included studies; therefore, high-quality large-scale sample RCTs are needed.

Conclusion

This meta-analysis suggests that TXA plus DEP has benefits in terms of total blood loss, hidden blood loss and the need for transfusion. Furthermore, TXA plus DEP had no influence on the occurrence of DVT or haematoma formation. Given all the shortcomings of this meta-analysis, further research and analysis are required to draw more reliable conclusions.

Abbreviations

CIs: Confidence intervals; DEP: Diluted epinephrine; DVT: Deep venous thrombosis; OA: Osteoarthritis; RCTs: Randomized controlled trials; RR: Risk ratio; THA: Total hip arthroplasty; TXA: Tranexamic acid; WMD: Weighted mean difference

Authors' contributions

ZW designed the study and developed the retrieval strategy. ZW and HJZ searched and screened the summaries and titles. HJZ and ZW drafted the article. Both authors read and approved the final draft.

Competing interests

Both authors declare that they have no competing interests.

Author details

[1]Department of Orthopedics, Jingjiang People's Hospital, Jingjiang, China. [2]Department of Orthopaedics, The 82rn Hospital of People's Liberation Army of China, No. 100, Jiankangdong Road, Huai'an, Jiangsu, China.

References

1. Guo H, Wang C, He Y. A meta-analysis evaluates the efficacy of intravenous acetaminophen for pain management in knee or hip arthroplasty. J Orthop Sci. 2018;23(5):793–800.
2. Kurtz S, Ong K, Lau E, Mowat F, Halpern M. Projections of primary and revision hip and knee arthroplasty in the United States from 2005 to 2030. J Bone Joint Surg Am. 2007;89(4):780–5.
3. Liu Q, Geng P, Shi L, Wang Q, Wang P. Tranexamic acid versus aminocaproic acid for blood management after total knee and total hip arthroplasty: a systematic review and meta-analysis. Int J Surg. 2018;54(Pt A): 105–12.
4. Li JF, Li H, Zhao H, Wang J, Liu S, Song Y, Wu HF. Combined use of intravenous and topical versus intravenous tranexamic acid in primary total knee and hip arthroplasty: a meta-analysis of randomised controlled trials. J Orthop Surg Res. 2017;12(1):22.
5. Li YJ, Xu BS, Bai SP, Guo XJ, Yan XY. The efficacy of intravenous aminocaproic acid in primary total hip and knee arthroplasty: a meta-analysis. J Orthop Surg Res. 2018;13(1):89.
6. Bloch EM, Ingram C, Hull J, Fawcus S, Anthony J, Green-Thompson R, Crookes RL, Ngcobo S, V Creel D, Courtney L, et al. Risk factors for peripartum blood transfusion in South Africa: a case-control study. Transfusion. 2018;[Epub ahead of print].
7. Gianakos AL, Hurley ET, Haring RS, Yoon RS, Liporace FA. Reduction of blood loss by tranexamic acid following total hip and knee arthroplasty: a meta-analysis. JBJS reviews. 2018;6(5):e1.
8. Sridharan K, Sivaramakrishnan G. Tranexamic acid in total hip arthroplasty: mixed treatment comparisons of randomized controlled trials and cohort studies. J Orthop. 2018;15(1):81–8.
9. Huang F, Wu Y, Yin Z, Ma G, Chang J. A systematic review and meta-analysis of the use of antifibrinolytic agents in total hip arthroplasty. Hip Int. 2015;25(6):502–9.
10. Wu Y, Zeng Y, Bao X, Xiong H, Fan X, Shen B. Application of tranexamic acid and diluted epinephrine in primary total hip arthroplasty. Blood Coagul Fibrinolysis. 2018;29(5):451–7.
11. Teng Y, Ma J, Ma X, Wang Y, Lu B, Guo C. The efficacy and safety of epinephrine for postoperative bleeding in total joint arthroplasty: a PRISMA-compliant meta-analysis. Medicine. 2017;96(17):e6763.
12. Tullavardhana T, Akranurakkul P, Ungkitphaiboon W, Songtish D. Efficacy of submucosal epinephrine injection for the prevention of postpolypectomy bleeding: a meta-analysis of randomized controlled studies. Annals of Medicine and Surgery. 2012;2017(19):65–73.
13. Knobloch K, Yoon U, Vogt PM. Preferred reporting items for systematic reviews and meta-analyses (PRISMA) statement and publication bias. J Craniomaxillofac Surg. 2011;39(2):91–2.
14. Gao F, Sun W, Guo W, Li Z, Wang W, Cheng L. Topical application of tranexamic acid plus diluted epinephrine reduces postoperative hidden blood loss in total hip arthroplasty. J Arthroplast. 2015;30(12):2196–200.
15. Jans O, Grevstad U, Mandoe H, Kehlet H, Johansson PI. A randomized trial of the effect of low dose epinephrine infusion in addition to tranexamic acid on blood loss during total hip arthroplasty. Br J Anaesth. 2016;116(3):357–62.
16. Liu JL, Zeng WN, Wang FY, Chen C, Gong XY, Yang H, Tan ZJ, Jia XL, Yang L. Effects of low-dose epinephrine on perioperative hemostasis and inflammatory reaction in major surgical operations: a randomized clinical trial. J. Thromb. Haemost. 2018;16(1):74–82.
17. Wang JW, Ren SH. The effects of topical tranexamic acid plus epinephrine for blood loss in total hip arthroplasty patients. J Pract Med. 2017;33(2):279–81.
18. Zhang JK, Liang PX, Liu Z. Effects of topical application of tranexamic acid plus adrenaline in total hip arthroplasty. Journal of Clinical Orthopaedics. 2017;20(1):58–61.
19. Zhang JZ, Zhu K. Hemostasis effect of local application of tranexamic acid and epinephrine for total hip arthroplasty. Journal of Clinical Orthopaedics. 2017;20(3):318–21.
20. Yu Z, Yao L, Yang Q. Tranexamic acid plus diluted-epinephrine versus tranexamic acid alone for blood loss in total joint arthroplasty: a meta-analysis. Medicine. 2017;96(24):e7095.
21. Alshryda S, Sukeik M, Sarda P, Blenkinsopp J, Haddad FS, Mason JM. A systematic review and meta-analysis of the topical administration of tranexamic acid in total hip and knee replacement. Bone Joint J. 2014;96-b(8):1005–15.
22. Wei Z, Liu M. The effectiveness and safety of tranexamic acid in total hip or knee arthroplasty: a meta-analysis of 2720 cases. Transfus Med. 2015;25(3):151–62.
23. Abdel MP, Chalmers BP, Taunton MJ, Pagnano MW, Trousdale RT, Sierra RJ, Lee YY, Boettner F, Su EP, Haas SB, et al. Intravenous versus topical tranexamic acid in total knee arthroplasty: both effective in a randomized clinical trial of 640 patients. J Bone Joint Surg Am. 2018;100(12):1023–9.
24. Wei W, Dang S, Duan D, Wei L. Comparison of intravenous and topical tranexamic acid in total knee arthroplasty. BMC Musculoskelet Disord. 2018; 19(1):191.
25. Luo ZY, Wang D, Meng WK, Wang HY, Pan H, Pei FX, Zhou ZK. Oral tranexamic acid is equivalent to topical tranexamic acid without drainage in primary total hip arthroplasty: a double-blind randomized clinical trial. Thromb Res. 2018;167:1–5.
26. von Kanel R, Dimsdale JE. Effects of sympathetic activation by adrenergic infusions on hemostasis in vivo. Eur J Haematol. 2000;65(6):357–69.
27. Bakovic D, Pivac N, Eterovic D, Breskovic T, Zubin P, Obad A, Dujic Z. The effects of low-dose epinephrine infusion on spleen size, central and hepatic circulation and circulating platelets. Clin Physiol Funct Imaging. 2013;33(1):30–7.
28. Lei Y, Huang Q, Huang Z, Xie J, Chen G, Pei F. Multiple-dose intravenous tranexamic acid further reduces hidden blood loss after total hip arthroplasty: a randomized controlled trial. J Arthroplast. 2018;33(9):2940–5.
29. Xie J, Hu Q, Ma J, Huang Q, Pei F. Multiple boluses of intravenous tranexamic acid to reduce hidden blood loss and the inflammatory response following enhanced-recovery primary total hip arthroplasty: a randomised clinical trial. Bone Joint J. 2017;99-b(11):1442–9.
30. Wu XD, Hu KJ, Sun YY, Chen Y, Huang W. Letter to the editor on "the safety of tranexamic acid in total joint arthroplasty: a direct meta-analysis". J Arthroplast. 2018;[Epub ahead of print].

20

Exploratory analysis of predictors of revision surgery for proximal junctional kyphosis or additional postoperative vertebral fracture following adult spinal deformity surgery in elderly patients: a retrospective cohort study

Hiroshi Uei[*] , Yasuaki Tokuhashi, Masafumi Maseda, Masahiro Nakahashi, Hirokatsu Sawada, Koji Matsumoto and Hiroyuki Miyakata

Abstract

Background: Proximal junctional kyphosis (PJK) following adult spinal deformity (ASD) surgery in elderly patients is markedly influenced by osteoporosis causing additional vertebral fracture and loosening of pedicle screws (PS). This study aimed to investigate the association between mean bone density represented in Hounsfield units (HU) on spinal computed tomography (CT) and revision surgery for PJK or postoperative additional vertebral fracture following ASD surgery in elderly patients.

Methods: The subjects were 54 ASD patients aged 65 years or older who were treated with correction and fusion surgery of four or more levels and could be followed for 2 years or longer. Bone density was measured before surgery using lumbar dual-energy X-ray absorptiometry (DXA) and spinal CT in all patients. The patients were divided into group A ($n = 14$) in which revision surgery was required for PJK or additional vertebral fracture and group B ($n = 40$) in which revision surgery was not required. We retrospectively investigated incidences of PJK, additional vertebral fracture, and PS loosening, perioperative parameters, radiographic parameters before and after surgery, and osteoporosis treatment administration rate.

Results: No significant difference was noted in young adult mean (YAM) on DXA between groups A and B, respectively ($P = 0.62$), but the mean bone densities represented in HU of the T8 ($P = 0.002$) and T9 ($P = 0.01$) vertebral bodies on spinal CT were significantly lower in group A, whereas those of the L4 ($P = 0.002$) and L5 ($P = 0.01$) vertebral bodies were significantly higher in group A. The incidence of PJK was not significantly different ($P = 0.07$), but the incidence of additional vertebral fracture was significantly higher in group A ($P < 0.001$). The incidences of uppermost PS loosening within 3 months after surgery were 71% and 40% in groups A and B, respectively ($P = 0.04$).

Conclusions: In elderly patients who required revision surgery, the mean bone densities of vertebral bodies at T8 and T9 were significantly lower. The mean bone density represented in HU on spinal CT may be useful for risk assessment of and countermeasures against revision surgery after ASD surgery in elderly patients.

Keywords: Mean bone density, adult spinal deformity, Pedicle screw loosening, Proximal junctional kyphosis, Upper instrumented vertebra

* Correspondence: uei.hiroshi@nihon-u.ac.jp
Department of Orthopaedic Surgery, Nihon University School of Medicine,
30-1 Oyaguchi Kami-cho, Itabashi-ku, Tokyo 173-8610, Japan

Background

The rates of revision surgery due to proximal junctional kyphosis/failure (PJK/PJF) following correction and fusion surgery for adult spinal deformity (ASD) is high, and its risk assessment and countermeasures are necessary but still insufficient [1–7]. The potentially modifiable risk factors are greater curvature correction, combined anterior-posterior spinal fusion, hybrid instrumentation (proximal hooks and distal pedicle screws), fusion to the sacro-pelvis, thoracoplasty procedure, and residual sagittal imbalance [4, 5, 7]. Non-modifiable risk factors include older age (> 55 years) and severe preoperative sagittal imbalance [4, 5, 7]. Other less well-established but likely risk factors of PJK/PJF following ASD surgery are low bone density, high body mass index, and presence of a comorbidity [4, 5], and the risk of revision surgery due to complications associated with not only PJK/PJF due to adjacent segment disease but also additional remote level vertebral fracture following posterior instrumentation fusion surgery has been a concern for elderly patients with low vertebral bone density [8, 9]. Bone density has been normally evaluated in an anteroposterior projection of the lumbar vertebra using dual-energy X-ray absorptiometry (DXA), but there are some problems with lumbar DXA in ASD patients. It is unclear whether it reflects the bone density of the lower thoracic vertebrae, in which upper instrumented vertebra (UIV) of ASD surgery is frequently present. Besides, no study in ASD patients on the bone density in the vertebrae around the UIV has been reported. The use of spinal CT substituting for lumbar DXA to complement this disadvantage has been reported, and a significant positive correlation between the T-score on DXA and Hounsfield units (HU) on spinal CT was reported [10]. Bone density on spinal CT can be measured at any vertebral level [10–13], and it can be investigated separately in the vertebral body and pedicle. In addition, accurate measurement is possible even in the presence of spinal deformity. Given the risk for possible neurological damage as well as severe back pain or impaired quality of life, PJK/PJF or additional remote level vertebral fracture is particularly serious complications for ASD patients. The etiology of PJK/PJF is multifactorial as no study has evaluated a single factor that strongly and consistently predicts their development. Furthermore, there remains conflicting evidence with regard to whether the number of levels fused, the UIV implant types, or the location of the UIV influence the risk of PJK/PJF development. Thus, we aimed to identify factors associated with revision surgery following correction and fusion surgery for ASD in elderly patients. Demographics, clinical data, and radiographic variables were analyzed.

Methods

Patient population

This study was a retrospective review of a prospectively collected data from 1654 consecutive patients who underwent spine surgery at our institution from January 2007 to December 2014. Ninety-six out of 1654 patients underwent ASD surgery. The inclusion criteria for the study were ASD patients aged 65 years or older who were treated with correction and fusion surgery of four or more levels and could be followed by our institution for 2 years or longer. We performed ASD surgery without the use of bone morphogenetic protein because it was not permitted by the Ministry of Health, Labour and Welfare in Japan. Regarding rod type, we used 6.0 titanium alloy dual rods from the same company for all cases. Patients with a past medical history of malignant cancer, Parkinson's disease, secondary osteoporosis, metabolic bone disease other than osteoporosis, or those taking medications such as chronic glucocorticoids that cause a decrease in bone strength were excluded. This decision was made prior to study initiation by both two surgeons (H.U. and Y.T.). Seventy-three patients were included in this study, and 19 out of 73 patients were excluded. Twelve patients were lost to follow up, 2 patients had malignant cancer, 2 patients had Parkinson's disease, 2 patients had secondary osteoporosis, and 1 patient had rheumatoid arthritis. The 54 patients were divided into two groups and retrospectively investigated: group A (n = 14) which required revision surgery due to severe pain, neurological deficits, or progressive sagittal deformity associated with PJK or additional vertebral fracture and group B (n = 40) which did not require revision surgery. Revision surgeries were performed for PJK in 12 and additional remote level vertebral fracture in 2. Postoperative follow-up was performed at 1, 3, 6, 9, and 12 months and every 6 months thereafter.

Evaluation of bone density

We performed both lumbar DXA and spinal CT as a standard practice on ASD patients within 3 months before surgery. To evaluate bone density on lumbar DXA, the mean values in an anteroposterior projection of the L2, L3, and L4 vertebral bodies were calculated and evaluated based on the young adult mean (YAM) values. In the evaluation of bone density represented in HU on spinal CT, the middle lower thoracic over the lumbosacral vertebrae and pelvis were imaged in all patients. The images were digitized, and the bone density was calculated using the software SYNAPSE Enterprise-PACS (FUJIFILM Corporation, Tokyo, Japan), employing the method reported by Schreiber et al. [10]. The vertebral body was divided into one third cranial, one third central, and one third caudal regions excluding the vertebral endplate in the sagittal section (Fig. 1a), and the bone density of cancellous bone excluding cortical bone was measured in an oval pattern (Fig. 1b, d). The bone density of pedicle was similarly measured on the bilateral sides excluding cortical bone (Fig. 1b, d) in the axial section at the center in the cranio-caudal direction of the pedicle in a parasagittal section on spinal CT (Fig. 1c).

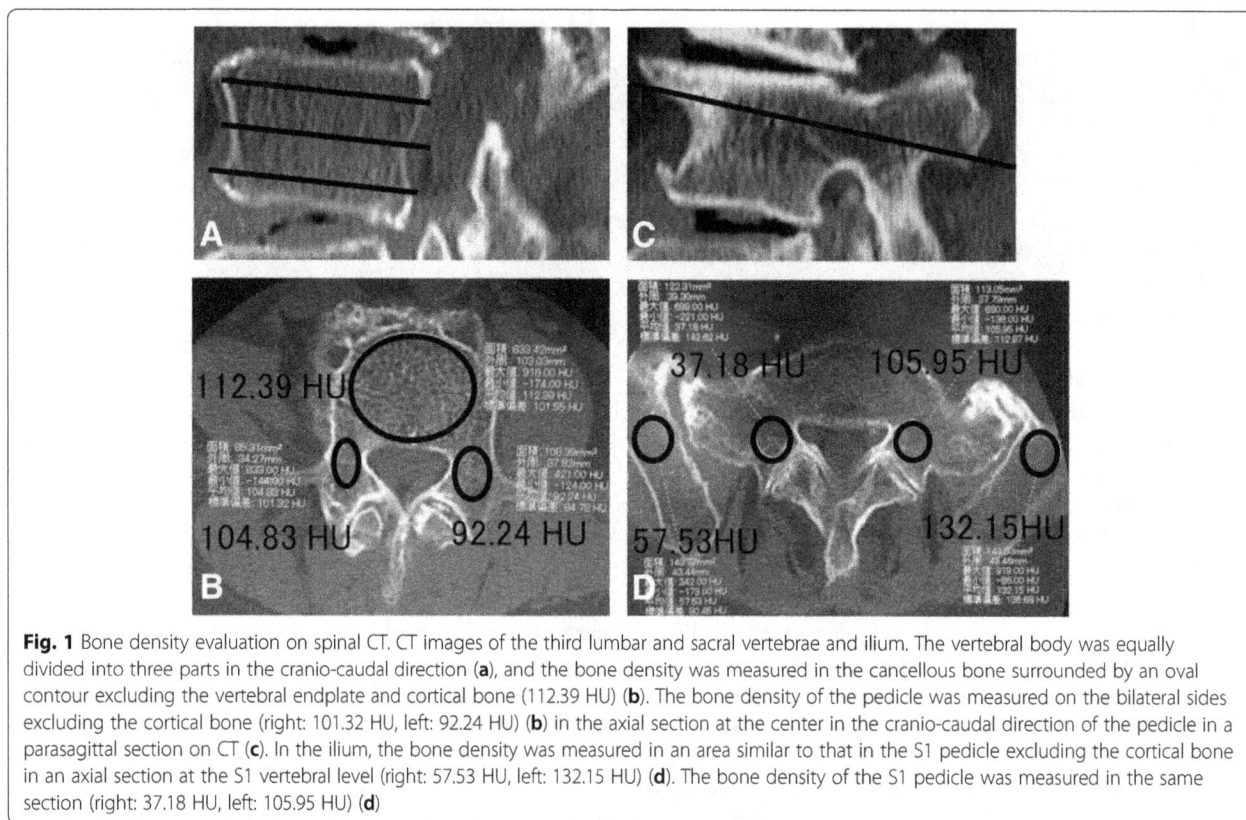

Fig. 1 Bone density evaluation on spinal CT. CT images of the third lumbar and sacral vertebrae and ilium. The vertebral body was equally divided into three parts in the cranio-caudal direction (**a**), and the bone density was measured in the cancellous bone surrounded by an oval contour excluding the vertebral endplate and cortical bone (112.39 HU) (**b**). The bone density of the pedicle was measured on the bilateral sides excluding the cortical bone (right: 101.32 HU, left: 92.24 HU) (**b**) in the axial section at the center in the cranio-caudal direction of the pedicle in a parasagittal section on CT (**c**). In the ilium, the bone density was measured in an area similar to that in the S1 pedicle excluding the cortical bone in an axial section at the S1 vertebral level (right: 57.53 HU, left: 132.15 HU) (**d**). The bone density of the S1 pedicle was measured in the same section (right: 37.18 HU, left: 105.95 HU) (**d**)

In the ilium, the bone density was measured in the region excluding cortical bone in the axial section at the S1 level (Fig. 1c). The mean values of each measured levels represented in HU were calculated in the vertebral body, pedicle and ilium, and regarded as the mean bone densities at the level.

Data collection

The demographic, clinical, and radiographic data collected included preoperative factors, perioperative factors, and postoperative factors. As preoperative factors, age, sex, body mass index (BMI), bone density (DXA and spinal CT), radiographic parameters, and presence or absence of preoperative treatment of osteoporosis were investigated. In bone density evaluation on spinal CT, the mean bone density was determined in T8, T9, T10, T11, T12, L1, L2, L3, L4, L5, S1, and ilium. The following radiographic parameters were measured: (1) sagittal vertical axis (SVA), the distance between the C7 plumb line and the posterosuperior corner of S1; (2) pelvic tilt (PT), the angle between the line connecting the midpoint of the sacral endplate to the middle axis of the femoral heads and the vertical; (3) thoracic kyphosis (TK), the angle between the upper endplate of T5 vertebra and the lower endplate of T12; (4) lumbar lordosis (LL), the angle between the lower endplate of T12 and the upper endplate of S1; (5) pelvic incidence (PI), the

angle between the line perpendicular to the sacral endplate at its midpoint and the line connecting the point to the middle axis of the femoral heads; (6) UIV + 2 angle, the angle between the caudal endplate of the upper instrumented vertebra and the cranial endplate of the two supra-adjacent vertebra; and (7) PI-LL. On the basis of the above radiographic parameters, patients were additionally stratified by the SRS-Schwab ASD classification [14].

As perioperative factors, operation time, intraoperative blood loss, number of levels fused, implant types of UIV, level of uppermost PS, and presence or absence of pedicle subtraction osteotomy (PSO) and sacral fusion were investigated, and SVA, PT, TK, LL, change in LL (Postoperative LL–preoperative LL), PI, PI-LL, and UIV + 2 angle were investigated as radiographic parameters immediately after surgery. We distinguished the UIV levels from uppermost pedicle screw or hook. For example, when we placed bilateral pedicle screws at UIV level of T10, the uppermost pedicle screw level was T10. When we placed bilateral hooks at UIV level of T10, the uppermost pedicle screw level was T11. When we placed unilateral pedicle screw and unilateral hook at UIV level of T10, the uppermost pedicle screw level was T10.

As postoperative factors, duration of follow-up, incidences of additional vertebral fracture, PJK, and PS loosening, and treatment of osteoporosis were investigated.

PJK was defined following the method reported by Glattes et al. [2]. The following conditions were regarded as PJK: (1) when the sagittal Cobb angle (UIV + 2 angle) formed by the caudal endplate of UIV and cephalad endplate of two vertebrae proximal (UIV + 2) was 10° or larger and (2) the UIV + 2 angle increased at least 10° greater than the preoperative measurement. Regarding PS loosening, the presence of a 1 mm or larger circumferential radiolucent zone around PS on plain radiographs acquired in two or more directions was judged as PS loosening [15].

Statistical analysis was performed using the SPSS 19.0 version software (SPSS Inc., Chicago, IL, USA). The chi-square test for independence was used for the nominal scales, the t test or Mann-Whitney U test was used for the data scales, and the significance level was set at 5%.

Results

Mean age at the time of surgery was 73.0 and 74.2 years old, respectively ($P = 0.55$) (Table 1). Groups A and B included 14 (100%) and 36 (90%) female patients, respectively ($P = 0.28$). Group B had a greater mean BMI ($P = 0.01$). Indication for the index surgical procedure included degenerative scoliosis in 4 and 12 patients, degenerative kyphosis in 4 and 8, degenerative kyphoscoliosis in 2 and 8, and posttraumatic kyphosis in 2 and 10, in groups A and B respectively, and posttraumatic kyphoscoliosis in 2 in group B, and iatrogenic kyphosis in 2 in groups A ($P = 0.18$). The

mean YAM value on DXA was 92.9% and 96.2%, respectively ($P = 0.62$). The number of patients with osteoporosis or osteopenia evaluated on lumbar DXA were 6 (42.9%) and 18 (45%), respectively ($P = 1.0$). The mean bone densities of T8 ($P = 0.002$) and T9 ($P = 0.01$) on spinal CT were significantly lower in group A (Fig. 2), whereas those of L4 ($P = 0.002$) and L5 ($P = 0.01$) were significantly higher in group A. The mean bone densities of the T8 ($P = 0.03$) and T9 ($P = 0.02$) pedicles were significantly lower in group A (Fig. 3), whereas that of the L3 pedicle ($P = 0.04$) was significantly higher in group A. Preoperative treatment of osteoporosis was performed in 6 (42.8%) and 22 patients (55%), respectively ($P = 0.54$). Regarding the radiographic parameters before surgery, no significant difference was noted in SVA, PT, TK, LL, PI, PI-LL, or UIV + 2 angle between the groups. The proportions of the SRS-Schwab ASD classification were not also significantly different between the groups (Table 2).

Regarding the perioperative factors, mean operation time were 282 and 304 min in groups A and B, respectively ($P = 0.37$), mean blood losses were 698 and 1128 mL, respectively ($P = 0.02$), mean number of levels fused were 6.9 and 7.6, respectively ($P = 0.24$), and UIV implant type was PS in more than half of the patients ($P = 0.30$) (Table 3). The level of uppermost PS was not significantly different between the groups ($P = 0.32$) (Fig. 4). PSO was applied to 14% and 30% in groups A and B, respectively

Table 1 Baseline characteristics in group A and group B

Characteristic	Group A ($n = 14$)	Group B ($n = 40$)	P value
Age at surgery, mean (SD), years	73.0 (5.5)	74.2 (6.0)	0.55
Female, n (%)	14 (100)	36 (90)	0.28
BMI, mean (SD), kg/m^2	20.5 (3.6)	23.6 (4.0)	0.01
Diagnosis, n (%)			0.18
Degenerative scoliosis	4 (28.6)	12 (30)	
Degenerative kyphosis	4 (28.6)	8 (20)	
Degenerative kyphoscoliosis	2 (14.3)	8 (20)	
Posttraumatic kyphosis	2 (14.3)	10 (25)	
Posttraumatic kyphoscoliosis	0	2 (5)	
Iatrogenic kyphosis	2 (14.3)	0	
BMD YAM, mean (SD), %	92.9 (21.6)	96.2 (21.0)	0.62
Osteopenia or osteoporosis, n (%)	6 (42.8)	18 (45)	1.0
No. of preoperative treatment for osteoporosis, n (%) preoperative radiographic parameters	6 (42.8)	22 (55)	0.54
Sagittal vertical axis, mean (SD), mm	103.4 (57.0)	90.0 (48.6)	0.39
Pelvic tilt, mean (SD), degrees	30.3 (9.7)	27.7 (8.3)	0.33
Thoracic kyphosis, mean (SD), degrees	15.0 (12.9)	25.0 (17.4)	0.07
Lumbar lordosis, mean (SD), degrees	8.9 (15.0)	20.7 (16.1)	0.09
Pelvic incidence, mean (SD), degrees	47.0 (3.3)	50.1 (7.8)	0.21
PI-LL, mean (SD), degrees	38.1 (12.8)	29.5 (14.8)	0.14
UIV + 2 angle, mean (SD), degrees	7.4 (5.2)	3.7 (7.0)	0.11

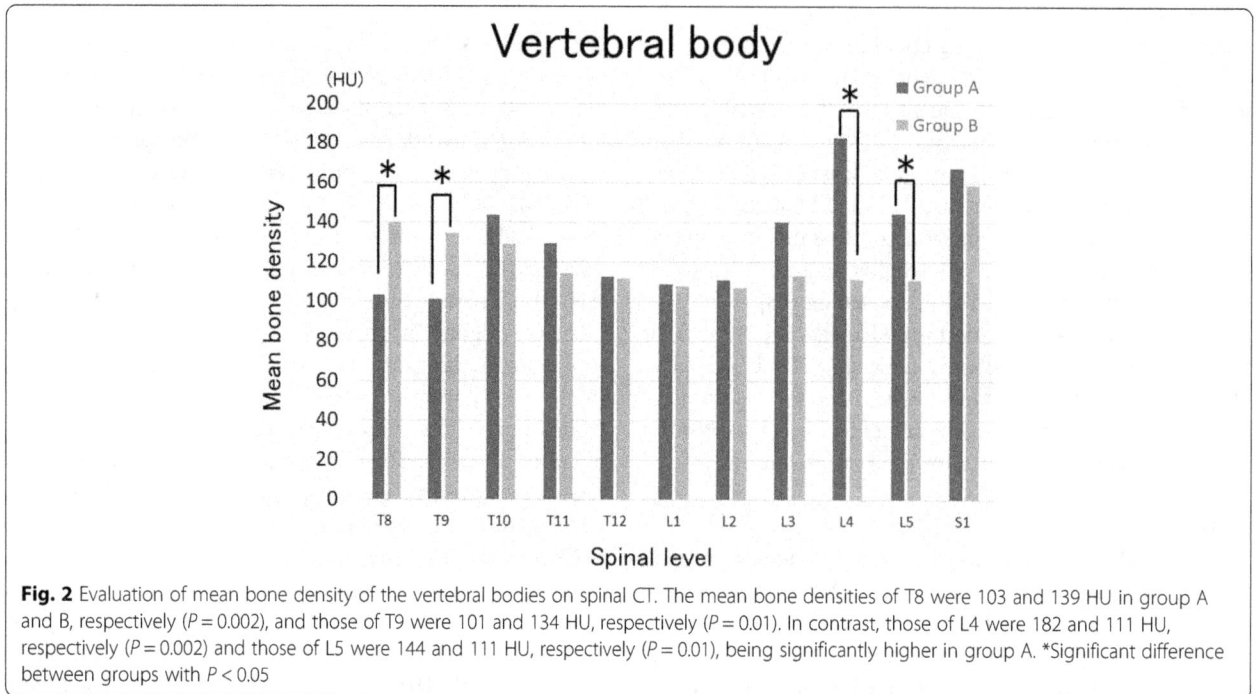

Fig. 2 Evaluation of mean bone density of the vertebral bodies on spinal CT. The mean bone densities of T8 were 103 and 139 HU in group A and B, respectively ($P = 0.002$), and those of T9 were 101 and 134 HU, respectively ($P = 0.01$). In contrast, those of L4 were 182 and 111 HU, respectively ($P = 0.002$) and those of L5 were 144 and 111 HU, respectively ($P = 0.01$), being significantly higher in group A. *Significant difference between groups with $P < 0.05$

($P = 0.21$), and sacral fusion was applied in 57% and 70%, respectively ($P = 0.28$). No significant difference was noted between the groups in any radiographic parameter immediately after surgery.

Regarding the postoperative factors, the mean durations of follow-up after surgery were 40 and 37 months in groups A and B, respectively ($P = 0.61$) (Table 4), additional vertebral fracture developed in 85% and 25%, respectively ($P < 0.001$), PJK developed in 85% and 60%, respectively ($P = 0.07$), and PS loosening occurred in 100% and 95%, respectively ($P = 0.54$). As for the PJK levels in revision surgeries, there were 1 case at T7, 2 cases at T8, 5 cases at T9, 2 cases at T10, and 2 cases at T12, respectively. Loosening of the uppermost PS occurred in 100% and 75%, respectively ($P = 0.04$), and it occurred within 3 months after surgery in 71% and 40%,

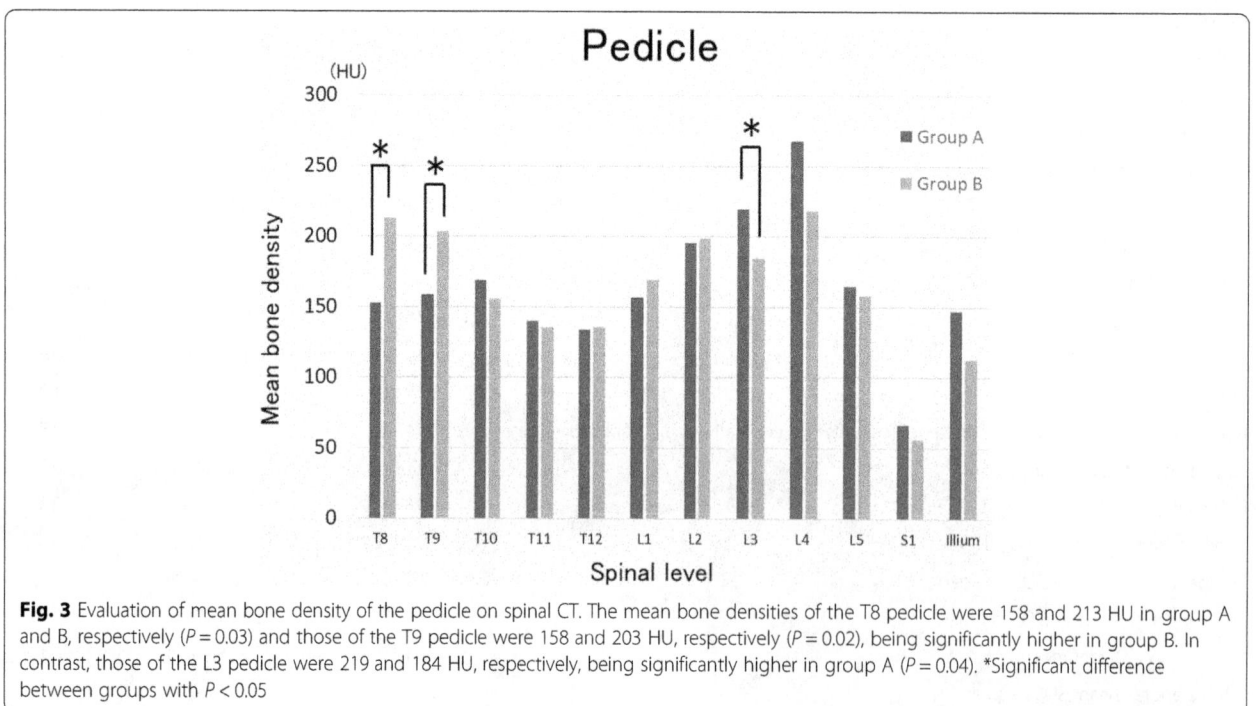

Fig. 3 Evaluation of mean bone density of the pedicle on spinal CT. The mean bone densities of the T8 pedicle were 158 and 213 HU in group A and B, respectively ($P = 0.03$) and those of the T9 pedicle were 158 and 203 HU, respectively ($P = 0.02$), being significantly higher in group B. In contrast, those of the L3 pedicle were 219 and 184 HU, respectively, being significantly higher in group A ($P = 0.04$). *Significant difference between groups with $P < 0.05$

Table 2 Baseline SRS-Schwab adult spinal deformity classification for group A and group B

	Group A (n = 14)	Group B (n = 40)	P value
Coronal curve type, n (%)			
T	0	0	0.37
L	4 (20)	8 (28.6)	
D	0	0	
N	10 (80)	32 (71.4)	
PI-LL, n (%)			
0	0	4 (10)	0.11
+	0	6 (15)	
++	14 (100)	30 (75)	
Global alignment, n (%)			
0	3 (21.4)	5 (12.5)	0.71
+	5 (35.7)	17 (42.5)	
++	6 (42.9)	18 (45)	
Pelvic tilt, n (%)			
0	2 (14.3)	7 (17.5)	0.74
+	5 (35.7)	10 (25)	
++	7 (50)	23 (57.5)	

PI-LL: 0, < 10°; +, 10–20°; ++, > 20°. Global alignment, based on C7 SVA value: 0, < 4 cm; +, 4–9.5 cm; ++, > 9.5 cm. Pelvic tilt: 0, < 20°; +, 20–30°; ++, > 30°

respectively ($P = 0.04$). Postoperative treatment of osteoporosis was performed in 100% and 77%, respectively ($P = 0.04$), and 14% and 40% of them were treated with teriparatide, respectively ($P = 0.07$).

Discussion

In this study, patients who required revision surgery due to complications associated with PJK or additional remote level vertebral fracture after ASD surgery had significantly lower mean bone densities of T8 and T9 vertebra and significantly higher mean bone densities of L4 and L5 vertebra. The rates of loosening of the uppermost PS within 3 months after surgery and additional vertebral fracture were significantly higher in patients who required revision surgery.

Since the sagittal alignment of the spine is often corrected largely in ASD surgery and this loads a large physical stress on the adjacent intervertebral segments, PJK is likely to develop [5, 7, 16]. PJK caused by bone failure and implant/bone interface failure are strongly influenced by the bone strength of UIV and nearby vertebrae. Bone strength is generally evaluated based on the bone density. Bredow et al. measured the mean bone density of vertebrae on spinal CT in 365 patients aged 59 years on average treated with PS fixation of one or two levels and observed that PS loosening occurred in the vertebrae with a mean bone density of 116 HU, but it did not occur in those with a mean bone density of 132 HU [12]. Kumano et al. reported that lower BMD assessed using HU values from preoperative CT is

Table 3 Comparison of perioperative parameters in group A and group B

Parameter	Group A (n = 14)	Group B (n = 40)	P value
Operation time, mean (SD), min	282.1 (82.7)	304.7 (79.4)	0.37
Blood loss, mean (SD), mL	698.6 (335.1)	1128.0 (949.1)	0.02
No. of levels fused, mean (SD)	6.9 (2.7)	7.6 (1.7)	0.24
UIV implant types, n (%)			0.30
Pedicle screws	9 (64.3)	22 (55)	
Hooks	3 (21.4)	16 (40)	
Unilateral pedicle screw and unilateral hook	2 (14.3)	2 (5)	
No. of pedicle subtraction osteotomy, n (%)	2 (14.2)	12 (30)	0.21
No. of fusion to sacrum, n (%)	8 (57.1)	28 (70)	0.28
Immediate postoperative radiographic parameters			
Sagittal vertical axis, mean (SD), (mm)	70.2 (29.6)	63.2 (24.8)	0.45
Pelvic tilt, mean (SD), (degrees)	30.2 (9.9)	25.4 (7.6)	0.08
Thoracic kyphosis, mean (SD), (degrees)	31.4 (16.8)	31.4 (13.4)	0.66
Lumbar lordosis, mean (SD), (degrees)	26.0 (11.7)	28.7 (11.3)	1.0
Change in LL, mean (SD), degrees	17.1 (17.0)	10.0 (13.0)	0.11
Pelvic incidence, mean (SD), degrees	46.7 (2.9)	49.5 (7.8)	0.32
PI-LL, mean (SD), (degrees)	22.2 (13.6)	21.9 (7.8)	0.94
UIV + 2 angle (SD), degrees	8.9 (5.6)	7.7 (7.9)	0.52

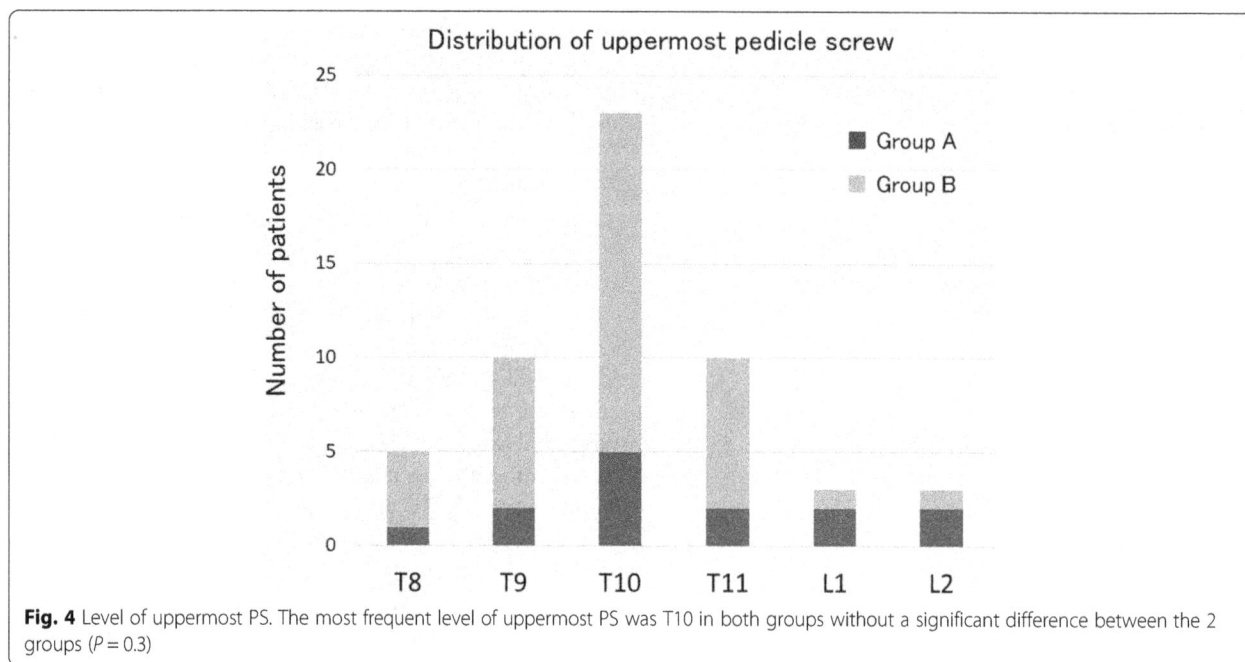

Fig. 4 Level of uppermost PS. The most frequent level of uppermost PS was T10 in both groups without a significant difference between the 2 groups (*P* = 0.3)

associated with adjacent segment fracture after spinal fusion surgery [8]. The present study clarified that in patients who required revision surgery due to complications associated with PJK or additional remote level vertebral fracture after ASD surgery, PS loosening occurred early and the mean bone density was low in the T8 and T9 vertebral bodies and high in the L4 and L5 vertebral bodies. For these patients, certain countermeasures may be necessary, such as strengthening of osteoporosis treatment and augmentation of PS.

The incidence of uppermost PS loosening was significantly higher in group A, and it occurred within 3 months after surgery in 71% and 40% in groups A and B, respectively, being significantly higher in group A. PS loosening does not necessarily cause PJK or additional vertebral fracture, but it was clarified that the probability of revision surgery is high when uppermost PS loosening occurs within 3 months after surgery. To prevent

uppermost PS loosening early after surgery, risk assessment and certain countermeasures are necessary. It has been reported that the threshold of the mean bone density of the vertebra for applying augmentation to prevent PS loosening is about 120 HU [12]. In our study, the most frequent level of the uppermost PS was T10 and the mean bone densities of the vertebral body were 143 and 129 HU in groups A and B, respectively, being not significantly different between the groups, and both values were higher than 120 HU. However, the mean bone densities of the T8 and T9 vertebral bodies were about 100 HU in group A whereas these were about 140 HU in group B, being significantly different. Besides, there were more than half of the patients whose PJK levels were at T8 (2cases) and T9 (5cases) out of the 12 cases in group A. These results clarified that PJK should be strongly influenced by the bone density of nearby UIV. Also, mean bone densities of the T8 and T9

Table 4 Comparison of postoperative clinical results in group A and group B

Parameter	Group A (n = 14)	Group B (n = 40)	P value
Follow up, mean (SD), (months)	40.4 (19.5)	37.4 (19.3)	0.61
No. of postoperative fracture, n (%)	12 (85.7)	10 (25)	< 0.001
No. of proximal junctional kyphosis, n (%)	12 (85.7)	24 (60)	0.07
No. of PS loosening, n (%)	14 (100)	38 (95)	0.54
No. of uppermost PS loosening, n (%)	14 (100)	30 (75)	0.04
No. of uppermost PS loosening within 3 months, n (%)	10 (71.4)	16 (40)	0.04
No. of lowermost PS loosening, n (%)	10 (71.4)	32 (80)	0.37
No. of postoperative treatment for osteoporosis, n (%)	14 (100)	34 (77.2)	0.04
No. of teriparatide use, n (%)	2 (14.2)	16 (40)	0.07

vertebral bodies whose uppermost PS levels except for T9 and T10 were 107 and 109 HU in group A, respectively, being significantly low. It was suggested that the risk of uppermost PS loosening early after ASD surgery is high in elderly patients regardless of the level of the uppermost PS when the mean bone densities of the T8 and T9 vertebral bodies are lower than about 140 HU.

Ohtori et al. reported the effect of drugs for treatment of osteoporosis on PS loosening [17]: PS loosening occurred in 26% and 25% of patients on CT in the oral risedronate treatment and control groups at 12 months after surgery, respectively, whereas the incidence was 13% in the teriparatide injection group, being significantly lower. In our study, no significant difference was noted in the incidence of PS loosening between patients with and without preoperative treatment of osteoporosis, and on the contrary, fewer patients received postoperative treatment of osteoporosis in group B. However, limited to teriparatide, the drug was more frequently used in group B, although the difference was not significant. To prevent uppermost PS loosening early after surgery, pre- and postoperative treatment with teriparatide or certain PS augmentation such as polymethylmethacrylate cement injection and/or expandable PS may be necessary [1, 6, 18].

The limitations of this study were the retrospective design, multiple factors associated with revision surgery to be tested, and small number of patients who were included in the study. In the baseline characteristics of SRS-Schwab ASD classification, there were more kyphosis patients in group A and more scoliosis patients in group B. Kyphosis patients tend to have highly degenerated lumbar vertebra, and sclerosed changes could occur in curved vertebra in scoliosis patients. Patients in group A could have more sclerosed lumbar vertebra, and patients in group B could have more sclerosed thoracic vertebra. The higher mean bone density of L4 and L5 in group A and T8 and T9 in group B could be caused by the sclerosed vertebra. Therefore, if we performed a matched pair analysis in each curve type, results could be different from the current study. However, baseline characteristics excluding BMI, preoperative parameters, and postoperative parameters excluding blood loss were not statistically different between the groups. Second, there were some biases in deciding to perform additional surgery. There were many patients who developed PJK in both group A (85%) and group B (60%) in the current study. Clinical symptoms of patients with PJK/PJF were variable, and patients who needed revision surgery could have not decided to have additional surgery. However, patients who received revision surgery had severe symptoms such as severe pain, neurological deficits, or progressive sagittal deformity. Thus, there were no patients with mild symptoms included in group A who needed

not have revision surgery. Another limitation was the diversity of UIV implant types, such as bilateral PS, bilateral hooks, and unilateral PS with unilateral hook, and this made the risk assessment of PS loosening based on the mean bone density of UIV difficult. Therefore, we compared the mean bone density of the extensive region from T8 to the ilium. Another limitation was the slightly broad range of the UIV level from lower thoracic to upper lumbar vertebrae. We considered that the inclusion of patients with UIV at an upper lumbar level is more practical because no significant bias was noted in the basic background between the groups.

Conclusions

We focused on the factors associated with revision surgery for proximal junctional kyphosis or additional postoperative vertebral fracture following correction and fusion surgery for ASD in elderly patients. In patients who required revision surgery, the mean bone densities of vertebral bodies and pedicles at T8 and T9 were significantly lower. The mean bone density represented in HU on spinal CT may be useful for risk assessment of and countermeasures against revision surgery after ASD surgery in elderly patients.

Abbreviations

ASD: Adult spinal deformity; BMI: Body mass index; CT: Computed tomography; DXA: Dual-energy X-ray absorptiometry; HU: Hounsfield units; LL: Lumbar lordosis; PI: Pelvic incidence; PJF: Proximal junctional failure; PJK: Proximal junctional kyphosis; PS: Pedicle screw; PSO: Pedicle subtraction osteotomy; PT: Pelvic tilt; SVA: Sagittal vertical axis; TK: Thoracic kyphosis; UIV: Upper instrumented vertebra; YAM: Young adult mean

Authors' contributions

HU performed the study design, analyzed the results, and contributed to the manuscript. YT, MM, MN, HS, KM, and HM contributed to the collection of the cases. YT made some meaningful suggestions. All authors reviewed and approved the final submitted version.

Competing interests

The authors declare that they have no competing interests.

References

1. Ghobrial GM, Eichberg DG, Kolcun JPG et al. Prophylactic vertebral cement augmentation at the uppermost instrumented vertebra and rostral adjacent vertebra for the prevention of proximal junctional kyphosis and failure following long segment fusion for adult spinal deformity. Spine J 2017, DOI: https://doi.org/10.1016/j.spinee.2017.05.015
2. Glattes RC, Bridwell KH, Lenke LG, et al. Proximal junctional kyphosis in adult spinal deformity following long instrumented posterior spinal fusion: incidence, outcomes, and risk factor analysis. Spine (Phila Pa 1976). 2005;30:1643–9.
3. Han S, Hyun SJ, Kim KJ, et al. Rod stiffness as a risk factor of proximal junctional kyphosis after adult spinal deformity surgery: comparative study between cobalt chrome multiple-rod constructs and titanium alloy two-rod constructs. Spine J. 2017;17:962–8. https://doi.org/10.1016/j.spinee.2017.02.005.
4. Liu FY, Wang T, Yang SD, et al. Incidence and risk factors for proximal

junctional kyphosis: a meta-analysis. Eur Spine J. 2016;25:2376–83. https://doi.org/10.1007/s00586-016-4534-0.

5. Park SJ, Lee CS, Chung SS, et al. Different risk factors of proximal junctional kyphosis and proximal junctional failure following long instrumented fusion to the sacrum for adult spinal deformity: survivorship analysis of 160 patients. Neurosurgery. 2017;80:279–86. https://doi.org/10.1227/neu.0000000000001240.

6. Park YS, Hyun SJ, Choi HY, et al. Association between bicortical screw fixation at upper instrumented vertebra and risk for upper instrumented vertebra fracture. J Neurosurg Spine. 2017;26:638–44. https://doi.org/10.3171/2016.10.spine16535.

7. Scheer JK, Osorio JA, Smith JS, et al. Development of validated computer-based preoperative predictive model for proximal junction failure (PJF) or clinically significant PJK with 86% accuracy based on 510 ASD patients with 2-year Follow-up. Spine. 2016;41:E1328–e1335. https://doi.org/10.1097/brs.0000000000001598.

8. Kumano K, Hirabayashi S, Ogawa Y, et al. Pedicle screws and bone mineral density. Spine (Phila Pa 1976). 1994;19:1157–61.

9. Pearson HB, Dobbs CJ, Grantham E, et al. Intraoperative biomechanics of lumbar pedicle screw loosening following successful arthrodesis. J Orthop Res. 2017;35:2673–81. https://doi.org/10.1002/jor.23575.

10. Schreiber JJ, Anderson PA, Rosas HG, et al. Hounsfield units for assessing bone mineral density and strength: a tool for osteoporosis management. J Bone Joint Surg Am. 2011;93:1057–63. https://doi.org/10.2106/jbjs.j.00160.

11. Pickhardt PJ, Pooler BD, Lauder T, et al. Opportunistic screening for osteoporosis using abdominal computed tomography scans obtained for other indications. Ann Intern Med. 2013;158:588–95. https://doi.org/10.7326/0003-4819-158-8-201,304,160-00003.

12. Bredow J, Boese CK, Werner CM, et al. Predictive validity of preoperative CT scans and the risk of pedicle screw loosening in spinal surgery. Arch Orthop Trauma Surg. 2016;136:1063–7. https://doi.org/10.1007/s00402-016-2487-8.

13. Meredith DS, Schreiber JJ, Taher F, et al. Lower preoperative Hounsfield unit measurements are associated with adjacent segment fracture after spinal fusion. Spine (Phila Pa 1976). 2013;38:415–8. https://doi.org/10.1097/BRS.0b013e31826ff084.

14. Schwab F, Ungar B, Blondel B, et al. Scoliosis Research Society-Schwab adult spinal deformity classification: a validation study. Spine (Phila Pa 1976). 2012;37:1077–82. https://doi.org/10.1097/BRS.0b013e31823e15e2.

15. Tokuhashi Y, Matsuzaki H, Oda H, et al. Clinical course and significance of the clear zone around the pedicle screws in the lumbar degenerative disease. Spine (Phila Pa 1976). 2008;33:903–8. https://doi.org/10.1097/BRS.0b013e31816b1eff.

16. Yagi M, Rahm M, Gaines R, et al. Characterization and surgical outcomes of proximal junctional failure in surgically treated patients with adult spinal deformity. Spine (Phila Pa 1976). 2014;39:E607–14. https://doi.org/10.1097/brs.0000000000000266.

17. Ohtori S, Inoue G, Orita S, et al. Comparison of teriparatide and bisphosphonate treatment to reduce pedicle screw loosening after lumbar spinal fusion surgery in postmenopausal women with osteoporosis from a bone quality perspective. Spine. 2013;38:E487–92. https://doi.org/10.1097/BRS.0b013e31828826dd.

18. Wu ZX, Gong FT, Liu L, et al. A comparative study on screw loosening in osteoporotic lumbar spine fusion between expandable and conventional pedicle screws. Arch Orthop Trauma Surg. 2012;132:471–6. https://doi.org/10.1007/s00402-011-1439-6.

21

Efficacy and safety of 3D print-assisted surgery for the treatment of pilon fractures: a meta-analysis of randomized controlled trials

Jianzhong Bai[1†], Yongxiang Wang[2†], Pei Zhang[1], Meiying Liu[1], Peian Wang[3], Jingcheng Wang[2*] and Yuan Liang[2*]

Abstract

Objective: To compare the effects of 3D print-assisted surgery and conventional surgery in the treatment of pilon fractures.

Methods: PubMed, Embase, Web of Science, CNKI, CBM, and WanFang data were searched until July 2018. Two reviewers selected relevant studies, assessed the quality of studies, and extracted data. For continuous data, a weighted mean difference (WMD) and 95% confidence intervals (CI) were used. For dichotomous data, a relative risk (RR) and 95% CI were calculated as the summary statistics.

Results: There were seven randomized controlled trials (RCT) enrolling a total of 486 patients, 242 patients underwent 3D print-assisted surgery and 244 patients underwent conventional surgery. The pooled outcomes demonstrate 3D print-assisted surgery was superior to conventional surgery in terms of operation time [WMD = − 26.16, 95% CI (− 33.19, − 19.14), $P < 0.001$], blood loss [WMD = − 63.91, 95% CI (− 79.55, − 48.27), $P < 0.001$], postoperative functional scores [WMD = 8.16, 95% CI (5.04, 11.29), $P < 0.001$], postoperative visual analogue score (VAS) [WMD = − 0.59, 95% CI (− 1.18, − 0.01), $P = 0.05$], rate of excellent and good outcome [RR = 1.20, 95% CI (1.07, 1.34), $P = 0.002$], and rate of anatomic reduction [RR = 1.35, 95% CI (1.19, 1.53), $P < 0.001$]. However, there was no significant difference between the groups regarding the rate of infection [RR = 0.51, 95% CI (0.20, 1.31), $P = 0.16$], fracture union time [WMD = − 0.85, 95% CI (− 1.79, 0.08), $P = 0.07$], traumatic arthritis [RR = 0.34, 95% CI (0.06, 2.09), $P = 0.24$], and malunion [RR = 0.34, 95% CI (0.06, 2.05), $P = 0.24$].

Conclusions: Our meta-analysis demonstrates 3D print-assisted surgery was significantly better than conventional surgery in terms of operation time, blood loss, postoperative functional score, postoperative VAS, rate of excellent and good outcome, and rate of anatomic reduction. Concerning postoperative complications, there were no significant differences between the groups.

Keywords: Three-dimensional, 3D printing, Computer-assisted, Pilon fractures, Surgery

* Correspondence: wangjcyangzhou@163.com; 464156241@qq.com
†Jianzhong Bai and Yongxiang Wang contributed equally to this work.
2Clinical Medical College, Yangzhou University, Yangzhou 225001, China
Full list of author information is available at the end of the article

Introduction

Pilon fractures are usually caused by high energy trauma, accompanied by multiple metaphyseal fragments, displaced intra-articular comminution, and severe soft tissue injuries: this is a substantial problem for experienced orthopedic surgeons [1, 2]. The purpose of surgical treatment is an anatomic reduction of the articular fragments, firm fixation, and early functional exercise [3, 4]. However, postoperative complications seriously affect the effects of surgery, such as severe pain, skin necrosis, malunion, implant failure, joint stiffness, and even post-traumatic arthritis [5, 6]. Therefore, it is necessary to seek a new method to reduce postoperative complications and improve the outcomes of surgery.

Recently, 3D printing technology has developed rapidly in the medical field [7], primarily using a 3D digital model to build a 1:1 fracture model based on the patient's imaging data. Furthermore, surgeons can perform a pre-operation to identify unforeseen problems during surgery that could assist in formulation of preoperative planning, simulation of the surgical procedure, and achievement of better surgical outcomes [8]. However, there are no relevant meta-analyses or clinical guides to assess the effects of 3D print-assisted surgery for the treatment of pilon fractures. It is unclear whether 3D print-assisted surgery can significantly improve the postoperative outcomes of patients compared to conventional surgery. Therefore, we performed this meta-analysis to identify the issue and then provided a better treatment strategy for clinicians.

Methods

We carried out this meta-analysis strictly according to the Preferred Reporting Items for Systematic Reviews and Meta-Analysis (PRISMA) statement [9] and the Cochrane Collaboration guidelines.

Search strategy

PubMed, Embase, Web of Science, CNKI, CBM, and WanFang data were searched until July 2018. Besides, we manually searched the reference lists of all included relevant publications to identify potential studies. We considered articles published in any language. The following keywords were adopted in the database search: "pilon fractures," "3D printing," "computer-assisted," and "surgery." The Boolean operators were used to combine them.

Study selection and eligibility criteria

The inclusion criteria were as follows: (1) pilon fractures diagnosed by validated screening or diagnostic instruments, (2) the study compared 3D print-assisted surgery with conventional surgery for the treatment of pilon fractures, (3) the study design was randomized controlled trial (RCT), (4) Chinese articles included must have title and abstract in English, and (5) the study contained at least one of the following indicators: operation time, blood loss, postoperative functional score, rate of excellent and good outcome, rate of anatomic reduction, or postoperative complications. The exclusion criteria were as follows: (1) other types of fractures, (2) studies provided insufficient data, and (3) case report, review, commentary, or study only included an abstract (Table 1).

Data extraction

Two reviewers performed data extraction. The following information was extracted from eligible studies: author, year, study design, sample size, age, postoperative outcomes, and classification of pilon fractures. Any disagreements were resolved by discussion to reach a consensus. All extracted data were entered into a predefined standardized Excel (Microsoft Corporation, USA) file carefully.

Quality assessment

We evaluated the quality of the RCTs according to the methods of the 12-item scale [10]. Each item was scored "Yes," "Unclear," or "No." A study with a score of more than 7 "Yes" response was considered as of high quality, 5–7 was considered as of moderate quality, and 0–4 was considered as of low quality.

Statistical analysis

Statistical analyses were performed by using Revman 5.3 software. For continuous outcomes, weighted mean difference (WMD) with 95% CI was used. For dichotomous data, relative risk (RR) with 95% CI was calculated as the summary statistics. $P \leq 0.05$ was regarded as statistically significant. The I^2 statistic assessed statistical heterogeneity, with I^2 value more than 50% indicating significant heterogeneity, the random-effects model was used to do the analysis; otherwise, the fixed-effects model was used. In addition, sensitivity analyses were conducted to insure the accuracy of the outcomes.

Results

Search result

A total of 84 potentially relevant references were found. We removed 39 duplicate studies. By scanning the titles and abstracts, 37 studies were excluded from the analysis. After full texts were carefully read according to eligibility, one study was excluded because it was not an RCT [11]. Finally, seven studies were included in quantitative synthesis [12–18]. The characteristics of all included studies are shown in Table 1. Details of the study selection process are shown in Fig. 1.

Table 1 Characteristics of included studies

Studies	Year	Study year	Groups	Sample size	Age ± mean (year)	Pilon fracture classification
Huang et al.	2015	2008–2013	3D	31	48.6	RA: I 9, II 12, III 10
			C	30	48.6	RA: I 7, II 15, III 8
Tang et al.	2015	2012–2014	3D	32	38.4 ± 2.8	RA: II 12, III 20
			C	32	37.2 ± 2.4	RA: II 15, III 17
Fan et al.	2016	2014–2015	3D	50	43.5 ± 3.5	RA: II 20, III 30
			C	50	43.5 ± 3.5	RA: II 21, III 29
Li et al.	2016	2013–2014	3D	30	34.8 ± 6.0	AO:13 C2, 17 C3
			C	30	35.8 ± 6.2	AO:12 C2, 18 C3
Gu et al.	2017	2011–2015	3D	36	38.9 ± 5.9	RA: II 15, III 21
			C	36	39.6 ± 5.5	RA: II 12, III 24
Ou et al.	2017	NR	3D	18	37.4 ± 3.7	RA: II 10, III 8
			C	18	38.4 ± 3.5	RA: II 9, III 9
Zheng et al.	2018	2013–2016	3D	45	41.2 ± 9.3	AO:5 C1, 14 C2, 26 C3
			C	48	42.5 ± 9.0	AO: 8 C1, 17 C2, 23 C3

3D 3D print-assisted surgery, *C* conventional surgery, *RA* Ruedi-Allgower, *NR* no report

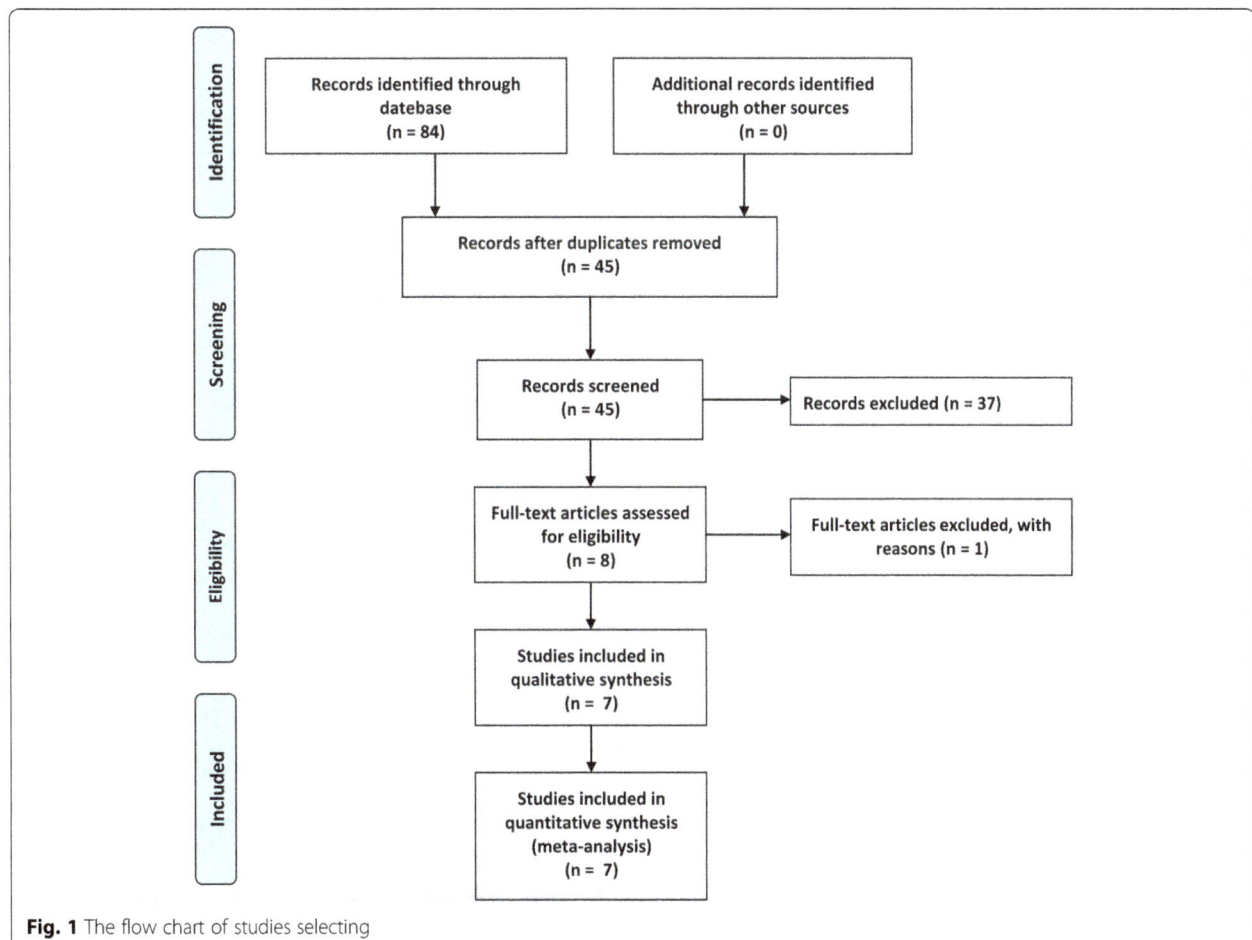

Fig. 1 The flow chart of studies selecting

Table 2 The 12-item appraisal scores for the RCTs

Studies	Randomized adequately[a]	Allocation concealed	Patient blinded	Care provider blinded	Outcome assessor blinded	Acceptable drop-out rate[b]	ITT analysis[c]	Avoided selective reporting	Similar baseline	Similar or avoided cofactor	Patient compliance	Similar timing	Quality[d]
Huang et al	Yes	Yes	Unclear	Unclear	Unclear	Yes	Yes	Yes	Yes	Unclear	Yes	Yes	High
Tang et al	Yes	Yes	Unclear	Unclear	Unclear	Yes	Yes	Yes	Yes	Unclear	Yes	Yes	High
Fan et al	Yes	Yes	Unclear	Unclear	Unclear	Yes	Yes	Yes	Yes	Unclear	Yes	Yes	High
Li et al	No	Unclear	Unclear	Unclear	Unclear	Yes	Yes	Yes	Yes	Unclear	Yes	Yes	Moderate
Gu et al	Yes	Yes	Unclear	Unclear	Unclear	Yes	Yes	Yes	Yes	Unclear	Yes	Yes	High
Ou et al	Unclear	Yes	Unclear	Unclear	Unclear	Yes	Yes	Yes	Yes	Unclear	Yes	Yes	Moderate
Zheng et al	Yes	Yes	Unclear	Unclear	Unclear	Yes	Yes	Yes	Yes	Unclear	Yes	Yes	High

[a] Only if the method of sequence made was explicitly introduced could get a "Yes"

[b] Drop-out rate < 20% could get a "Yes," otherwise "No"

[c] ITT intention-to-treat, only if all randomized participants were analyzed in the group, they were allocated to could receive a "Yes"

[d] "Yes" items more than 7 means "High"; more than 4 but no more than 7 means "Moderate"; no more than 4 means "Low"

Quality assessment

The details of the quality assessment of included studies are shown in Table 2. Five studies [12, 13, 15, 17, 18] were of high quality, and two studies [14, 16] were of moderate quality. The randomization methods were explicitly introduced in five studies [12, 13, 15, 17, 18]. No study reported blinding of outcome assessment. However, all of the included studies were reported with complete outcome data.

Clinical outcomes

Operation time (mins)

The operation time was reported in seven studies [12–18], and the pooled results demonstrated that the 3D print-assisted surgery group had a significantly shorter operation time than did the conventional surgery group [WMD = − 26.16, 95% CI (− 33.19, − 19.14), $P < 0.001$, $I^2 = 95\%$, Fig. 2].

Blood loss (ml)

Five studies [12, 13, 15–17] provided available data, and the pooled results demonstrated that the 3D print-assisted surgery group had a significantly less blood loss than the conventional surgery group [WMD = − 63.91, 95% CI (− 79.55, − 48.27), $P < 0.001$, $I^2 = 93\%$, Fig. 3].

Postoperative functional scores

Five studies [12, 13, 15–17] provided available data, and the pooled results demonstrated that the 3D print-assisted surgery group had a significantly higher functional score than did the conventional surgery group [WMD = 8.16, 95% CI (5.04, 11.29), $P < 0.001$, $I^2 = 64\%$, Fig. 4].

The rate of excellent and good outcomes

Four studies [14, 15, 17, 18] provided available data, and the pooled results demonstrated that the 3D print-assisted surgery group had a higher rate of excellent and good outcomes than did the conventional surgery group [RR = 1.20, 95% CI (1.07, 1.34), $P = 0.002$, $I^2 = 0\%$, Fig. 5].

The rate of anatomic reduction

Three studies [12, 13, 17] provided available data, and the pooled results demonstrated that the 3D print-assisted surgery group had a higher rate of anatomic reduction than the conventional surgery group [RR = 1.35, 95% CI (1.19, 1.53), $P < 0.001$, $I^2 = 14\%$, Fig. 5].

Fracture union time (month)

Three studies [15–17] provided available data concerning fracture union time, and the pooled outcomes demonstrated that there was no significant difference between the groups [WMD = − 0.85, 95% CI (− 1.79, 0.08), $P = 0.07$, $I^2 = 96\%$, Fig. 6].

Postoperative VAS

Two studies [15, 17] provided available data, and the pooled outcomes demonstrated that 3D print-assisted surgery group had a lower VAS than the conventional surgery group [WMD = − 0.59, 95% CI (− 1.18, − 0.01), $P = 0.05$, $I^2 = 71\%$, Fig. 6].

Traumatic arthritis

Two studies [17, 18] provided available data, and the pooled results demonstrated that two surgical methods have a similar effect regarding the rate of traumatic arthritis [RR = 0.34, 95% CI (0.06, 2.09), $P = 0.24$, $I^2 = 0\%$, Fig. 7].

Malunion

Two studies [17, 18] provided available data regarding malunion, and the pooled results demonstrated there was no significant difference between the groups [RR = 0.34, 95% CI (0.06, 2.05), $P = 0.24$, $I^2 = 3\%$, Fig. 7].

Infection rate

Three studies [14, 15, 17] provided available data concerning infection rate, and the pooled results demonstrated

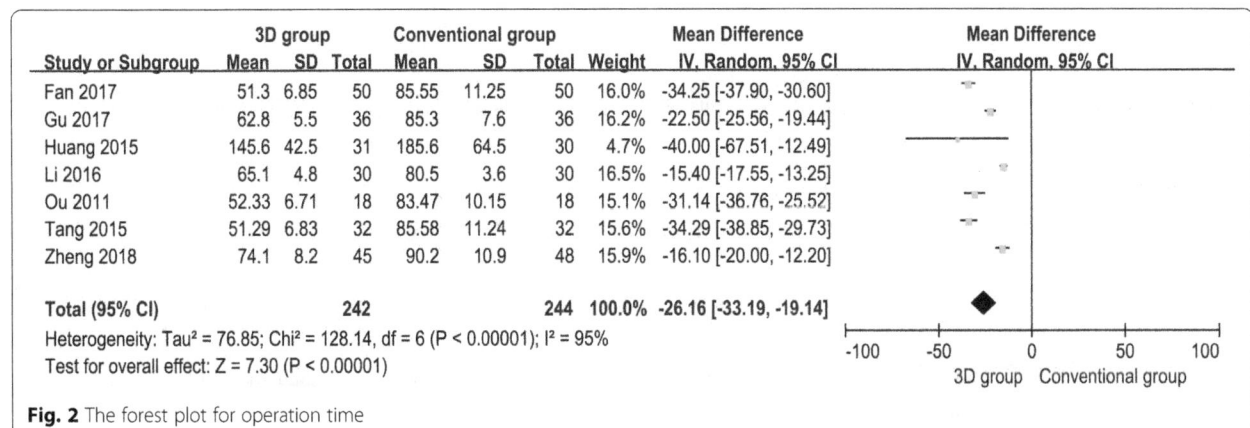

Study or Subgroup	3D group Mean	SD	Total	Conventional group Mean	SD	Total	Weight	Mean Difference IV, Random, 95% CI	Mean Difference IV, Random, 95% CI
Fan 2017	51.3	6.85	50	85.55	11.25	50	16.0%	-34.25 [-37.90, -30.60]	
Gu 2017	62.8	5.5	36	85.3	7.6	36	16.2%	-22.50 [-25.56, -19.44]	
Huang 2015	145.6	42.5	31	185.6	64.5	30	4.7%	-40.00 [-67.51, -12.49]	
Li 2016	65.1	4.8	30	80.5	3.6	30	16.5%	-15.40 [-17.55, -13.25]	
Ou 2011	52.33	6.71	18	83.47	10.15	18	15.1%	-31.14 [-36.76, -25.52]	
Tang 2015	51.29	6.83	32	85.58	11.24	32	15.6%	-34.29 [-38.85, -29.73]	
Zheng 2018	74.1	8.2	45	90.2	10.9	48	15.9%	-16.10 [-20.00, -12.20]	
Total (95% CI)			**242**			**244**	**100.0%**	**-26.16 [-33.19, -19.14]**	

Heterogeneity: Tau² = 76.85; Chi² = 128.14, df = 6 (P < 0.00001); I² = 95%
Test for overall effect: Z = 7.30 (P < 0.00001)

Fig. 2 The forest plot for operation time

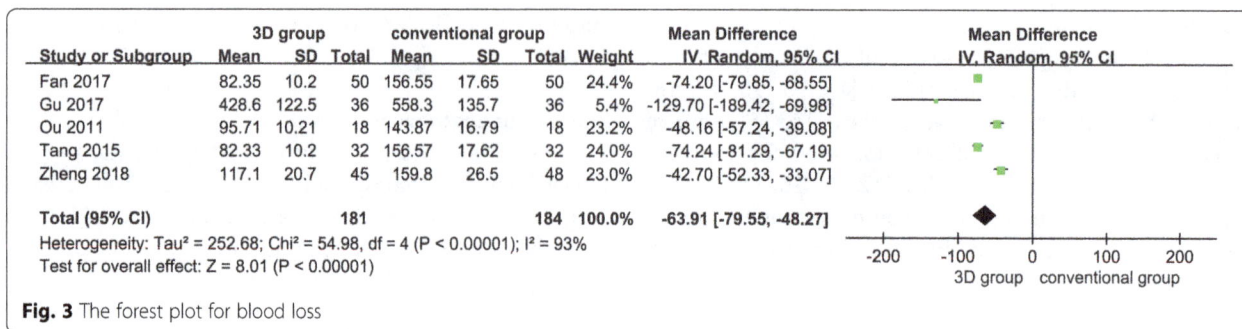

| Study or Subgroup | 3D group | | | conventional group | | | Weight | Mean Difference IV, Random, 95% CI | Mean Difference IV, Random, 95% CI |
	Mean	SD	Total	Mean	SD	Total			
Fan 2017	82.35	10.2	50	156.55	17.65	50	24.4%	-74.20 [-79.85, -68.55]	
Gu 2017	428.6	122.5	36	558.3	135.7	36	5.4%	-129.70 [-189.42, -69.98]	
Ou 2011	95.71	10.21	18	143.87	16.79	18	23.2%	-48.16 [-57.24, -39.08]	
Tang 2015	82.33	10.2	32	156.57	17.62	32	24.0%	-74.24 [-81.29, -67.19]	
Zheng 2018	117.1	20.7	45	159.8	26.5	48	23.0%	-42.70 [-52.33, -33.07]	
Total (95% CI)			**181**			**184**	**100.0%**	**-63.91 [-79.55, -48.27]**	

Heterogeneity: Tau² = 252.68; Chi² = 54.98, df = 4 (P < 0.00001); I² = 93%
Test for overall effect: Z = 8.01 (P < 0.00001)

Fig. 3 The forest plot for blood loss

that the 3D print-assisted surgery group had a lower infection rate than the conventional surgery group, but there is no significant difference between the groups [RR = 0.51, 95% CI (0.20, 1.31), P = 0.16, I² = 0%, Fig. 7].

Sensitivity analysis

Due to fewer studies were included in some outcomes, we only performed sensitivity analysis on the results of operation time, blood loss, and postoperative functional score. These outcomes all remained stable after the exclusion of each study once a time.

Discussion

Main findings

Our meta-analysis demonstrated that the 3D print-assisted surgery was significantly better than the conventional surgery concerning operation time, blood loss, postoperative functional score, postoperative VAS, rate of excellent and good outcome, and rate of anatomic reduction. Although the 3D print-assisted surgery group had a lower incidence rate than the conventional surgery group concerning infection rate, traumatic arthritis, and malunion, there were no significant differences between the groups.

It is approximated that pilon fractures constitute 1% of all lower extremity fractures and 5–10% of tibia fractures [19]. Most pilon fractures require surgery, and the main purpose is to firmly fix the intra-articular fragments and restore the length and alignment, allowing for earlier weight bearing and functional exercise [20]. Orthopedists usually formulate surgical plans based on X-ray, CT, or other examination outcomes with conventional surgery [21]. However, pilon fractures are severely comminuted fractures, and the ankle joints are often accompanied by severe collapse and loss of bone. Conventional imaging outcomes cannot directly display the specific shape of the fracture, and even sometimes omit occult fractures. The surgeon continues surgery based on clinical experience when the intraoperative condition is not consistent with the expected situation during surgery, which possibly leads to change of the surgical plan, prolong the operation time, increase the blood loss, aggravate the soft tissue injury, and even cause the failure of the operation. Therefore, it is critical for surgeons to perform a pre-surgery based on 3D printing model. They can predict the problems that may be encountered during the operation, such as the optimal surgical approach, matched implant. Therefore, this surgical method shortens the operation time and improves the effects of surgery [22]. In addition, the surgeon can adequately communicate with patients using this vivid fracture model [23].

Although 3D printing technology promotes the development of orthopedic surgery, it has some certain limitations, such as increasing the economic burden of patients. Besides, 3D printing technology requires high

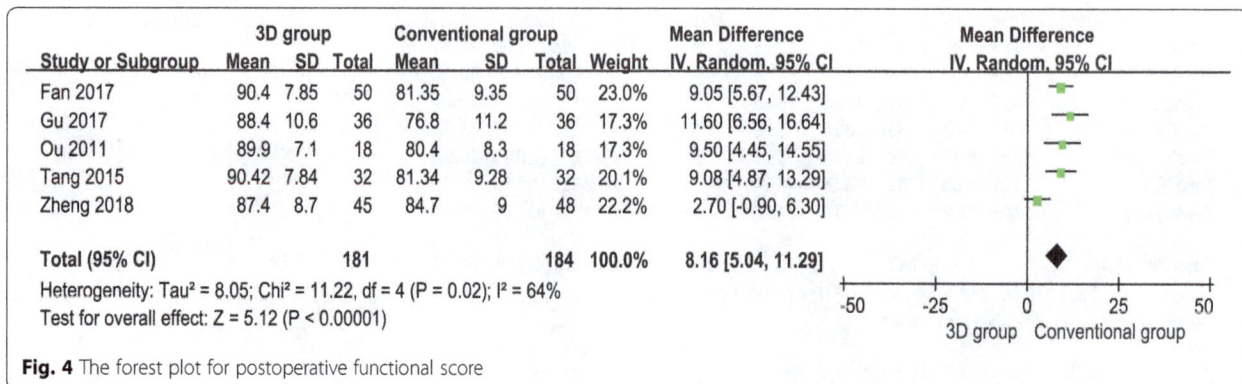

| Study or Subgroup | 3D group | | | Conventional group | | | Weight | Mean Difference IV, Random, 95% CI | Mean Difference IV, Random, 95% CI |
	Mean	SD	Total	Mean	SD	Total			
Fan 2017	90.4	7.85	50	81.35	9.35	50	23.0%	9.05 [5.67, 12.43]	
Gu 2017	88.4	10.6	36	76.8	11.2	36	17.3%	11.60 [6.56, 16.64]	
Ou 2011	89.9	7.1	18	80.4	8.3	18	17.3%	9.50 [4.45, 14.55]	
Tang 2015	90.42	7.84	32	81.34	9.28	32	20.1%	9.08 [4.87, 13.29]	
Zheng 2018	87.4	8.7	45	84.7	9	48	22.2%	2.70 [-0.90, 6.30]	
Total (95% CI)			**181**			**184**	**100.0%**	**8.16 [5.04, 11.29]**	

Heterogeneity: Tau² = 8.05; Chi² = 11.22, df = 4 (P = 0.02); I² = 64%
Test for overall effect: Z = 5.12 (P < 0.00001)

Fig. 4 The forest plot for postoperative functional score

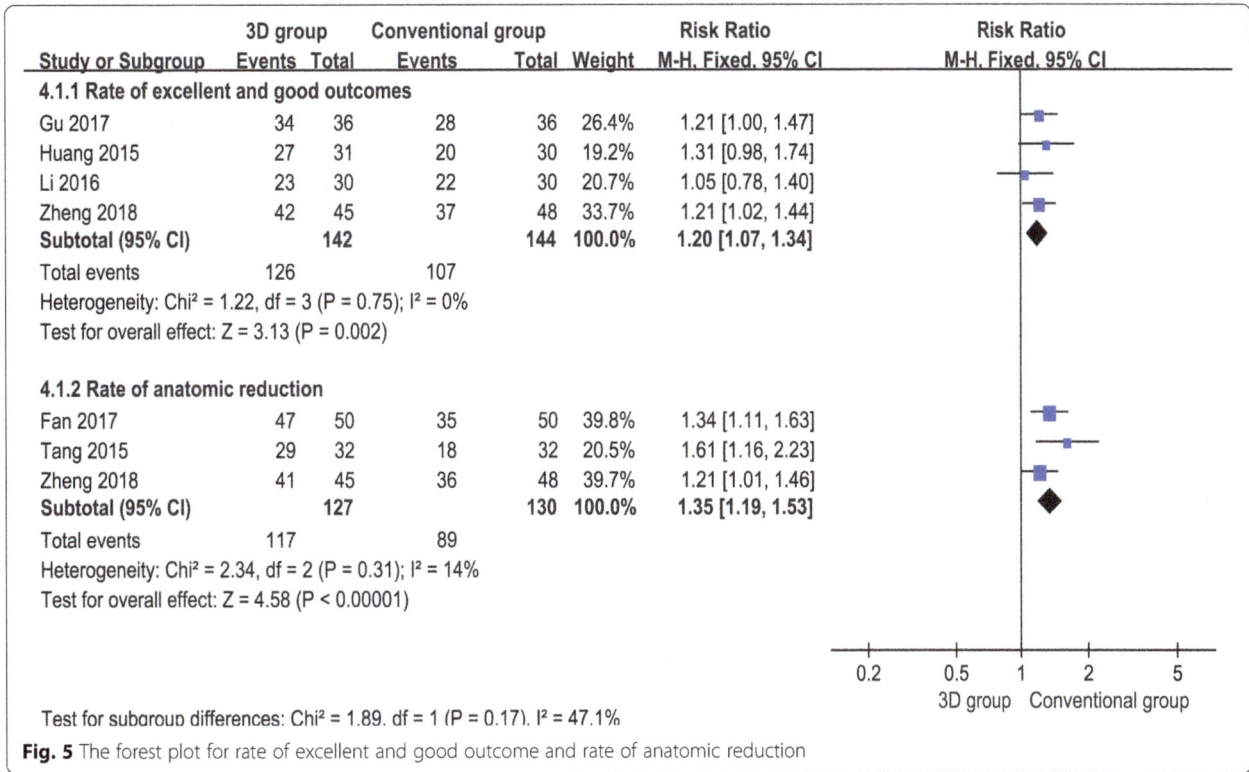

Fig. 5 The forest plot for rate of excellent and good outcome and rate of anatomic reduction

requirements, complicated operating technique, and expensive 3D printing instruments that limit the promotion of this technology. Furthermore, for some complex intra-articular fractures, reconstruction and printing of 3D models increase preoperative preparation time, so this technique is not suitable for emergency surgery. Another disadvantage of 3D printing technology is that it cannot be displayed for soft tissues, such as vasculars and nerves.

Currently, there remains a lack of attention to the treatment of pilon fractures with 3D print-assisted surgery, and to the best of our knowledge, there has been no meta-analysis of the comparison between the methods. Our meta-analysis demonstrated that 3D print-assisted

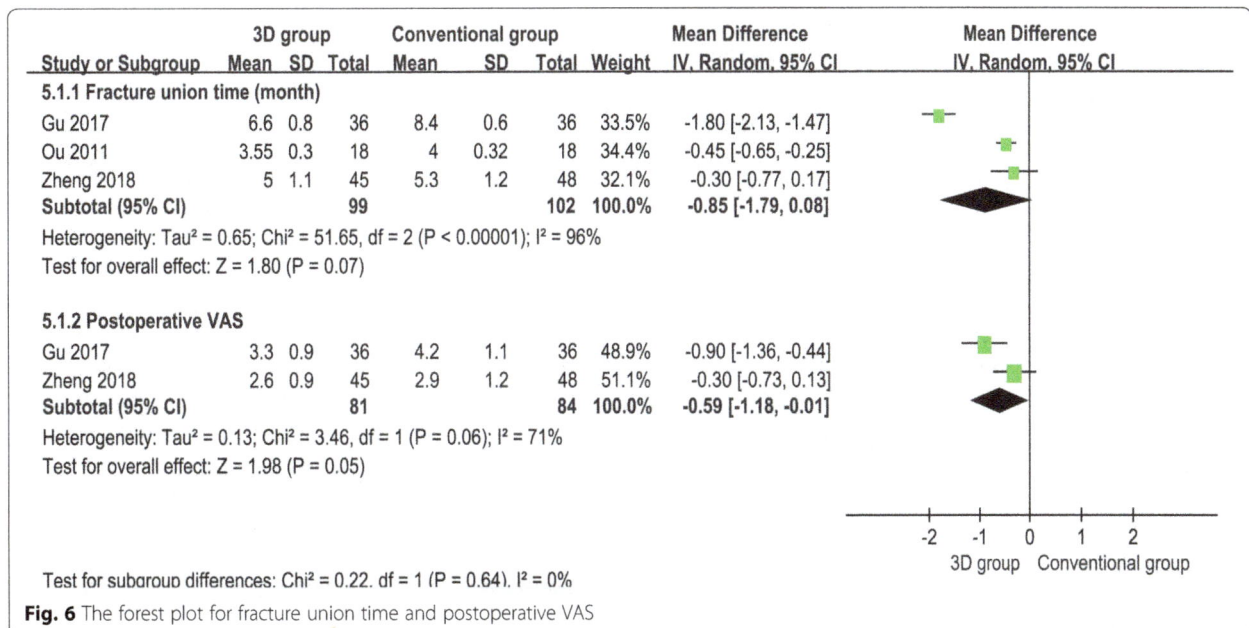

Fig. 6 The forest plot for fracture union time and postoperative VAS

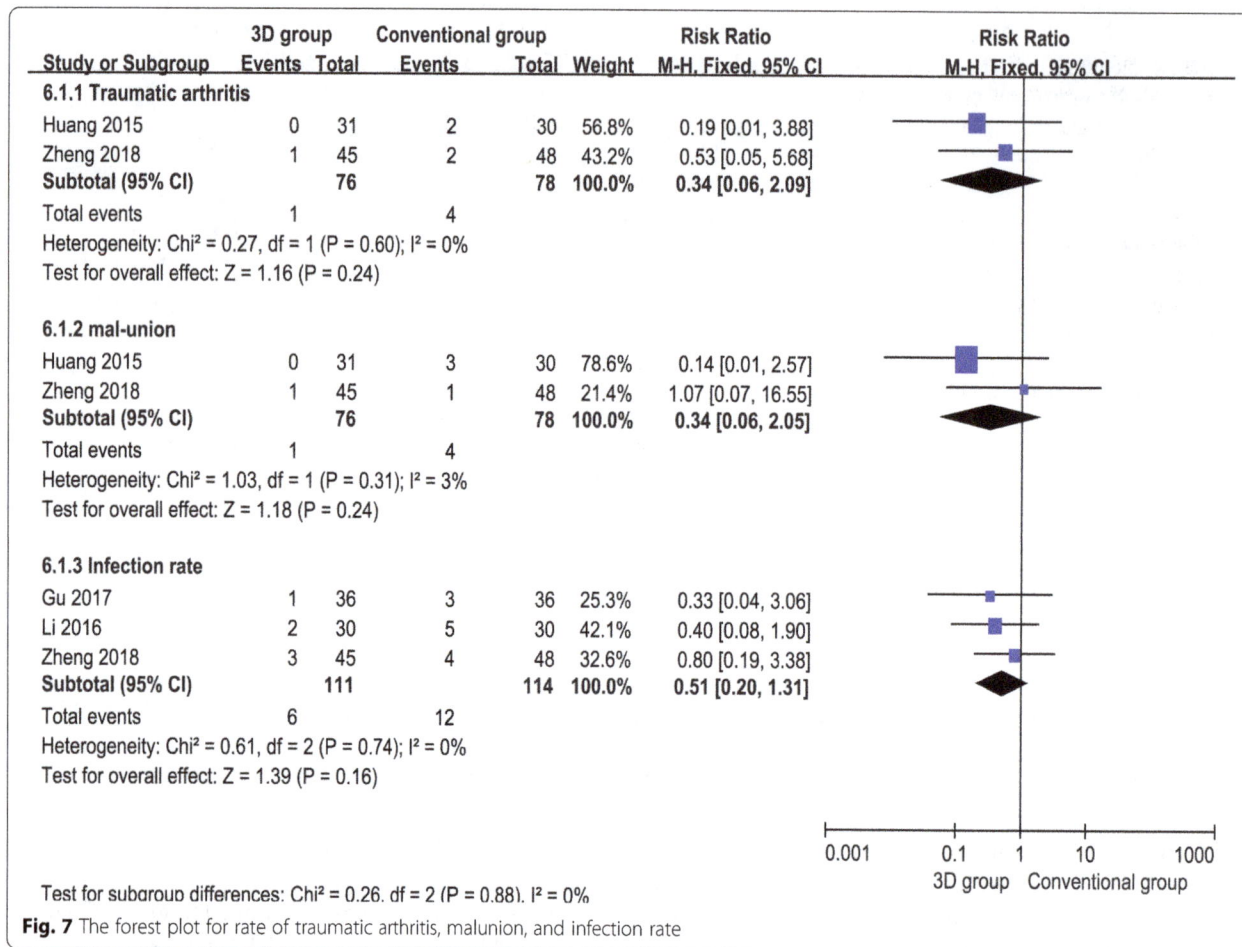

Fig. 7 The forest plot for rate of traumatic arthritis, malunion, and infection rate

surgery has advantages in terms of operation time, blood loss, and functional scores, similar to the previous studies [12–17]. However, both groups had similar infection rates, the pooled results consistent with the results of Li et al. and Zheng et al. [14, 17]. In theory, 3D print-assisted surgery has shorter operative time and less blood loss, so the infection rate should be lower, which requires a large sample of RCTs to update this conclusion.

Limitations

Although this was the first meta-analysis to compare 3D print-assisted surgery with conventional surgery for the treatment of pilon fractures based on seven RCTs, there was a small sample size of included studies, possibly affecting the accuracy of our conclusions. Besides, this meta-analysis had a higher heterogeneity in some pooled outcomes; unequal levels of regional medical care, varying follow-up time, different levels of the operators, and degree of patient injury may contribute it.

Conclusions

Our meta-analysis demonstrates 3D print-assisted surgery was significantly better than the conventional surgery in

terms of operation time, blood loss, postoperative functional score, postoperative VAS, rate of excellent and good outcome, and rate of anatomic reduction. Although the 3D print-assisted surgery group had a lower incidence rate than the conventional surgery group concerning infection rate, traumatic arthritis, and malunion, there were no significant differences between the groups. Future large-volume, well-designed RCTs with extensive follow-up are awaited to confirm and update the findings of this analysis.

Abbreviations

3D: Three-dimensional; CI: Confidence interval; RCT: Randomized controlled trial; RR: Relative risk; VAS: Visual analogue score; WMD: Weighted mean difference

Acknowledgements

We thank the authors of the included studies for their help.

Funding

This study was supported by the project foundation of Northern Jiangsu People's Hospital: (yzucms201623), (fcjs201715); National Natural Science Foundation of China: (81772332); Natural Science Foundation of Jiangsu Province (BK20141281), Special Foundation Project on the Prospective Study of Social Development in Jiangsu Province (BE2013911); Jiangsu Six Categories of Talent Summit Fund (WSW-133); Social Development of Science and Technology Research Project in Yangzhou (YZ2011082); and Jiangsu Province 333 talent Project (BRA2016159).

Authors' contributions

JCW, YL, YXW, and JZB conceived of the design of the study. JZB and PZ participated in the literature search, study selection, data extraction, and quality assessment. MYL and PAW performed the statistical analysis. JZB finished the manuscript. All authors read and approved the final manuscript.

Competing interests

The authors declare that they have no competing interests.

Author details

[1]Dalian Medical University, Dalian 116044, Liaoning, China. [2]Clinical Medical College, Yangzhou University, Yangzhou 225001, China. [3]Heze Mudan People's Hospital, Heze 274000, China.

References

1. Bacon S, Smith WR, Morgan SJ, et al. A retrospective analysis of comminuted intra-articular fractures of the tibial plafond: open reduction and internal fixation versus external Ilizarov fixation. Injury. 2008;39(2):196–202.
2. Patterson MJ, Cole JD. Two-staged delayed open reduction and internal fixation of severe pilon fractures. J Orthop Trauma. 1999;13(2):85–91.
3. Bonar SK, Marsh JL. Unilateral external fixation for severe pilon fractures. Foot Ankle. 1993;14(2):57–64.
4. d'Heurle A, Kazemi N, Connelly C, et al. Prospective randomized comparison of locked plates versus nonlocked plates for the treatment of high-energy pilon fractures. J Orthop Trauma. 2015;29(9):420–3.
5. Sirkin M, Sanders R, DiPasquale T, Herscovici D Jr. A staged protocol for soft tissue management in the treatment of complex pilon fractures. J Orthop Trauma. 1999;13(2):78–84.
6. McFerran MA, Smith SW, Boulas HJ, Schwartz HS. Complications encountered in the treatment of pilon fractures. J Orthop Trauma. 1992;6(2):195–200.
7. Chana-Rodriguez F, Mananes RP, et al. 3D surgical printing and pre contoured plates for acetabular fractures. Injury. 2016;47(11):2507–11.
8. Azuma M, Yanagawa T, Ishibashi-Kanno N, et al. Mandibular reconstruction using plates prebent to fit rapid prototyping 3-dimensional printing models ameliorates contour deformity. Head Face Med. 2014;10:45.
9. Moher D, Liberati A, Tetzlaff J, Altman DG. Preferred reporting items for systematic reviews and meta-analyses: the PRISMA statement. Int J Surg. 2010;8(5):336–41.
10. Furlan AD, Pennick V, Bombardier C, van Tulder M. 2009 updated method guidelines for systematic reviews in the Cochrane Back Review Group. Spine. 2009;34(18):1929–41.
11. Zhang GY, Peng Y, Peng LL, et al. The clinical research of 3D printing technology in treatment of high-energy Pilon fractures. J Minim Invasive Med. 2017;12(01):19–21.
12. Tang SH, Sun YJ, Zhao HM, et al. Clinical application of three-dimensional printing technique for the treatment of tibial Pilon fractures caused by high-energy. Orthop J China. 2015;23(22):2042–6.
13. Fan LJ. Clinical efficacy of 3D printing technology in the treatment of high energy Pilon fractures. World Latest Med Inf. 2016;16(19):27–8.
14. Li Y, Yuan Z. Application of rapid prototype and 3D printing in therapy of complex pilon fractures. Chin J Orthop trauma. 2016;18(1):42–6.
15. Gu H, Zhang Y, Lv XF, et al. 3D printing technology in applicatoin of tibial PILON fractures. Chin J Trauma Disabil Med. 2017;24:8–10.
16. Ou Yang HW, Zhao XD, Shi KM, et al. Clinical application of 3D printing technique in the treatment of high energy Pilon fracture. Chin Cont Med Edu. 2017;9(17):130–1.
17. Zheng W, Chen C, Zhang C, et al. The feasibility of 3D printing technology on the treatment of pilon fracture and its effect on doctor-patient communication. Biomed Res Int. 2018;8054698:1–10.
18. Huang J, Wang XP, Deng ZC, et al. Application of three-dimensional reconstruction using mimics software to repair of pilon fracture. J Clin Tis Eng Res. 2015;19(44):7167–71.
19. Vidyadhara S, Rao SK. Ilizarov treatment of complex tibial pilon fractures. Int Orthop. 2006;30(2):113–7.
20. Lomax A, Singh A, M NJ KCS. Complications and early results after operative fixation of 68 pilon fractures of the distal tibia. Scott Med J. 2015;60(2):79–84.
21. Badillo K, Pacheco JA, Padua SO, Gomez AA, Colon E, Vidal JA. Multidetector CT evaluation of calcaneal fractures. Radiographics. 2011;31(1):81–92.
22. Bagaria V, Deshpande S, Rasalkar DD, Kuthe A, Paunipagar BK. Use of rapid prototyping and three-dimensional reconstruction modeling in the management of complex fractures. Eur J Radiol. 2011;80(3):814–20.
23. Yang L, Shang XW, Fan JN, et al. Application of 3D printing in the surgical planning of trimalleolar fracture and doctor-patient communication. Biomed Res Int. 2016;2016:2482086.

22

A novel scoring system to guide prognosis in patients with pathological fractures

Xiang Salim[1]*(iD), Peter D'Alessandro[2,5], James Little[2], Kulvir Mudhar[3], Kevin Murray[4], Richard Carey Smith[1] and Piers Yates[2,5]

Abstract

Background: The most appropriate treatment of pathological fractures from metastatic disease depends on several factors, one of the most important being predicted life expectancy. The aim of this study was to identify the variables that influence prognosis and utilise these to develop a novel scoring system to better predict life expectancy post-pathological fracture.

Methods: The records of all patients that presented with metastatic pathological fractures over a 10-year period from the only tertiary orthopaedic departments in Western Australia were retrospectively examined. Variables assessed were primary cancer type, fracture site, fixation method, cement augmentation, pre-morbid level of physical functioning, complication rate, treatment with chemotherapy or radiotherapy and appendicular, spinal and visceral metastatic load.

Results: A total of 233 patients were included. Median survival from fracture to death was 4.1 months. Median time from cancer diagnosis to pathological fracture was 14.2 months. There was a statistically significant association between patient survival and primary cancer type, physical functional score, spinal metastatic burden and use of chemotherapy or radiotherapy.

Conclusion: A novel scoring system has been developed that offers a survival probability based on patient's individual circumstances. This can guide specialist management and offer patients a more accurate expectation of functional outcome and survival time.

Keywords: Pathological fracture, Metastases, Scoring system, Survival probability

Background

As the average life expectancy has increased, so too has the prevalence of cancer [1, 2]. Recent advances in diagnostic and therapeutic capabilities have resulted in a better prognosis in many cancer patients [3]. Approximately 10% of patients with bony metastases will suffer a pathological fracture at some point during their clinical course [1, 4, 5]. Pathological fractures have significant implications for patient morbidity and mortality and are often considered a marker of end-stage cancer. The literature suggests a 1-year survival rate in the range of 30–40% [6–9].

A number of studies have identified significant variables in patients with metastatic lesions and how they relate to patient prognosis [4, 8–12]. However, this study differs by identifying the significant variables at time of pathological fracture, which is often the point at which the surgical team are first involved.

When considering surgical management of a pathological fracture, the key operative goals include pain relief, early mobilisation and minimal morbidity and complications [2, 5, 13]. The chosen implant and construct should be able to withstand the patient's expected level of activity and appropriately match their expected survival [2, 5].

Although important, the documented ability of clinicians to predict prognosis in patients with metastatic bone disease is poor, with reported accuracy of only 18% reported in the literature [11]. In response to this, we sought to develop a novel scoring system based on the statistically significant variables identified at the time of pathological fracture that can be utilised to more accurately predict prognosis and overall survival. Such a scoring system has never before been developed in patients who

* Correspondence: xiangsalim1@gmail.com
[1]Department of Orthopaedics, Sir Charles Gairdner Hospital, 55 Viewway Nedlands, Perth, WA 6009, Australia
Full list of author information is available at the end of the article

suffer a pathological fracture, and has the potential to guide surgical management and provide a more evidence-based patient expectation.

Methods

All records from patients admitted with a pathological fracture over a 10-year period (2002–2012) to Fremantle, Sir Charles Gairdner and Royal Perth Hospital in Western Australia were retrospectively analysed. Inclusion criteria were pathological fractures secondary to metastatic bone disease. Exclusion criteria were primary bone tumours, spinal pathological fractures, paediatric patients (< 18 years) and peri-prosthetic fractures. Two hundred thirty-three patients that met these criteria were identified.

Recorded variables included age, sex, primary cancer, fracture site, method of fixation, use of cement augmentation, appendicular metastatic load, spinal metastatic load, presence of visceral metastases, co-morbidities, functional scoring before and after the fracture has occurred (Eastern Cooperative Oncology Group (ECOG) score) [14], post-operative complications and use of chemotherapy and radiotherapy. ECOG score was obtained by review of allied health notes and recording pre-injury and best post-operative functional score. The metastatic load was measured through review of existing imaging including plain film, computed tomography (CT), magnetic resonance imaging (MRI), bone scan and positron emission tomography (PET). Metastatic lesions were counted and recorded as 0, 1, 2 or 3 or more to axial and appendicular skeleton as well as viscera.

Statistical analysis of time to death from fracture and the time between cancer diagnosis and fracture was carried out using Cox proportional hazards modelling. Multivariate hazard ratios (HRs) and 95% confidence intervals (CIs) are presented for only those variables that were retained and statistically significant in the final model. Change in ECOG scores (pre- to post-operatively) was analysed using multiple linear regression. In all models, model selection was carried out retaining significant predictors in the final model using a 0.05 significance level. The Cox proportional hazards regression model was used to construct a nomogram, providing a visual representation of our scoring system. All data was analysed using the R environment for statistical computing [15].

Results

Analysis of the combined hospital database identified 233 patients from Sir Charles Gairdner Hospital ($n = 89$), Fremantle Hospital ($n = 72$) and Royal Perth Hospital ($n = 72$). Table 1 provides an outline of the basic demographics and a breakdown of several key variables investigated in this group. Primary cancer type was predominantly breast and lung (29% and 21% respectively). The majority

Table 1 Demographics and distribution of study group

Variable	Category	Number (%)
Age	< 60	53 (23)
	60–74	94 (40)
	75+	86 (37)
Gender	Female	124 (53)
	Male	109 (47)
Primary cancer	Breast	69 (29)
	Lung	49 (21)
	Other	56 (24)
	Prostate	32 (14)
	Renal	27 (12)
Spinal metastases	0	70 (30)
	1, 2, 3	163 (70)
Appendicular metastases	0, 1, 2	106 (45)
	3	127 (55)
Visceral metastases	Missing	11 (5)
	No	71 (30)
	Yes	151 (65)
Fracture site	Humerus	58 (25)
	Proximal femur	131 (56)
	Distal femur	24 (10)
	Other	20 (9)
Treatment	Non-operative	25 (11)
	Plate fixation	27 (12)
	Intramedullary nail	114 (49)
	Arthroplasty	67 (29)
Chemotherapy	Missing	14 (6)
	No	75 (32)
	Yes	144 (62)
Radiotherapy	Missing	13 (6)
	No	64 (27)
	Yes	156 (67)

of fractures were at the proximal femur and humerus (56% and 25% respectively).

Diagnosis to fracture

The median time from cancer diagnosis to pathological fracture was 14.2 months (IQR 1.8–57.3). For 40 patients (17.1%), the pathological fracture itself was the presenting event for a malignant diagnosis. When examining the time from diagnosis to fracture, primary cancer type was a statistically significant variable with lung cancer having the worst prognosis and breast cancer the best (HR for lung to breast = 5.70, 95% CI 3.66–8.88). After adjusting for cancer type distribution, gender was also statistically significant with males having a higher event risk compared to females (HR 1.69, 95% CI 1.28–2.25). Treatment with chemotherapy was statistically significant in delaying time from cancer diagnosis to pathological fracture (HR, 1.46 95% CI 1.09–1.95) while radiotherapy was not. The overall median follow-up time from cancer diagnosis to death was 26.6 months (IQR 6.7–72.8).

Fracture to death

The median time from fracture to death in all comers was 4.1 months (IQR 1.6–12.7). When examining the time to death from fracture, the variables primary cancer type ($P < 0.001$), ECOG pre-fracture score ($P = 0.004$), chemotherapy ($P = 0.003$), radiotherapy ($P < 0.001$) and spinal bone metastases ($P = 0.004$) were all statistically significant in the final multivariate model.

Breast cancer had the best survival outcome and lung cancer the worst (HR lung to breast = 4.29, 95% CI 2.74–6.71) ($P < 0.001$). Between fracture and death, the median survival duration for breast cancer was 7 months (IQR 4–24), which compares well against lung cancer with a median survival 1.87 months (IQR 0.8–4). Figure 1 shows a Kaplan-Meier analysis of the survival rates of each primary cancer. All patients with lung cancer were deceased 17 months after fracture.

ECOG

Pre-fracture ECOG score was statistically significant when analysing time from fracture to death ($P = 0.004$). An ECOG score of 0 suggests that a disease process does not alter physical functioning whilst a score of 4 implies that the patient is completely disabled and bound to bed or chair [14]. Patients with a higher pre-fracture ECOG had a poorer prognosis when compared to those with a score of 0 (HR 1.58, CI 95% 1.16–2.14).

Figure 2 shows the distribution of ECOG score pre-fracture and post-operation. As expected, the majority of subjects had an increase in ECOG score (75.7%), indicating a worse post-operative level of functioning. Noticeably, nine cases (4.1%) moved from an ECOG score of 0 to a score of 4. A statistical analysis on change in ECOG score (while adjusting for pre-treatment score) found that the statistically significant predictors of a worsening in ECOG score included fracture site ($P = 0.008$) and treatment with chemotherapy ($P = 0.009$), with those receiving chemotherapy having a smaller change in ECOG. When examining fracture site, those with a humeral fracture had a smaller loss of function than those with a fracture at proximal or distal femur ($P = 0.001$ and $P = 0.017$ respectively).

Spinal, appendicular and visceral metastases

There were no spinal metastases in 30% of cases; however, 53.7% of cases had three or more. The number of spinal metastases was shown to be statistically significant in predicting time from fracture to death ($P = 0.004$). Those who had any spinal metastases had a shorter survival time when compared to those who had none (HR 1.65, 95% CI 1.18–2.31).

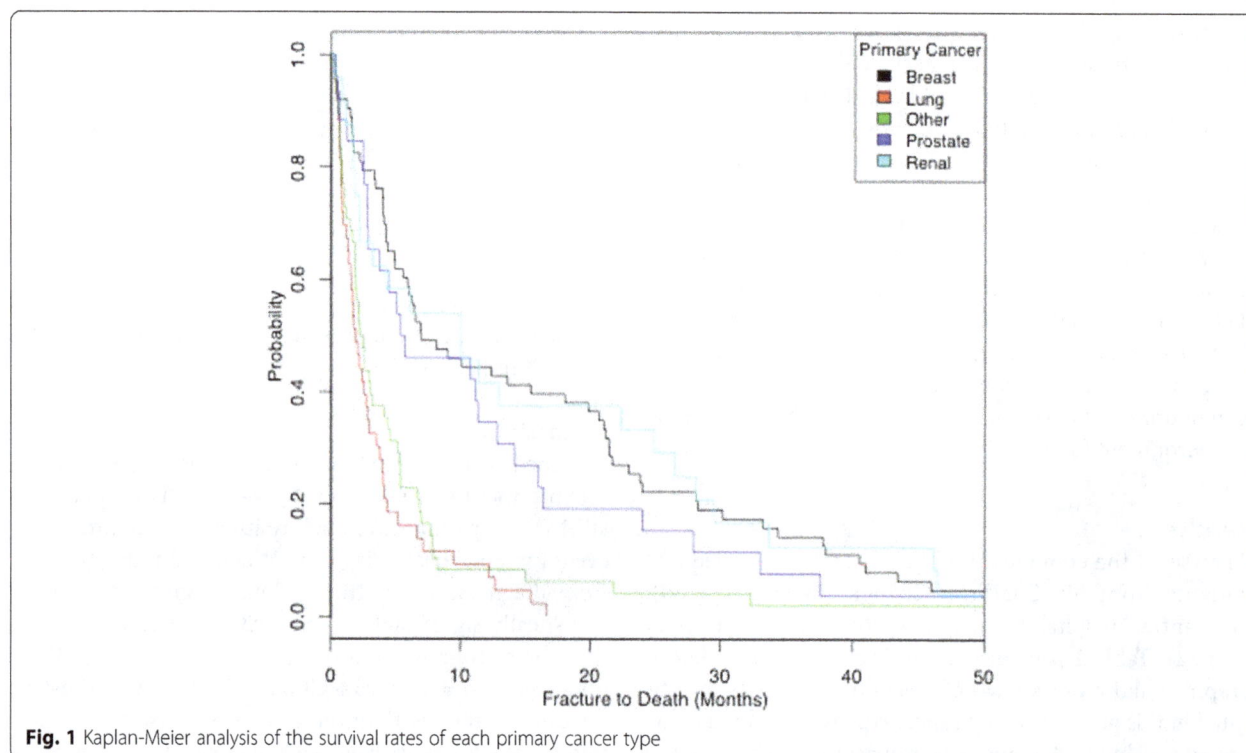

Fig. 1 Kaplan-Meier analysis of the survival rates of each primary cancer type

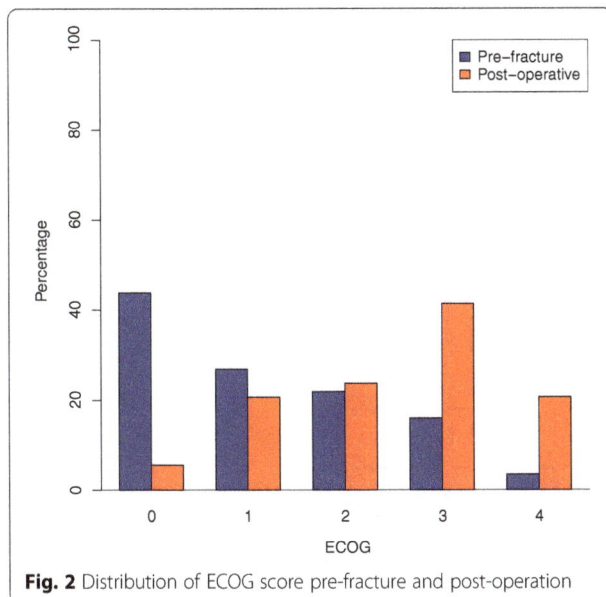

Fig. 2 Distribution of ECOG score pre-fracture and post-operation

A large proportion (54.5%) of cases had three additional appendicular bone metastases, while 14.2% had zero. There was no statistically significant relationship between appendicular or visceral metastatic load and survival rate post-fracture.

Fracture site, method of fixation and use of cement augment

Fracture site was predominantly proximal femur and humerus (56% and 25% respectively). Treatment included intramedullary nail, plate fixation and arthroplasty (49%, 12% and 29% respectively) with 10% of patients were managed non-operatively. Fracture site, method of fixation and use of cement augmentation did not have a statistically significant impact on survival post-fracture.

Chemotherapy and radiotherapy

Chemotherapy and radiotherapy treatment was present in 61.8% and 66.95% of patients. Patients who did not receive chemotherapy had a higher risk of mortality than those who did (HR 1.74, 95% CI 1.21–2.49) ($P = 0.003$). Similarly, radiotherapy was also protective in survival post-fracture (HR 1.79, 95% CI 1.27–2.51) ($P < 0.001$). Median extended survival duration with use of chemotherapy and radiotherapy was 3.56 and 3.78 months respectively.

Survival probability score

With our large sample size drawn across an entire population base along with the incorporation of statistically significant variables, our team was able to develop a novel and unique scoring system for these patients. This has never before been available for patients at time of pathological fracture and can be used to provide a more accurate assessment of prognosis and survival. This is

depicted in Fig. 3 where a nomogram gives a visual representation of our scoring system which provides different survival probabilities for a range of survival times based on individual patient characteristics. This is yet to be validated as our team elected to use all 233 available cases to generate a sufficiently powered scoring system, rather than divide the group into a subset for generating and a subset for validating.

To use the nomogram, each variable is identified on the left and the individual patient's characteristic circled. A vertical line is then drawn up to intersect the 'points' axis to determine the point score for each variable. The total sum of points is then calculated. This total sum value is located on the 'total points' axis, and a vertical line is drawn down. Survival probability at each time period (2/6/12/24 months) is determined by the point at which this line intersects it. As an example, Fig. 4 shows the process for a patient with a pathological fracture of breast cancer origin, with spinal metastases, a pre-injury ECOG of 1, who has had chemotherapy and radiotherapy treatment.

Discussion

During the natural course of the disease process, malignancies commonly metastasise to the bone [1, 4]. Many studies have examined the variables that influence progression of metastatic lesions to pathological fracture [1, 4, 5, 7]; however, few studies have investigated the factors that impact morbidity and mortality once the pathological fracture has occurred.

This study is a state-wide expansion on the pilot paper published by our institution [13]. Our preceding pilot article was the first to document survival time following pathological fracture and was able to identify variables that significantly influenced prognosis [13]. However, until now, there has been no conclusive scoring system available to help predict prognosis at time of pathological fracture. This is an important and novel development, as better insight into prognosis would help treating clinicians identify patients with poorer or favourable survival prospects and therefore guide surgical treatment options.

Our study found that the primary cancer type had a statistically significant impact on time from cancer diagnosis to pathological fracture. Demographic primary cancer type was mainly of breast and lung origin which is consistent with existing literature [6, 10, 11]. Breast and prostate had the longest time to pathological fracture with a median delay of 49.2 (IQR 11.7–115.6) and 29 months (IQR 12.2–59.4) respectively. In contrast, lung cancer had the shortest time to fracture with a median of just 2.1 months (IQR 0–6.8). Given the shorter period from diagnosis to fracture, we recommend more frequent screening in this subgroup so as to detect significant metastatic bone lesions before they fracture. This is especially important given the poor prognosis

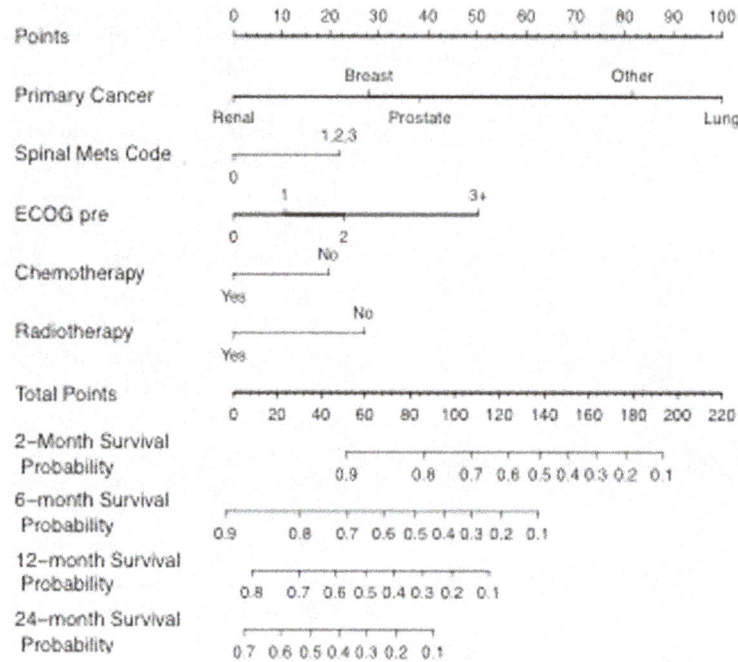

Fig. 3 Nomogram representation of our scoring system which provides different survival probabilities for a range of survival times based on individual patient characteristics

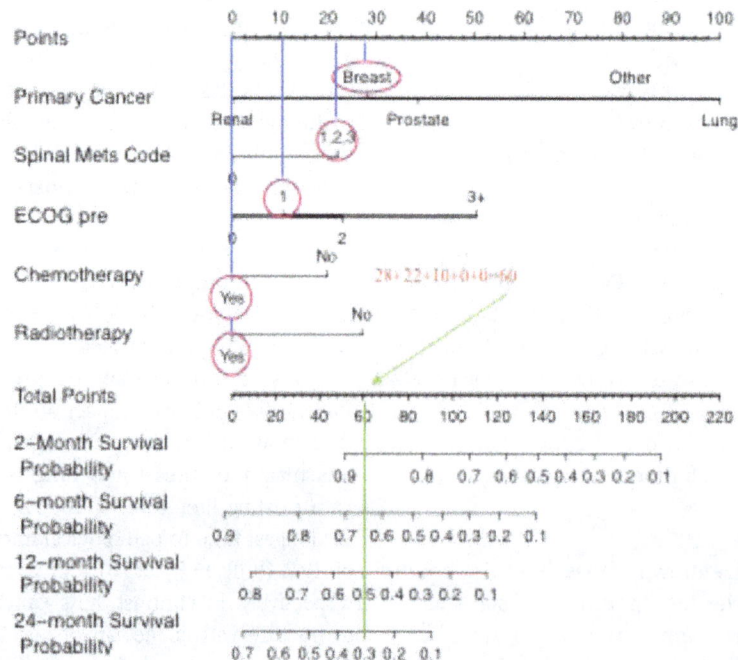

Fig. 4 Example case of a pathological fracture of breast cancer origin, with spinal metastases, a pre-injury ECOG of 1, who has had chemotherapy and radiotherapy treatment. Circle relevant variable (red). Draw line up to attribute point (blue). Add each variable point to find the sum (orange). Find total point value and draw line down to identify the survival probability at each time (green)

following a fracture in this subgroup. After adjusting for primary cancer type distribution, gender was also statistically significant with males having a higher event risk compared to females in time from diagnosis to fracture. This is difficult to interpret, but may be related to males typically seeking medical attention later in a disease course which may result in a delay to cancer diagnosis.

Median survival post-fracture in our expanded cohort was 4.1 months with a 1-year survival rate across all patients of 27%. While slightly better than the survival described in our pilot paper (3.3 months), this is still a group of patients with an incredibly poor overall prognosis that has perhaps been underestimated in previous literature [6–9]. Lung cancer median survival was much worse at 1.87 months when compared to breast (7 months), prostate (5.24 months) and renal (10.09 months) median survival. This variability of prognosis in different primary cancers is well recognised in existing literature [1, 5, 8, 10, 11, 16, 17]; however, it has never been incorporated into a scoring system to predict patient prognosis post-pathological fracture as it has in this paper.

Negative prognostic factors in patients with metastatic bone disease include primary lung cancer, metastatic load, visceral metastases, pathological fracture and poor functional performance score [8, 10, 11]. Katagiri et al. developed a scoring system for patients with bony metastases [18]. This differed from our team's goal of identifying prognostic factors post-pathological fracture. Their team found that primary cancer site, ECOG score, presence of visceral and cerebral metastases, any previous chemotherapy and multiple skeletal metastases were significant prognostic factors. Interestingly, their team found chemotherapy to be a negative prognostic factor, which likely represents a treatment selection bias. Furthermore, their findings suggested that pathological fractures are not a negative prognostic factor in patients with metastatic bone disease, which differs from what most evidence suggests [8, 10, 11].

An article by Nathan et al. also examined the biochemical factors surrounding prognosis and found that low pre-operative haemoglobin, albumin and white cell count were all independent negative prognostic factors [11]. This paper emphasised the difficulty in estimating mortality rate in patients with metastatic bone disease, as only 18% of clinician estimates were accurate in predicting actual survival [11].

Multiple scoring systems exist for patients with spinal metastases, which attempt to predict post-operative prognosis so as to rationalise management decisions [10, 12, 19]. The sentinel paper by Tokuhashi et al. that first developed a scoring system in patients with spinal metastases was the initial inspiration for our study into appendicular pathological fracture prognosis and guided the choice of variables we would investigate [12]. A more recent paper by Dardic et al. evaluated these scoring systems and corroborated that

visceral metastases, primary tumour type, functional performance score and number of spinal metastases all significantly influenced survival [20]. The prognostic relevance of spinal metastatic burden in patients with an appendicular pathological fracture has not been previously studied.

Tsuda et al. recently conducted an investigation assessing the factors affecting post-operative complications and short-term mortality after surgery specific to femoral pathological fractures [2]. They found that post-operative complications were significantly associated with older age, primary tumour type, higher Charlson Comorbidity Index and blood transfusion [2]. In addition, they concluded that 30-day mortality was significantly higher in patients with rapid-rapid growth tumours, visceral metastases, internal fixation method and no post-operative chemotherapy [2].

Our study found that primary cancer type, pre-fracture ECOG score, spinal metastatic burden and treatment with chemotherapy and radiotherapy were statistically significant variables in the survival rate post-pathological fracture. Age, complications, gender, fixation method, fracture site and visceral and appendicular metastases were not found to be significant factors.

Spinal metastases had a statistically significant effect on patient outcome following pathological fracture. Our pilot study was the first to describe the spinal metastatic burden as a prognostic variable in patients with appendicular bony metastases. Our expanded study has also found it to be a significant predictive variable and one that should be considered in patients with appendicular pathological fractures.

Visceral and appendicular metastatic load was not a statistically significant prognostic factor in our study. This is in contrast to existing evidence in patients with metastatic bone disease that suggest a greater appendicular or visceral metastatic burden to be a negative prognostic factor [1, 4, 8–11]. We believe this finding reflects the different points on the pathological spectrum, where pathological fractures are further progressed and are often considered end-stage markers. Our results suggest that at point of pathological fracture, as the disease process is so advanced, the number of visceral or appendicular metastasis are not relevant to survival prognosis.

The use of chemotherapy and radiotherapy was found to have a significantly positive effect on survival rate following a pathological fracture. Interestingly, it was observed that use of chemotherapy also prolonged the time between diagnosis and pathological fracture, whereas use of radiotherapy did not. This likely reflects the systemic nature of chemotherapy as oppose to the targeted local effects of radiotherapy. It was also observed that patients who received chemotherapy had a significantly smaller change in ECOG post-operatively. These findings corroborate existing evidence advocating use of adjuvant chemotherapy and radiotherapy. In Australia, these adjuvant therapies are commonly available; however, not all patients receive adjuvant treatment. In our study, a surprising 32.19% and 27.47% did not receive chemotherapy and radiotherapy respectively. Furthermore, in certain developing countries, these treatments are less available due to financial and logistical reasons. For these reasons, use of adjuvant therapy is included in our prognosticating scoring system.

Pre-fracture ECOG score statistically significantly influenced prognosis as patients with a better functional score prior to pathological fracture lived longer following surgery. These findings are consistent with existing literature supporting the impact of pre-morbid physical function on post-operative function and survival time [1, 8, 9, 11, 16]. This is intuitive; however, it emphasises the importance of optimising and maintaining cancer patients' functional mobility and independence at both the pre-injury and post-operative stage.

Our study's limitations reflect the nature of the retrospective audit design. Our collection of ECOG score was dependent on the assessment and documentation of several different occupational therapists. Similarly, the operation itself was performed by different surgeons of differing levels of experience across three hospital sites. Finally, the heterogeneity of our cohort and their primary tumour type means a wide variety of chemotherapy and radiotherapy regimes prescribed of which the binary yes/no analysis likely oversimplifies. Despite these limitations, we have found a statistically significant relationship between prognosis following pathological fracture and several variables including primary cancer type, pre-fracture ECOG score, spinal metastatic burden and use of chemotherapy and radiotherapy. Using these significant variables, we have developed a novel scoring system which can be used to estimate survival probability at time of pathological fracture.

Conclusion

This expanded study has included a large cohort of patients, with more than triple the number of patients described in the original pilot paper within the same 10-year time frame. It is adequately powered to find statistical significance in several of our key variables of interest. Due to the relative geographical isolation of Western Australia and the inclusion of every tertiary referral centre in the state, it is likely that the vast majority of patients presenting with pathological fractures in this community have been included.

We have been able to develop a novel scoring system that can be utilised to estimate survival probability based on these statistically significant variables. This will enable treating clinicians to more accurately estimate survival time, which is often a source of great anxiety to both the patient and their family. An important principle in the management of patients with a pathological fracture is that the patient should live longer than the time needed to recover and rehabilitate from the operation. A more evidence-based estimate of prognosis will be an invaluable tool in guiding the treating team in management decisions. This paper will fill a significant void in the literature; as to our knowledge, there is no existing scoring system of this nature currently available.

Funding

Funding is from Orthopaedic Research Foundation of Western Australia for the publication cost. No other funding sources.

Authors' contributions

XGS is the primary author and contributed in drafting and revising the manuscript. KM/JL contributed to the data collection and drafting of the manuscript. KM contributed to the data analysis and interpretation. PD/RCS/PY contributed to the conception of the article and manuscript revision. All authors read and approved the final manuscript.

Competing interests

The authors declare that they have no competing interests.

Author details

[1]Department of Orthopaedics, Sir Charles Gairdner Hospital, 55 Viewway Nedlands, Perth, WA 6009, Australia. [2]Department of Orthopaedics, Fiona Stanley Fremantle Hospital Groups, Perth, Australia. [3]Department of Orthopaedics, Royal Perth Hospital, Perth, Australia. [4]Centre for Applied Statistics, University of Western Australia, Perth, Australia. [5]Orthopaedic Research Foundation of Western Australia (ORFWA), Perth, Australia.

References

1. Coleman RE. Skeletal complications of malignancy. Cancer. 1997;80:1588–94.
2. Tsuda Y, Yasunaga H, Horiguchi H, et al. Complications and postoperative mortality rate after surgery for pathological femur fracture related to bone metastasis: analysis of a nationwide database. Ann Surg Oncol. 2015;23(3): 801–10. https://doi.org/10.1245/s10434-015-4881-9.
3. Santini D, Tampellini M, Vincenzi B, et al. Natural history of bone metastasis in colorectal cancer: final results of a large Italian bone metastases study. Ann Oncol. 2012;23(8):2072–7.
4. Böhm P, Huber J. The surgical treament of bony metastases of the spine and limbs. J Bone Joint Surg Br. 2002;84:521–9.
5. Ruggieri P, Mavrogenis AF, Casadei R, et al. Protocol of surgical treatment of long bone pathological fractures. Injury. 2010;41:1161–7.
6. Sorensen MS, Gregersen KG, Gum-Schwensen T, et al. Patient and implant survival following joint replacement because of metastatic bone disease. Acta Orthop. 2013;84:301–6.
7. Harvey N, Ahlmann ER, Allison DC, et al. Endoprosthesis last longer than intramedullary devices in proximal femur metastases. Clin Orthop Relat Res. 2012;470:684–91.
8. Hansen BH, Keller J, Laitinen M, et al. The Scandanavian sarcoma group skeletal metastasis register survival after surgery for bone metastases in the pelvis and extremities. Acta Orthop Scand Suppl. 2004;75:11–5.
9. Wedin R, Hansen BH, Laitinen M, et al. Complications and survival after surgical treatment of 214 metastatic lesions of the humerus. J Shoulder Elb Surg. 2012;21:1049–55.
10. Bauer HC, Wedin R. Survival after surgery for spinal and extremity metastases: prognostication in 241 patients. Acta Orthop. 1995;66(2):143–6.

11. Nathan SS, Healey JH, Mellano D, et al. Survival in patients operated on for pathological fracture: implications for end-of-life orthopaedic care. J Clin Oncol. 2005;23:6072–82.

12. Tokuhashi Y, Matsuzaki H, Toriyama S. Scoring system for the preoperative evaluation of metastatic spine tumour prognosis. Spine. 1990;15(11):1110–3.

13. Hill T, D'Alessandro P, Murray K, et al. Prognostic factors following pathological fractures. ANZ J Surg. 2015;85:159–63.

14. Oken M, Creech R, Tormey D, et al. Toxicity and response criteria of the eastern cooperative oncology group. Am J Clin Oncol. 1982;5:649–55.

15. R Core Team. R: a language and environment for statistical computing. R Foundation for Statistical Computing 2015, Vienna, Austria. URL http://www.R-project.org/.

16. Forsberg JA, Eberhardt J, Boland PJ, et al. Estimating survival in patients with operable skeletal metastases: an application of a bayesian belief network. PLoS One. 2011;6:e19956.

17. Coleman RE. Clinical features of metastatic bone disease and risk of skeletal morbidity. Clin Cancer Res. 2006;12:6243s–9s.

18. Katagiri H, Takahashi M, Wakai K, et al. Prognostic factors and a scoring system for patients with skeletal metastasis. J Bone Joint Surg. 2005;87-B:698–703.

19. Leithner A, Radl R, Gruber G, et al. Predictive value of seven preoperative prognostic scoring systems for spinal metastases. Eur Spine J. 2008;17(11):1488–95.

20. Dardic M, Wibmer C, Berhold A, et al. Evaluation of prognostic scoring systems for spinal metastases in 196 patients treated during 2005-2010. Eur Spine J. 2015;24(10):2133–41.

23

Clinical application of the pedicle in vitro restorer in percutaneous kyphoplasty

Yimin Qi[1], Yiwen Zeng[2]* ⓘ, Dalin Wang[2], Jisheng Sui[2] and Qiang Wang[2]

Abstract

Background: Percutaneous kyphoplasty (PKP) is widely applied for the treatment of osteoporotic vertebral compression fractures (OVCFs) and has achieved satisfactory clinical results. With the accumulation of clinical cases and prolonged follow-up times, the inability to reconstruct vertebral height defects has attracted more and more attention. A comparison of clinical effects was retrospectively reviewed in 72 patients who underwent simple PKP or pedicle in vitro restorer (PIVR) combined with PKP to discuss the clinical application of self-developed PIVR used in PKP.

Methods: From August 2013 to August 2016, 72 patients with OVCFs were treated surgically, with 30 patients undergoing PKP (group A) and 42 undergoing PIVR combined with PKP (group B). Operation-related situations, radiological data, and related scores were compared between the two groups by corresponding statistical methods.

Results: Bone cement was successfully injected into 72 vertebral bodies. Sixty-three cases were followed up for an average of 14 months. There were significant differences between the two groups in the improvement of the height of the vertebral body, sagittal Cobb angle, and visual analogue scale (VAS) 1 week after the operation ($P < 0.05$), and the improvements of group B were better than those in group A. The cement leakage ratio was significantly different between the two groups ($P < 0.05$). The Oswestry Disability Index (ODI) at last follow-up was significantly different between the two groups ($P < 0.05$). There was no significant difference in the incidence of recurrent vertebral fractures between the two groups at the last follow-up ($P > 0.05$).

Conclusion: PIVR combined with PKP can overcome the limitations of PKP alone, that is, hardly restoring vertebral height and height being easily lost again with balloon removal. The combined method can also restore the vertebral fractures to a satisfactory height and effectively maintain the stability of the spine, which improves the long-term quality of life of patients. Thus, PIVR combined with PKP is a better choice for patients with OVCFs.

Keywords: Percutaneous kyphoplasty, Osteoporotic vertebral compression fractures, Restorer, Distraction, Reduction, Reconstruction

Background

With the aging of the population, the incidence of osteoporotic vertebral compression fractures (OVCFs) is getting higher and higher in clinics around the world, seriously threatening the life and health of elderly patients. OVCFs always cause chronic pain, depression, insomnia, and even loss of ability to perform daily activities [1]. At present, percutaneous kyphoplasty (PKP) is widely used for the treatment of OVCFs [2, 3]. PKP has the advantages of being minimally invasive and safe, providing rapid pain relief, and being a simple manipulation technique [4]. However, there are still some drawbacks, including unsatisfactory reduction, postoperative long-term loss of height, and kyphosis, especially for patients with severe OVCFs [5–7]. In order to achieve a better vertebral restorative effect, some scholars [8] have used open surgery with pedicle screws for distraction and fixation combined with vertebroplasty to treat OVCFs and have achieved satisfactory recovery of the collapsed vertebral body. However, the surgical trauma is substantial, and due to the poor bone quality of the patients, the holding force of the internal fixation is often insufficient, and the risk of postoperative failure is high. At the same time, the retention of the

* Correspondence: 654468946@qq.com
[2]Department of Orthopaedic Surgery, Nanjing First Hospital, Nanjing Medical University, #68 Changle Rd, Qinhuai District, Nanjing 210000, Jiangsu, China
Full list of author information is available at the end of the article

pedicle screw not only affects spinal activity but also may cause fractures of the adjacent vertebrae [9]. How to perfectly integrate the advantages of vertebral restoration and vertebroplasty is still a problem to be solved.

Therefore, we have developed a device to solve the above problems. This device has obtained a national invention patent. The current study was to compare the clinical effects of pedicle in vitro restorer (PIVR) combined with PKP with simple PKP surgery for the treatment of OVCFs. We hypothesized that the application of PIVR combined with PKP would perfectly restore the height of the vertebral body and correct kyphosis by using the method's unique reduction technique.

Materials and methods
Clinical data
From August 2013 to August 2016, 72 patients with a single osteoporotic thoracic or lumbar vertebral compression fracture treated at Nanjing First Hospital, Nanjing Medical University, were selected. Seventy-two patients with OVCFs were treated surgically, with 30 patients undergoing PKP (group A) and 42 undergoing PIVR combined with PKP (group B). The procedures followed were in accordance with the ethical standards of Nanjing First Hospital's committee, and consent was obtained from each patient (Permit Number KY20130201-02). All patients met the following inclusion criteria: (1) single vertebral fracture; (2) T10 and below vertebral fractures; (3) loss of vertebral body anterior column height of 30% or more, with no significant lesion to the middle and/or posterior columns; (4) age between 55 and 75 years old; (5) disease duration less than 3 weeks; and (6) bone mineral density value -4.0 SD $< T < -2.5$ SD. Patients with multi-segmental fractures, non-osteoporotic compression fractures, burst fractures, and fractures with spinal stenosis or spinal cord injury were excluded. In group A, there were 6 males and 24 females, and the ages ranged from 58 to 73 years, with an average age of 66.83 ± 4.90 years. In group B, there were 8 males and 34 females, and the ages ranged from 58 to 75 years, with an average age of 65.74 ± 4.65 years. The locations of the collapsed vertebrae were 58 lumbar vertebrae and 14 thoracic vertebrae, including 2 cases at T10, 4 cases at T11, 8 cases at T12, 22 cases at L1, 16 cases at L2, 13 cases at L3, and 7 cases at L4. In group A, the locations of the collapsed vertebrae were 5 thoracic vertebrae and 25 lumbar vertebrae. In group B, the locations of the collapsed vertebrae were 9 thoracic vertebrae and 33 lumbar vertebrae. The reasons for injuries were 16 cases of sprains, 12 cases of car accident injuries, 36 cases of tumbling injuries, and 8 cases of falling injuries. There were no significant differences in sex, age, and location of the collapsed vertebrae between the two groups ($P > 0.05$).

Equipment and instruments
The minimally invasive equipment and the balloon were manufactured by the Kyphon Company of America, and the Flexiview 8800 C-type arm X-ray machine was manufactured by the GE Company of America. The PIVR was self-developed and has been awarded a national invention patent (Fig. 1 patent number: ZL200810123915.6).

Surgical technique
For the group A procedure, patients were placed in the prone position with two pads for abdominal hanging, and the procedures were performed under local anesthesia with electrocardiogram monitoring; at the same time, fluoroscopy was used throughout the procedure. A small 8-mm incision was placed on the skin at the pedicle level, and the accurate incision position was on the outer edge of the pedicle's projection under the anteroposterior view of the image. The needle was placed into the pedicle, and the needle pin was removed. Next, the guide pin was inserted into the first two thirds of the vertebral body in the lateral view; subsequently, a cannula was placed through the guide pin. The guide pin was pulled out, and the drill was inserted through the cannula to establish a surgical tunnel. The length of the tunnel in the vertebral body should be 3 mm larger than the length of the balloon after expansion. The balloon was inserted through the cannula and placed into the anterior three fourths of the vertebral body from a lateral view. The balloon was slowly inflated by injecting contrast media through the high-pressure pump. When the Cobb angle and vertebra's height were satisfactory compared to preoperative radiographs (Fig. 2), the operator extracted the contrast media and withdrew the balloon. The same volume of bone cement, which became doughy, was injected into the collapsed vertebral body. When the bone cement was spread near the posterior wall of the vertebral body or

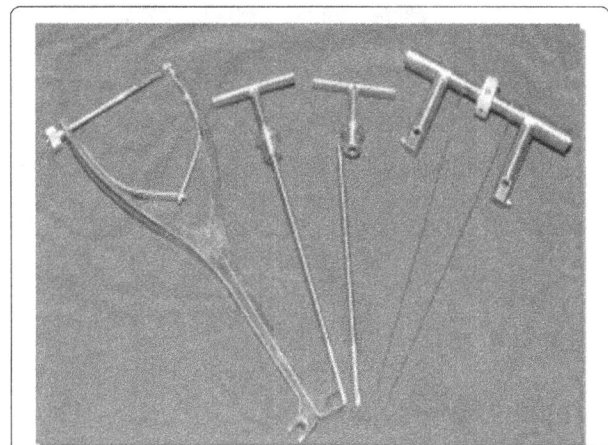

Fig. 1 Picture of the PIVR

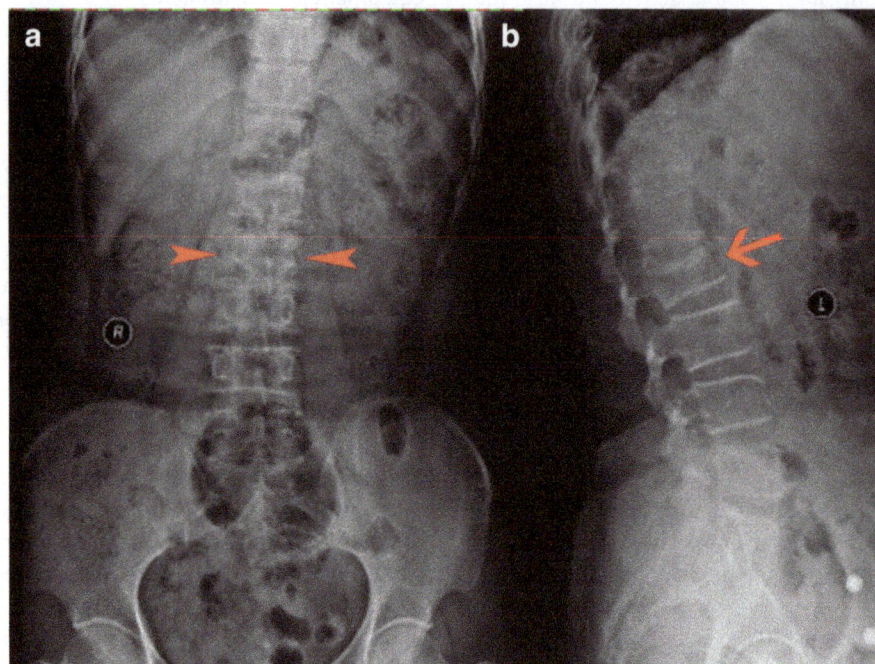

Fig. 2 Typical radiographic views. **a**, **b** Preoperative anteroposterior and lateral radiographs showing a compression fracture of the second lumbar vertebra

appeared to leak, the procedure was stopped immediately. Contralateral puncture was performed simultaneously. Patients stayed in bed for 24 h.

For the group B procedure, the patients were fixed in the prone position. PIVR was used to perform distraction on the side of the severe fracture of the vertebral body. If the collapse of the vertebral body was only in front and there was no significant difference in the bilateral height, the operation was performed on the left or right side according to the operator's habits. Pedicle needles were implanted into the adjacent vertebral bodies around the collapsed vertebral body through minimally invasive percutaneous implantation under fluoroscopy (Fig. 3a). Subsequently, hollow pedicle screws were inserted one third of the way into the vertebral body along the positioning needle, and the distraction device was placed below the extension rod. Next, the distraction device was used to restore the vertebra (Figs. 3b and 4a); at the same time, the hex rotator of the positive and reverse threads was tightened to prevent the restorer

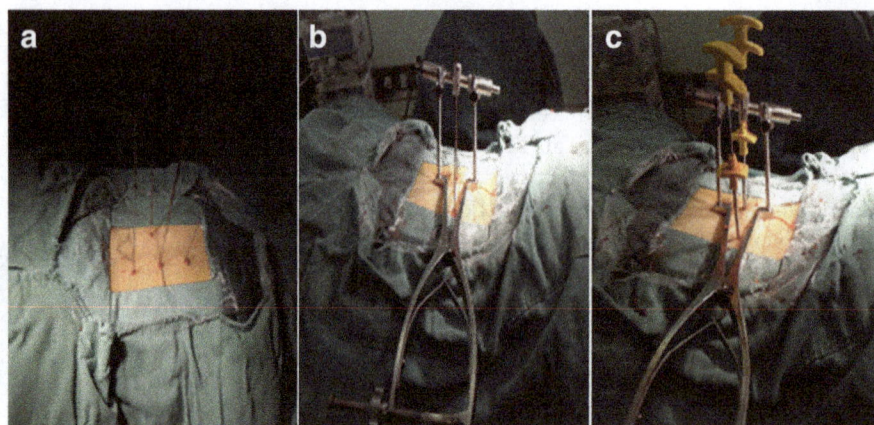

Fig. 3 Three intraoperative photographs showing the operation process using PIVR. **a** Four pedicle screw guide pins are inserted into the pedicles via a minimally invasive percutaneous incision. **b** The restorer was used for distraction and restored the vertebral body. **c** PKP combined with PIVR

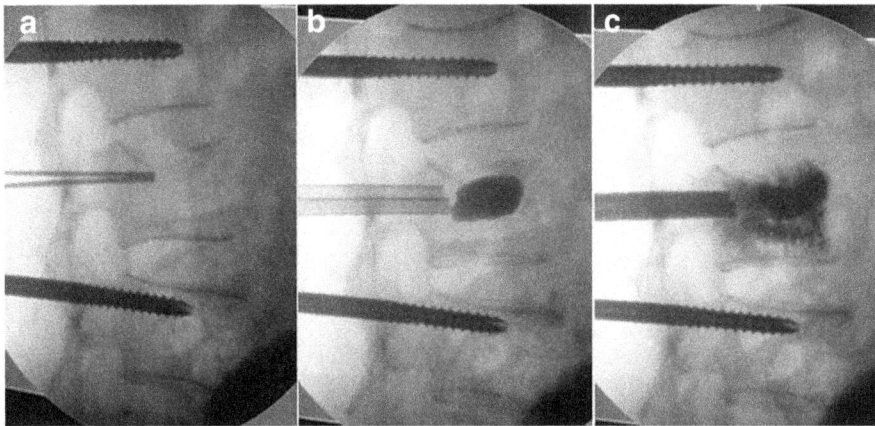

Fig. 4 Intraoperative radiographs. **a** Distracting reduction using PIVR. **b** The balloon slowly inflates by injecting contrast media. **c** Bone cement being injected into the collapsed vertebral body

from retreating. Under fluoroscopy, when the vertebral body reset was satisfactory or a screw-cutting phenomenon occurred, the reset procedure was terminated, and PKP was performed (Figs. 3c and 4b, c) with the application of a bilateral puncture technique; then, the restorer was removed. Patients stayed in bed for 24 h.

Clinical and radiographic assessment

The improvement of anterior and mid-vertebral heights and the sagittal Cobb angle, which was defined as the crossing angle of the vertical lines parallel to the collapsed vertebral superior and inferior endplates in the lateral X-ray image, were the observed indices of the effect of restoration. A visual analogue scale (VAS) [10] was used to assess back pain control, and the Oswestry Disability Index (ODI) [11] was used to estimate the activities of daily living. Sexual life was deleted; as a result, the remaining 9 items totaled 45 points, according to living habits and age. Considering that there may be a mechanical imbalance in the unilateral distraction of the restorer, the lateral wall height improvement ratio on the distraction side of the restorer was compared with that of the non-distraction side. Lateral wall height improvement ratio = (postoperative height − preoperative height)/postoperative height × 100%.

Statistical analysis

Statistical analyses were performed using SPSS version 19.0 statistical software (IBM SPSS, Chicago). Quantitative data are displayed in the form of $\bar{x} \pm s$. The values between groups were analyzed by independent sample T test. Preoperative and postoperative values between different subgroups were compared using the paired T test. Enumeration data between groups were analyzed by chi-square test. The results were considered significant at $P < 0.05$.

Results

Seventy-two vertebrae were successfully injected with bone cement, with negligible blood loss, no deaths, no spinal cord injuries, and no pulmonary embolisms or postoperative infections. Sixty-three patients were followed up. Two patients were followed up for 3 months and actively withdrew from follow-up. Five patients actively withdrew from follow-up at 6 months. Two patients withdrew from follow-up due to relocation. Eight asymptomatic extravasations of vertebral bone cement occurred, including 2 cases of intervertebral space, 2 cases of paravertebral vein, and 3 cases of paravertebral soft tissue in group A and 1 case of paravertebral vein in group B. There were significant differences in the ratio of cement leakage between the two groups ($P < 0.05$). The anterior and mid-vertebral body heights for group A increased from 18.23 ± 1.11 mm and 19.80 ± 1.05 mm preoperatively to 22.61 ± 1.21 mm and 23.88 ± 1.05 mm 1 week postoperatively, respectively. The anterior and mid-vertebral body heights for group B increased from 17.67 ± 1.18 mm and 19.17 ± 1.04 mm preoperatively to 23.32 ± 1.14 mm and 24.34 ± 0.97 mm 1 week postoperatively, respectively. Cobb angles between group A and group B improved from $20.87° \pm 1.32°$ and $22.60° \pm 1.43°$ before surgery to $10.84° \pm 1.03°$ and $10.51° \pm 0.77°$ 1 week after surgery, respectively; VAS between the two groups decreased from 8.03 ± 0.40 and 8.01 ± 0.37 before surgery to 3.01 ± 0.35 and 2.35 ± 0.28 1 week after surgery, respectively. ODI at the last follow-up in group A ($17.69\% \pm 4.60\%$) was significantly different than that in group B ($11.71\% \pm 2.20\%$) ($P < 0.05$). There was no significant difference in the incidence of recurrent vertebral fractures between the two groups at last follow-up ($P > 0.05$) (Tables 1 and 2). There was no significant difference in the improvement ratio of the height of the lateral wall of the vertebral body between the distraction side and non-distraction side of the restorer ($P < 0.05$) (Table 3).

Table 1 Preoperative and postoperative characteristics of the two groups

Characteristic	Group A	Group B	t/χ^2	P
No. (male:female)	30 (6:24)	42 (8:34)	0.010	> 0.05
Mean age, year	66.83 ± 4.90	65.74 ± 4.65	0.964	> 0.05
Mean improvement of anterior height, mm	4.38 ± 0.59	5.66 ± 0.64	− 8.549	< 0.05
Mean improvement of mid height, mm	4.09 ± 0.27	5.17 ± 0.49	− 11.938	< 0.05
Mean improvement of VAS	5.01 ± 0.22	5.66 ± 0.29	− 10.353	< 0.05
Mean improvement of Cobb angle, deg	10.03 ± 0.52	11.08 ± 1.12	− 10.380	< 0.05
The ratio of bone cement leakage, %	23.33	2.38	5.802	< 0.05

No. number, *deg* degrees, *VAS* visual analogue scale

Discussion

PKP has opened up a new way for the treatment of OVCFs in the elderly. However, the dilator expands in the collapsed vertebral body with greater resistance, and there is limited space for expansion. In addition, the height of vertebral body cannot be completely maintained under the compression of the adjacent upper and lower vertebral bodies after the balloon is withdrawn from the vertebral body, and the height of the vertebral body is easily lost again. PKP may also be associated with paraspinal muscle tension and traction because of local anesthesia [12]. The above factors have an influence on the height of collapsed vertebrae, which cannot be fully restored. So, kyphosis of the spine can only be partially rectified. Therefore, we developed a set of special equipment, named PIVR.

The principle of PIVR is a hollow elongated pedicle screw and its self-locking compression-distraction device, with large arms. The pedicle screw is 15 cm long, with a hollow diameter of 1.2 mm and outer diameter of 6.5 mm, 6.0 mm, 5.5 mm, or 5.0 mm. The self-locking compression-distraction device includes a screw-tail prolonged rod and a distraction prolonged rod. The hollow structure of the pedicle screw allows easy implantation of the minimally invasive percutaneous needle and hollow taps; the hollow screw is longer than common screws used for internal fixation. Moreover, the rod at the screw tail prolongs the length of the extension arm. The hollow pedicle screw is located at the adjacent vertebrae and can exert its powerful distraction and compression effect through its long arm, resetting the collapsed vertebrae according to the principle of ligament reconstruction [13]. The distraction and compression effects are mediated via distraction and compression devices, which are equipped with positive and reverse screw threads (thread bar); the thread bar is vertically connected to the prolonged rod. The hex rotator

is fixed on the thread bar, and rotation of the hex rotator can shorten the distance between the two prolonged rods, thus functioning for distraction and reduction.

Reconstruction of the vertebral body by balloon during PKP surgery has a very limited effect on restoration, which may be related to the following factors: (1) the direction of balloon expansion is difficult to control, (2) the volume and expansion capacity of the balloon itself is limited (the working tension of the balloon is generally less than 300 psi), and (3) after the balloon is removed from the vertebral body during the operation, fracture reduction is difficult to maintain. However, PIVR, through the self-locking distraction device to maintain the distraction state, can overcome easy loss of vertebral body height after withdrawal of the balloon and can effectively restore the height and correct the kyphosis. There were significant differences between the two groups in the improvement of the height of the vertebral body and Cobb angle 1 week postoperatively ($P < 0.05$), and the improvements in group B were better than those in group A. Some patients undergoing PKP surgery suffer from "stress concentration" due to poor reduction of vertebral fractures caused by collapsed fractures and adjacent vertebrae, which may lead to long-term complications of low back pain and affect quality of life. However, PIVR can effectively maintain the stability of the spine, which improves the long-term quality of life of patients. ODI at the last follow-up in group A (17.69% ± 4.60%) was significantly different than that in group B (11.71% ± 2.20%) ($P < 0.05$). It showed that the long-term clinical effect for group B was significantly better than that for group A.

PVP and PKP can effectively reduce pain. He et al. [3] reported the follow-up results of an average of 58 months (24.1–98.9) in 11 cases of PVP, and all patients were significantly relieved of pain, with significant long-term

Table 2 Characteristics of the two groups at last follow-up

Characteristic	Group A	Group B	t/χ^2	P
Mean ODI, %	17.69 ± 4.60	11.71 ± 2.20	6.157	< 0.05
No. (refracture:normal)	26(2:24)	37(1:36)	0.099	> 0.05

No. number, *ODI* Oswestry Disability Index

Table 3 Comparison of the lateral wall height improvement ratio by the restorer

Group B	n	Lateral wall height improvement ratio, %	t	P
Distraction side	42	22.75 ± 2.10	1.18	0.24
Non-distraction side	42	22.20 ± 2.22		

pain relief and no restriction of daily activities. In our study, the pain in each group was alleviated to different degrees, and the improvement of VAS in group A postoperatively was less than that in group B. PIVR had a good reduction effect on the collapsed vertebrae; as a result, bone cement fully infiltrated. Additionally, bone cement filling can effectively block blood supply and lead to nerve ending necrosis, which results in a more satisfactory analgesic effect [14].

Bone cement leakage and adjacent vertebral fractures are the common complications of PKP. Zhan et al. [15] concluded that the leakage rate of bone cement in PVP and PKP was 54.7% and 18.4%, respectively, through 22 meta-analyses of 2872 cases. Lieberman [16] reported 70 cases of PKP in 30 patients where the incidence of bone cement leakage was 8.6%. Xie et al. believed that the leakage of bone cement may be related to patient age, bone density, vertebral cortical defect, bone cement viscosity, bone cement injection speed, and time [17]. In our study, the bone cement leakage rate in group A (23.33%) was higher than that in group B (2.38%). There was a significant difference in the ratio of bone cement leakage between the two groups ($P < 0.05$). PIVR has a powerful distraction effect on collapsed vertebra. It promotes the reduction of the compressed height and increases the volume of the compressed bone tissue, restoring bone density of the compression zone to normal. The increase in bone tissue volume reduces the pressure during the injection of bone cement, which leads to a decrease in the bone cement leakage rate. Although the recovery of vertebral body stiffness is closely related to the amount of bone cement, it is controversial whether more bone cement injections will result in better treatment outcomes [18, 19]. Some scholars believe that excessive bone cement injection can cause fractures in adjacent vertebrae. Similarly, different scholars hold different perspectives on the factors that cause fractures in adjacent vertebral bodies [20–23]. Yang et al. [24] showed that the injection of a large amount of bone cement, bone cement leakage, and severe osteoporosis in patients were risk factors for adjacent vertebral fracture. In our study, there were no significant differences in the incidence of recurrent vertebral fractures between the two groups at the last follow-up ($P > 0.05$).

Considering that there may be a mechanical imbalance in unilateral distraction, this study specifically compared the improvement ratio of the height of the lateral wall of the vertebral body on the side of the restorer as compared with that of the non-distraction side, and the results showed that there was no statistically significant difference between the two sides (Table 3). There are three possible reasons. (1) Intraoperative adjustment was based on the reduction of the restorer. If the height of the non-distraction side was found to be poorly reset, the balloon should be inflated as much as possible to reduce the angulation of the vertebral body. In addition, if lateral compression of the vertebral body was found to be uneven intraoperatively, the severe side wall was selected to distract. (2) OVCFs were mostly low-energy injuries, even if they were unilaterally stretched, and the fractures were easily reset. (3) In the case that the middle and posterior columns were relatively intact, under the action of the tensile stress of the annulus fibrosus and the anterior and posterior longitudinal ligaments, the collapsed vertebral body was more evenly balanced; generally, no lateral angulation occurred.

PIVR combined with PKP should avoid the cutting effect of screws because of excessive distraction, which causes iatrogenic fractures. There were various reasons for the absence of iatrogenic vertebral fractures in group B. First, the process of resetting was under X-ray to observe whether there was a light zone between the screws and the vertebral body; the reset should be stopped immediately once a light zone is observed. Second, patients with severe osteoporosis ($T < -4.0$ SD) were not included in the study. Lastly, the sample size of this study was small, and more studies need to be conducted with PIVR to observe its complications.

There are some limitations in the application of PIVR combined with PKP. Only thoracic and lumbar segmental vertebral fractures can be treated because thoracic protection of the vertebrae above T10 is not required for reduction. The course of illness after injury is less than 3 weeks; otherwise, it is difficult to recover from surgery. The operation requires another two punctures in the adjacent vertebral body, which increases new trauma, but postoperative VAS did not show an increase in pain. For the case of multiple vertebral fractures, PIVR is difficult to operate, and multiple vertebral fractures require multiple operations. For patients with severe osteoporosis, the nail rod is easily made unstable, and the holding force of pedicle screws is insufficient; as a result, the effect of distraction is poor. Additionally, it is easy to form iatrogenic fractures due to the screw-cutting effects of severe osteoporosis.

Conclusion

PIVR has great fatigue performance regarding the biomechanics in PKP and can restore physiological curvature and mechanical strength of the spine effectively, overcoming the weaknesses of PKP restoring the vertebral height and easily losing the height of the vertebral body after withdrawal of the balloon. Especially for patients with significant compression of the vertebral body (more than 1/3), the effect of the surgery is obvious. PIVR can restore the vertebral fractures to a satisfactory height, effectively maintaining the stability of the spine and significantly improving the quality of life of patients. PIVR combined with PKP is a better treatment option.

Abbreviations

ODI: Oswestry Disability Index; OVCFs: Osteoporotic vertebral compression fractures; PIVR: Pedicle in vitro restorer; PKP: Percutaneous kyphoplasty; VAS: Visual analogue scale

Acknowledgements

We are grateful to Yan Ni from Nanjing First Hospital for her help in compiling the data from the patient records. And we thank the company named American Journal Experts for the language help on the manuscript.

Funding

This study was supported by a grant from the Nanjing Medical Science and Technology Development Project (Grant number YKK07028).

Authors' contributions

YZ and YQ were involved with the design of the research. DW and YZ performed all the surgeries. QW participated in the evaluations of clinical and radiographic parameters. JS and YQ assembled and analyzed the data. YQ wrote the manuscript. All authors read and approved the final manuscript.

Competing interests

The authors declare that they have no competing interests.

Author details

[1]Nanjing Medical University, Nanjing, China. [2]Department of Orthopaedic Surgery, Nanjing First Hospital, Nanjing Medical University, #68 Changle Rd, Qinhuai District, Nanjing 210000, Jiangsu, China.

References

1. Svensson HK, Olofsson EH, Karlsson J, et al. A painful, never ending story: older women's experiences of living with an osteoporotic vertebral compression fracture. Osteoporos Int. 2016;27(5):1729–36.
2. Boonen S, Wahl DA, Nauroy L, et al. Balloon kyphoplasty and vertebroplasty in the management of vertebral compression fractures. Osteoporos Int. 2011;22(12):2915–34.
3. He SC, Zhong BY, Zhu HD, et al. Percutaneous vertebroplasty for symptomatic Schmorl's nodes: 11 cases with long-term follow-up and a literature review. Pain Physician. 2017;20(2):69–76.
4. Klazen CA, Lohle PN, de Vries J, et al. Vertebroplasty versus conservative treatment in acute osteoporotic vertebral compression fractures (Vertos II): an open-label randomised trial. Lancet. 2010;376(9746):1085–92.
5. Kan SL, Yuan ZF, Chen LX, et al. Which is best for osteoporotic vertebral compression fractures: balloon kyphoplasty, percutaneous vertebroplasty or non-surgical treatment? A study protocol for a Bayesian network meta-analysis. BMJ Open. 2017;7(1):e012937.
6. Wang H, Sribastav SS, Ye F, et al. Comparison of pullout strength of the thoracic pedicle screw between intrapedicular and extrapedicular technique: a meta-analysis and literature review. Int J Clin Exp Med. 2015; 8(12):22237–45.
7. Lu J, Jiang G, Lu B, et al. The positive correlation between upper adjacent vertebral fracture and the kyphosis angle of injured vertebral body after percutaneous kyphoplasty: an in vitro study. Clin Neurol Neurosurg. 2015; 139:272–7.
8. Zhang L, Wang JC, Feng XM, et al. Pedicle screw fixation combined with vertebroplasty for single-level thoracolumbar osteoporotic burst fractures. Chinese Journal of Tissue Engineering Research. 2014;78(77):2722–7.
9. Nakashima H, Kawakami N, Tsuji T, et al. Adjacent segment disease after posterior lumbar interbody fusion: based on cases with a minimum of 10 years of follow-up. J.Spine(Phila Pa 1976). 2015;40(14):831–41.
10. Feldmann I, List T, Feldmann H, et al. Pain intensity and discomfort following surgical placement of orthodontic anchoring units and premolar extraction: a randomized controlled trial. Angle Orthod. 2007;77(4):578–85.
11. Shah S, Balaganapathy M. Reliability and validity study of the Gujarati version of the Oswestry Disability Index 2.1a. J Back Musculoskelet Rehabil. 2017;30(5):1103–9.
12. Bonnard E, Foti P, Kastler A, et al. Percutaneous vertebroplasty under local anaesthesia: feasibility regarding patients' experience. Eur Radiol. 2017;27(4): 1512–6.
13. Hashimoto T, Kaneda K, Abumi K. Relationship between traumatic spinal canal stenosis and neurologic deficits in thoracolumbar burst fractures. Spine (Phila Pa 1976). 1988;13(11):1268–72.
14. Tekaya R, Yaich S, Rajhi H, et al. Percutaneous vertebroplasty for pain relief in patients with osteoporotic spine fractures. Tunis Med. 2012;90(5):370–4.
15. Zhan Y, Jiang J, Liao H, et al. Risk factors for cement leakage after vertebroplasty or kyphoplasty: a meta-analysis of published evidence. World Neurosurg. 2017;101:633–42.
16. Lieberman IH, Dudeney S, Reinhardt MK, et al. Initial outcome and efficacy of "kyphoplasty" in the treatment of painful osteoporotic vertebral compression fractures. Spine (Phila Pa 1976). 2001;26(14):1631–8.
17. Xie W, Jin D, Ma H, et al. Cement leakage in percutaneous vertebral augmentation for osteoporotic vertebral compression fractures: analysis of risk factors. Clin Spine Surg. 2016;29(4):E171–6.
18. Liebschner MA, Rosenberg WS, Keaveny TM. Effects of bone cement volume and distribution on vertebral stiffness after vertebroplasty. Spine (Phila Pa 1976). 2001;26(14):1547–54.
19. Li YA, Lin CL, Chang MC, et al. Subsequent vertebral fracture after vertebroplasty: incidence and analysis of risk factors. Spine (Phila Pa 1976). 2012;37(3):179–83.
20. Syed MI, Patel NA, Jan S, et al. New symptomatic vertebral compression fractures within a year following vertebroplasty in osteoporotic women. AJNR Am J Neuroradiol. 2005;26(6):1601–4.
21. Yoo CM, Park KB, Hwang SH, et al. The analysis of patterns and risk factors of newly developed vertebral compression fractures after percutaneous vertebroplasty. J Korean Neurosurg Soc. 2012;52(4):339–45.
22. Lu K, Liang CL, Hsieh CH, et al. Risk factors of subsequent vertebral compression fractures after vertebroplasty. Pain Med. 2012;13(3):376–82.
23. Villarraga ML, Bellezza AJ, Harrigan TP, et al. The biomechanical effects of kyphoplasty on treated and adjacent nontreated vertebral bodies. J Spinal Disord Tech. 2005;18(1):84–91.
24. Yang S, Liu Y, Yang H, et al. Risk factors and correlation of secondary adjacent vertebral compression fracture in percutaneous kyphoplasty. Int J Surg. 2016;36(Pt A):138–42.

24

Using anatomical landmarks to calculate the normal joint line position in Chinese people: an observational study

Aoyuan Fan[1,2], Tianyang Xu[1,2], Xifan Li[2,3], Lei Li[1,4], Lin Fan[1,2], Dong Yang[1,2] and Guodong Li[1,2*]

Abstract

Background: Restoring the normal joint line (JL) is an important goal to achieve in total knee arthroplasty (TKA). We intended to study the veracity of several landmarks used to level the normal JL in Chinese people.

Methods: Two hundred fifteen standard CT scans of knee joint were included to measure the distances from landmarks to distal JL (DJL) and posterior JL (PJL), along with femoral width (FW) in order to calculate the ratios. Landmarks included adductor tubercle (AT), medial epicondyle (ME), lateral epicondyle (LE), tibial tubercle (TT), fibular head (FH) and the inferior pole of the patella (IPP). Ratios were calculated between distances and FW (e.g. FHDJL/FW). Linear regression analysis and t test were used to determine the accuracy and the differences amongst sides of the leg, genders and races.

Results: The average of IPPDJL/FW, TTDJL/FW, FHDJL/FW, LEDJL/FW, LEPJL/FW, MEDJL/FW, MEPJL/FW, ATDJL/FW and ATPJL/FW were 0.165, 0.295, 0.232, 0.297, 0.281, 0.327, 0.3PJL, 0.558 and 0.313, respectively. No significant difference had been found between the left and right leg. A gender difference was only found statistically on the ratio of IPP, and also, no linear correlation was observed only between IPP and FW. Most of the difference values lain in a 4-mm threshold for MEDJL (95.81%), LEDJL (94.88%), MEPJL (97.21%), LEPJL (94.88%), ATPJL (93.49%) and ATDJL (100%). Significant differences were observed amongst different races.

Conclusions: AT, ME and LE can be used as reliable landmarks to locate the normal JL in Chinese population intraoperatively. It is meaningful to come up with a set of ratios to different races.

Keywords: Knee joint line position, Total knee arthroplasty, Landmark, Computed tomography, Chinese population

Background

Restoring the normal joint line (JL) is an important yet challenging goal for surgeons to achieve in total knee arthroplasty (TKA) [1]. Malposition of the JL in the coronal plane happened frequently to primary and especially revision TKAs [2]. That malposition could cause relatively patella alta or patella baja [3], which may lead to unpleasant clinic outcomes. Researches showed that coronal changes of JL position may alter the patellar strain and the patellofemoral contact forces [3, 4]. Even 4–8 mm

elevation or descent to the normal JL position could generate midrange flexion laxity, decrease to the patellofemoral contact area, which may lead to a lower total range of movement, postoperative knee pain, premature component wear and lower Knee Society Score [1, 5–8]. These outcomes may result in another revision TKA.

Anatomical landmarks such as adductor tubercle, medial epicondyle and lateral epicondyle were studied previously by many investigators. The absolute distances were measured from landmarks to JL, yet the distances may bias by different genders, heights or races [9]. In order to avoid those deviations, researchers began to use the ratios of absolute distances and femoral width [10]. Studies showed no statistical difference in ratios of different genders and heights [10, 11], yet we still need diverse ratios for various races. Literatures had proved

---

* Correspondence: litrue2004@163.com

Aoyuan Fan, Tianyang Xu and Xifan Li are co-first authors.

Aoyuan Fan, Tianyang Xu and Xifan Li are contributed equally to this work.

[1]Department of Orthopedics, Shanghai Tenth People's Hospital of Tongji University, 301 Yanchang Rd, Shanghai 200072, China

[2]Tongji University School of Medicine, Shanghai, China

Full list of author information is available at the end of the article

that the Chinese population showed a modicum of anatomical difference [12–14], yet no study fully analyzes the usage of landmarks in the Chinese population.

With the benefits of ratios, studies showed a slight difference between different races [9, 15]. And several studies have already proved the distinction between the Chinese population and other countries [12–14]. Nevertheless, to our knowledge, no accuracy comparison amongst those osteal anatomical landmarks in Chinese population using computed tomography (CT) scan was published before. The purposes of our study were to (1) verify the non-gender otherness of ratios to Chinese people and compare whether left or right knee biased the ratios, (2) compare the accuracy of these landmarks in Chinese population, (3) provide ratios for surgeons to calculate the distance from several landmarks to JL and verify these veracity and (4) look out whether there is a difference amongst Chinese and other different races.

Methods

A total of 215 standard CT scans(GE Medical Systems/ LightSpeed VCT, Siemens, New York, USA) of knee joint from 194 patients(102 male and 92 female) examined in our hospital from January 2013 to July 2017 were collected in this study. No CT was performed solely for our study and no information which could be used to identify the patient was collected in our study. Our study was approved by the institutional review board of Shanghai Tenth Hospital Affiliated to Tongji University. CT scans that showed evidence of knee fracture, history of knee surgery, degeneration or malformation was excluded. Imaging data was derived from the PACS system along with patients' age and gender. Patients younger than 18 or older than 40 years old were excluded from our study (average 30.56). Distances were measured by mimics 17.0 and analyzed by SPSS 20.0.

JL was defined as the tangent that connects two most distal points of the femoral condyles, but we used a plane to represent the JL so that measurement could take place on three-dimensional reconstruction. During measurements, we created a plane (distal JL, DJL) that crossed the JL and was vertical to the coronal plane as a reference to JL at full extension of the leg. We then created a plane (posterior JL, PJL) that is vertical to DJL and cross the two most posterior points of the femoral condyles as the reference to femoral JL under PJL degrees flexion of the knee for femoral landmarks. Selected anatomical landmarks were adductor tubercle (AT), medial epicondyle (ME), lateral epicondyle (LE), tibial tubercle (TT), fibular head (FH) and the inferior pole of the patella (IPP) (Fig. 1). In order to gather more accurate data, we came up with a bunch of methods based on previous researches [9, 16] and our pre-measurement. AT was measured at its most anterior and medial point where adductor muscle contacted with bone, which can be identified with the coronal plane reconstruction of the CT data. ME and LE were identified as the most prominent point of medial and lateral epicondyle, which can be located on transverse sections of CT. And landmarks were verified on computer-aided design (CAD) model created by three-dimensional reconstruction again (Fig. 1). TT is a rather large landmark, so after the pre-measurement, we decided to use the most proximal point of the slope of TT (Fig. 1). FH and IPP were measured on the most superior and inferior point and were easy to identify with the CAD model on three-dimensional reconstruction (Fig. 1). The perpendicular lines made from those landmarks to DJL were measured as the distance (mm), marked as ATDJL, MEDJL, LEDJL, TTDJL, FHDJL and IPPDJL. And we only measured the perpendicular distances from femoral landmarks to PJL, marked as ATPJL, MEPJL and LEPJL. The distance between the most prominent points of medial and lateral epicondyles was defined as the femoral width (FW). The ratios of distances between the landmarks to JL and FW were calculated respectively. We randomly chose 40 CT scans to measured the distances twice (day 1 and 2 weeks later) by two observers so as to determine

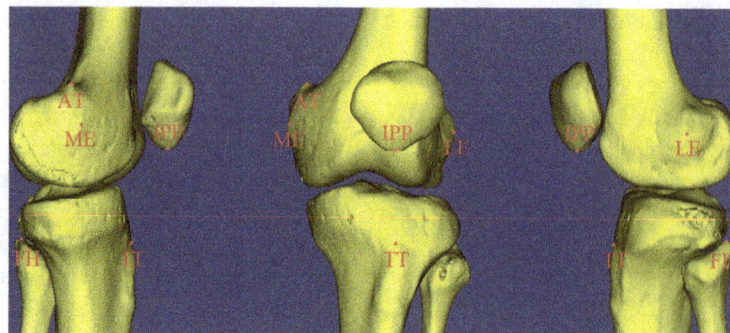

Fig. 1 Positions of the knee joint landmarks. Landmarks were marked and verified on three-dimensional reconstruction. AT adductor tubercle, ME medial epicondyle, LE lateral epicondyle, TT tibial tubercle, FH fibular head, IPP the inferior pole of the patella

intraobserver and interobserver variability before the measurements of all patients took place.

Statistical analysis

Firstly, we used the data of those who underwent bilateral CT scan to determine whether there's a difference between the two sides of the leg by paired t test. And then amongst all data, the unpaired t test was used to determine the difference between different genders and sides of leg again. Linear regression analysis was performed between FW and those distances separately. The average ratios were used to estimate the distance (e.g. ATDJL), and the difference value between the measured distance and estimate distance was calculated to verify the veracity of those ratios. Moreover, our data were compared with other investigators to determine the difference between Chinese and other populations using Student's t test. A p value < 0.05 was considered statistically significant in this study.

Results

Intraobserver and interobserver variability

The measurements amongst intraobserver and interobserver did not statistically differ, demonstrating the methods' reproducibility (Tables 1 and 2).

Measured distances

Mean measurements of FW and the distances from landmarks to JL were given in Table 3. Measurements from different genders or sides of the leg were listed in Tables 3, 4 and 5 respectively. Data of both 21 patients who underwent bilateral knee CT scan and all 215 CT scans (116 left and 99 right) showed that there is no significant difference between the left and right legs on all the measurements (Tables 4 and 5). Compared with all the distances, the statistical difference had been found amongst different genders for except IPPDJL ($p = 0.916$).

Ratios

The average ratios of all data and different genders were given in Table 6. No gender-specific difference had been found apart from IPPDJL/FW ($p = 0.008$).

Linear regression analysis

ATDJL showed the best linear co-relationship with FW ($R^2 = 0.8205$), followed by MEDJL ($R^2 = 0.5544$) and LEDJL ($R^2 = 0.5015$). As for PJL degrees flexion of the knee, MEPJL showed the best linear co-relationship with FW ($R^2 = 0.6422$), followed by ATPJL ($R^2 = 0.4193$) and LEPJL ($R^2 = 0.4049$). A not good co-relationship was showed for TTDJL ($R^2 = 0.2438$) and FHDJL ($R^2 = 0.1003$). No co-relationship between IPPDJL and FW had been found ($p = 0.3746$) (Fig. 2).

Estimated distances

All difference values between measured distances and estimated distances from reliable landmarks (LE, ME, AT) lain in a 8-mm threshold, except for one value from MEPJL (99.53%). Most of the difference values lain in a 4-mm threshold for MEDJL (95.81%), LEDJL (94.88%), MEPJL (97.21%), LEPJL (94.88%) and ATPJL (93.49%) except for ATDJL (100%) (Fig. 3).

Difference between races

Ratios from different races were listed in Table 7. Unpaired t test was used to verify the differences between Chinese and other races and the results showed significant differences between the Chinese and other countries' researches ($p < 0.001$). No statistical difference has been found amongst the Chinese population when compared with another research based on Chinese people.

Discussion

The current study gave answers as follows: (1) no side of the leg difference lain in these methods of determining

Table 1 Intraobserver measurements

	Measurements at day 1 ($n = 40$) (mm)	Measurements at day 14 ($n = 40$) (mm)	p
FW	82.39 ± 6.37	82.43 ± 6.33	0.668
IPPDJL	12.68 ± 6.55	12.88 ± 6.76	0.420
TTDJL	25.16 ± 2.68	25.06 ± 2.64	0.086
FHDJL	18.54 ± 4.25	18.85 ± 3.94	0.134
LEDJL	24.59 ± 2.87	24.70 ± 2.79	0.504
LEPJL	23.28 ± 2.29	23.44 ± 2.20	0.256
MEDJL	27.32 ± 2.71	27.48 ± 2.49	0.444
MEPJL	32.11 ± 2.63	32.15 ± 2.41	0.780
ATDJL	45.40 ± 3.36	44.86 ± 4.21	0.328
ATPJL	26.32 ± 2.18	26.20 ± 2.2	0.428

FW femoral width, *AT* adductor tubercle, *ME* medial epicondyle, *LE* lateral epicondyle, *TT* tibial tubercle, *FH* fibular head, *IPP* the inferior pole of the patella, *DJL* distance from landmarks to the distal joint line, *PJL* distance from landmarks to posterior joint line

Table 2 Interobserver measurements

	First measurer ($n = 40$) (mm)	Second measurer ($n = 40$) (mm)	p
FW	82.79 ± 6.26	82.63 ± 6.44	0.883
IPPDJL	11.59 ± 6.83	13.58 ± 6.31	0.245
TTDJL	25.23 ± 2.56	25.19 ± 2.76	0.739
FHDJL	18.07 ± 4.18	18.71 ± 3.99	0.432
LEDJL	24.96 ± 2.42	25.13 ± 3.18	0.787
LEPJL	23.28 ± 2.24	23.03 ± 2.24	0.497
MEDJL	27.82 ± 2.92	27.17 ± 2.19	0.253
MEPJL	32.31 ± 2.56	32.15 ± 2.49	0.702
ATDJL	45.59 ± 3.25	45.68 ± 4.30	0.902
ATPJL	26.41 ± 2.32	26.71 ± 2.09	0.396

FW femoral width, *AT* adductor tubercle, *ME* medial epicondyle, *LE* lateral epicondyle, *TT* tibial tubercle, *FH* fibular head, *IPP* the inferior pole of the patella, *DJL* distance from landmarks to the distal joint line, *PJL* distance from landmarks to posterior joint line

JL positions amongst Chinese people, and gender differences were not found to be significant (except for IPP). (2) AT may be the best landmark to locate JL positions at full extension with the ratio of 0.558 in the Chinese population followed by ME (0.327) and LE (0.297). As for PJL degrees flexion, ME (0.390) may be the best choice for Chinese people followed by AT (0.313) and LE (0.281). (3) There are significant differences between the ratios of the Chinese population and other races.

Although restoring normal JL is necessary for either primary and revision TKAs, there is still no consensus on how to approach the normal JL [9]. During primary TKAs, surgeons could estimate the normal JL position based on the thickness of the femoral osteotomy. But when it comes to revision TKAs, normal anatomy had already been affected by primary TKA so surgeons cannot directly use the tangent line of the distal medial and lateral femoral condyles as JL. Leveling the position of the femoral prosthesis from primary TKA intraoperatively is inappropriate by reasons for loosening or the

situation that JL position was already altered in primary TKA, which happened a lot [2]. Additionally, with the help of probably bone loss while removing the components from primary TKA or two stages of revision TKA after infection, reliable references to locate JL is needed during revision TKA. Using anatomical landmarks to locate JL position is well accepted during clinical practice [10]. Landmarks can be divided into two kinds, osteal landmarks and soft tissue landmarks. Soft tissue landmarks such as meniscal scar can be variable and not so distinct intraoperatively [17], whereas osteal landmarks are more reliable during surgery. Famously used osteal landmarks included adductor tubercle, medial and lateral epicondyles, tibial tubercle, fibular head and inferior patellar pole [10, 16, 18]. Surgeons can evaluate these landmarks in imageological examinations preoperatively and palpation intraoperatively.

With the help of those reliable landmarks, surgeons can measure the distance between the landmarks and JL from imageological examinations taken before the

Table 3 Mean measurements and gender difference

	Total ($n = 215$) (mm)	Male ($n = 110$) (mm)	Female ($n = 105$) (mm)	p
FW	79.61 ± 6.60	85.05 ± 3.84	73.92 ± 3.19	< 0.001
IPPDJL	13.04 ± 5.16	13.01 ± 5.90	13.08 ± 4.26	0.916
TTDJL	23.45 ± 3.74	25.32 ± 3.90	21.50 ± 2.31	< 0.001
FHDJL	18.48 ± 3.89	19.59 ± 4.34	17.32 ± 2.95	< 0.001
LEDJL	23.62 ± 2.70	25.12 ± 2.43	22.05 ± 1.97	< 0.001
LEPJL	22.37 ± 2.58	23.80 ± 2.31	20.86 ± 1.92	< 0.001
MEDJL	26.04 ± 2.83	27.65 ± 2.42	24.34 ± 2.18	< 0.001
MEPJL	31.05 ± 2.99	33.08 ± 2.26	28.93 ± 2.03	< 0.001
ATDJL	44.40 ± 3.76	47.39 ± 2.41	41.27 ± 1.91	< 0.001
ATPJL	24.89 ± 2.89	26.39 ± 2.64	23.31 ± 2.23	< 0.001

p was compared between genders

FW femoral width, *AT* adductor tubercle, *ME* medial epicondyle, *LE* lateral epicondyle, *TT* tibial tubercle, *FH* fibular head, *IPP* the inferior pole of the patella, *DJL* distance from landmarks to the distal joint line, *PJL* distance from landmarks to posterior joint line

Table 4 Mean measurements of 21 bilateral CT and sides of leg difference

	Total (n = 42) (mm)	Left (n = 21) (mm)	Right (n = 21) (mm)	p
FW	78.16 ± 5.71	78.07 ± 5.68	78.24 ± 5.88	0.338
IPPDJL	12.19 ± 4.59	12.36 ± 4.96	12.02 ± 4.31	0.602
TTDJL	21.12 ± 1.85	21.10 ± 1.90	21.15 ± 1.84	0.889
FHDJL	16.74 ± 3.80	16.84 ± 3.66	16.63 ± 4.03	0.526
LEDJL	22.74 ± 2.39	22.45 ± 2.50	23.04 ± 2.30	0.268
LEPJL	21.18 ± 2.41	21.10 ± 2.48	21.26 ± 2.39	0.640
MEDJL	25.40 ± 2.95	25.19 ± 3.28	25.61 ± 2.64	0.506
MEPJL	30.28 ± 2.42	30.19 ± 2.55	30.38 ± 2.34	0.421
ATDJL	43.18 ± 3.26	43.19 ± 3.38	43.16 ± 3.23	0.880
ATPJL	24.47 ± 2.54	24.57 ± 2.48	24.37 ± 2.66	0.367

p was compared between sides of the leg

FW femoral width, AT adductor tubercle, ME medial epicondyle, LE lateral epicondyle, TT tibial tubercle, FH fibular head, IPP the inferior pole of he patella, DJL distance from landmarks to the distal joint line, PJL distance from landmarks to posterior joint line

primary TKA, or from the contralateral knee if it is still intact with no TKA or fracture. But apparently, the usage of this method is limited when the images of previous examinations could not be found. Several credos like "two fingerbreadths of the tibial tubercle", "20 mm above the fibular head" and "at the inferior patellar pole in extension" were used by some surgeons [19, 20], but with no literature to support those. And with the concept of slight changes in JL position could cause much worse outcomes in mind [3, 19, 20], these credos are too obscure to be used intraoperatively. So, we call for accurate methods that can apply to mostly (hopefully all) of the knee undergoing revision TKA. In order to achieve that goal, several studies measure the absolute distance from landmarks to JL [18, 21], but their results showed a variation in different ages, genders, body mass indices and races [10, 16, 18]. Servien et al. described a ratio between FW and the distances from LE or ME to JL and discovered a much smaller variation [10]. The usage of ratio had been proved to be more reliable [22]

and negate those variations caused by age, body mass index and gender and showed reproducibility both from imageological examinations and intraoperative measurements [11, 23, 24]. However, differences still exist between different races, and previous studies had shown differences in anatomy between Chinese people and others [12–14]. Under this circumstance, we decided to provide methods to locate JL position in TKAs that suit the Chinese population.

The reason we chose CT scans for this study was that we could do the measurement based on a CAD model created by three-dimensional reconstruction, which should be the most similar way using imageological examination to stimulate measurement intraoperatively. Although researches showed no difference in radiographic MRI and CT measurements [25, 26], we preferred measuring the distance from the CAD model better. Based on our experiences with those measurements, landmarks may not lie in the same plane that parallels to the coronal plane according to JL. Under this

Table 5 Mean measurements of all CT and sides of leg difference

	Total (n = 215) (mm)	Left (n = 116) (mm)	Right (n = 99) (mm)	p
FW	79.61 ± 6.60	79.72 ± 6.99	79.49 ± 6.15	0.793
IPPDJL	13.04 ± 5.16	13.18 ± 5.18	12.88 ± 5.15	0.676
TTDJL	23.45 ± 3.74	23.52 ± 3.50	23.38 ± 4.02	0.787
FHDJL	18.48 ± 3.89	18.58 ± 3.82	18.36 ± 3.98	0.685
LEDJL	23.62 ± 2.70	23.82 ± 2.86	23.38 ± 2.49	0.223
LEPJL	22.37 ± 2.58	22.53 ± 2.79	22.18 ± 2.31	0.309
MEDJL	26.04 ± 2.83	26.01 ± 3.09	26.07 ± 2.51	0.862
MEPJL	31.05 ± 2.99	31.04 ± 3.19	31.07 ± 2.74	0.940
ATDJL	44.40 ± 3.76	44.72 ± 3.91	44.03 ± 3.57	0.177
ATPJL	24.89 ± 2.89	25.01 ± 2.92	24.75 ± 2.87	0.514

p was compared between sides of the leg

FW femoral width, AT adductor tubercle, ME medial epicondyle, LE lateral epicondyle, TT tibial tubercle, FH fibular head, IPP the inferior pole of the patella, DJL distance from landmarks to the distal joint line, PJL distance from landmarks to posterior joint line

Table 6 Mean ratios and gender difference

	Total ($n = 215$)	Male ($n = 110$)	Female ($n = 105$)	p
IPPDJL/FW	*0.165 ± 0.066*	*0.154 ± 0.071*	*0.177 ± 0.058*	*0.008*
TTDJL/FW	0.295 ± 0.040	0.298 ± 0.047	0.291 ± 0.031	0.199
FHDJL/FW	0.232 ± 0.046	0.231 ± 0.051	0.234 ± 0.040	0.526
LEDJL/FW	0.297 ± 0.024	0.295 ± 0.024	0.298 ± 0.024	0.371
LEPJL/FW	0.281 ± 0.025	0.280 ± 0.025	0.282 ± 0.025	0.464
MEDJL/FW	0.327 ± 0.024	0.325 ± 0.024	0.329 ± 0.024	0.209
MEPJL/FW	0.390 ± 0.022	0.389 ± 0.022	0.391 ± 0.023	0.431
ATDJL/FW	0.558 ± 0.020	0.557 ± 0.021	0.559 ± 0.019	0.710
ATPJL/FW	0.313 ± 0.028	0.310 ± 0.029	0.315 ± 0.026	0.203

p was compared between genders

FW femoral width, *AT* adductor tubercle, *ME* medial epicondyle, *LE* lateral epicondyle, *TT* tibial tubercle, *FH* fibular head, *IPP* the inferior pole of the patella, *DJL* distance from landmarks to the distal joint line, *PJL* distance from landmarks to posterior joint line

circumstance, measurements took place on MRI may not be equal to the real distances. No statistical difference had been found amongst the measurements of intraobserver and interobserver (Tables 1 and 2), demonstrating the methods' reproducibility. As for ratios calculation, some researchers may prefer femoral diameter rather than FW [24]. However, research based on Chinese population showed that FW had a better linear correlation with ATDJL than femoral diameter [14], so we decided to use FW to calculate the ratios.

No difference was found between distances between the left and right knee amongst bilateral CT scan and total samples. Our results came in line with Havet et al. [18]. By the help of this statistical evidence, the measurement could be used in revision TKAs while the contralateral knee is free from TKA, fracture or osteoarthritis.

Gender differences were found to be significant on absolute distances except for IPPDJL, taking together with

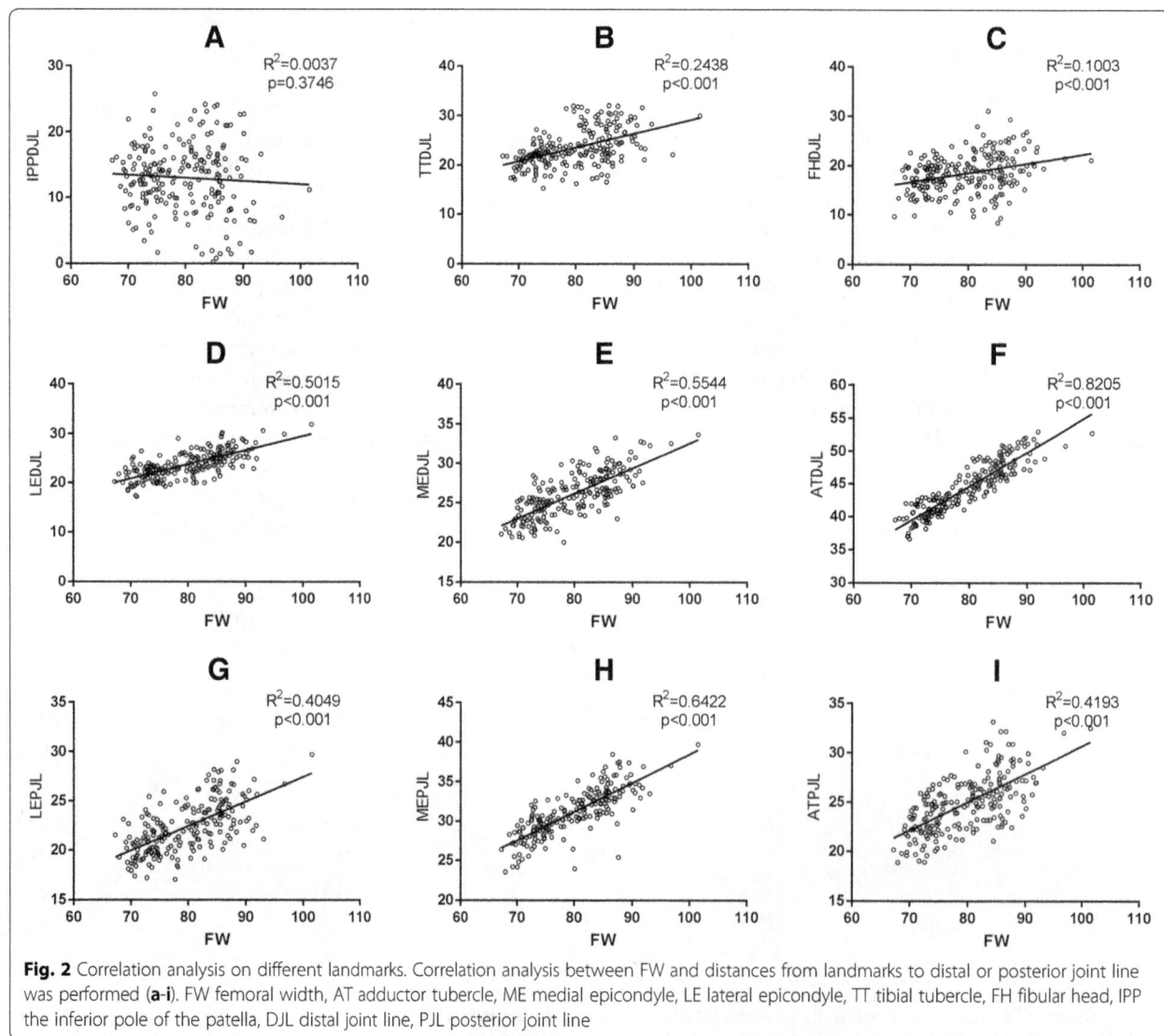

Fig. 2 Correlation analysis on different landmarks. Correlation analysis between FW and distances from landmarks to distal or posterior joint line was performed (**a-i**). FW femoral width, AT adductor tubercle, ME medial epicondyle, LE lateral epicondyle, TT tibial tubercle, FH fibular head, IPP the inferior pole of the patella, DJL distal joint line, PJL posterior joint line

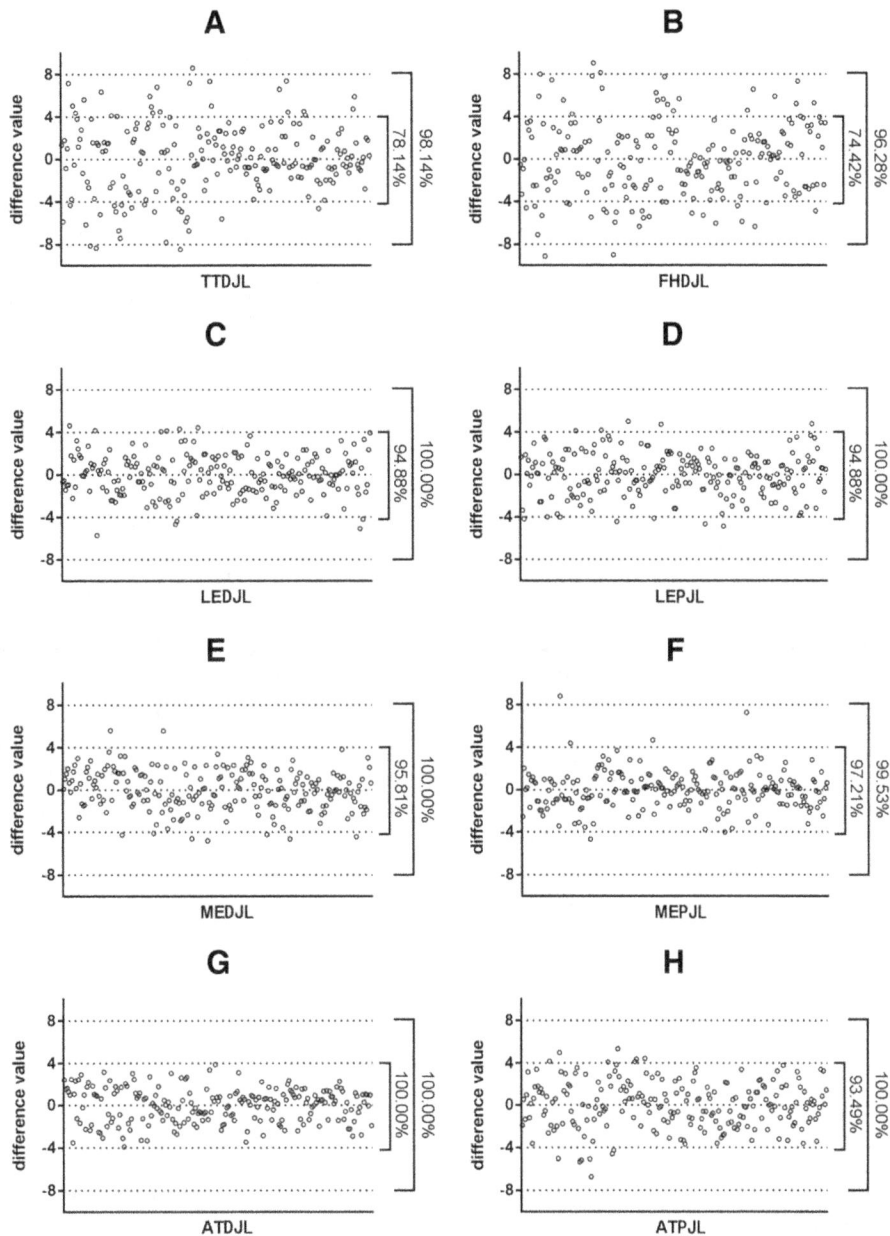

Fig. 3 Difference between the measured distance and the estimated distance calculated by ratios. Difference values between the measured distance from landmarks to the joint line, and the estimated distance calculated from FW and mean ratios were calculated. Percentages of difference value within 4 mm or 8 mm were given on the graphs (**a-h**). FW femoral width, AT adductor tubercle, ME medial epicondyle, LE lateral epicondyle, TT tibial tubercle, FH fibular head, IPP the inferior pole of the patella, DJL distal joint line, PJL posterior joint line

statistical gender difference in the ratio of IPPDJL, which may probably be explained by the variability of patella position [3, 4, 27]. In this case, we believed that IPP may not be a good reference to locate JL in the Chinese population. Most of the other researches showed no gender discrepancy in ratios of landmarks and JL [10, 11]. We came in line with those researchers. There is still a need for further research to rectify our results.

AT is the attachment point of the adductor muscle and is easy to be found during revision surgeries. Iacono et al.

firstly used AT as landmarks to determine the JL and demonstrate its repeatability and accuracy preoperatively and intro-operatively [16, 28]. Recently, Xiao et al. proved that AT is a reliable landmark in the Chinese population [14]. In our study, we drew the same conclusion. ATDJL/FW showed the highest R^2 (0.8205) above all those landmarks, which indicates AT may be the most precise landmarks in locating JL on full extension knee in Chinese people. Putting these all together, AT may be the first choice for surgeons to determine the level of the JL.

Table 7 Ratios difference on races

	Our data ($n = 215$)	Servien et al. [10]	Ozkurt et al. [11]	Luyckx et al. [31]	Iacono et al. [28]	Xiao et al. [14]
TTDJL/FW	0.295 ± 0.040	0.27 ± 0.03				
LEDJL/FW	0.297 ± 0.024	0.28 ± 0.02	0.28 ± 0.02	0.32 ± 0.029		
LEPJL/FW	0.281 ± 0.025	0.29 ± 0.03	0.29 ± 0.03			
MEDJL/FW	0.327 ± 0.024	0.34 ± 0.02	0.35 ± 0.03	0.32 ± 0.027		
MEPJL/FW	0.390 ± 0.022	0.34 ± 0.03	0.34 ± 0.02			
ATDJL/FW	0.558 ± 0.020			0.52 ± 0.029	0.53 ± 0.03	0.56 ± 0.03

p was compared between ratios from different races. The significant difference had been found except for the ratio from the study of Xiao et al
FW femoral width, *AT* adductor tubercle, *ME* medial epicondyle, *LE* lateral epicondyle, *TT* tibial tubercle, *FH* fibular head, *IPP* the inferior pole of the patella, *DJL* distance from landmarks to the distal joint line, *PJL* distance from landmarks to posterior joint line

ME and LE had been used for years as landmarks in researches [2, 19]. Researchers used the most prominent point of the LE to measure the distance but as for ME, there are two methods. One is the most prominent point of medial epicondyle while the other is the sulcus of the medial epicondyle. The sulcus of medial epicondyle may be less accurate in an arthritic deformed knee [29], so we chose to use the most prominent point. In another way, we believed that the most prominent point may be easier to locate and more accurate during palpation intro-operatively. Our data showed ME and LE are less precise than AT based on relatively lower R^2, but still they had a relatively strong correlation amongst distances to distal JL and FW in the Chinese population. These results are consistent with previous researches [9, 16]. Hence, ME and LE may serve as second choices while AT is not available.

TT is the attachment point of the patellar tendon and is palpable during surgery. Many investigators have studied this landmark and came out with different conclusions. Servien et al. [10] believed that TT is a precise landmark while as Bieger et al. [22] and Mason et al. [19] hold discordant thoughts. In normal Chinese population, our data revealed $R^2 = 0.2438$, which means that TT may not be a preferred landmark to level the distal normal JL. Nevertheless, TT is more like a small area rather than a precise point due to the cover of the patellar tendon, which undoubtedly limited its usage.

FH may not be a precise landmark in locating femoral JL, which had been proved by several investigators recently [15, 18]. In Chinese people, FH may not serve as a reliable landmark either ($R^2 = 0.1003$). Otherwise, the anatomical position of the FH is always various [10] and untouchable during revision surgeries unless surgeons would like to take the risk of damaging the surrounding structure, not alone primary TKA.

During revision TKAs, surgeons always need to locate the tibial JL at PJL degrees first. In our study, with the difficulty to get CT data while knee joint is in PJL degrees flexion, we decided to use posterior femoral JL to represent tibial JL just like other researchers did [10, 11].

Regression analyses based on our data showed that AT, ME and LE have good pertinence during the leveling of the PJL degrees flexion JL. No study reported the usage to locate the posterior JL by the help of AT, but investigators had already proved that ME and LE can be used to level the posterior JL amongst other races [10, 11]. We held the same thoughts with these investigators.

JL positions altered within 4–8 mm may lead to post-operative complications like pain or lack of range of movement [5, 8, 30]. In order to further verify the accuracy of those landmarks, we used the ratios and FW to calculate the distance between JL and those landmarks. And if the deviations from one landmark are within 8 mm, 4 mm even better, then this landmark should be considered accurate. After data processing, using ratios of AT to calculate JL position proved to be the most accurate method of Chinese people. Other landmarks (ME and LE) could satisfy the surgical need in most situations.

When compared with the ratios of other races' researches, significant differences had been found amongst our data based on the Chinese population and other races' data [10, 11, 14, 28, 31]. Otherwise, we found no statistical difference that exists on our data onto ATDJL and ratios from Xiao et al. based on the Chinese population. In a way, our data may prove that it is necessary to come up with a set of ratios for different races.

Conclusions

Our study has demonstrated that AT, ME and LE can be used as veracity and reliable landmarks to locate the normal JL. Differences should be noticed between different races, and it may serve better effect using ratios based on the Chinese population when TKA was operated on Chinese people.

Abbreviations

AT: Adductor tubercle; CT: Computed tomography; FH: Fibular head; FW: Femoral width; IPP: The inferior pole of the patella; JL: Joint line; LE: Lateral epicondyle; ME: Medial epicondyle; TKA: Total knee arthroplasty; TT: Tibial tubercle

Authors' contributions

AYF and GDL conceived and designed the study. TYX and XFL collected and processed the data. AYF and TYX wrote the paper. AYF, TYX, LL, LF and DY reviewed and edited the manuscript. All authors read and approved the final manuscript.

Competing interests

The authors declare that they have no competing interests.

Author details

[1]Department of Orthopedics, Shanghai Tenth People's Hospital of Tongji University, 301 Yanchang Rd, Shanghai 200072, China. [2]Tongji University School of Medicine, Shanghai, China. [3]Department of Radiology, Shanghai Tenth People's Hospital of Tongji University, Shanghai, China. [4]Department of Neurosurgery, Shanghai Tenth People's Hospital of Tongji University, Shanghai, China.

References

1. Clave A, Le Henaff G, Roger T, Maisongrosse P, Mabit C, Dubrana F. Joint line level in revision total knee replacement: assessment and functional results with an average of seven years follow-up. Int Orthop. 2016;40(8):1655–62. https://doi.org/10.1007/s00264-015-3096-9.
2. Romero J, Seifert B, Reinhardt O, Ziegler O, Kessler O. A useful radiologic method for preoperative joint-line determination in revision total knee arthroplasty. Clin Orthop Relat Res. 2010;468(5):1279–83. https://doi.org/10.1007/s11999-009-1114-1.
3. Singerman R, Heiple KG, Davy DT, Goldberg VM. Effect of tibial component position on patellar strain following total knee arthroplasty. J Arthroplast. 1995;10(5):651–6.
4. Singerman R, Davy DT, Goldberg VM. Effects of patella alta and patella infera on patellofemoral contact forces. J Biomech. 1994;27(8):1059–65.
5. Martin JW, Whiteside LA. The influence of joint line position on knee stability after condylar knee arthroplasty. Clin Orthop Relat Res. 1990;259:146–56.
6. Fornalski S, McGarry MH, Bui CN, Kim WC, Lee TQ. Biomechanical effects of joint line elevation in total knee arthroplasty. Clin Biomech (Bristol, Avon). 2012;27(8):824–9. https://doi.org/10.1016/j.clinbiomech.2012.05.009.
7. Hofmann AA, Kurtin SM, Lyons S, Tanner AM, Bolognesi MP. Clinical and radiographic analysis of accurate restoration of the joint line in revision total knee arthroplasty. J Arthroplast. 2006;21(8):1154–62. https://doi.org/10.1016/j.arth.2005.10.026.
8. Partington PF, Sawhney J, Rorabeck CH, Barrack RL, Moore J. Joint line restoration after revision total knee arthroplasty. Clin Orthop Relat Res. 1999;367:165–71.
9. Pereira GC, von Kaeppler E, Alaia MJ, Montini K, Lopez MJ, Di Cesare PE, Amanatullah DF. Calculating the position of the joint line of the knee using anatomical landmarks. Orthopedics. 2016;39(6):381–6. https://doi.org/10.3928/01477447-20160729-01.
10. Servien E, Viskontas D, Giuffre BM, Coolican MR, Parker DA. Reliability of bony landmarks for restoration of the joint line in revision knee arthroplasty. Knee Surg Sports Traumatol Arthrosc. 2008;16(3):263–9. https://doi.org/10.1007/s00167-007-0449-y.
11. Ozkurt B, Sen T, Cankaya D, Kendir S, Basarir K, Tabak Y. The medial and lateral epicondyle as a reliable landmark for intra-operative joint line determination in revision knee arthroplasty. Bone Joint Res. 2016;5(7):280–6. https://doi.org/10.1302/2046-3758.57.bjr-2016-0002.r1.
12. Tang Q, Zhou Y, Yang D, Tang J, Shao H. The knee joint line position measured from the tibial side in Chinese people. J Arthroplast. 2011;26(7):989–93. https://doi.org/10.1016/j.arth.2011.02.027.
13. Xiao JL, Zuo JL, Liu P, Qin YG, Li XZ, Liu T, Gao ZL. Cross-sectional anatomy of ilium for guiding acetabular component placement using high hip center technique in Asian population. Chin Med J. 2015;128(12):1579–83. https://doi.org/10.4103/0366-6999.158298.
14. Xiao J, Wang S, Chen W, Yang Y, Liu T, Zuo J. A study to assess the accuracy

15. of adductor tubercle as a reliable landmark used to determine the joint line of the knee in a Chinese population. J Arthroplast. 2017;32(4):1351–5. https://doi.org/10.1016/j.arth.2016.10.002.
15. Gurbuz H, Cakar M, Adas M, Tekin AC, Bayraktar MK, Esenyel CZ. Measurement of the knee joint line in Turkish population. Acta Orthop Traumatol Turc. 2015;49(1):41–4. https://doi.org/10.3944/aott.2015.14.0050.
16. Iacono F, Lo Presti M, Bruni D, Raspugli GF, Bignozzi S, Sharma B, Marcacci M. The adductor tubercle: a reliable landmark for analysing the level of the femorotibial joint line. Knee Surg Sports Traumatol Arthrosc. 2013;21(12):2725–9. https://doi.org/10.1007/s00167-012-2113-4.
17. Khan WS, Bhamra J, Williams R, Morgan-Jones R. "Meniscal" scar as a landmark for the joint line in revision total knee replacement. World J Orthop. 2017;8(1):57–61. https://doi.org/10.5312/wjo.v8.i1.57.
18. Havet E, Gabrion A, Leiber-Wackenheim F, Vernois J, Olory B, Mertl P. Radiological study of the knee joint line position measured from the fibular head and proximal tibial landmarks. Surg Radiol Anat. 2007;29(4):285–9. https://doi.org/10.1007/s00276-007-0207-3.
19. Mason M, Belisle A, Bonutti P, Kolisek FR, Malkani A, Masini M. An accurate and reproducible method for locating the joint line during a revision total knee arthroplasty. J Arthroplast. 2006;21(8):1147–53. https://doi.org/10.1016/j.arth.2005.08.028.
20. Laskin RS. Joint line position restoration during revision total knee replacement. Clin Orthop Relat Res. 2002;404:169–71.
21. Stiehl JB, Abbott BD. Morphology of the transepicondylar axis and its application in primary and revision total knee arthroplasty. J Arthroplast. 1995;10(6):785–9.
22. Bieger R, Huch K, Kocak S, Jung S, Reichel H, Kappe T. The influence of joint line restoration on the results of revision total knee arthroplasty: comparison between distance and ratio-methods. Arch Orthop Trauma Surg. 2014;134(4):537–41. https://doi.org/10.1007/s00402-014-1953-4.
23. Rajagopal TS, Nathwani D. Can interepicondylar distance predict joint line position in primary and revision knee arthroplasty? Am J Orthop (Belle Mead, NJ). 2011;40(4):175–8.
24. Sadaka C, Kabalan Z, Hoyek F, Abi Fares G, Lahoud JC. Joint line restoration during revision total knee arthroplasty: an accurate and reliable method. SpringerPlus. 2015;4:736. https://doi.org/10.1186/s40064-015-1543-0.
25. Herzog RJ, Silliman JF, Hutton K, Rodkey WG, Steadman JR. Measurements of the intercondylar notch by plain film radiography and magnetic resonance imaging. Am J Sports Med. 1994;22(2):204–10. https://doi.org/10.1177/036354659402200209.
26. Sarmah SS, Patel S, Hossain FS, Haddad FS. The radiological assessment of total and unicompartmental knee replacements. J Bone Joint Surg Br. 2012;94(10):1321–9. https://doi.org/10.1302/0301-620x.94b10.29411.
27. Weale AE, Murray DW, Newman JH, Ackroyd CE. The length of the patellar tendon after unicompartmental and total knee replacement. J Bone Joint Surg Br Vol. 1999;81(5):790–5.
28. Iacono F, Raspugli GF, Bruni D, Filardo G, Zaffagnini S, Luetzow WF, Lo Presti M, Akkawi I, Marcheggiani Muccioli GM, Marcacci M. The adductor tubercle as an important landmark to determine the joint line level in total knee arthroplasty: from radiographs to surgical theatre. Knee Surg Sports Traumatol Arthrosc. 2014;22(12):3034–8. https://doi.org/10.1007/s00167-013-2809-0.
29. Yoshino N, Takai S, Ohtsuki Y, Hirasawa Y. Computed tomography measurement of the surgical and clinical transepicondylar axis of the distal femur in osteoarthritic knees. J Arthroplast. 2001;16(4):493–7. https://doi.org/10.1054/arth.2001.23621.
30. Figgie HE 3rd, Goldberg VM, Heiple KG, Moller HS 3rd, Gordon NH. The influence of tibial-patellofemoral location on function of the knee in patients with the posterior stabilized condylar knee prosthesis. J Bone Joint Surg Am. 1986;68(7):1035–40.
31. Luyckx T, Beckers L, Colyn W, Vandenneucker H, Bellemans J. The adductor ratio: a new tool for joint line reconstruction in revision TKA. Knee Surg Sports Traumatol Arthrosc. 2014;22(12):3028–33. https://doi.org/10.1007/s00167-014-3211-2.

25

Bioinformatics analysis of differentially expressed genes in rotator cuff tear patients using microarray data

Yi-Ming Ren[†], Yuan-Hui Duan[†], Yun-Bo Sun[†], Tao Yang and Meng-Qiang Tian[*]

Abstract

Background: Rotator cuff tear (RCT) is a common shoulder disorder in the elderly. Muscle atrophy, denervation and fatty infiltration exert secondary injuries on torn rotator cuff muscles. It has been reported that satellite cells (SCs) play roles in pathogenic process and regenerative capacity of human RCT via regulating of target genes. This study aims to complement the differentially expressed genes (DEGs) of SCs that regulated between the torn supraspinatus (SSP) samples and intact subscapularis (SSC) samples, identify their functions and molecular pathways.

Methods: The gene expression profile GSE93661 was downloaded and bioinformatics analysis was made.

Results: Five hundred fifty one DEGs totally were identified. Among them, 272 DEGs were overexpressed, and the remaining 279 DEGs were underexpressed. Gene ontology (GO) and pathway enrichment analysis of target genes were performed. We furthermore identified some relevant core genes using gene–gene interaction network analysis such as GNG13, GCG, NOTCH1, BCL2, NMUR2, PMCH, FFAR1, AVPR2, GNA14, and KALRN, that may contribute to the understanding of the molecular mechanisms of secondary injuries in RCT. We also discovered that GNG13/calcium signaling pathway is highly correlated with the denervation atrophy pathological process of RCT.

Conclusion: These genes and pathways provide a new perspective for revealing the underlying pathological mechanisms and therapy strategy of RCT.

Keywords: Rotator cuff muscle, Satellite cells, Differentially expressed genes, Bioinformatics analysis, Calcium signaling, Denervation

Introduction

The rotator cuff muscle complex of the shoulder is comprised of four distinct muscles (supraspinatus, infraspinatus, teres minor, and subscapularis), which controls essential shoulder movements [1, 2]. The rotator cuff tear (RCT) is a common cause of impact pain, nocturnal pain and shoulder joint dysfunction, which seriously affect the life and working ability of patients, and reduce the quality of life of patients [3, 4]. Most tears require reparative surgery; however, recurrence of tears following surgery is common, with failure rates ranging from 30 to 94% [5]. Rotator cuff tendon tears are accompanied by secondary changes in the rotator cuff muscles, including muscle

atrophy, denervation, and fatty infiltration, which may explain the progressive loss of function after an acute injury and also the high rate of surgical failure. However, the underlying mechanism is not well understood.

Satellite cells (SCs) are mitotically quiescent muscle stem cells located between the basal lamina and the muscle membrane, which are known to play a key role in the adaptive response of muscle to exercise, and in the maintenance of the regenerative capacity of muscle. Hepatocyte growth factor (HGF) and nitric oxide (NO) could regulate transit of a SC from the quiescent G0 state into the G1 (activated) stage of the cell cycle [6]. Recently, Deanna et al. discovered possible supraspinatus denervation in RCT and suggested NO-donor treatment combined with stretching has potential to promote growth in atrophic supraspinatus muscle after RCT and improve functional outcome [7, 8]. Lundgreen et al.

---

* Correspondence: tmqjoint@126.com
[†]Yi-Ming Ren, Yuan-Hui Duan and Yun-Bo Sun contributed equally to this work.
Department of Joint and Sport Medicine, Tianjin Union Medical Center, Jieyuan Road 190, Hongqiao District, Tianjin 300121, People's Republic of China

showed patients with full-thickness tears had a reduced density of SCs, fewer proliferating cells, and atrophy of myofibers [9]. With muscle atrophy, fatty infiltration into skeletal muscles is thought to cause muscle degeneration by impairing the myogenic function of SCs [10].

Here, we downloaded the gene expression profile GSE93661 from the Gene Expression Omnibus database (GEO) and made bioinformatics analysis to investigate differentially expressed genes (DEGs) of SCs that regulated between torn supraspinatus (SSP) samples and intact subscapularis (SSC) samples from RCT patients. By doing this, we hope that the key target genes and pathways involved in the pathological process of RCT could be identified and existing molecular mechanisms could be revealed.

Materials and methods

Gene expression microarray data

The gene expression profile GSE93661 was downloaded from the Gene Expression Omnibus (GEO, www.ncbi.nlm. nih.gov/geo/). GSE93661 was based on Agilent-026652 Whole Human Genome Microarray 4x44K v2 platform. GSE93661 dataset contained four samples, including two torn SSP samples, and two intact SSC samples.

DEGs in torn SSP and intact SSC samples

The raw data files used for the analysis included TXT files. The analysis was carried out using GEO2R, which can perform comparisons on original submitter-supplied processed data tables using the GEO query and limma R packages from Bioconductor project. The P value < 0.05 and log fold change (FC) > 2.0 or log FC < -2.0 were used as the cut-off criteria. The DEGs with statistical significance between the torn SSP samples and intact SSC samples were selected and identified.

GO and KEGG analysis of DEGs

Target genes list were submitted to the DAVID 6.8 (https://david.ncifcrf.gov/tools.jsp) and ClueGO version 2.33 (based on Cytoscape software version 3.4.0 (www.cy toscape.org)) to identify overrepresented GO categories and pathway categories. Gene ontology (GO) analysis was used to predict the potential functions of the DEGs in biological process (BP), molecular function (MF), and cellular component (CC). The Kyoto Encyclopedia of Genes and Genomes (KEGG) is a knowledge base for systematic analysis of gene functions, linking genomic information with higher-level systemic functions. Finally, the overrepresented pathway categories were considered statistically significant using KEGG pathway enrichment analysis.

Gene interaction network construction

A large number of DEGs we obtained may be RCT-associated genes, and it is suggested that these DEGs in torn SSP samples may participate in the progression of RCT. Firstly, DEGs list was submitted to the Search Tool for the Retrieval of Interacting Genes (STRING) database (http://www.string-db.org/), and an interaction network chart with a combined score > 0.4 was saved and exported. Subsequently, the interaction regulatory network of RCT-associated genes was visualized using Cytoscape software version 3.4.0. The distribution of core genes in the interaction network was made by NetworkAnalyzer in Cytoscape. Then, the plugin Molecular Complex Detection (MCODE) was applied to screen the modules of the gene interaction network in Cytoscape. Venn diagram was drawn using Venny 2.1 (http://bioinfogp.cnb.csic.es/tools/venny/).

Result

Identification of DEGs

The gene expression profile GSE93661 was downloaded from the GEO, and the GEO2R method was used to identify DEGs in torn SSP samples compared with intact SSC samples. P value < 0.05, log FC > 2.0, or log FC < -2.0 were used as the cut-off criteria. After analyzing, differentially expression gene profiles were obtained. Totally, 551 DEGs were identified including 272 upregulated DEGs and 279 downregulated DEGs screened in torn SSP samples compared with intact SSC samples. Parts of DEGs were listed in Table 1.

GO term enrichment analysis of DEGs

Functional annotation of the 551 DEGs was clarified using the DAVID 6.8 online tool. GO analysis indicated that these DEGs were significantly enriched in muscle contraction, aging, regulation of ion transmembrane transport, mesenchymal cell development, and other biological processes (Fig. 1). For MF, the DEGs were enriched in ion channel activity, calcium ion binding, structural molecule activity, and others. In addition, GO CC analysis also showed that the DEGs were significantly enriched in keratin filament, integral component of plasma membrane, axon, cornified envelope, cortical cytoskeleton, and others.

KEGG pathway analysis of DEGs

The result of KEGG pathway analysis revealed that target genes were enriched in butanoate metabolism, ABC transporters, notch signaling pathway, arachidonic acid metabolism, hedgehog signaling pathway, cell adhesion molecules (CAMs), prolactin signaling pathway, neuroactive ligand-receptor interaction, dopaminergic synapse, GABAergic synapse, calcium signaling pathway, cGMP-PKG signaling pathway, drug metabolism, B cell receptor signaling pathway, NF-kappa B signaling pathway, estrogen signaling pathway, cAMP signaling pathway, and others. These key pathways were showed in Fig. 2.

Table 1 The top 10 Regulated DEGs in SCs of torn rotator cuff muscle with *P* value< 0.05

ID	*P* value	logFC	Gene symbol
Upregulated			
9522	0.0024644	5.71	FAM196B
39,990	0.0031637	5.05	SCN2A
8187	0.0000663	4.91	NNT
41,585	0.0035824	4.74	TDRD3
8204	0.0040603	4.46	LOC100131129
28,406	0.0002489	4.42	C8orf42
8118	0.0041306	4.42	KIAA1751
12,220	0.0043186	4.32	LRRC2
7774	0.0044309	4.27	CYP2E1
37,687	0.0007211	4.24	CUBN
Downregulated			
32,273	0.0024714	− 4.62	PTPRC
45,097	0.0037977	− 4.61	TCF7L2
12,505	0.0016694	− 4.49	tcag7.1023
35,725	0.0001639	− 4.11	FAM101A
45,093	0.0083048	− 4.08	C8orf67
8427	0.0005044	− 3.84	PTCH2
38,947	0.0004951	− 3.6	PLLP
31,098	0.0001216	− 3.55	TRPV5
31,980	0.0064577	− 3.54	SPNS3
29,856	0.0004283	− 3.52	ACP2

SCs satellite cells, *DEGs* differentially expressed genes, *FC* fold change

Besides, these core pathways and their associated genes found were summarized in Table 2. The first-ranking butanoate metabolism signaling pathway had the 10.71% associated genes, which included ACSM2B, ACSM4, and ACSM6. The second-placed ABC transporters signaling pathway had the 8.89% associated genes, which included ABCA3, ABCD1, ABCG2, and ABCG4. The third-placed notch signaling pathway had the 8.33% associated genes, which included JAG2, MAML3, MFNG, and NOTCH1.

Interaction network of DEGs and core genes in the interaction network

Based on the information in the STRING database, the gene interaction network contained 386 nodes and 440 edges. The nodes indicated the DEGs, and the edges indicated the interactions between the DEGs. NetworkAnalyzer in Cytoscape software was used to analyze these genes, and core genes were ranked according to the predicted scores. The top 10 high-degree hub nodes included GNG13, GCG, NOTCH1, BCL2, NMUR2, PMCH, FFAR1, AVPR2, GNA14, and KALRN. Among these genes, GNG13 showed the highest node degree which was 32. The core genes and their corresponding degree were shown in Table 3. The distribution of core genes in the interaction network was revealed in Fig. 3. The correlation between the data points and corresponding points on the line is approximately 0.993. The R^2 value is 0.902, giving a relatively high confidence that the underlying model is indeed linear. Then, we used MCODE to screen the modules of the gene interaction network, and eight modules were showed in Fig. 4.

The score of top 1 module including GCG, GNG13, NMUR2, and KALRN was 14, which had 14 nodes and 91 edges. The score of top 2 module including BCL2 and CD22 was 6, which had 6 nodes and 15 edges. The

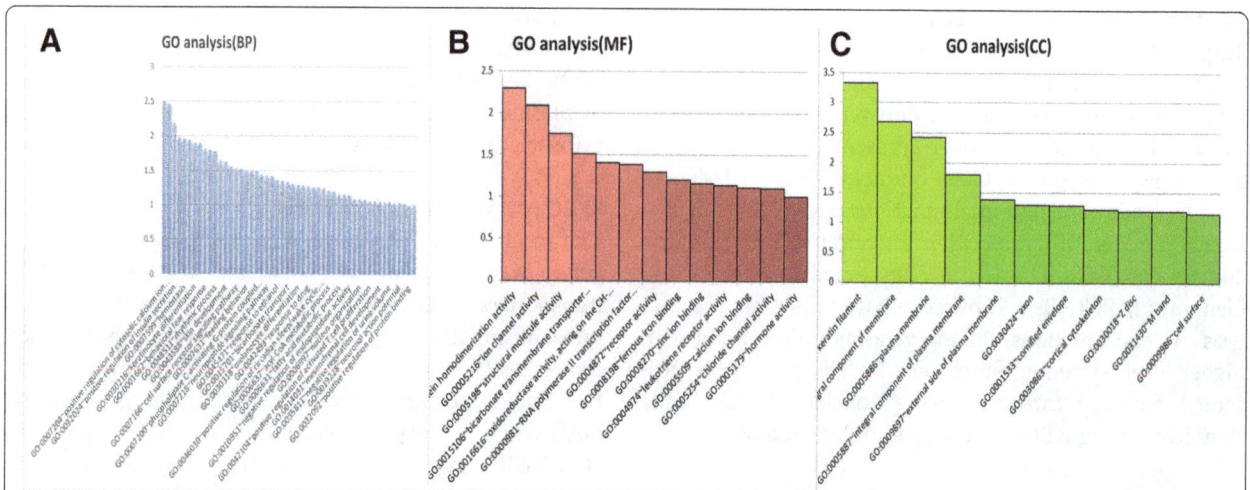

Fig. 1 Gene ontology (GO)-enrichment analysis of biological processes (**a**) molecular functions (**b**) and cellular components (**c**). The labels in *Y* axis mean enrichment score (−log$_{10}$ *P* value), and labels in *X* axis mean GO terms

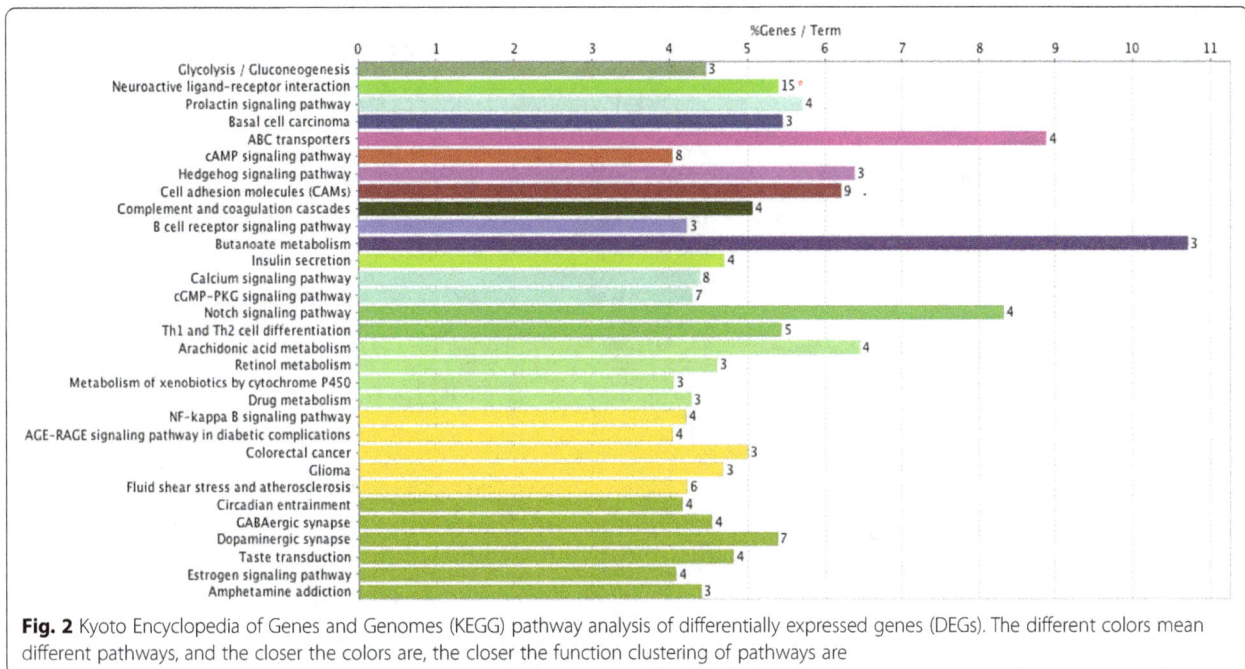

Fig. 2 Kyoto Encyclopedia of Genes and Genomes (KEGG) pathway analysis of differentially expressed genes (DEGs). The different colors mean different pathways, and the closer the colors are, the closer the function clustering of pathways are

score of top 3 module including CBLB, RNF6, TRIM9, and FBXO44 was 6, which had 6 nodes and 15 edges. Lastly, the interaction network of the top 10 high-degree hub nodes (core genes) was made by STRING database in Fig. 5. GNG13, GCG, NOTCH1, BCL2, NMUR2, PMCH, FFAR1, AVPR2, GNA14, and KALRN, which regulate 7, 7, 2, 2, 6, 6, 6, 3, 6, and 7 targets, respectively, showed the good connectivity.

Interestingly, Chaudhury et al. [9, 11] reported that gene expression profiles of different-sized human rotator cuff tendon tears versus normal rotator cuff tendons. In order to seek the possibly common target genes, we pooled together the top 10 high-degree core genes as mentioned earlier and the 77 significantly DEGs of Chaudhury's research using Venn diagram [9, 11]. GNG13 was discovered as the only common target gene in Fig. 6.

Discussion
RCT is common and painful. Even after surgery, joint stability and function may not recover [11]. SCs play a major role in muscle regeneration. However, human SCs in muscles with atrophy, denervation, and fatty infiltration are unclear due to the difficulty in isolating from small samples, and the mechanism has not been elucidated [12–14]. In the present study, the gene expression profile of GSE93661 was downloaded and a bioinformatics analysis was performed. The results showed that there were 551 DEGs in SCs of torn rotator cuff tendons and normal rotator cuff tendons. Furthermore, GO, KEGG pathway, and gene–gene interaction network analysis were performed to obtain the biomarkers or the major genes related to pathogenicity mechanism of RCT.

In order to disclose the underlying molecular mechanisms between SCs and RCT, we characterized the possible GO functional terms and signaling pathways of DEGs. Considering the results of GO function analysis, we linked the DEGs with aging, regulation of ion transmembrane transports, ion channel activity, and calcium ion binding, which are very important for the development process of RCT. When muscle is injured, exercised, overused, or mechanically stretched, SCs are activated to enter the cell cycle, divide, differentiate, and fuse with the adjacent muscle fiber. In this way, SCs are responsible for regeneration and work-induced hypertrophy of muscle fibers. Ryuichi's results suggested that the activation mechanism is a cascade of molecular events including an influx of calcium ions and their binding to calmodulin, nitric oxide synthase (NOS) activation, NO radical production by cNOS, matrix metalloproteinase activation, HGF release from the matrix, and presentation of HGF to the signaling receptor c-met. Understanding the mechanisms of SC activation is essential when planning procedures that could enhance muscle growth and repair [15].

As previous articles reported, our KEGG pathway analysis showed that notch signaling pathway, hedgehog signaling pathway, dopaminergic synapse, GABAergic synapse, calcium signaling pathway, NF-kappa B signaling pathway, and estrogen signaling pathway were among the most relevant pathways for SCs in RCT. Pasut et al. found that in normal muscle, high levels of notch signaling is required to maintain the uncommitted state of SCs. Notch signaling plays a role in SC fate as activation of Notch1 strongly promotes the lineage

Table 2 Core pathways and their associated genes found

GOID	GO term	Term P value	% associated genes	Associated genes found
GO:0000650	Butanoate metabolism	0.02	10.71	[ACSM2B, ACSM4, ACSM6]
GO:0002010	ABC transporters	0.01	8.89	[ABCA3, ABCD1, ABCG2, ABCG4]
GO:0004330	Notch signaling pathway	0.02	8.33	[JAG2, MAML3, MFNG, NOTCH1]
GO:0000590	Arachidonic acid metabolism	0.04	6.45	[CYP2B6, CYP2E1, PTGS1, TBXAS1]
GO:0004340	Hedgehog signaling pathway	0.07	6.38	[BCL2, IHH, PTCH2]
GO:0004514	Cell adhesion molecules (CAMs)	0.00	6.21	[CD22, CD226, CD86, CLDN15, ITGAM, NCAM2, NLGN1, PTPRC, VCAM1]
GO:0004917	Prolactin signaling pathway	0.05	5.71	[CISH, MAPK10, PRL, TH]
GO:0005217	Basal cell carcinoma	0.10	5.45	[PTCH2, TCF7L2, WNT10A]
GO:0004658	Th1 and Th2 cell differentiation	0.04	5.43	[IL12RB1, JAG2, MAML3, MAPK10, NOTCH1]
GO:0004080	Neuroactive ligand-receptor interaction	0.00	5.40	[AVPR2, CHRNB3, CHRNE, CYSLTR1, EDNRB, GABBR1, GIPR, GLP2R, HRH3, LTB4R, NMUR2, NPY2R, NPY4R, OPRL1, PRL]
GO:0004728	Dopaminergic synapse	0.02	5.38	[CACNA1C, CALML6, GNG13, KCNJ6, MAPK10, SCN1A, TH]
GO:0004610	Complement and coagulation cascades	0.07	5.06	[F7, ITGAM, MASP2, VWF]
GO:0005210	Colorectal cancer	0.12	5.00	[BCL2, MAPK10, TCF7L2]
GO:0004742	Taste transduction	0.09	4.82	[CACNA1C, GABBR1, GNG13, SCN2A]
GO:0004911	Insulin secretion	0.09	4.71	[CACNA1C, FFAR1, GCG, KCNU1]
GO:0005214	Glioma	0.14	4.69	[CALML6, PDGFB, PLCG2]
GO:0000830	Retinol metabolism	0.14	4.62	[ADH6, CYP2B6, DHRS4L1]
GO:0004727	GABAergic synapse	0.10	4.55	[CACNA1C, GABBR1, GNG13, KCNJ6]
GO:0000010	Glycolysis/gluconeogenesis	0.15	4.48	[ACSS1, ADH6, LDHC]
GO:0005031	Amphetamine addiction	0.16	4.41	[CACNA1C, CALML6, TH]
GO:0004020	Calcium signaling pathway	0.03	4.40	[ATP2A1, ATP2B3, CACNA1C, CALML6, CYSLTR1, EDNRB, GNA14, PLCG2]
GO:0004022	cGMP-PKG signaling pathway	0.05	4.29	[ATP2A1, ATP2B3, CACNA1C, CALML6, EDNRB, KCNU1, NPPB]
GO:0000982	Drug metabolism	0.17	4.29	[ADH6, CYP2B6, CYP2E1]
GO:0004662	B cell receptor signaling pathway	0.17	4.23	[CD22, PLCG2, RASGRP3]
GO:0005418	Fluid shear stress and atherosclerosis	0.07	4.23	[BCL2, CALML6, MAPK10, PDGFB, PIAS4, VCAM1]
GO:0004064	NF-kappa B signaling pathway	0.12	4.21	[BCL2, PIAS4, PLCG2, VCAM1]
GO:0004713	Circadian entrainment	0.13	4.17	[CACNA1C, CALML6, GNG13, KCNJ6]
GO:0004915	Estrogen signaling pathway	0.14	4.08	[CALML6, GABBR1, HSPA6, KCNJ6]
GO:0000980	Metabolism of xenobiotics by cytochrome P450	0.19	4.05	[ADH6, CYP2B6, CYP2E1]
GO:0004024	cAMP signaling pathway	0.06	4.04	[ATP2B3, CACNA1C, CALML6, FXYD1, GABBR1, GHRL, GIPR, MAPK10]
GO:0004933	AGE-RAGE signaling pathway in diabetic complications	0.14	4.04	[BCL2, MAPK10, PLCG2, VCAM1]

Table 3 The core genes and their corresponding degree

Gene	Degree	Gene	Degree	Gene	Degree	Gene	Degree
GNG13	32	PMCH	18	PTPRC	14	MPO	13
GCG	22	FFAR1	15	CYSLTR1	14	OPN4	13
NOTCH1	21	AVPR2	15	EDNRB	14	GNRHR2	13
BCL2	21	GNA14	15	UTS2D	13	LTB4R	13
NMUR2	18	KALRN	15	UTS2	13	PRL	13

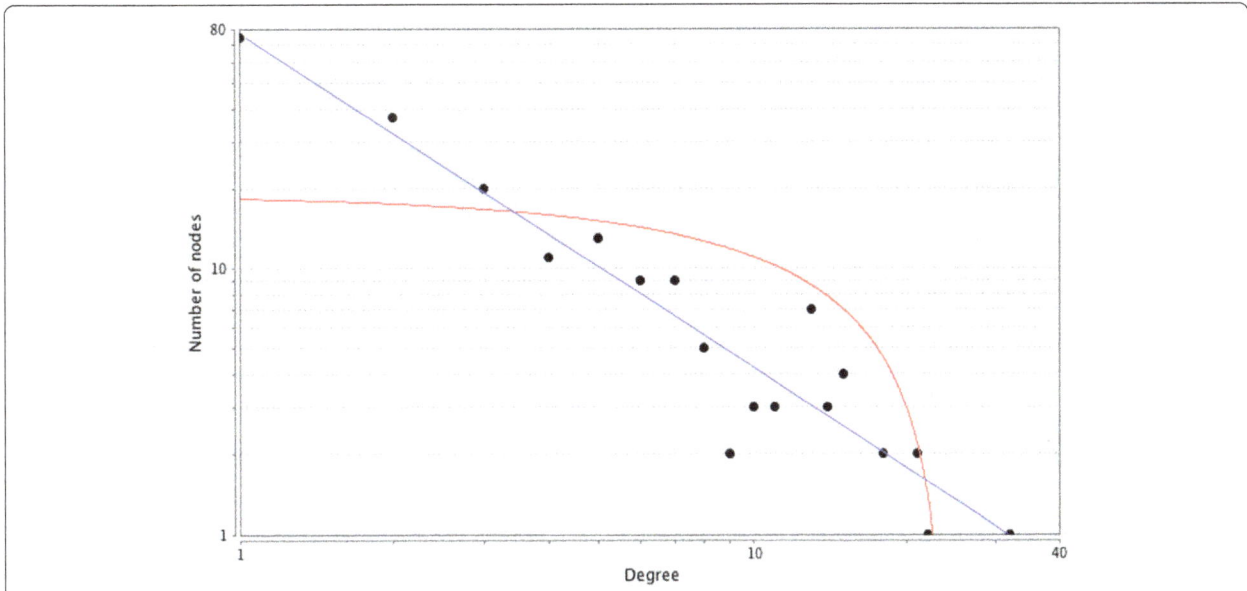

Fig. 3 The distribution of core genes in the interaction network. The black node means the core gene. The red line mans the fitted line, and the blue line means the power law. The correlation between the data points and corresponding points on the line is approximately 0.993. The R^2 value is 0.902, giving a relatively high confidence that the underlying model is indeed linear

switch from myogenic towards brown adipogenic fate [16]. Khayrullin et al. reported that upregulation of Notch signaling suppresses myogenesis and maintains muscle SC quiescence and miRNAs targeting Notch are likely to play important roles in alcohol-related myopathy in zebrafish model [17]. SC self-renewal is an essential process to maintaining the robustness of skeletal muscle regenerative capacity. Ogura's study demonstrates that TNF-like weak inducer of apoptosis cytokine suppresses SC self-renewal through activating NF-kappa B and repressing Notch signaling [18]. Kamizaki's findings indicate that Ror1 has a critical role in regulating

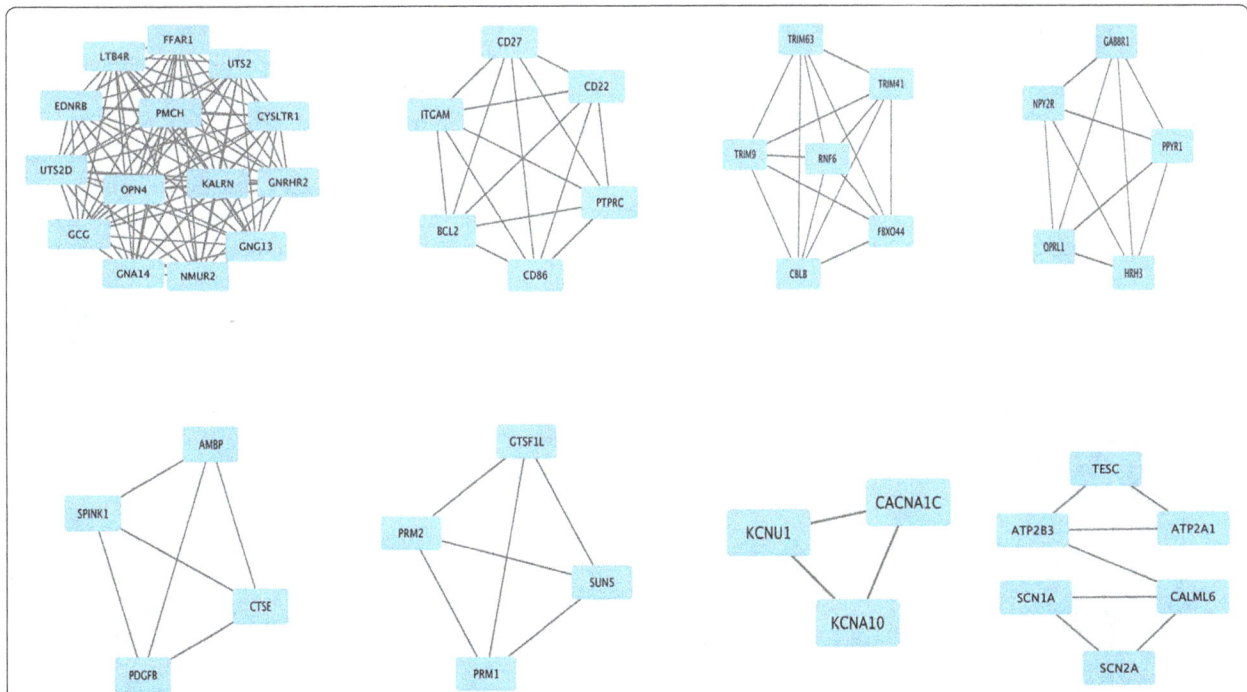

Fig. 4 The top 8 modules from the gene–gene interaction network. The squares represent the differentially expressed genes (DEGs) in modules, and the lines show the interaction between the DEGs

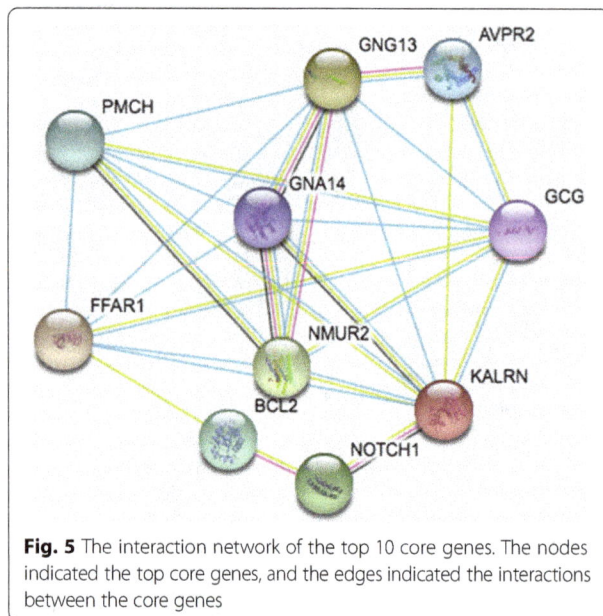

Fig. 5 The interaction network of the top 10 core genes. The nodes indicated the top core genes, and the edges indicated the interactions between the core genes

SC proliferation via NF-kappa B activation during skeletal muscle regeneration of injured muscle [19]. In addition, estrogen regulates myosin heavy chain expression in SCs related to muscle function mainly through an estrogen receptor α-mediated pathway [20]. In Voronova's study, the formation of skeletal muscle during embryogenesis and adult muscle regeneration is regulated by myocyte enhancer factors and myogenic regulatory factors (such as MyoD). Hedgehog signaling could regulate MyoD expression during embryogenesis and adult muscle regeneration in SCs [21].

The gene interaction network analysis revealed top 10 high-degree hub nodes of DEGs including GNG13, GCG, NOTCH1, BCL2, NMUR2, PMCH, FFAR1, AVPR2, GNA14, and KALRN. Most of them were not reported in SCs and RCT research. Only NOTCH1, who is a receptor that mediates intercellular signaling through a pathway conserved across the metazoan, had be studied [22].

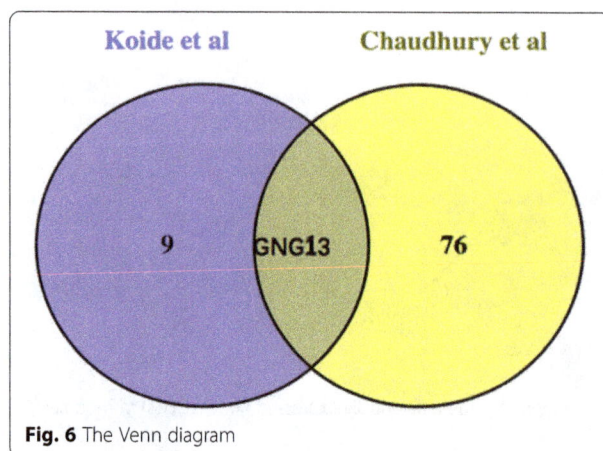

Fig. 6 The Venn diagram

Rando et al. found that activation of Notch1 signaling stimulates the proliferation of SCs and leads to the expansion of proliferating myoblasts. And, inhibition of Notch1 signaling abolishes SC activation and impairs muscle regeneration [23]. Also, recent studies found Notch1 is active in quiescent muscle SCs, and Notch1 signaling is critical for maintaining the quiescence of muscle SCs [24, 25]. As a supplement, Fujimaki et al. indicated that Notch1 and Notch2 coordinately maintain the SC pool in the quiescent state by preventing activation and regulate SC-fate decision in the activated state, governing adult muscle regeneration [26]. To sum up, upregulation of Notch1 may result in SC proliferation and self-renewal in the activated state, controlling muscle regeneration and improving muscle atrophy in RCT.

Furthermore, we analyzed the top 10 high-degree core genes and the 77 significantly DEGs of different-sized human rotator cuff tendon tears versus normal rotator cuff tendons in Chaudhury's research using Venn diagram [27]. GNG13 was discovered as the only common core gene. Heterotrimeric G proteins, which consist of alpha, beta, and gamma subunits, function as signal transducers for the 7-transmembrane-helix G protein-coupled receptors. GNG13 is a gamma subunit that is expressed in taste, retinal, and neuronal tissues, and plays a key role in taste transduction [28]. Through KEGG pathway results, we discovered that GNG13 acts as an important node in dopaminergic synapse signaling, and targets PLC and AC5 in calcium signaling pathway. Many previous studies had emphasized the importance of calcium signaling pathway and skeletal muscle development, homeostasis, and regeneration. Calcium-ion is an important component of the signaling promoting muscle formation, muscle homeostasis, and regeneration. In particular, calcium-ion changes may direct muscle SCs to maintain their quiescent state, proliferate, or differentiate into functional muscle [29]. What is more, we are still learning how calcium signaling pathway and neuromuscular connections are restored on regenerating muscle. The establishment of connections between the motor nerve terminal and a post-synaptic region of membrane on regenerating fibers is essential to re-innervation and functional contractility, which is important for clarifying denervation atrophy pathological process of injured rotator cuff muscle. Recent researches have implicated SC signaling in the process of muscle re-innervation. SC have potential to influence axon growth and the reappearance of neuromuscular connections by their secretion of semaphorin 3A (Sema3A). Sema3A is a neural chemorepellent that is thought to coordinate the reconnection of motor axons with a differentiating fiber in a regenerating muscle. These direct proofs encourage a possible implication of SCs in the spatiotemporal regulation of extracellular Sema3A concentrations, which potentially ensures coordinating a delay in neurite sprouting and re-attachment of motoneuron terminals onto damaged muscle fibers early in muscle regeneration in synchrony with recovery of muscle-fiber integrity [30–32]. In addition, calcium signaling pathway is also linked with the activation of neuromuscular connections, and calcium-ion influx through voltage-gated calcium channels regulates the neuron's responsiveness to Sema2A-dependent chemorepulsion exerted by the muscle [33]. Our research highlights the crucial role of nerve–muscle interaction in restoring innervation after RCT, and hypothesizes that SC-mediated GNG13 could affect neuromuscular connections and cause denervation atrophy via calcium signaling after rotator cuff muscle injured.

Conclusions

In summary, 551 DEGs were identified including 272 upregulated DEGs and 279 downregulated DEGs screened in SCs of torn SSP samples compared with intact SSC samples. GO and KEGG pathway analysis provided a series of related key genes and pathways to contribute to the understanding of the molecular mechanisms between SCs and RCT, thus yielding clues to speculate the GNG13/calcium signaling pathway is highly correlated with the denervation atrophy pathological process of RCT. Furthermore, further experimental validation should be made in future studies.

Abbreviations

BP: Biological process; CAMs: Cell adhesion molecules; CC: Cellular component; FC: Fold change; GEO: Gene Expression Omnibus database; GO: Gene ontology; HGF: Hepatocyte growth factor; KEGG: Kyoto Encyclopedia of Genes and Genomes; MCODE: Molecular Complex Detection; MF: Molecular function; NO: Nitric oxide; NOS: Nitric oxide synthase; RCT: Rotator cuff tear; SCs: Satellite cells; Sema3A: Semaphorin 3A; SSC: Subscapularis; SSP: Supraspinatus; STRING: Search Tool for the Retrieval of Interacting Genes

Acknowledgements
None.

Funding
This research is supported by Foundation of Tianjin Union Medical Center (2017YJ018).

Authors' contributions
YMR, YHD, and YBS conceived the design of the study. TY and YMR performed and collected the data, and contributed to the design of the study. TY and YMR analyzed the data. YMR and MQT prepared and revised the manuscript. All authors read and approved the final content of the manuscript.

Competing interests
The authors declare that they have no competing interests.

References

1. Yamaguchi K, Ditsios K, Middleton WD, et al. The demographic and morphological features of rotator cuff disease. J Bone Joint Surg (Am Vol). 2006;88(8):1699–704.
2. Liu X, Ravishankar B, Ning A, et al. Knocking-out matrix metalloproteinase-13 exacerbates rotator cuff muscle fatty infiltration. Muscles Ligaments Tendons J. 2017;7(2):202–7.
3. Schmidt CC, Jarrett CD, Brown BT. Management of rotator cuff tears. J Hand Surg. 2015;40(2):399–408.
4. Liu X, Ning AY, Chang NC, et al. Investigating the cellular origin of rotator cuff muscle fatty infiltration and fibrosis after injury. Muscles Ligaments Tendons J. 2016;6(1):6.
5. Isaac C, Gharaibeh B, Witt M, et al. Biologic approaches to enhance rotator cuff healing after injury. J Shoulder Elb Surg. 2012;21(2):181–90.
6. Dhawan J, Rando TA. Stem cells in postnatal myogenesis: molecular mechanisms of satellite cell quiescence, activation and replenishment[J]. Trends in Cell Biology. 2005;15(12):666–673.
7. Deanna G, Leiter JRS, Macdonald PB, et al. Altered satellite cell responsiveness and denervation implicated in progression of rotator-cuff injury. PLoS One. 2016;11(9):e0162494.
8. Gigliotti D, Leiter JR, Macek B, et al. Atrophy, inducible satellite cell activation and possible denervation of supraspinatus muscle in injured human rotator-cuff muscle. Am J Physiol Cell Physiol. 2015;309(6):C383.
9. Lundgreen K, Lian OB, Engebretsen L, et al. Lower muscle regenerative potential in full-thickness supraspinatus tears compared to partial-thickness tears. Acta Orthop. 2013;84(6):565.
10. Pisani DF, Clement N, Loubat A, et al. Hierarchization of myogenic and adipogenic progenitors within human skeletal muscle. Stem Cells. 2010; 28(12):2182–94.
11. Cofield RH, Parvizi J, Hoffmeyer PJ, et al. Surgical repair of chronic rotator cuff tears. A prospective long-term study. J Bone Joint Surg Am. 2001;83-A(1):71–7.
12. Zammit PS, Partridge TA, Yablonkareuveni Z. The skeletal muscle satellite cell: the stem cell that came in from the cold. J Histochem Cytochem. 2006; 54(11):1177–91.
13. Oliva F, Piccirilli E, Bossa M, et al. I.S.Mu.L.T - Rotator Cuff Tears Guidelines. Muscles Ligaments Tendons J. 2016;5(4):227.
14. Hall KE, Sarkissian EJ, Sharpe O, et al. Identification of differentially expressed micro-RNA in rotator cuff tendinopathy. Muscles Ligaments Tendons J. 2018;8:8–14.
15. Ryuichi T, Ronalde A. Mechano-biology of resident myogenic stem cells: molecular mechanism of stretch-induced activation of satellite cells. Anim Sci J. 2008;79(3):279–90.
16. Pasut A, Chang NC, Rodriguez UG, et al. Notch signaling rescues loss of satellite cells lacking Pax7 and promotes brown adipogenic differentiation. Cell Rep. 2016;16(2):333–43.
17. Khayrullin A, Smith L, Mistry D, et al. Chronic alcohol exposure induces muscle atrophy (myopathy) in zebrafish and alters the expression of microRNAs targeting the Notch pathway in skeletal muscle. Biochem Biophys Res Commun. 2016;479(3):590–5.
18. Ogura Y, Mishra V, Hindi SM, et al. Proinflammatory cytokine tumor necrosis factor (TNF)-like weak inducer of apoptosis (TWEAK) suppresses satellite cell self-renewal through inversely modulating notch and NF-kappa B signaling pathways. J Biol Chem. 2013;288(49):35159–69.
19. Kamizaki K, Doi R, Hayashi M, et al. The Ror1 receptor tyrosine kinase plays a critical role in regulating satellite cell proliferation during regeneration of injured muscle. J Biol Chem. 2017;292(38):15939.
20. Guo T, Liu W, Konermann A, et al. Estradiol modulates the expression pattern of myosin heavy chain subtypes via an ERu03b1-mediated pathway in muscle-derived tissues and satellite cells. Cell Physiol Biochem. 2014;33(3):681–91.
21. Voronova A, Coyne E, Madhoun AA, et al. Hedgehog signaling regulates MyoD expression and activity. J Biol Chem. 2013;288(6):4389–404.
22. Conboy IM, Conboy MJ, Smythe GM, et al. Notch-mediated restoration of regenerative potential to aged muscle. Science. 2003;302(5650):1575–7.
23. 9Luo D, Renault VM, Rando TA. The regulation of notch signaling in muscle stem cell activation and postnatal myogenesis. Semin Cell Dev Biol. 2005;16(5): 612–22.
24. Mourikis P, Sambasivan R, Castel D, et al. A critical requirement for notch signaling in maintenance of the quiescent skeletal muscle stem cell state. Stem Cells. 2012;30(2):243–52.

25. Bjornson CRR, Cheung TH, Liu L, et al. Notch signaling is necessary to maintain quiescence in adult muscle stem cells. Stem Cells. 2012;30(2):232–42.

26. Fujimaki S, Seko D, Kitajima Y, et al. Notch1 and Notch2 Coordinately Regulate Stem Cell Function in the Quiescent and Activated States of Muscle Satellite Cells[J]. Stem Cells. 2018;36(2):278–285.

27. Chaudhury S, Xia Z, Thakkar D, et al. Gene expression profiles of changes underlying different-sized human rotator cuff tendon tears. J Shoulder Elbow Surg. 2016;25(10):1561–70.

28. Blake BL, Wing MR, Zhou JY, et al. G beta association and effector interaction selectivities of the divergent G gamma subunit G gamma(13). J Biol Chem. 2001;276(52):49267–74.

29. Tu MK, Levin JB, Hamilton AM, et al. Calcium signaling in skeletal muscle development, maintenance and regeneration. Cell Calcium. 2016;59(2–3):91–7.

30. Anderson JE, Do MQ, Daneshvar N, et al. The role of semaphorin3A in myogenic regeneration and the formation of functional neuromuscular junctions on new fibres[J]. Biological Reviews. 2016;92(3):1389-1405.

31. Sato Y, Do MK, Suzuki T, et al. Satellite cells produce neural chemorepellent semaphorin 3A upon muscle injury. Anim Sci J Nihon chikusan Gakkaihō. 2013;84(2):185–9.

32. Tatsumi R, Sankoda Y, Anderson JE, et al. Possible implication of satellite cells in regenerative motoneuritogenesis: HGF upregulates neural chemorepellent Sema3A during myogenic differentiation. Am J Physiol Cell Physiol. 2009;297(2):C238.

33. Vonhoff F, Keshishian H. In vivo calcium signaling during synaptic refinement at the Drosophila neuromuscular junction. J Neurosci. 2017; 37(22):5511–26.

Balloon kyphoplasty versus percutaneous vertebroplasty for osteoporotic vertebral compression fracture

Bo Wang, Chang-Ping Zhao, Lian-Xin Song and Lian Zhu[*]

Abstract

Background: This meta-analysis was aimed to explore the overall safety and efficacy of balloon kyphoplasty versus percutaneous vertebroplasty for osteoporotic vertebral compression fracture (OVCF) based on qualified studies.

Methods: By searching multiple databases and sources, including PubMed, Cochrane, and Embase by the index words updated to January 2018, qualified studies were identified and relevant literature sources were also searched. The qualified studies included randomized controlled trials, prospective or retrospective comparative studies, and cohort studies. The meta-analysis was performed including mean difference (MD) or relative risk (RR) and 95% confidence interval (95% CI) to analyze the main outcomes.

Results: A total of 16 studies were included in the meta-analysis to explore the safety and efficacy of kyphoplasty versus vertebroplasty for the treatment of OVCF. The results indicated that kyphoplasty significantly decreased the kyphotic wedge angle (SMD, 0.98; 95% CI 0.40–1.57), increased the postoperative vertebral body height (SMD, − 1.27; 95% CI − 1.86 to − 0.67), and decreased the risk of cement leakage (RR, 0.62; 95% CI 0.47–0.80) in comparison with vertebroplasty. However, there was no statistical difference in visual analog scale (VAS) scores (WMD, 0.04; 95% CI − 0.28–0.36) and Oswestry Disability Index (ODI) scores (WMD, − 1.30; 95% CI − 3.34–0.74) between the two groups.

Conclusions: Kyphoplasty contributes especially to decreasing the mean difference of kyphotic wedge angle and risk of cement leakage and increasing the vertebral body height when compared with vertebroplasty. But radiographic differences did not significantly influence the clinical results (no significant difference was observed in VAS scores and ODI scores between the two groups); thus, kyphoplasty and vertebroplasty are equally effective in the clinical outcomes of OVCF. In addition, more high-quality multi-center RCTs with a larger sample size and longer follow-up are warranted to confirm the current findings.

Keywords: Meta-analysis, Balloon kyphoplasty, Percutaneous vertebroplasty, Osteoporotic vertebral compression fracture

* Correspondence: superzhu118@126.com
Department of Orthopedic Trauma Centre, 3rd Hospital of Hebei Medical University, No. 139 ZiQiang Road, Qiaoxi District, Shijiazhuang 050051, China

Background

Osteoporotic vertebral compression fracture (OVCF), one of the most common healthcare issues worldwide, commonly occurs after ankle, wrist, or hip fractures. Its incidence and severity have been steadily increasing over the last decades among elderly patients. In the USA, approximately 750,000 adults suffer from OVCFs each year [1], including 8% of women older than 50 years of age and 27% of men and women older than 65 years of age [2]. However, only about one third of patients with fractures are symptomatic, with compromised quality of life. OVCF occurs due to insufficient anterior vertebral height and causes spinal deformities, reduced pulmonary function, restriction of the abdominal and thoracic contents, impaired mobility, and depression [3–5]. Moreover, it prolongs hospitalization, affects quality of life, increases morbidity, and inflicts a heavy burden on the society.

Different approaches are available for the treatment of OVCFs, including standard medical and surgical therapy. The standard medical therapy contains bed rest, analgesia, bracing, external fixation, rehabilitation, and a combination of these treatments [6]. However, there are several limitations in the standard therapy: long-term bed rest can lead to subsequent demineralization and OVCF recurrence; anti-inflammatory drugs and certain types of analgesics cause intolerable side effects for older patients; and medical management does not reverse kyphotic deformity. Surgical treatment involves surgical stabilization via dorsal instrumentation, which is available for patients with OVCFs who are refractory to medical therapy [7]. Due to the poor quality of the osteoporotic bone, classical open surgery with metal implants often fails and leads to persistent back pain, neurological symptoms, and limited functions [8, 9]. Vertebroplasty was introduced by Galibert and Deramend in 1984 in France for treating hemangiomas at the C2 vertebra [10]. Balloon kyphoplasty was first performed in 1998. It is a minimally invasive surgical technique that corrects kyphosis secondary to collapsed vertebral bodies using a balloon (an inflation bone tamp) [9].

Therefore, in this meta-analysis, we assessed the existing evidence on the safety and effect of balloon kyphoplasty versus vertebroplasty in the treatment of OVCFs based on qualified trials.

Methods

Search strategy

The Cochrane Library, PubMed, and Embase databases were searched updated to January 2018 for all the qualified studies in order to analyze the effect of balloon kyphoplasty versus vertebroplasty in the treatment of OVCF. Literature was also identified by tracking reference lists from papers and Internet searches. Two investigators independently extracted data, and a third investigator was involved when a disagreement occurred.

Study selection

To be included in the meta-analysis, studies should meet the following criteria: (1) comparative studies: randomized controlled trails, prospective or retrospective case-control study, or cohort study; (2) the included patients had OVCF; (3) the test group were treated with balloon kyphoplasty the control group were treated with vertebroplasty; (4) the clinical outcomes included the visual analog scale (VAS) scores, Oswestry Disability Index (ODI), kyphotic wedge angle, vertebral body height restoration, and incidence of cement leakage; and (5) the publications were available in English and Chinese.

The following studies were excluded from the review: (1) repeat published articles or articles having the same content and result; (2) case report, theoretical research, conference report, systematic review, meta-analysis, expert comment, and economic analysis; (3) the outcomes were not relevant.

Data extraction

Two reviewers determined study eligibility independently. A third investigator was involved to reach an agreement. The analyzed data were extracted from all the included studies and consisted of two parts: basic information and main outcomes. The first part was about the basic information: the authors' name, the publication year, study design, country, sample size, age, and percentage of male. The second part was the clinical outcomes: the VAS scores, ODI, kyphotic wedge angle, vertebral body height restoration, and incidence of cement leakage. The studies were performed by two reviewers independently. Any arising difference was resolved by discussion.

Statistical analysis

All statistical analyses were performed in the STATA 10.0 (TX, USA). Chi-squared and I^2 tests were used to assess heterogeneity of clinical trial results and determine the analysis model (fixed-effects model or random-effects model). When the chi-squared test P value was ≤ 0.05 and I^2 tests value was $> 50\%$, it was defined as high heterogeneity and assessed by the random-effects model. When the chi-squared test P value was > 0.05 and I^2 tests value was $\leq 50\%$, it was defined as an acceptable heterogeneity data and assessed by the fixed-effects model. Continuous variables were expressed as mean $\pm$ standard deviation and analyzed by mean difference (MD). Categorical data were presented as percentages and analyzed by relative risk (RR) or odds ratio (OR). VAS, ODI, the kyphotic wedge angle, and the vertebral body height were analyzed by MD and 95% confidence interval (CI). The incidence of cement leakage was analyzed by RR and 95% CI.

Results

Characteristics of the included studies

By searching multiple databases and sources, we identified 937 articles by the index words. After screening titles and abstracts, 869 articles were excluded, leaving 68 articles for further evaluation. During full-text screening, 52 articles were excluded due to the following criteria: for having no clinical outcomes ($n = 21$), no qualified outcomes ($n = 8$), diagnostic analysis ($n = 15$), and theoretical research or review ($n = 8$). Finally, 16 studies [11–26] were included in the meta-analysis with 647 subjects in the kyphoplasty group and 758 subjects in the vertebroplasty group. The selection process is presented in Fig. 1.

The main characteristics of the included studies are summarized in Table 1, with one prospective randomized comparative study, four prospective comparative studies, five prospective cohort studies, two retrospective comparative studies, and four retrospective cohort studies. The patients were from Israel, Australia, Japan, Canada, Italy, Slovenia, the USA, Spain, Germany, China, and Korea. The age of patients in the kyphoplasty group and the vertebroplasty group was all more than 60 years. Other information included the number of patients and gender.

VAS

Ten studies on 769 patients provided preoperative and postoperative VAS scores. Based on the chi-squared test P value ($P = 0.000$) and I^2 test value ($I^2 = 80.5\%$), we chose the random-effects model to analyze the MD of VAS scores between kyphoplasty and vertebroplasty. The pooled results showed no significant difference in changes in VAS scores between kyphoplasty and vertebroplasty (WMD, 0.04; 95% CI – 0.28–0.36, Fig. 2).

ODI

Three studies on 263 patients had preoperative and postoperative ODI scores. Based on the chi-squared test P value ($P = 0.284$) and I^2 test value ($I^2 = 20.5\%$), we chose the fixed-effects model to analyze the MD of ODI scores between kyphoplasty and vertebroplasty. The pooled results showed no significant difference in changes in ODI scores between kyphoplasty and vertebroplasty (WMD, – 1.30; 95% CI – 3.34–0.74, Fig. 3).

Kyphotic wedge angle

Nine studies on 761 patients had preoperative and postoperative kyphotic wedge angles. Based on the chi-squared test P value ($P = 0.000$) and I^2 test value ($I^2 = 92.5\%$), we chose the random-effects model to analyze the MD of the kyphotic wedge angle. The pooled results showed that compared with vertebroplasty, kyphoplasty significantly decreased the kyphotic wedge angle (SMD, 0.98; 95% CI 0.40–1.57, Fig. 4).

Vertebral body height

Six studies on 489 patients had preoperative and postoperative vertebral body heights. Based on the chi-squared test P value ($P = 0.000$) and I^2 test value ($I^2 = 92.4\%$), we chose the random-effects model to analyze the MD of vertebral body height. The pooled results showed that compared with vertebroplasty, kyphoplasty significantly increased postoperative vertebral body height (SMD, – 1.27; 95% CI – 1.86 to – 0.67, Fig. 5).

Cement leakage

Eleven studies on 1057 patients provided data on the incidence of cement leakage after the operation. Based on the chi-squared test P value ($P = 0.088$) and I^2 test value ($I^2 = 39.4\%$), we chose the fixed-effects model to analyze the incidence of cement leakage. The pooled results showed that compared with vertebroplasty, kyphoplasty significantly decreased the risk of cement leakage (RR, 0.62; 95% CI 0.47–0.80, Fig. 6).

Quality assessment and potential bias

Based on the inclusion and exclusion criteria, 16 articles were included in the meta-analysis. Quality and potential bias were assessed by funnel plot, Begg's and Mazumdar's rank test, and Egger's test. The funnel plot for log WMD in VAS scores of the included studies was notably symmetrical, suggesting no significant publication bias (Fig. 7). In addition, significant symmetry was detected by Begg's and Mazumdar's rank test ($Z = 0.36$, $P = 0.721$). However, Egger's test result showed no significant publication bias ($P = 0.677$).

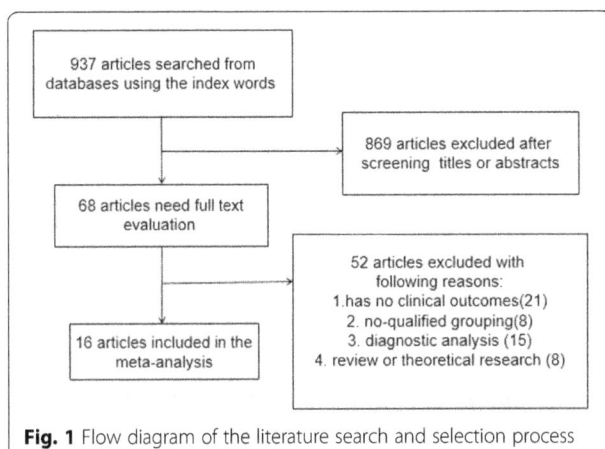

Fig. 1 Flow diagram of the literature search and selection process

Table 1 The basic characteristics description of included studies

Study	Study design	Country	No. of patients		Age		Gender	
			KP	VP	KP	VP	KP	VP
Yoram Folman 2011 [11]	Prospective cohort	Israel	31	14	70.74	75.57	9 M	5 M
Grohs JG 2005 [12]	Prospective comparative study	Australia	28	23	70		7 M	5 M
A. Hiwatashi 2009 [13]	Retrospective cohort	Japan	40	66	75	77	11 M	21 M
Krishna Kumar 2010 [14]	Prospective cohort	Canada	24	48	73	78	7 M	9 M
J. T. Liu 2009 [31]	Prospective randomized comparative study	Taiwan	50	50	72.3	74.3	11 M	12 M
Alessio Lovi 2009 [16]	Prospective cohort	Italy	36	118	67.6		98 M	
I. Movrin 2010 [17]	Prospective cohort	Slovenia	46	27	67.8	72.9	10 M	5 M
M. Rollinghoff 2009 [18]	Prospective comparative study	USA	53	52	68.9		20 M	
Fernando Ruiz Santiago 2010 [19]	Prospective cohort	Spain	30	30	65.9	73	9 M	5 M
Markus Dietmar Schofer 2009 [20]	Prospective comparative study	Germany	30	30	72.5	73.8	8 M	6 M
Denglu Yan 2011 [21]	Retrospective cohort	China	98	94	76.9	77.2	41 M	39 M
Zhou Jianlin 2008 [22]	Retrospective cohort	China	42	56	64	62	17 M	21 M
Hu Chunhua 2016 [23]	Retrospective cohort	China	30	30	67.44	68.73	18 M	18 M
Du Junhua 2014 [24]	Prospective comparative study	China	44	42	75.6	72.1	8 M	9 M
Wu Yao 2014 [25]	Retrospective comparative study	China	20	20	65.12	66.37	9 M	12 M
Kyung-Hyun Kim 2012 [26]	Retrospective comparative study	Korea	45	58	72.5	74.6	10 M	13 M

Discussion

Moderate evidence has been collected with funnel plot, Begg's and Mazumdar's rank test, and Egger's test, showing no publication bias in the included studies; therefore, the results are credible. In this study, the outcomes include two categories, the radiographic difference and the clinical difference. The indexes of radiographic difference include kyphotic wedge angle, vertebral body height, and cement leakage. We found that compared with vertebroplasty, kyphoplasty could significantly increase postoperative vertebral body height and decrease the risk of cement leakage. The clinical outcomes include VAS scores and ODI scores. However, we did not find any significant difference in changes in VAS scores and ODI scores between the two groups.

Admittedly, there are several limitations in this analysis: (1) differences in the inclusion criteria and exclusion criteria for patients; (2) different patients with

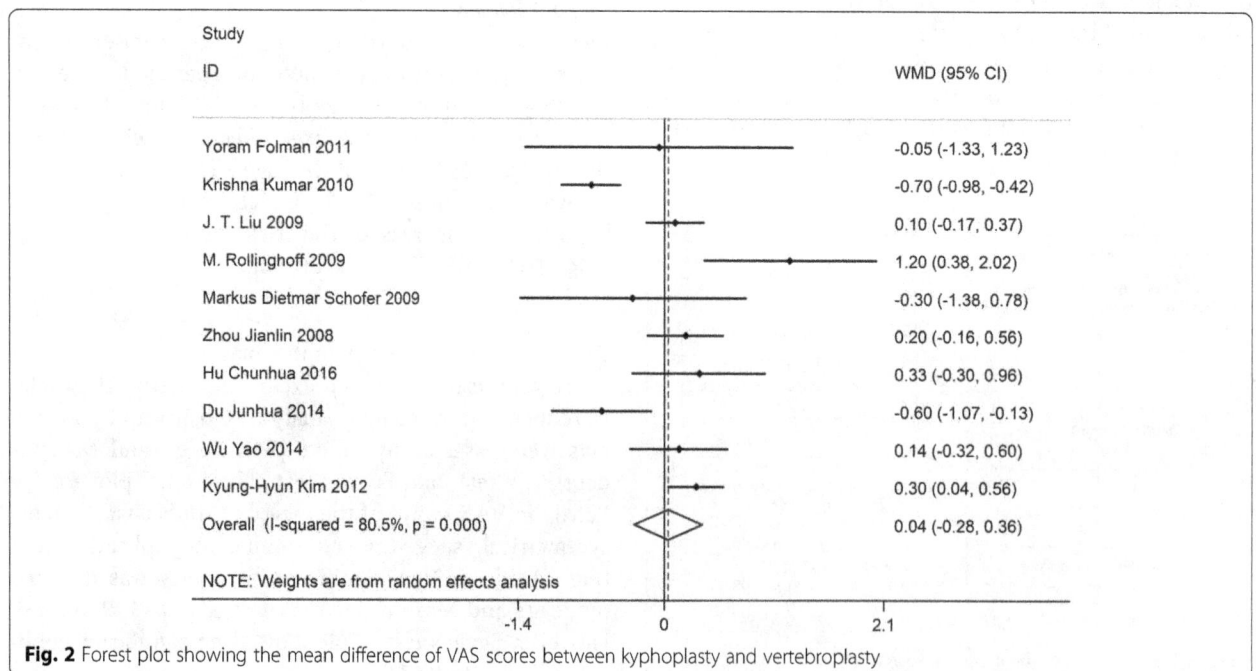

Study ID	WMD (95% CI)
Yoram Folman 2011	-0.05 (-1.33, 1.23)
Krishna Kumar 2010	-0.70 (-0.98, -0.42)
J. T. Liu 2009	0.10 (-0.17, 0.37)
M. Rollinghoff 2009	1.20 (0.38, 2.02)
Markus Dietmar Schofer 2009	-0.30 (-1.38, 0.78)
Zhou Jianlin 2008	0.20 (-0.16, 0.56)
Hu Chunhua 2016	0.33 (-0.30, 0.96)
Du Junhua 2014	-0.60 (-1.07, -0.13)
Wu Yao 2014	0.14 (-0.32, 0.60)
Kyung-Hyun Kim 2012	0.30 (0.04, 0.56)
Overall (I-squared = 80.5%, p = 0.000)	0.04 (-0.28, 0.36)

NOTE: Weights are from random effects analysis

-1.4   0   2.1

Fig. 2 Forest plot showing the mean difference of VAS scores between kyphoplasty and vertebroplasty

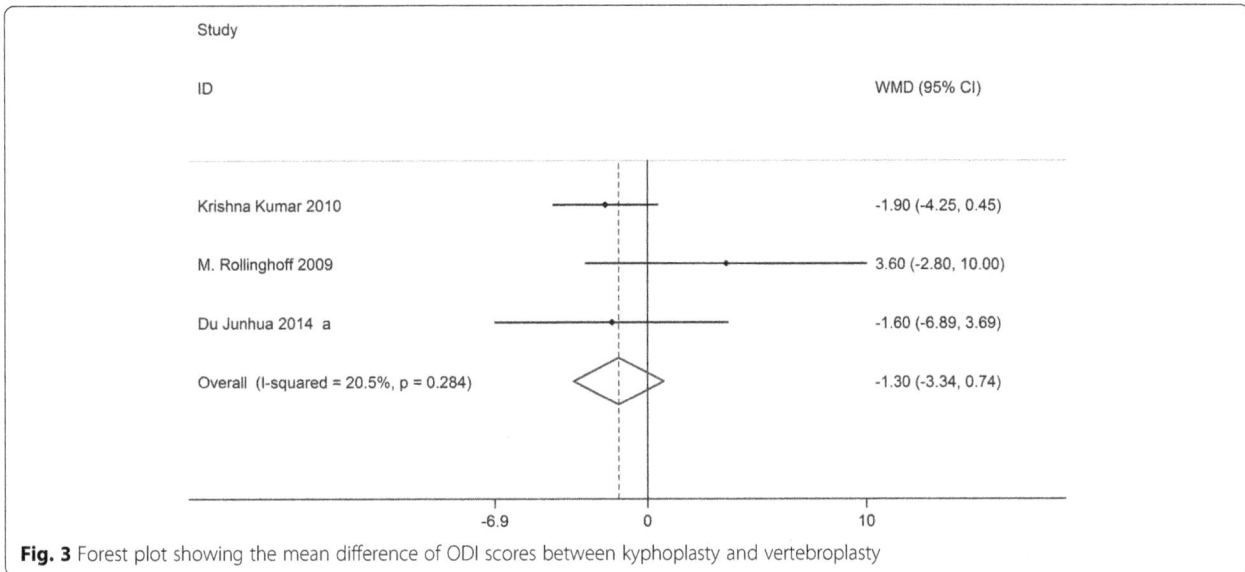

Fig. 3 Forest plot showing the mean difference of ODI scores between kyphoplasty and vertebroplasty

previous disease and treatments were unavailable; (3) all the included studies were English and Chinese publications being the source of bias; (4) the operating techniques in different studies were varied; (5) the low quality of included studies and the number of included studies is limited; (6) different types studies were included in the study; and (7) pooled data were used for analysis and individual patients' data were unavailable, which limited more comprehensive analyses.

Several studies have been published in the past few years that performed similar meta-analysis of the efficacy of kyphoplasty versus vertebroplasty in the treatment of OVCF. Ma et al. [27] found that in the RCT subgroup,

there were significant differences between the two procedures in short-term VAS, long-term kyphosis angles, operative times, and anterior vertebrae heights. In the cohort study subgroup, there were significant differences between the two procedures in short- and long-term VAS and ODI, cement leakage rates, short- and long-term kyphosis angles, operative times, and anterior vertebrae heights. Both kyphoplasty and vertebroplasty appeared to be safe and effective surgical procedures for the treatment of OVCF. Kyphoplasty tended to have more favorable outcomes than vertebroplasty for patients with large kyphosis angles, vertebral fissures, fractures in the posterior edge of the vertebral body, or

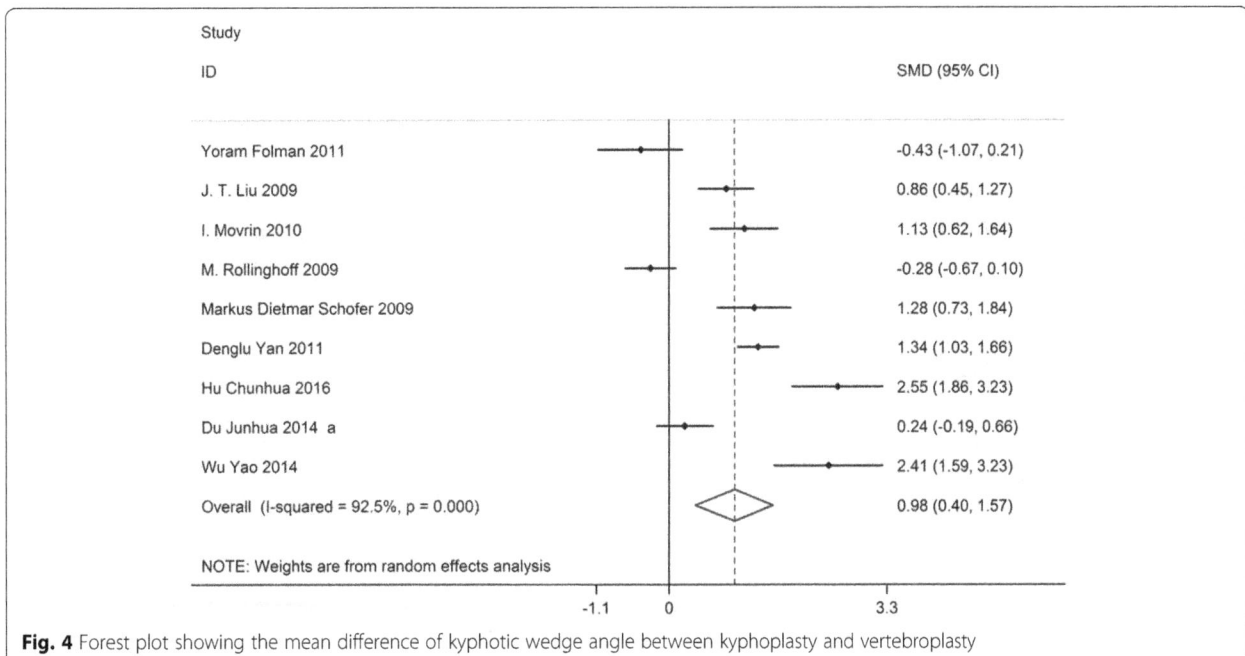

Fig. 4 Forest plot showing the mean difference of kyphotic wedge angle between kyphoplasty and vertebroplasty

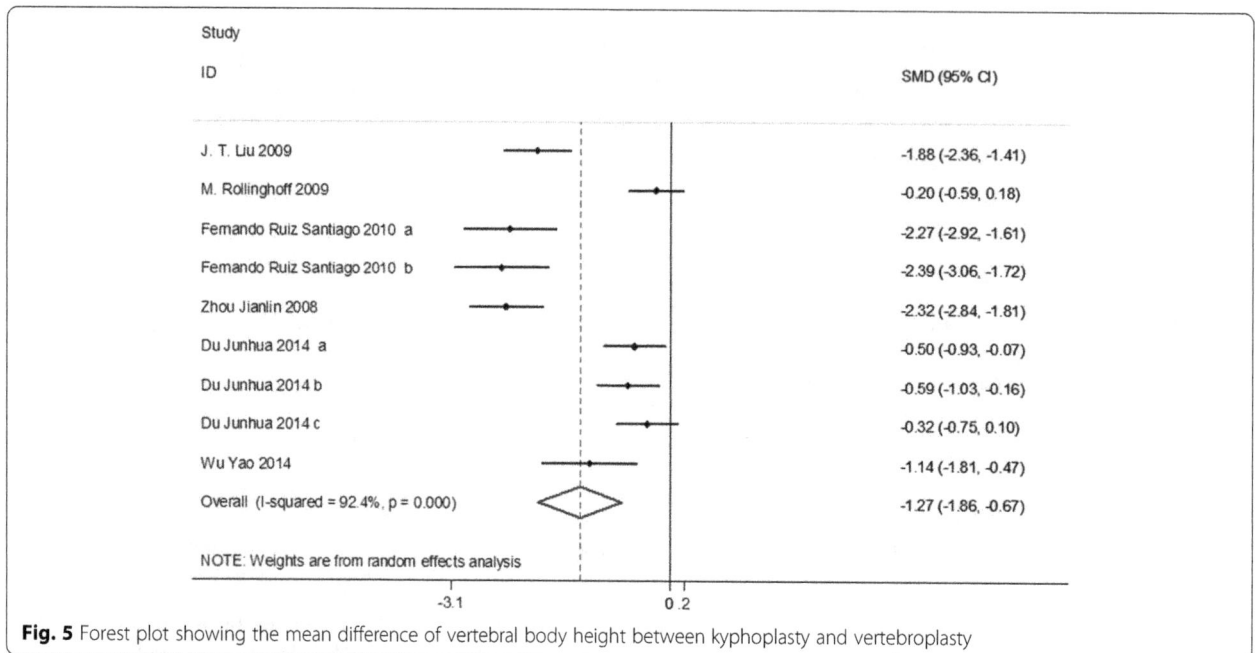

Fig. 5 Forest plot showing the mean difference of vertebral body height between kyphoplasty and vertebroplasty

significant height loss in the fractured vertebrae. Han et al. [1] reported that vertebroplasty is more effective in the short-term (no more than 7 days) pain relief. Kyphoplasty had a superior capability for intermediate-term (around 3 months) functional improvement. As for long-term pain relief and functional improvement, there was no significant difference between these two interventions. Consistently, both interventions were considered to have similar risks with subsequent fracture and

cement leakage. Wang et al. [28] concluded that kyphoplasty and vertebroplasty are both safe and effective surgical procedures for the treatment of OVCF. Kyphoplasty has similar long-term pain relief, function outcomes (short-term ODI scores, short- and long-term SF-36 scores), and new adjacent VCFs in comparison to vertebroplasty. Kyphoplasty appears to be superior to vertebroplasty for the injected cement volume, the short-term pain relief, the improvement of short- and

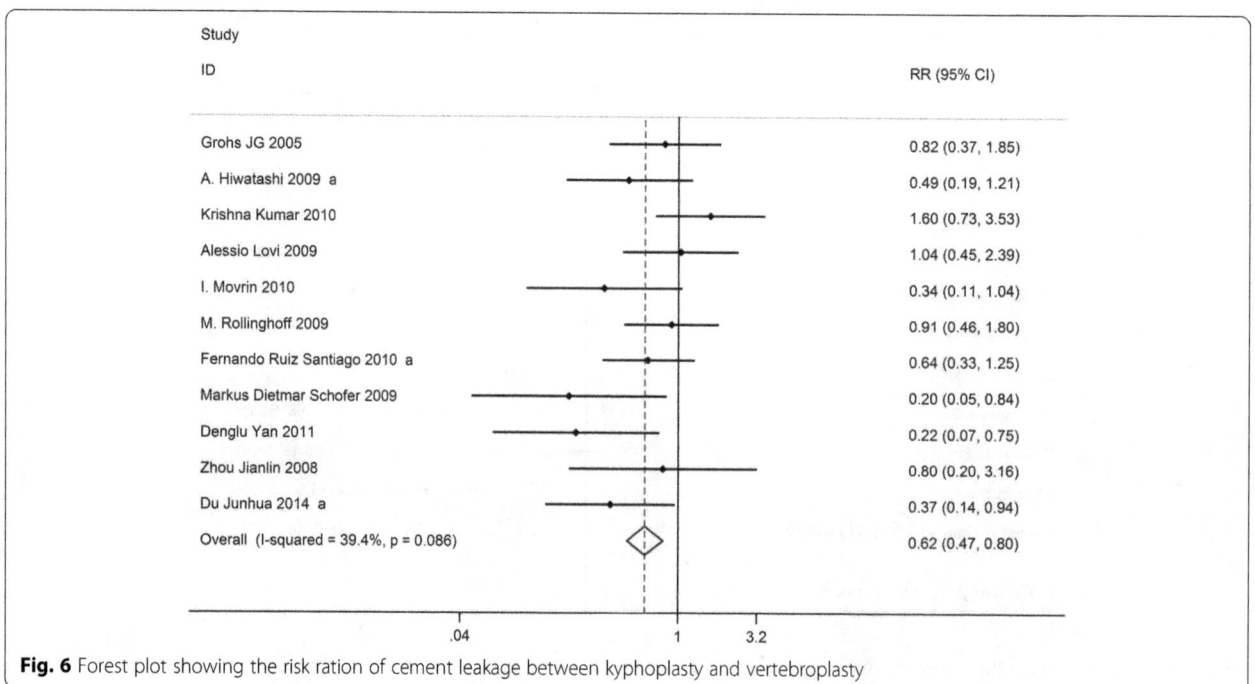

Fig. 6 Forest plot showing the risk ration of cement leakage between kyphoplasty and vertebroplasty

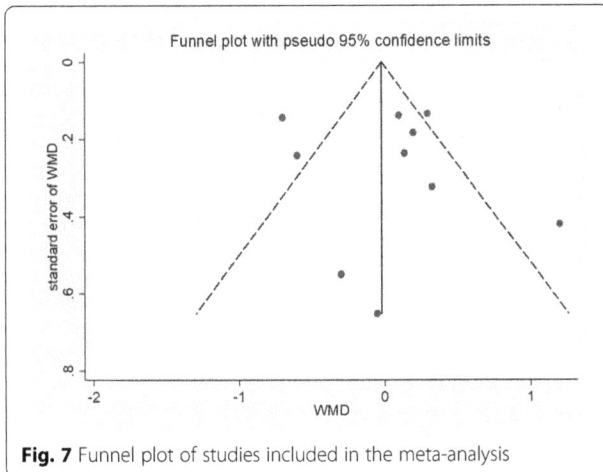

Fig. 7 Funnel plot of studies included in the meta-analysis

long-term kyphotic angle, and lower cement leakage rate. However, kyphoplasty needs longer operation time and higher material cost compared with vertebroplasty.

Longo et al. [29] reviewed conservative management of patients with VCFs, and found that no conclusions can be drawn on the superiority of cementoplasty techniques over conservative management. Denaro et al. [30] compared vertebroplasty with kyphoplasty in the treatment of VCFs and reminded us not to forget that for many years successful conservative management of vertebral fractures has been the standard of care. These conclusions are consistent with our findings that vertebroplasty and kyphoplasty had no significant difference in VAS scores, ODI scores, OVCF, and radiographic differences. Compared with the previous studies, some conclusions are consistent with Ma et al. [27] and Wang et al. [28]: kyphoplasty has some advantage in decreeing the kyphotic wedge angle, increasing the vertebral body height, and decreasing the risk of cement leakage than vertebroplasty. However, the conclusions about VAS scores and ODI scores were consistent with the studies of Vincenzo Denaro et al. [30].

Conclusion

This systematic review and meta-analysis suggest that kyphoplasty confers benefits in decreasing the MD of kyphotic wedge angle and the risk of cement leakage, increasing the mean difference of vertebral body height. In addition, kyphoplasty has no statistical influence on the VAS scores and ODI scores compared with vertebroplasty. Therefore, kyphoplasty and vertebroplasty are equally effective in the clinical outcomes of OVCF, and radiographic differences do not make significant influence on the clinical results. Considering the limitations of this meta-analysis (different types of studies were included, and some studies were of low quality), more high-quality RCTs with larger sample size, multi-centric, and longer follow-up are warranted to confirm the current findings.

Abbreviations
CI: Confidence interval; KP: Kyphoplasty; MD: Mean difference; OVCF: Osteoporotic vertebral compression fracture; RR: Relative risk; VP: Vertebroplasty

Authors' contributions
BW and LZ have made substantial contributions to the conception and design of the study. CPZ and LXS searched literature, extracted data from the collected literature, and analyzed the data. BW wrote the manuscript. LZ revised the manuscript. All authors approved the final version of the manuscript.

Competing interests
The authors declare that they have no competing interests.

References
1. Han S, Wan S, Ning L, Tong Y, Zhang J, Fan S. Percutaneous vertebroplasty versus balloon kyphoplasty for treatment of osteoporotic vertebral compression fracture: a meta-analysis of randomised and non-randomised controlled trials. Int Orthop. 2011;35:1349–58.
2. Kumar K, Verma AK, Wilson J, LaFontaine A. Vertebroplasty in osteoporotic spine fractures: a quality of life assessment. Can J Neurol Sci Le journal canadien des sciences neurologiques. 2005;32:487–95.
3. Frankel BM, Monroe T, Wang C. Percutaneous vertebral augmentation: an elevation in adjacent-level fracture risk in kyphoplasty as compared with vertebroplasty. Spine J : official journal of the North American Spine Society. 2007;7:575–82.
4. Leech JA, Dulberg C, Kellie S, Pattee L, Gay J. Relationship of lung function to severity of osteoporosis in women. Am Rev Respir Dis. 1990;141:68–71.
5. Schlaich C, Minne HW, Bruckner T, Wagner G, Gebest HJ, Grunze M, Ziegler R, Leidig-Bruckner G. Reduced pulmonary function in patients with spinal osteoporotic fractures. Osteoporos Int : a journal established as result of cooperation between the European Foundation for Osteoporosis and the National Osteoporosis Foundation of the USA. 1998;8:261–7.
6. Harris ST, Watts NB, Genant HK, McKeever CD, Hangartner T, Keller M, Chesnut CH 3rd, Brown J, Eriksen EF, Hoseyni MS, Axelrod DW, Miller PD. Effects of risedronate treatment on vertebral and nonvertebral fractures in women with postmenopausal osteoporosis: a randomized controlled trial. Vertebral Efficacy with Risedronate Therapy (VERT) study group. JAMA. 1999;282:1344–52.
7. Dickman CA, Fessler RG, MacMillan M, Haid RW. Transpedicular screw-rod fixation of the lumbar spine: operative technique and outcome in 104 cases. J Neurosurg. 1992;77:860–70.
8. Phillips FM. Minimally invasive treatments of osteoporotic vertebral compression fractures. Spine. 2003;28:S45–53.
9. Garfin SR, Yuan HA, Reiley MA. New technologies in spine: kyphoplasty and vertebroplasty for the treatment of painful osteoporotic compression fractures. Spine. 2001;26:1511–5.
10. Galibert P, Deramond H, Rosat P, Le Gars D. Preliminary note on the treatment of vertebral angioma by percutaneous acrylic vertebroplasty. Neuro-Chirurgie. 1987;33:166–8.
11. Folman Y, Shabat S. A comparison of two new technologies for percutaneous vertebral augmentation: confidence vertebroplasty vs. sky kyphoplasty. Isr Med Assoc J : IMAJ. 2011;13:394–7.
12. Grohs JG, Matzner M, Trieb K, Krepler P. Minimal invasive stabilization of osteoporotic vertebral fractures: a prospective nonrandomized comparison of vertebroplasty and balloon kyphoplasty. J Spinal Disord Tech. 2005;18:238–42.
13. Hiwatashi A, Westesson PL, Yoshiura T, Noguchi T, Togao O, Yamashita K, Kamano H, Honda H. Kyphoplasty and vertebroplasty produce the same degree of height restoration. AJNR Am J Neuroradiol. 2009;30:669–73.
14. Kumar K, Nguyen R, Bishop S. A comparative analysis of the results of vertebroplasty and kyphoplasty in osteoporotic vertebral compression fractures. Neurosurgery. 2010;67:ons171–88 discussion ons88.
15. Liu JT, Liao WJ, Tan WC, Lee JK, Liu CH, Chen YH, Lin TB. Balloon kyphoplasty versus vertebroplasty for treatment of osteoporotic vertebral

compression fracture: a prospective, comparative, and randomized clinical study. Osteoporos Int: a journal established as result of cooperation between the European Foundation for Osteoporosis and the National Osteoporosis Foundation of the USA. 2010;21:359–64.

16. Lovi A, Teli M, Ortolina A, Costa F, Fornari M, Brayda-Bruno M. Vertebroplasty and kyphoplasty: complementary techniques for the treatment of painful osteoporotic vertebral compression fractures. A prospective non-randomised study on 154 patients. Eur Spine J : official publication of the European Spine Society, the European Spinal Deformity Society, and the European Section of the Cervical Spine Research Society. 2009;18(Suppl 1):95–101.

17. Movrin I, Vengust R, Komadina R. Adjacent vertebral fractures after percutaneous vertebral augmentation of osteoporotic vertebral compression fracture: a comparison of balloon kyphoplasty and vertebroplasty. Arch Orthop Trauma Surg. 2010;130:1157–66.

18. Rollinghoff M, Siewe J, Zarghooni K, Sobottke R, Alparslan Y, Eysel P, Delank KS. Effectiveness, security and height restoration on fresh compression fractures--a comparative prospective study of vertebroplasty and kyphoplasty. Minim Invasive Neurosurg : MIN. 2009;52:233–7.

19. Santiago FR, Abela AP, Alvarez LG, Osuna RM, Garcia Mdel M. Pain and functional outcome after vertebroplasty and kyphoplasty. A comparative study. Eur J Radiol. 2010;75:e108–13.

20. Schofer MD, Efe T, Timmesfeld N, Kortmann HR, Quante M. Comparison of kyphoplasty and vertebroplasty in the treatment of fresh vertebral compression fractures. Arch Orthop Trauma Surg. 2009;129:1391–9.

21. Yan D, Duan L, Li J, Soo C, Zhu H, Zhang Z. Comparative study of percutaneous vertebroplasty and kyphoplasty in the treatment of osteoporotic vertebral compression fractures. Arch Orthop Trauma Surg. 2011;131:645–50.

22. Zhou JL, Liu SQ, Ming JH, Peng H, Qiu B. Comparison of therapeutic effect between percutaneous vertebroplasty and kyphoplasty on vertebral compression fracture. Chin J Traumatol = Zhonghua chuang shang za zhi. 2008;11:42–4.

23. Hu CH, Li QP, Wang C, Liu QP, Long HG. Analysis of clinical effects of three operative methods for osteoporotic vertebral compression fracture. Zhongguo Gu Shang = China journal of orthopaedics and traumatology. 2016;29:619–24.

24. Du J, Li X, Lin X. Kyphoplasty versus vertebroplasty in the treatment of painful osteoporotic vertebral compression fractures: two-year follow-up in a prospective controlled study. Acta Orthop Belg. 2014;80:477–86.

25. Wu Y, Wang F, Zhou JQ, Liu CY, Wu RX. Analysis of clinical effects of percutaneous vertebroplasty and percutaneous kyphoplasty in treating osteoporotic vertebral compression fracture. Zhongguo Gu Shang = China journal of orthopaedics and traumatology. 2014;27:385–9.

26. Kim KH, Kuh SU, Chin DK, Jin BH, Kim KS, Yoon YS, Cho YE. Kyphoplasty versus vertebroplasty: restoration of vertebral body height and correction of kyphotic deformity with special attention to the shape of the fractured vertebrae. J Spinal Disord Tech. 2012;25:338–44.

27. Ma XL, Xing D, Ma JX, Xu WG, Wang J, Chen Y. Balloon kyphoplasty versus percutaneous vertebroplasty in treating osteoporotic vertebral compression fracture: grading the evidence through a systematic review and meta-analysis. Eur Spine J : official publication of the European Spine Society, the European Spinal Deformity Society, and the European Section of the Cervical Spine Research Society. 2012;21:1844–59.

28. Wang H, Sribastav SS, Ye F, Yang C, Wang J, Liu H, Zheng Z. Comparison of percutaneous vertebroplasty and balloon kyphoplasty for the treatment of single level vertebral compression fractures: a meta-analysis of the literature. Pain Physician. 2015;18:209–22.

29. Longo UG, Loppini M, Denaro L, Maffulli N, Denaro V. Conservative management of patients with an osteoporotic vertebral fracture: a review of the literature. J Bone Joint Surg Br. 2012;94:152–7.

30. Denaro V, Longo UG, Maffulli N, Denaro L. Vertebroplasty and kyphoplasty. Clinical cases in mineral and bone metabolism: the official journal of the Italian Society of Osteoporosis, Mineral Metabolism, and Skeletal Diseases. 2009;6:125–30.

31. Liu JT, Liao WJ, Tan WC, Lee JK, Liu CH, Chen YH, Lin TB. Balloon kyphoplasty versus vertebroplasty for treatment of osteoporotic vertebral compression fracture: a prospective, comparative, and randomized clinical study. Osteoporos Int. 2010;21:359–64.

27

Measurement of scoliosis Cobb angle by end vertebra tilt angle method

Jing Wang[1][†], Jin Zhang[1][†], Rui Xu[2], Tie Ge Chen[1], Kai Sheng Zhou[1] and Hai Hong Zhang[1][*] ⓘ

Abstract

Background: Scoliosis is a common deformity, and its severity is usually assessed by measuring the Cobb angle on the spinal X-ray film. The measurement of the Cobb angle is an important basis for selecting therapeutic methods and evaluating therapeutic effects. To measure and calculate the scoliosis Cobb angle by end vertebra tilt angle method (tilt angle method) and assess its accuracy and usability.

Methods: It is deduced that the Cobb angle is the sum of upper and lower end vertebra tilt angles through the law of plane geometry. The project included 32 patients with scoliosis who have received treatment in our hospital from June 2011 to July 2016, whose Cobb angles were measured at various segments (total 50). The measuring results of the tilt angle method and the classical method were compared, and the time spent for the measurement of the two groups was respectively recorded with an electronic stopwatch for comparison. The interference of line marking in imaging data pixel in the two groups was compared using Beyond Compare software.

Results: The measuring results through PACS (picture archiving and communication systems) were regarded as the reference standard. There was no statistical difference for measuring the Cobb angle between the PACS method, end vertebra tilt angle method, and classical method. The end vertebra tilt angle method takes less measuring time than the classical method. The measuring error between the classical method and the tilt angle method showed no statistical significance for the difference.

Conclusion: The scoliosis Cobb angle can be measured accurately and rapidly using the principle of the Cobb angle being equal to the sum of tilt angles of the upper and lower end vertebra, where in the film data of imaging will not be easily contaminated. Under special conditions, the average measuring error is ± 3°.

Keywords: End vertebra, Tilt angle, Scoliosis, Cobb angle

Background

The scoliosis Cobb angle is an important index of disease assessment. The classical method is used to determine the upper/lower end vertebras (UEV/LEV) on the whole spine anteroposterior X-ray film; then, draw a vertical line respectively at the upper/lower end vertebra endplate lines (UEVEL/LEVEL), and the included angle of the two vertical lines is the Cobb angle [1] (Fig. 1). Manually drawing a line on the image film for measurement is needed in this method and hence is slightly cumbersome, and the line markings can easily contaminate the image data. This study

deduced the geometry law of the classical measurement method to calculate the Cobb angle by the end vertebra tilt angle measurement method (tilt angle method) and assess its accuracy, quickness, and contaminated interference in the image data.

Methods
General data

This group of patients included 10 males and 22 females, aged 11~24 with an average age of 16. Among which, 22 patients suffered from idiopathic scoliosis, 8 patients suffered from congenital scoliosis, and 2 patients suffered from neuromuscular scoliosis. There were 50 scoliosis segments totally including 24 main thoracic scoliosis segments, 18

---

* Correspondence: m13519698516_1@163.com
[†]Jing Wang and Jin Zhang contributed equally to this work.
[1]Department Of Orthopedics, Orthopedics Key Laboratory of Gansu Province, Lanzhou University Second Hospital, Cuiyingmen, Lanzhou 730030, Gansu province, China
Full list of author information is available at the end of the article

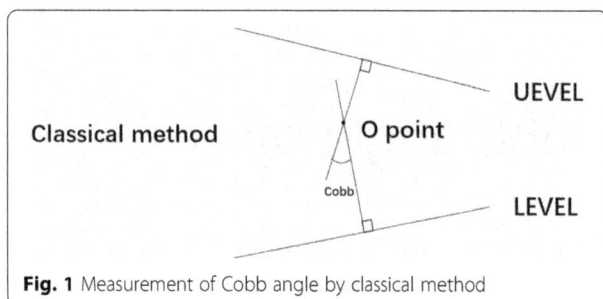

Fig. 1 Measurement of Cobb angle by classical method

thoracolumbar scoliosis segments, and 8 lumbar scoliosis segments.

Measurement of Cobb angle by PACS

Anteroposterior X-ray of the whole spine was performed on patients to determine the UEV and LEV of scoliosis segments; then, UEVEL and LEVEL were marked on the film using the PACS (picture archiving and communication systems) built-in measuring procedure, and the Cobb angle was automatically calculated. The measurement was made by the same physician. To reduce the self-measuring deviation of the observer, the angle data of each patient was measured three times every 2 weeks and then the average value was taken as the final result.

End vertebra tilt angle measurement method

The classical method for measuring the Cobb angle is to draw a vertical line respectively at UEVEL and LEVEL, and the included angle between the two vertical lines is the Cobb angle. The following auxiliary lines are drawn: the horizontal lines AB and CD. The angle of AB with UEVEL is α, and the angle of CD with LEVEL is β, which are respectively the upper/lower end vertebra tilt angles (UEVTA/LEVTA) (Fig. 2a). The parallel line AB is drawn through the vertex of Cobb angle O (Fig. 2b). The sideline of the Cobb angle that extended to line AB intersects at E, the parallel line CD is drawn through the vertex of Cobb angle O, and the sideline of the Cobb angle that extended to line CD intersects at F (Fig. 2c). It can be deduced in accordance with parallelogram law and supplementary angle law that:

$$\angle\text{Cobb} = 180^\circ - \angle\text{AEO} - \angle\text{CFO}$$
$$= 180^\circ - (90^\circ - \alpha) - (90^\circ - \beta) = \alpha + \beta$$

The Cobb angle is the sum of upper and lower end vertebra tilt angles. The included angle of the upper vertebra endplate line with the horizontal line is measured on the imaging data (Fig. 2d), and the included angle of the lower vertebra endplate line with the horizontal line is measured on the imaging data (Fig. 2e). And then, the

sum of two measured included angles is the Cobb angle (Fig. 2f).

Time spent on measurement by end vertebra tilt angle

PACS spinal imaging pictures of this group of patients were exported and printed in A4 paper. After the upper and lower end vertebras and top vertebra were determined, three spine surgeons directly marked and measured the Cobb angle of the same scoliosis segment of the same patient using the classical method and tilt angle method, respectively, and then recorded the time spent on each measurement method using an electronic stopwatch and calculated the average value.

Occupied pixel space marked by the end vertebra tilt angle measurement method

The patient's whole spine anteroposterior X-ray film was scanned and made into a figure with a resolution of 654×1024 pixels. The drawing tool in the same computer was used to simulate the line markings of the classical method and the tilt angle method to measure the Cobb angle, and the stroke parameters of all drawings were kept the same. The line markings for the same Cobb angle should meet the following requirements to facilitate quantitative comparison: (1) The EVEL line ends with both lateral margins of the vertebra endplate (Fig. 3a). (2) Two EVEL vertical lines of the classical method are intersected into an angle, and one fifth of the EVEL length is extended from the intersection point (Fig. 3b). (3) The starting point of the horizontal line of the tilt angle method is intersected with the starting point of the EVEL line, and the vertical line drawn at ending point could be exactly intersected with the ending point of the EVEL line (Fig. 3c). Figures marked with a line were imported, and the line markings of the two measurement methods were compared with Beyond Compare for Mac software. The occupied pixel space value and the difference value of the two groups were automatically calculated. Then, the visual interference degree of line markings of the two groups in the whole imaging data was compared (Fig. 3d–g).

Statistical processing

Analysis was performed using SPSS 23.0 for Mac statistical software; data were expressed in mean value $\pm$ standard deviation. Complete random one-way ANOVA is used to test the results of the angle of the three methods whether there is any error. We select t test to compare whether there is a difference between the tilt angle method and the classical method in measuring time. To compare the measuring error between the tilt angle method and the classical method, whether there is statistical difference, we chose to use the Mann-Whitney

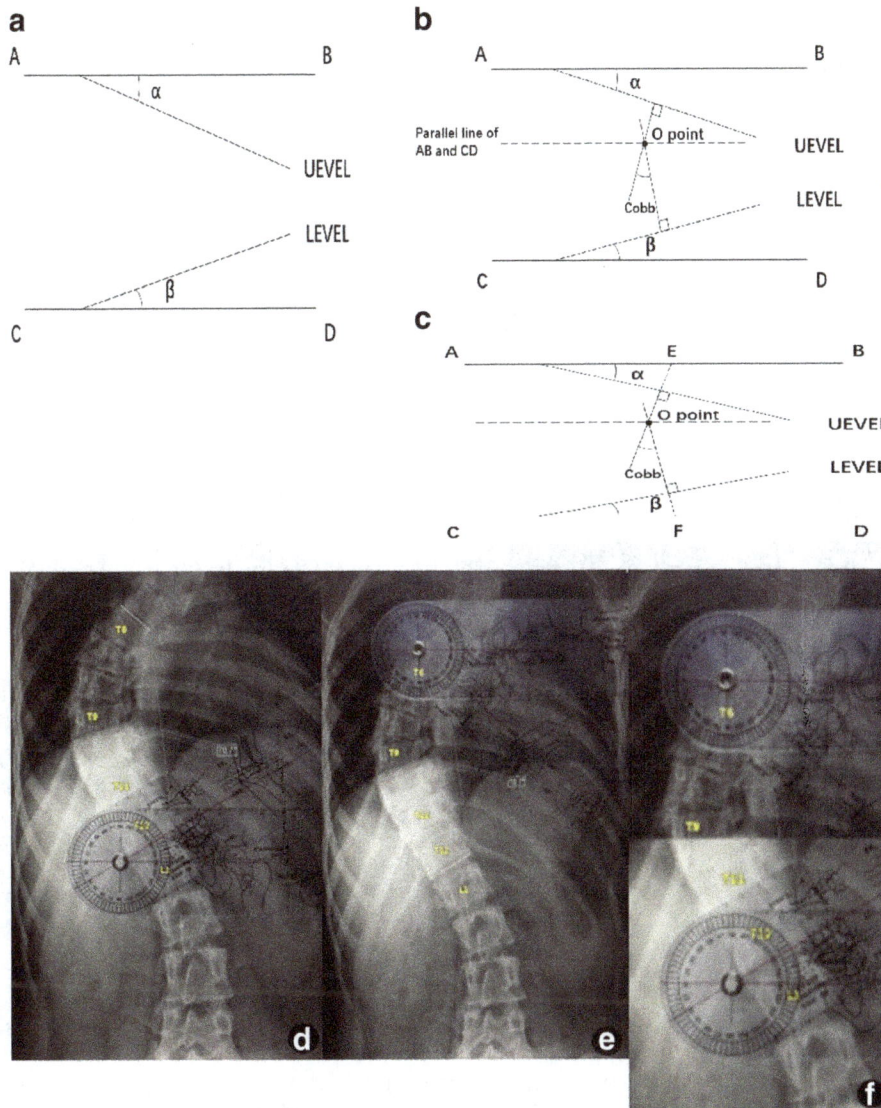

Fig. 2 a, **b**, **c** Measuring process of the Cobb angle by the end vertebra tilt angle method. **d** Measurement of the upper end vertebra tilt angle. **e** Measurement of the lower end vertebra tilt angle. **f** The upper end vertebra tilt angle $a = 41°$, the lower end vertebra tilt angle $\beta = 30°$, and the Cobb angle $= a + \beta = 71°$

U test. $p < 0.05$ means there is statistical significance for the difference.

Results

The PACS measuring result regarded as the reference standard [2] was rounded to an integer to conform to an actual clinical application. To compare the results of the angle of the three methods (PACS method, end vertebra tilt angle method, classical method), whether there is any error, a complete random one-way ANOVA is used to test.

In the test, we also need pairwise comparison; we choose the Bonferroni method and homogeneity test of variance. The following results were obtained:

1. In the homogeneity test of variance, significant $p > 0.1$ was obtained, which indicated that the same variance could be used for single-factor ANOVA.

2. Adjust $\alpha' = \alpha/m = 2 \times 0.05/3 \times (3 - 1) = 0.167$

3. Result of the PACS method: The range of Cobb angles for 50 cases was $25\sim125°$, the median was $60°$, the average value was $60.96 \pm 21.08°$, and 95% confidence interval was $54.9°$, $66.7°$. The tilt angle method result average was $61.34 \pm 21.24°$, and 95% confidence interval was $55.4°$, $67.5°$. The classical method result average was $61.90 \pm 21.34°$ and 95% confidence interval was $55.9°$, $67.9°$. The results of single-factor analysis of variance showed $F = 0.033$,

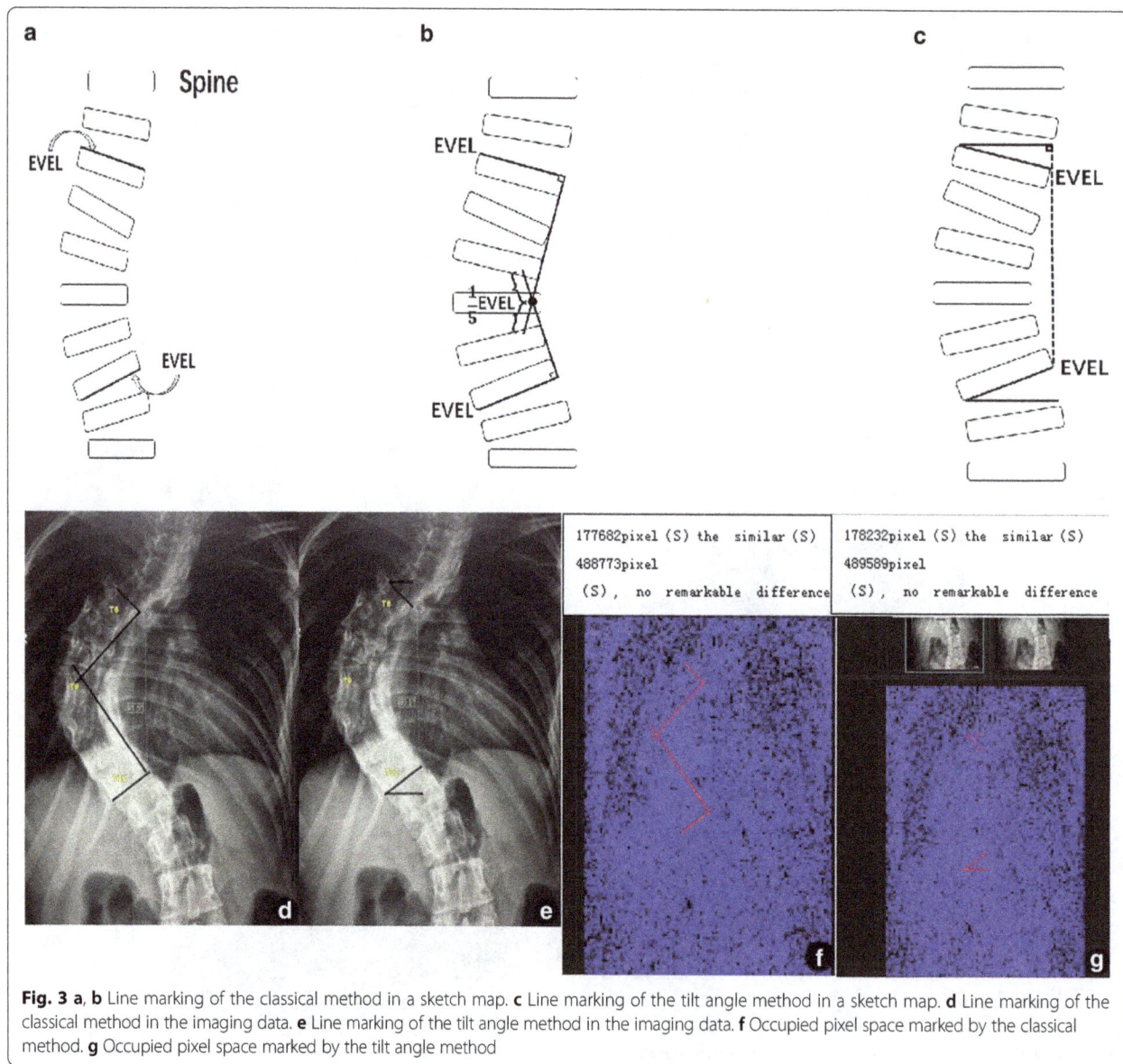

Fig. 3 a, b Line marking of the classical method in a sketch map. **c** Line marking of the tilt angle method in a sketch map. **d** Line marking of the classical method in the imaging data. **e** Line marking of the tilt angle method in the imaging data. **f** Occupied pixel space marked by the classical method. **g** Occupied pixel space marked by the tilt angle method

$p = 0.967$, indicating that there was no statistical difference between the three methods.

4. The Bonferroni method was used for pairwise comparison of the three methods ($p > 0.05$), and there was no statistical difference between the three methods, indicating that there was no difference in measuring the angle.

To compare whether there is a difference between the tilt angle method and the classical method in measuring time, we select t test and obtained the following results:

1. Correlation coefficient was 0.284 ($p < 0.05$).
2. We got $p < 0.05$ through t test. The average time spent for the tilt angle method was 12.98 ± 2.14 s with 95% confidence intervals of 12.37 s, 13.59 s.

The average time spent for the classical method was 18.96 ± 2.65 s with 95% confidence intervals of 18.20s, 19.71 s, which indicated that the measuring time of the two methods was different.

3. We got the mean difference of the measuring angle time between the tilt angle method and the classical method which is − 5.98, indicating that the time required to measure the angle by the tilt angle method is faster.

To compare the measuring error between the tilt angle method and classical method, whether there is statistical difference, we chose to use the Mann-Whitney U test. The measuring error range was − 15° to approximately + 6° through the classical method with an average error of ± 3.67° and − 9° to approximately + 5° through the tilt angle method with an average error of ± 3.19°, which showed no statistical significance for the difference ($Z = -0.430$; $p = 0.667$) (Fig. 4).

The software analysis of the pixel difference performed on picture results showed that the average pixel marked by the line drawing of the classical method was 3680 ± 533 pixels, accounting for 0.46~1.13% of total pixels, while the average pixel marked by the line drawing of the tilt angle method was 1539 ± 320 pixels, accounting for 0.12~0.32% of total pixels. Therefore, we can conclude that the pixel marked by the line drawing of the tilt angle method is less than that of the classical method, so the imaging data is less polluted.

Discussion

Scoliosis is a three-dimensional deformity of the spine. No matter how complicated the scoliosis is, the measurement of the Cobb angle is based on the coronal or sagittal plane of imaging [3]. The Cobb angle is closely related to the spinous process angle of the coronal plane and rotation of the apical vertebra [4]. As for the bigger bending deformity of the spine coronal plane, the Cobb angle is the included angle of the upper end vertebra endplate line directly intersected with the lower end vertebra endplate line. For the smaller deformity of the spine, the intersected point of two endplate lines is outside of the X-ray film, so the vertical line of the upper end vertebra endplate line and that of the lower end vertebra endplate line shall be drawn to perform the measurement. In recent years, new measurement methods have been reported, such as the smartphone software [5, 6], PACS, and other computer software, and those methods are reliable and convenient and can replace

the classical method to measure the Cobb angle [7–9]. In modern medical healthcare systems with digital radiographs and analyses, the idea of reducing drawing artifacts on an X-ray film is somewhat redundant. In developing countries, such as China, that still analyze radiographs on conventional X-ray films, steps for classical Cobb angle measurement are as follows: (1) Draw an endplate line between the two intersections of the end vertebra endplate and lateral margins on the film or a straight line drawn between the upper tangent of pedicles' eyes in the same vertebra. (2) Measure the rectangle angle of the upper endplate line to draw the vertical line, and measure the rectangle angle of the lower endplate line to draw the vertical line. (3) Measure the included angle between two vertical lines (Cobb angle). The classical Cobb method needs a line drawn in a large range, and this will easily contaminate imaging data. In addition, limited by conditions of radiology departments of different hospitals and imaging film size, it is hard to include the whole spine segments into one film, and films shall be taken segment by segment. Thus, the measurement of the Cobb angle shall be performed by manually splicing the films into one figure, so there are inconveniences and figure angle deviations.

According to the geometry law, it can be deduced that the Cobb angle is the sum of upper and lower end vertebra tilt angles, so the Cobb angle can be calculated by measuring end vertebra tilt angles. No matter how serious the curvature of scoliosis is, and whether the scoliosis segments are in one imaging film, the Cobb angle can be calculated accurately and rapidly just by determining the two end vertebras and measuring the tilt angles. The measuring steps of the tilt angle method are as

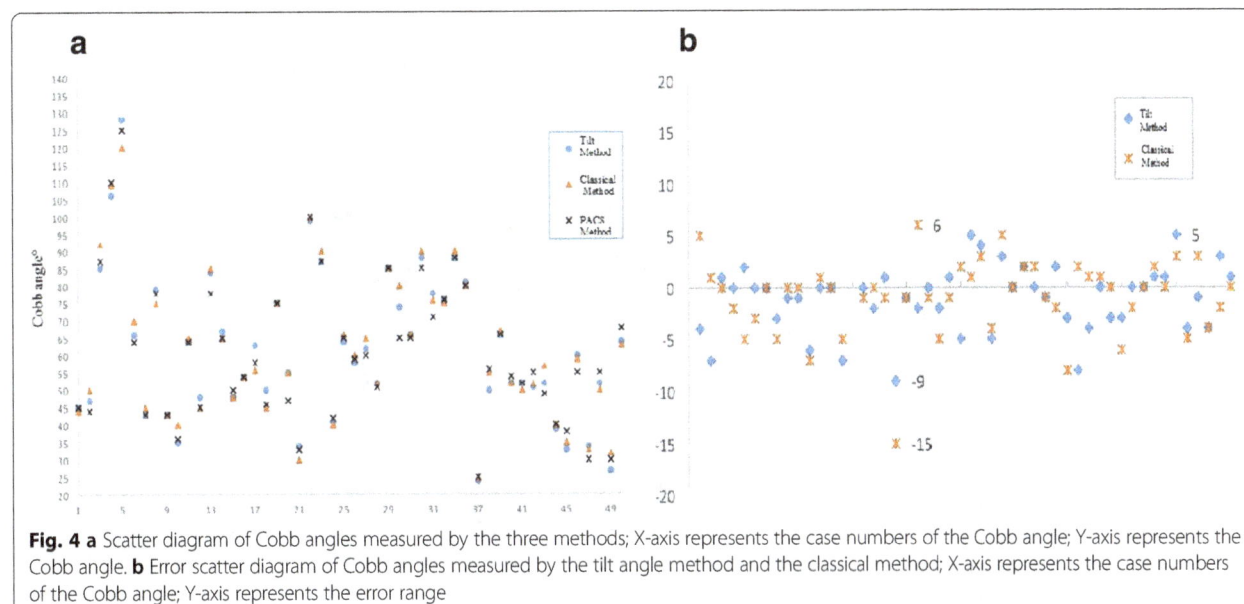

Fig. 4 a Scatter diagram of Cobb angles measured by the three methods; X-axis represents the case numbers of the Cobb angle; Y-axis represents the Cobb angle. **b** Error scatter diagram of Cobb angles measured by the tilt angle method and the classical method; X-axis represents the case numbers of the Cobb angle; Y-axis represents the error range

follows: (1) Draw the upper and lower end vertebra endplate connecting line on the film. (2) Measure the tilt angles of the upper and lower endplates. (3) Add the two measured results to get the Cobb angle. Obviously, the tilt method reduces one measurement step, so it can reduce the measuring time. In this study, the average time spent when using tilt angle to measure an angle is about 6 s less than that of the classical method. If you are skilled in the method, you can utilize the rectangular structure of a measuring ruler to fast determine the horizontal line and measure the end vertebra tilt angle in combination with the straight edge of the figure on the imaging film, which is more fast and convenient than the classical method in which the two vertical lines shall be additionally drawn for measurement. If the endplate connecting line develops clearly, the marker line of a measuring ruler can be directly utilized to perform overlap measurement, which can be free from the line drawing step.

When judging the interference and containment degree of line marking in imaging data, the figure treatment and analysis can be used to compare the difference of pixels marked by lines, which is more precise than visual observation and judgment [10]; the interference in pixels marked by the tilt angle is only 23.9~28.3% of that by the classical method, greatly lowering the contamination of line on imaging data.

A previous study has suggested that the Cobb measurement method has several sources of errors [11]: non-standard position of patients or/and devices in imagological examination. To confirm the correct marker lines in the scoliosis segments which have anatomical variation of the vertebrae, different observers identify the different upper and lower end vertebrae. For those reasons, the measuring error range for the classical Cobb method was 6~9° [11, 12]. The tilt method is a methodological improvement based on the Cobb method, which has the same measuring errors as the former one. The efficacy and effectiveness of the tilt

method were observed and compared by the same observers via using the same medical images. Therefore, the most common errors are intrinsic to the measurement method. The tilt method needs to draw two horizontal lines on the X-ray film. It is hard to make an accurate judgment about the reference points associated with the horizontal line of the actual torso. In addition, when the film is placed on the table or on the radiographic view box, the horizontal plane judgment will deviate from the real plane when the film is tilted, and the horizontal line is not the same as the horizontal of the actual torso. It is easy to make measuring error. But we found through computer simulation measurements that even though the film was tilted or the real horizontal plane was difficult to determine, there was no obvious measuring error. As shown, it is exactly the same case of scoliosis X-ray image data (Fig. 5a, b). We tilted the film to simulate the actual film placed on the table or on the film viewing illuminator, so the drawing line may deviate from the horizontal line. The green line is a horizontal line based on the entire imaging data, and it was given by the computer automatically. The red line was respectively at the upper/lower end vertebra endplate line. The angle between the red and green lines is an end vertebra tilt angle. The angle is completely consistent according to the geometry law and the actual observation (Fig. 5a, b).

Even though there is no statistical difference between the measurement error of the tilt method and the classical method, there are still some procedures to avoid the measurement error as far as possible. For instance, the shape of the imaging film is a rectangle, and the ruler line on the film is standard vertical or horizontal; it was given by the computer. We can use it as a reference point (Fig. 5c). On the other hand, we use the ruler as a measuring tool. The shape of the ruler is a rectangular structure, so we can make full use of the rectangular structure of the ruler and the rectangular outline of the imaging film as the reference point of the horizontal

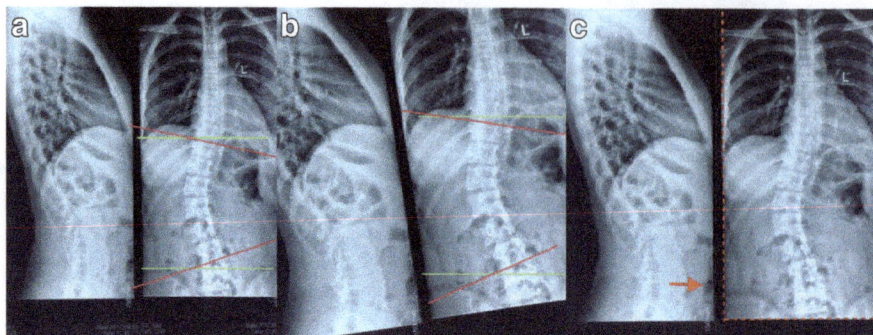

Fig. 5 a Normally placed film. **b** Tilted placed film. **c** Red dotted line: the rectangular structure of the imaging data itself, and the ruler line (arrow) is vertical to the real horizontal plane

line. For example, the wide edge of the ruler overlaps with the edge of the film, and the line drawn on the long edge of the ruler must be the true horizontal line of the imaging data.

Cobb angle > 10° means that scoliosis exists, 10~25° means regular recheck shall be performed, and 25~45° means orthosis shall be needed. Cobb angle > 45° means surgical interference is needed. Cobb angle > 5° in two X-ray examinations indicates the scoliosis deformity progress [13]. Therefore, the measuring error for Cobb angle > 5° will possibly interfere with the diagnosis and treatment results. There is always a difference existing in the measurement of the Cobb angle of the same patient, and it is related to the patient position and photography angle. The manual line drawing and artificial observation are still the main reasons for measuring error. This study took the Cobb angle measured by PACS as the reference standard; the measuring error range for the classical method was − 15~ 6° with an average error of ± 3.67°, and the measuring error range for the tilt angle method was − 9~5° with the average error of ± 3.19°. The first reason for error is that the cases with complicated scoliosis we included were less; the second reason is that the imaging data included in the study were made into pictures of the same resolution and size in advance and printed and then UEV and LEV were determined uniformly for measurement and comparison [14], which could statistically reduce the measurer's judgment bias and inter-group error.

Conclusions
The scoliosis Cobb angle can be measured accurately and rapidly by the principle of the Cobb angle being equal to the sum of tilt angles of upper and lower end vertebra, wherein the film data of imaging will not be easily contaminated. Under special conditions, the average measuring error is ± 3°.

Abbreviations
EVEL: End vertebra endplate lines; EVTA: End vertebra tilt angle method; LEV: Lower end vertebras; LEVEL: Lower end vertebra endplate lines; LEVTA: Lower end vertebra tilt angles; PACS: Picture archiving and communication systems; UEV: Upper end vertebras; UEVEL: Upper end vertebra endplate lines; UEVTA: Upper end vertebra tilt angles

Authors' contributions
JW and JZ contributed in the conception and design, analysis and interpretation, and writing of the manuscript. RX, TC, and KZ contributed to the data collection and material support. HZ contributed to the critical revision of the manuscript and supervision. All authors read and approved the final manuscript.

Competing interests
The authors declare that they have no competing interests.

Author details
[1]Department Of Orthopedics, Orthopedics Key Laboratory of Gansu Province, Lanzhou University Second Hospital, Cuiyingmen, Lanzhou 730030, Gansu province, China. [2]Radiology Department, Lanzhou University Second Hospital, Cuiyingmen, Lanzhou 730030, Gansu province, China.

References
1. Cobb J. Outline for the study of scoliosis. Instr Course Lect. 1947;5:261–75.
2. He J, Yan Z, Zhi Y, et al. The study of the reliability in Cobb measurement on PACS workstation. Zhongguo ji zhu ji sui za zhi. 2006;16(10):732–4.
3. Sangole AP, Aubin CE, Labelle H, et al. Three-dimensional classification of thoracic scoliotic curves. Spine. 2009;34(1):91–9.
4. Morrison DG, Chan A, Hill D, et al. Correlation between Cobb angle, spinous process angle (SPA) and apical vertebrae rotation (AVR) on posteroanterior radiographs in adolescent idiopathic scoliosis (AIS). Euro Spine J. 2014;24(2): 306–12.
5. Qiao J, Liu Z, Xu L, et al. Reliability analysis of a smartphone-aided measurement method for the Cobb angle of scoliosis. J Spinal Disord Tech. 2012;25(4):88–92.
6. Shaw M, Adam CJ, Izatt MT, et al. Use of the iPhone for Cobb angle measurement in scoliosis. Euro Spine J. 2012;21(6):1062–8.
7. Wang C, Lao L, Niu W, et al. Computer-assisted versus traditional Cobb angle measurement on digital radiograph in scoliosis. Zhonghua Yi Xue Za Zhi. 2010;90(19):1300–3.
8. Aubin CE, Bellefleur C, Joncas J, et al. Reliability and accuracy analysis of a new semiautomatic radiographic measurement software in adult scoliosis. Spine. 2011;36(12):780–90.
9. Zhang J, Lou E, Le LH, et al. Automatic Cobb measurement of scoliosis based on fuzzy Hough transform with vertebral shape prior. J Digit Imaging. 2009;22(5):463–72.
10. Thakkar SC, Mears SC. Visibility of surgical site marking: a prospective randomized trial of two skin preparation solutions. J Bone Joint Surg Am. 2012;94(2):97–102.
11. Capasso G, Maffulli N, Testa V. The validity and reliability of measurements in spinal deformities: a critical appraisal. Acta Orthop Belg. 1992;58(2):126–35.
12. Dickson RA, Lawton JO, Archer IA, et al. The pathogenesis of idiopathic scoliosis. Biplanar spinal asymmetry. J Bone Joint Surg Br. 1984;66(1):8–15.
13. Lonstein JE. Adolescent idiopathic scoliosis. Lancet. 1994;344(8934):1407–12.
14. Morrissy RT, Goldsmith GS, Hall EC, et al. Measurement of the Cobb angle on radiographs of patients who have scoliosis. Evaluation of intrinsic error. J Bone Joint Surg. 1990;72(3):320–7.

28

A new method of measuring the thumb pronation and palmar abduction angles during opposition movement using a three-axis gyroscope

Tomoyuki Kuroiwa[1], Koji Fujita[1]* ⓘ, Akimoto Nimura[2], Takashi Miyamoto[2], Toru Sasaki[1] and Atsushi Okawa[1]

Abstract

Background: Thumb opposition is vital for hand function and involves pronation and palmar abduction. The improvement of pronation is often used as one of the evaluation items of the opponensplasty method for severe carpal tunnel syndrome. However, most of the studies used substitution evaluation methods for measurement of the pronation angle. Thus, there is still no appropriate method for measuring thumb pronation angle accurately in carpal tunnel syndrome patients.

In recent reports, a wearable gyroscope was used to evaluate upper extremity motions and it can be possibly used for accurate measurement of the thumb pronation angle along the three-dimensionally moving bone axis.

Thus, we investigated the reliability of measuring thumb pronation using a gyroscope and evaluated whether this method can be used to detect opposition impairment.

Methods: The participants were volunteers with unaffected upper limbs (32 hands) and patients with carpal tunnel syndrome (27 hands). The pronation and palmar abduction angles during opposition movements were measured using a three-axis gyroscope that included a three-axis accelerometer. The gyroscope was fixed onto the first metacarpal bone and the thumb phalanx.

Results: The pronation and palmar abduction angles of the metacarpal bone and the palmar abduction angles of the phalanx significantly decreased in the carpal tunnel syndrome group. The pronation angle of the metacarpal bone during opposition movement peaked later than the palmar abduction angle in all hands.

Conclusions: We were able to measure the thumb pronation and palmar abduction angles using the three-axis gyroscope, and this tool was able to detect impairments of thumb opposition due to carpal tunnel syndrome. This could be a tool for measuring thumb and finger angles and for detecting impairments caused by various diseases.

Keywords: Gyroscope, Motion analysis, Thumb opposition, Thumb pronation, Carpal tunnel syndrome

Background

The thumb is vitally important for hand function and accounts for 40–50% of hand function [1–5]. The most significant factor contributor to the hand's function is opposition [6, 7]. Opposition movement plays a key role in hand motions such as pulp pinch, grip, and grasp [2, 8–10]. Thumb opposition movement includes two elements, namely, pronation and palmar abduction [1, 11, 12]. Of these, pronation is essential for grasp and pulp pinch [13]. Carpal tunnel syndrome (CTS) is a disease that causes weakness of the thumb's muscle because of thenar atrophy, resulting in opposition impairment [11, 14–16]. Hence, the extent of improvement in pronation was often used as one of the evaluation items of the opponensplasty method which is aimed to regain the opposition function equivalent to that of healthy subjects [13, 17–21]. Nevertheless, in

* Correspondence: fujiorth@tmd.ac.jp; fujita.orth@tmd.ac.jp
[1]Department of Orthopaedic and Spinal Surgery, Graduate School of Medical and Dental Sciences, Tokyo Medical and Dental University, 1-4-5, Yushima, Bunkyo-ku, Tokyo 113-8519, Japan
Full list of author information is available at the end of the article

these reports, nail tip angle, spatial angle, or Kapandji score were used in the substitution evaluation method for the measurement of the pronation angle. Indeed, these methods can be adapted longitudinal evaluation of a single patient; however, they have a number of shortcomings. The first two are not three-dimensional evaluation methods, and the last one is not an accurate quantitative evaluation method but is a numerical categorized method; therefore, even if thenar atrophy increases because of increasing severity, it does not reflect clearly in the numerical value [22]. Thus, despite the decrease in the pronation of the thumb in CTS patients in actual clinical practice, the lack of an appropriate assessment method to evaluate the patients' function remains.

Various motion analyses of the lower extremities using a gyroscope and accelerometer have been reported [23–26]. In some recent reports, a gyroscope was used to evaluate upper extremity motions in patients with neuromuscular disorders, such as Parkinson's disease [27, 28] or Duchenne muscular dystrophy [29]. A gyroscope is small, wearable, and easy to handle [30, 31]; hence, we hypothesized that we could measure the thumb pronation angle along the three-dimensionally moving bone axis using a gyroscope.

Therefore, we devised a method for measuring the angles of thumb pronation using a gyroscope and measured the angles in volunteers and patients with CTS during opposition movements. The purposes of this study were to investigate the reliability of measuring thumb pronation using a gyroscope and to evaluate whether this method can be used to detect opposition impairments.

Methods

This comparative study to investigate the validity of measuring thumb pronation using a new sensor was approved by the institutional review board of our institution, and all participants provided written informed consent.

Participants

We recruited 16 patients with CTS and thenar atrophy before surgery (CTS group, 27 hands) and 16 healthy volunteers (control group, 32 hands) between June 2017 and June 2018. Upon recruitment, we obtained information from the patients regarding their chief complaint and the trauma history of their hands. We performed medical interview and physical examination such as CTS induction tests and took X-ray images of the hands of all patients.

As the CTS group, patients were included if they were primarily diagnosed with CTS and planned to undergo carpal tunnel release. The diagnostic criteria for primary CTS included finger numbness; the

physical findings of CTS, such as Tinel's sign or positive results on a compression test and the Phalen test; and an abnormal nerve conduction velocity (NCV) value, based on Padua's classification [32]. We excluded patients with a history of hand surgery or injury, recurrence after carpal tunnel release, positive physical and imaging findings indicative of first carpometacarpal (CM) or thumb metacarpophalangeal (MP) osteoarthritis that could affect the motion of thumb, suspicion of cervical spine disease, or positive magnetic resonance imaging findings of compression because of a space-occupying lesion.

As the control group, volunteers were included if they had undergone total hip arthroplasty in our hospital and if their age and sex matched those of patients in the CTS group. We excluded patients from the control group if they had a history of wrist, hand, or finger surgery or injury; thumb pain; finger numbness; positive physical findings of CTS; or positive imaging findings of osteoarthritis of the first CM or thumb MP. The reason for recruiting patients who underwent total hip arthroplasty for the control group was that these patients underwent routine X-ray of the hand preoperatively to assess the effect on T cane use; therefore, additional radiation exposure was unnecessary.

Physical examination and NCV testing

To diagnose CTS and evaluate the extent of impairment of thumb opposition, we obtained the following data before this study was performed. All physical findings were obtained through a physical examination by experienced hand surgeons. The degree of atrophy was evaluated in four stages with a visual inspection. The scores of a manual muscle test were evaluated using the Medical Research Council's Muscle Scale [33]. Experienced neurologists performed all NCV tests and evaluated these data.

Apparatus

The thumb's angular velocities and accelerations were measured using a three-axis gyroscope with a three-axis accelerometer (MP-M6-02/500C, angular velocity range ± 500°/s; sampling rate 70 Hz, acceleration range ± 20 m/s^2; sampling rate 200 Hz, size 12 mm in width; 23 mm in depth; 5 mm in height, weight 3 g, MicroStone, Nagano, Japan) during the participants' opposition movements. The gyroscope was fixed with tape at the dorsal side of the first metacarpal bone or on the middle of the thumb phalanx along the bone axis (Fig. 1a). The gyroscope was connected to a data logger (MVP-RF8, size 45 mm in width; 45 mm in depth; 18.5 mm in height, weight 60 g, MicroStone). The accuracy of this data acquisition method was confirmed in a previous study using

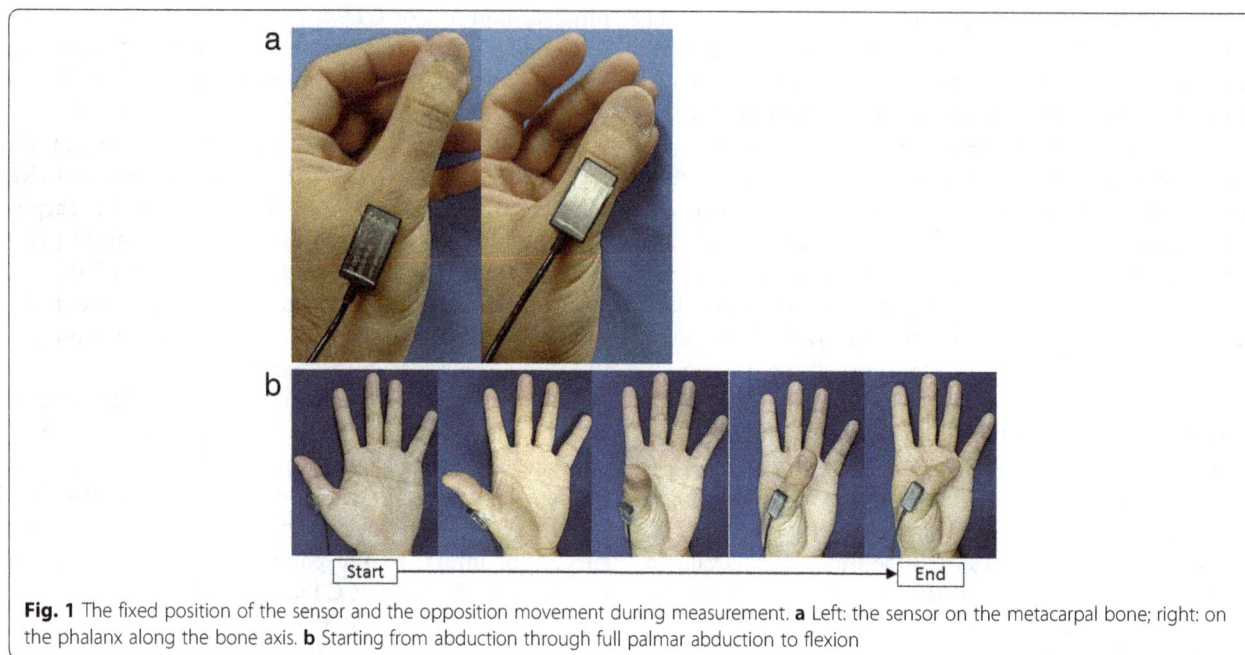

Fig. 1 The fixed position of the sensor and the opposition movement during measurement. **a** Left: the sensor on the metacarpal bone; right: on the phalanx along the bone axis. **b** Starting from abduction through full palmar abduction to flexion

the same type of sensor [34]. The gyroscope was calibrated statically against gravity before the measurements were made. The thumb's angular velocities and accelerations were sampled at 200 Hz, and these signals were synchronized. After analog-to-digital transformation (10-bit resolution), the signals were collected in the logger and immediately transferred to a laptop PC (HP ProBook 450 G2, Hewlett-Packard, Boeblingen, Germany) via a Bluetooth Personal Area Network. It was possible to simultaneously measure the inclination angle of the horizontal plane and the rotation angles of the three axes, and these were calculated with data processing. The working range of the gyroscope to the PC was approximately 80 cm. Signals were processed using commercially available software (MVP-DA2-S, MicroStone).

Measurement

Participants were instructed to oppose their thumb by drawing as large a semicircle as possible and to move their thumb five times in 45 s. The angles of rotation and inclination of each bone axis were measured during five continuous reciprocating opposition movements, which were from the position of full radial abduction through full palmar abduction to full flexion of the MP and interphalangeal joints (Fig. 1b). These angles were first measured on the thumb phalanx and then on the metacarpal bone. During measurement, the examiner maintained the participant's wrist and MP joint of fingers in a stationary position.

We regarded the rotation angle as pronation/supination and the inclination angle as palmar abduction (Fig. 2). Angle data were evaluated using a system in which the

direction of pronation and palmar abduction was considered positive. The difference between the maximum and minimum values was calculated for one opposition movement (Fig. 3). After excluding the first and last opposition movements from the five repeated measurements, we considered the average of these values as the range of motion during one opposition movement. Moreover, we evaluated which peak (pronation or palmar abduction) occurred earlier during one opposition movement.

Statistical analysis

Data regarding age and the motion angle are presented as the median with an interquartile range. The Mann-Whitney U test was used to compare differences. A power analysis was performed on the basis of the pronation angles. To evaluate the intra-tester reliability, the standard deviation of three measurements was calculated for all trials, and the average value was calculated. Using the value, the coefficient of variation (CV) was also calculated. We performed all statistical analyses using EZR (EasyR, version 1.36). $P < 0.05$ was considered statistically significant. We estimated that a sample size of 16 participants per group would be required to achieve 80% power to detect a 10° difference in the aggregated angle for the two groups, assuming an overall standard deviation of 10°, similar to what was observed in a previous study [35].

Results
Patient characteristics
The median age was 67.5 (62–76.5) and 68 (54.8–75.5) years in the control and CTS group, respectively. All the participants were female. The physical findings and

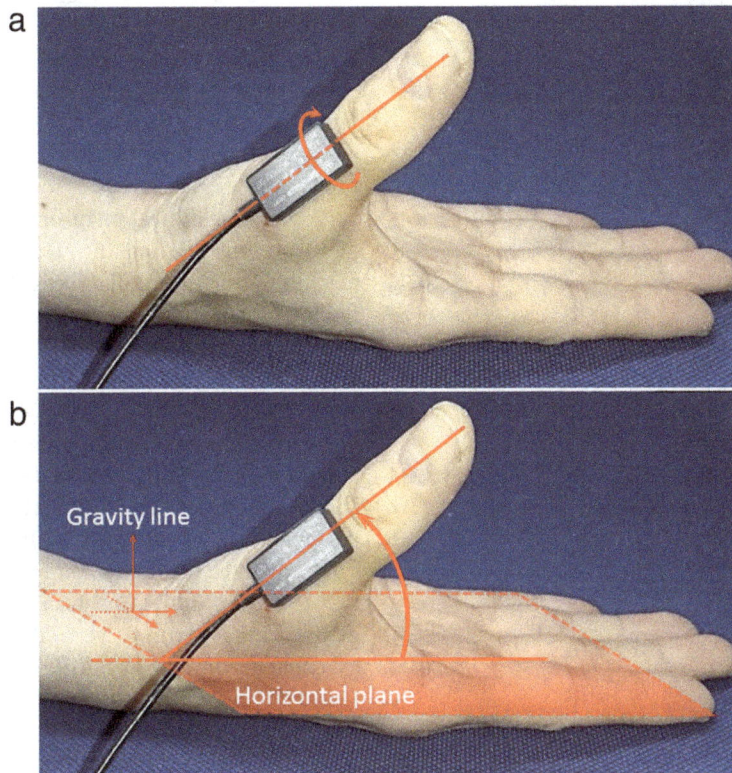

Fig. 2 The measured angle during opposition movement. **a** Pronation angle: the rotation angle around the longitudinal axis of the sensor. **b** Palmar abduction angle: the inclination angle of the longitudinal axis of the sensor to the horizontal plane

NCV tests in the CTS group are shown in Table 1. The physical examination showed moderate or severe thenar atrophy in 15 hands, and muscle strength less than good in 13 hands. In nearly all of the patients, CTS was classified as moderate or worse as per Padua's classification, and only one had mild CTS.

Measurement data

The median pronation angle on the first metacarpal was 31° in the control group and 20° in the CTS group. Median

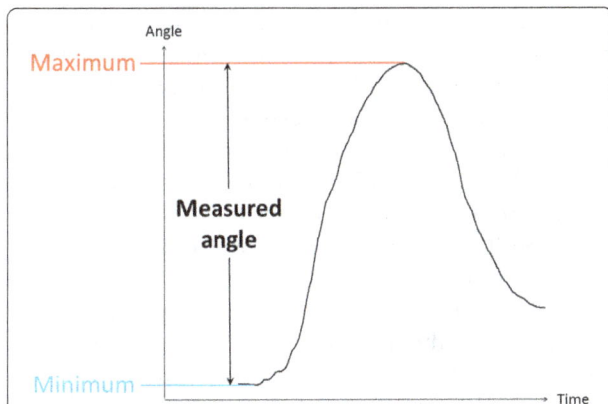

Fig. 3 The measured angle. Subtracting the minimum value from the maximum value of the obtained graph

pronation angle on the phalanx was 21.5° in the control group and 23° in the CTS group. The median palmar abduction angle on the first metacarpal was 25° in the control group and 18° in the CTS group. The median palmar abduction angle on the phalanx was 55° in the control group and 43° in the CTS group (Table 2). The pronation angle of the metacarpal bone and the palmar abduction angle of the metacarpal bone and phalanx decreased significantly in patients in the CTS group. The average standard deviation of pronation angles of the metacarpal bone and phalanx were 1.3° and 2.4° respectively, and palmar abduction angles of the metacarpal bone and phalanx were 1.3° and 1.9° respectively. The CV of the pronation angles of the metacarpal bone and phalanx were 0.051 and 0.1, and the palmar abduction angles of the metacarpal bone and phalanx were 0.059 and 0.04 respectively (Table 2).

We obtained transition graphs of the measured angles (Fig. 4). Most of the graphs of the pronation angle of phalanx showed a peak near the palmar abduction position during the opposition movement. However, the pronation angle of the metacarpal bone of 19 thumbs in the CTS group and 17 in the control group peaked when the thumb was in the full flexion position. Moreover, in all hands, the pronation angle peaked later than the palmar abduction angle did. The actual measurement time per participant was less than 10 min.

Table 1 Data of physical findings and NCV tests in the CTS group

	CTS ($n = 27$)
Thenar atrophy	
Absent	12
Mild	0
Moderate	8
Severe	7
Opposition MMT	
5 (normal)	8
4 (good)	6
3 (fair)	10
2 (poor)	2
1 (trace)	1
0 (zero)	0
Padua's classification	
Normal	0
Minimal	0
Mild	1
Moderate	16
Severe	6
Extreme	4

NCV nerve conduction velocity, *CTS* carpal tunnel syndrome, *MMT* manual muscle test

Discussion

First, we investigated the reliability of measuring the thumb pronation and palmar abduction angles using a small sensor with a three-axis gyroscope and accelerometer. Previous studies have evaluated the pronation angle of the first metacarpal bone using CT in healthy volunteers and yielded various values for the average pronation angle. Cheema et al. and Kimura et al. reported that the pronation angles were 56° and 57° respectively [36, 37]. We considered that the researchers only evaluated the thumb pronation, which was projected into two dimensions using CT imaging; therefore, the thumb pronation angle was overestimated as

Table 2 The range of motion during opposition movement

	Control ($n = 32$)	CTS ($n = 27$)	P value	CV
Pronation (°)				
Metacarpal bone	31 (22.8–36.3)	20 (16.5–24.5)	< 0.001	0.051
Phalanx	21.5 (15.3–30)	23 (23.5–33.5)	0.76	0.1
Palmar abduction (°)				
Metacarpal bone	25 (21.8–29.3)	18 (13.5–24)	0.004	0.059
Phalanx	55 (46.5–62.3)	43 (33–49)	< 0.001	0.04

Data are presented as the median (IQR). Statistical significance was determined with the Mann-Whitney *U* test
CTS carpal tunnel syndrome, *IQR* interquartile range, *CV* coefficient of variation

the palmar abduction angle became closer to 90°. By contrast, Goto et al. and Kawanishi et al. reported that the pronation angle was 14.8° and 22.3° respectively using three-dimensional evaluation method [38, 39]. However, since the former showed the angle from the adduction position to the full flexion position as the pronation angle, it is reasonable that the numerical value becomes lower than ours. Moreover, their report had only one participant. The latter evaluated the differences from the radial abduction position to the full flexion position as the pronation angle using not dynamic CT but the static one. Therefore, it is reasonable that they underestimated the maximum pronation angles of the participants whose thumb pronation angle became maximum slightly later than the palmar abduction position. Moreover, most classical studies showed that the arc of pronation of the first metacarpal bone was less than 30° [40].

Meanwhile, there are many reports of CV measurement of the range of motion of finger and wrist previously. Most of these were about 0.05–0.06 using the gyroscope, optical motion capture, and goniometer [41–43], and almost all the results of our study were similar values.

Hence, we considered that our method to measure the thumb pronation three-dimensionally using a gyroscope is sufficiently reliable.

We believe that measuring thumb pronation angle using a gyroscope has many advantages. Kapandji scores [44] are widely used to evaluate thumb opposition in clinical practice [20, 45–52]. However, it is not an accurate quantitative evaluation method but only a numerical categorized method; moreover, there were reports that almost all healthy subject and even CTS patients with thenar atrophy were able to obtain 9 or 10 points of this score [22, 53]. Although three-dimensional CT was able to measure the angle accurately, it is costly, requires time and effort, and above all, it is very invasive. Optical motion capture systems are dynamic, three-dimensional, and non-invasive but complicated and also require time, effort, and, moreover, a large specialized apparatus. In contrast, a gyroscope is compact, wearable, economical, easy to handle [30, 31], three-dimensional, and non-invasive.

Second, we were able to measure the pronation as well as the palmar abduction angles of the thumb during opposition movements in patients in the control and CTS groups. As expected, there was a significant decrease in the pronation angle of the metacarpal bone and palmar abduction angle of the metacarpal bone and phalanx in patients in the CTS group.

There is only one report of the comparison of thumb pronation angle along the three-dimensionally moving bone axis between healthy subjects and CTS patients

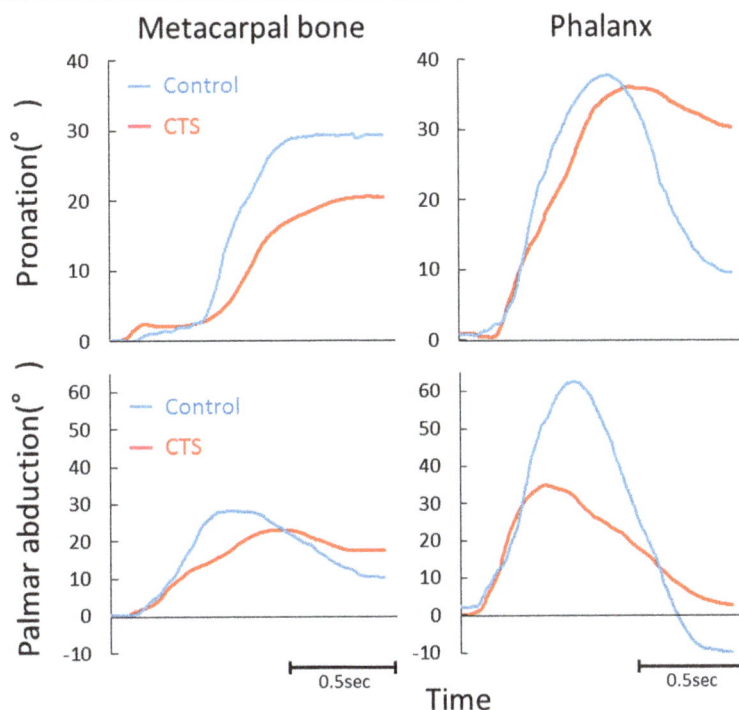

Fig. 4 Four representative examples of transition graphs. The measured angles in the CTS (red) and control (blue) groups. Upper: pronation angle; lower: palmar abduction angle; left: metacarpal bone; right: phalanx. CTS: carpal tunnel syndrome

using an optical motion capture system [35]. However, the pronation angle in the CTS group decreased, but not significantly. Conversely, our study showed a significant decrease in this angle in patients with CTS. We considered that the discrepancy in these results was because of the difference in the severity of CTS between patients in the previous study and those in ours. In our study, we recruited only CTS patients with thenar atrophy before they underwent surgery, and the disease in almost all of these patients was classified as moderate or worse according to Padua's classification. By contrast, it is reasonable to assume that the CTS group in the previous study included patients with minimal or mild CTS or patients without a motor disorder. This is because previous reports included (i) only patients with abnormal NCV values, while the threshold was not mentioned and (ii) those with a score of at least 1.5 on the Severity Scale [54]. Furthermore, our study had more than twice the number of cases that this previous study did. These differences in the characteristics of participants may account for the differences in results.

Interestingly, in this study, we also demonstrated a decrease in the angle on metacarpal bone. As CTS causes atrophies of the abductor pollicis brevis muscle and opponens pollicis muscle [55], the result is anatomically feasible. Furthermore, the fact that this method was able to measure the pronation of the metacarpal bone may suggest the applicability of the method to diseases other than CTS, such as osteoarthritis of the CM.

The advancement and importance of our method are anchored on two points. First, by miniaturization of gyroscopes, we succeeded in measuring the thumb pronation angle, which had not been previously measured with a gyroscope. Second, our method allowed the detection of the pronation angle impairment due to CTS easily, non-invasively, and three-dimensionally and represented it numerically.

This study has several limitations. First, it is possible that stretching of the skin while the sensor was applied affected the results. However, this effect should have reduced the measured angle, thereby making it more difficult to obtain any significant outcome. Second, we did not measure the angles of the metacarpal bone and phalanx simultaneously; therefore, we were not able to evaluate the phalanx angle independently. Third, six patients who used canes or walkers were included because the control group consisted of patients with hip osteoarthritis rather than healthy volunteers. Thus, the mechanical effect of a T cane on the first web may have affected the results.

We plan to perform further studies involving simultaneous measurement of the first metacarpal bone and phalanx of the participants and to apply this measurement technique in patients with mild CTS and those with other diseases such as osteoarthritis of the CM.

Furthermore, we plan to use this method to evaluate the differences in the pre- and post-opponensplasty pronation angles. In the future, we intend to establish this method as a diagnostic tool for CTS clinically.

Conclusion

We were able to apply a gyroscope as a new measurement method of pronation and palmar abduction angles of thumb. It was easy, quick, and non-invasive. Furthermore, we were able to demonstrate the significant decrease in the pronation angle of the metacarpal bone and palmar abduction angle of the metacarpal bone and phalanx in patients in the CTS group using the method.

Abbreviations
CM: Carpometacarpal; CT: Computed tomography; CTS: Carpal tunnel syndrome; CV: Coefficient of variation; MP: Metacarpophalangeal; NCV: Nerve conduction velocity

Acknowledgements
We would like to thank Editage (www.editage.jp) for English-language editing.

Funding
The study was funded by Hitachi, Ltd.

Authors' contributions
TK performed all experiments and analyses and prepared the first draft of the paper. KF designed the study, collected patient data, and supervised the project. He is the guarantor. AN and TM collected the patients' data and provided advice about the experimental conditions. TS and AO provided advice about the experimental conditions. All authors read and approved the final manuscript.

Competing interests
The authors declare that they have no competing interests.

Author details
[1]Department of Orthopaedic and Spinal Surgery, Graduate School of Medical and Dental Sciences, Tokyo Medical and Dental University, 1-4-5, Yushima, Bunkyo-ku, Tokyo 113-8519, Japan. [2]Department of Functional Joint Anatomy, Graduate School of Medical and Dental Sciences, Tokyo Medical and Dental University, 1-4-5, Yushima, Bunkyo-ku, Tokyo 113-8519, Japan.

References
1. Aubin PM, Sallum H, Walsh C, Stirling L, Correia A. A pediatric robotic thumb exoskeleton for at-home rehabilitation: the Isolated Orthosis for Thumb Actuation (IOTA). In: IEEE International Conference on Rehabilitation Robotics: [proceedings], vol. 2013; 2013. p. 6650500.
2. Berger AJ, Meals RA. Management of osteoarthrosis of the thumb joints. J Hand Surg Am. 2015;40:843–50.
3. Kurtzman LC, Stern PJ, Yakuboff KP. Reconstruction of the burned thumb. Hand Clin. 1992;8:107–19.
4. Swanson AB, Hagert CG, Swanson GD. Evaluation of impairment of hand function. J Hand Surg Am. 1983;8:709–22.
5. Winzeler S, Rosenstein BD. Occupational injury and illness of the thumb. Causes and solutions. AAOHN J. 1996;44:487–92.
6. Edmunds JO. Current concepts of the anatomy of the thumb trapeziometacarpal joint. J Hand Surg Am. 2011;36:170–82.
7. Olafsdottir H, Zatsiorsky VM, Latash ML. Is the thumb a fifth finger? A study of digit interaction during force production tasks. Exp Brain Res. 2005;160:203–13.
8. Lee DH, Oakes JE, Ferlic RJ. Tendon transfers for thumb opposition: a biomechanical study of pulley location and two insertion sites. J Hand Surg Am. 2003;28:1002–8.
9. Plata Bello J, Modrono C, Marcano F, Gonzalez-Mora JL. The effect of motor familiarity during simple finger opposition tasks. Brain Imaging Behav. 2015;9:828–38.
10. Tas S, Top H. Bilateral congenital absence of the opponens pollicis muscle: a case report. Hand (N Y). 2015;10:143–6.
11. Geere J, Chester R, Kale S, Jerosch-Herold C. Power grip, pinch grip, manual muscle testing or thenar atrophy - which should be assessed as a motor outcome after carpal tunnel decompression? A systematic review. BMC Musculoskelet Disord. 2007;8:114.
12. Li T, Hua XY, Zheng MX, Wang WW, Xu JG, Gu YD, et al. Different cerebral plasticity of intrinsic and extrinsic hand muscles after peripheral neurotization in a patient with brachial plexus injury: a TMS and fMRI study. Neurosci Lett. 2015;604:140–4.
13. Foucher G, Malizos C, Sammut D, Braun FM, Michon J. Primary palmaris longus transfer as an opponensplasty in carpal tunnel release. A series of 73 cases. J Hand Surg (Edinb.). 1991;16:56–60.
14. Gelberman RH, Pfeffer GB, Galbraith RT, Szabo RM, Rydevik B, Dimick M. Results of treatment of severe carpal-tunnel syndrome without internal neurolysis of the median nerve. J Bone Joint Surg Am. 1987;69:896–903.
15. Kaymak B, Inanici F, Ozcakar L, Cetin A, Akinci A, Hascelik Z. Hand strengths in carpal tunnel syndrome. J Hand Surg Eur Vol. 2008;33:327–31.
16. Nolan WB 3rd, Alkaitis D, Glickel SZ, Snow S. Results of treatment of severe carpal tunnel syndrome. J Hand Surg Am. 1992;17:1020–3.
17. Bertelli JA, Soldado F, Rodrigues-Baeza A, Ghizoni MF. Transfer of the motor branch of the abductor digiti quinti for thenar muscle reinnervation in high median nerve injuries. J Hand Surg Am. 2018;43:8–15.
18. Kato N, Yoshizawa T, Sakai H. Simultaneous modified Camitz opponensplasty using a pulley at the radial side of the flexor retinaculum in severe carpal tunnel syndrome. J Hand Surg Eur Vol. 2014;39:632–6.
19. Park IJ, Kim HM, Lee SU, Lee JY, Jeong C. Opponensplasty using palmaris longus tendon and flexor retinaculum pulley in patients with severe carpal tunnel syndrome. Arch Orthop Trauma Surg. 2010;130:829–34.
20. Poy-Gual C, Puente-Alonso C, Cano-Rodriguez G. Modified Camitz opponensplasty for treatment of severe carpal tunnel syndrome. J Hand Surg Eur Vol. 2018. https://doi.org/10.1177/1753193418787666.
21. Rymer B, Thomas PB. The Camitz transfer and its modifications: a review. J Hand Surg Eur Vol. 2016;41:632–7.
22. Dilokhuttakarn T, Naito K, Kinoshita M, Sugiyama Y, Goto K, Iwase Y, et al. Evaluation of thenar muscles by MRI in carpal tunnel syndrome. Exp Ther Med. 2017;14:2025–30.
23. Allseits E, Agrawal V, Lucarevic J, Gailey R, Gaunaurd I, Bennett C. A practical step length algorithm using lower limb angular velocities. J Biomech. 2018;66:137–44.
24. Allseits E, Kim KJ, Bennett C, Gailey R, Gaunaurd I, Agrawal V. A novel method for estimating knee angle using two leg-mounted gyroscopes for continuous monitoring with mobile health devices. Sensors (Basel). 2018;18:2759.
25. Holl S, Blum A, Gosheger G, Dieckmann R, Winter C, Rosenbaum D. Clinical outcome and physical activity measured with StepWatch 3 Activity Monitor after minimally invasive total hip arthroplasty. J Orthop Surg Res. 2018;13:148.
26. Staab W, Hottowitz R, Sohns C, Sohns JM, Gilbert F, Menke J, et al. Accelerometer and gyroscope based gait analysis using spectral analysis of patients with osteoarthritis of the knee. J Phys Ther Sci. 2014;26:997–1002.

27. Salarian A, Russmann H, Wider C, Burkhard PR, Vingerhoets FJ, Aminian K. Quantification of tremor and bradykinesia in Parkinson's disease using a novel ambulatory monitoring system. IEEE Trans Biomed Eng. 2007;54:313–22.

28. Summa S, Tosi J, Taffoni F, Di Biase L, Marano M, Rizzo AC, et al. Assessing bradykinesia in Parkinson's disease using gyroscope signals. In: IEEE International Conference on Rehabilitation Robotics : [proceedings], vol. 2017; 2017. p. 1556–61.

29. Le Moing AG, Seferian AM, Moraux A, Annoussamy M, Dorveaux E, Gasnier E, et al. A movement monitor based on magneto-inertial sensors for non-ambulant patients with Duchenne muscular dystrophy: a pilot study in controlled environment. PLoS One. 2016;11:e0156696.

30. Boonstra MC, van der Slikke RM, Keijsers NL, van Lummel RC, de Waal Malefijt MC, Verdonschot N. The accuracy of measuring the kinematics of rising from a chair with accelerometers and gyroscopes. J Biomech. 2006;39:354–8.

31. Camomilla V, Bergamini E, Fantozzi S, Vannozzi G. Trends supporting the in-field use of wearable inertial sensors for sport performance evaluation: a systematic review. Sensors (Basel). 2018;18:873.

32. Padua L, LoMonaco M, Gregori B, Valente EM, Padua R, Tonali P. Neurophysiological classification and sensitivity in 500 carpal tunnel syndrome hands. Acta Neurol Scand. 1997;96:211–7.

33. Bunnell S. Peripheral Nerve Injuries by the Nerve Injuries Committee of the Medical Research Council. Edited by H. J. Seddon. (Privy Council. Medical Research Council Special Report Series. No. 282.) London, Her Majesty's Stationery Office, 1954. 2 pounds, 15 shillings. JBJS 1955;37:895.

34. Doi T, Makizako H, Shimada H, Yoshida D, Ito K, Kato T, et al. Brain atrophy and trunk stability during dual-task walking among older adults. J Gerontol A Biol Sci Med Sci. 2012;67:790–5.

35. Marquardt TL, Nataraj R, Evans PJ, Seitz WH Jr, Li ZM. Carpal tunnel syndrome impairs thumb opposition and circumduction motion. Clin Orthop Relat Res. 2014;472:2526–33.

36. Cheema TA, Cheema NI, Tayyab R, Firoozbakhsh K. Measurement of rotation of the first metacarpal during opposition using computed tomography. J Hand Surg Am. 2006;31:76–9.

37. Kimura T, Takai H, Azuma T, Sairyo K. Motion analysis of the trapeziometacarpal joint using three-dimensional computed tomography. J Hand Surg Asian Pac Vol. 2016;21:78–84.

38. Goto A, Leng S, Sugamoto K, Cooney WP 3rd, Kakar S, Zhao K. In vivo pilot study evaluating the thumb carpometacarpal joint during circumduction. Clin Orthop Relat Res. 2014;472:1106–13.

39. Kawanishi Y, Oka K, Tanaka H, Okada K, Sugamoto K, Murase T. In vivo 3-dimensional kinematics of thumb carpometacarpal joint during thumb opposition. J Hand Surg Am. 2018;43:182 e1-.e7.

40. Coert JH, van Dijke HG, Hovius SE, Snijders CJ, Meek MF. Quantifying thumb rotation during circumduction utilizing a video technique. J Orthop Res. 2003;21:1151–5.

41. Ancillao A, Savastano B, Galli M, Albertini G. Three dimensional motion capture applied to violin playing: a study on feasibility and characterization of the motor strategy. Comput Methods Prog Biomed. 2017;149:19–27.

42. Lewis E, Fors L, Tharion WJ. Interrater and intrarater reliability of finger goniometric measurements. Am J Occup Ther. 2010;64:555–61.

43. O'Flynn B, Sanchez JT, Tedesco S, Downes B, Connolly J, Condell J, et al. Novel smart glove technology as a biomechanical monitoring tool. Sens Transducers. 2015;193:23–32.

44. Kapandji A. Clinical test of apposition and counter-apposition of the thumb. Ann Chir Main. 1986;5:67–73.

45. Durban CM, Antolin B, Sau CY, Li SW, Ip WY. Thumb function and electromyography result after modified Camitz tendon transfer. J Hand Surg Asian Pac Vol. 2017;22:275–80.

46. Goubier JN, Teboul F. Management of hand palsies in isolated C7 to T1 or C8, T1 root avulsions. Tech Hand Up Extrem Surg. 2008;12:156–60.

47. Hutchinson DT, Sueoka S, Wang AA, Tyser AR, Papi-Baker K, Kazmers NH. A prospective, randomized trial of mobilization protocols following ligament reconstruction and tendon interposition. J Bone Joint Surg Am. 2018;100:1275–80.

48. Lefevre-Colau MM, Poiraudeau S, Oberlin C, Demaille S, Fermanian J, Rannou F, et al. Reliability, validity, and responsiveness of the modified Kapandji index for assessment of functional mobility of the rheumatoid hand. Arch Phys Med Rehabil. 2003;84:1032–8.

49. Lemoine S, Wavreille G, Alnot JY, Fontaine C, Chantelot C. Second generation GUEPAR total arthroplasty of the thumb basal joint: 50 months follow-up in 84 cases. Orthop Traumatol Surg Res. 2009;95:63–9.

50. Pradier JP, Oberlin C, Bey E. Acute deep hand burns covered by a pocket flap-graft: long-term outcome based on nine cases. J Burns Wounds. 2007;6:e1.

51. van Rijn J, Gosens T. A cemented surface replacement prosthesis in the basal thumb joint. J Hand Surg Am. 2010;35:572–9.

52. Zhang YX, Wang D, Zhang Y, Ong YS, Follmar KE, Tahernia AH, et al. Triple chimeric flap based on anterior tibial vessels for reconstruction of severe traumatic injuries of the hand with thumb loss. Plast Reconstr Surg. 2009; 123:268–75.

53. Barakat MJ, Field J, Taylor J. The range of movement of the thumb. Hand (N Y). 2013;8:179–82.

54. Levine DW, Simmons BP, Koris MJ, Daltroy LH, Hohl GG, Fossel AH, et al. A self-administered questionnaire for the assessment of severity of symptoms and functional status in carpal tunnel syndrome. J Bone Joint Surg Am. 1993;75:1585–92.

55. Rhoades CE, Mowery CA, Gelberman RH. Results of internal neurolysis of the median nerve for severe carpal-tunnel syndrome. J Bone Joint Surg Am. 1985;67:253–6.

29

Reverse shoulder arthroplasty vs BIO-RSA: clinical and radiographic outcomes at short term follow-up

Nathan Kirzner[1]* [iD], Eldho Paul[2] and Ash Moaveni[3]

Abstract

Background: Bony increased-offset reverse shoulder arthroplasty (BIO-RSA) may address issues such as inferior scapular notching, prosthetic instability and limited postoperative shoulder rotation; all of which have been reported with the standard RSA and attributed to the medialized design. We hypothesised that this lateralization may increase the rate of scapular stress fractures.

Methods: A retrospective review of prospectively collected data was performed on patients who had undergone a RSA between January 2013 and October 2016. A comparative cohort study was designed to compare patients with a standard Grammont-style RSA to those with a BIO-RSA using the same implant. Functional outcome was measured by the American Shoulder and Elbow Surgeons (ASES) Shoulder Score, the Subjective Shoulder Value (SSV), the Western Ontario Osteoarthritis of the Shoulder (WOOS) index and pain scores. Radiographs were obtained for all patients and examined for the presence of scapular fracture as well as scapular notching and graft incorporation.

Results: A total of forty patients (22 patients in the standard RSA cohort and 18 with BIO-RSA) were included in the study. Patient characteristics (including age, gender, length of follow-up, dominant side and osteoporosis) were similar in both groups ($p > 0.05$). The average postoperative follow-up was 20 months (range 12–48 months). There was bone graft incorporation in all BIO-RSA patients at the final radiological follow-up, with no evidence of graft resorption. The overall scapular stress fracture rate was 12.5% (9.1% in the standard RSA and 16.7% in the BIO-RSA). The rates were similar in both cohorts ($p = 0.64$). All fractures were managed conservatively. To determine whether the presence of a scapular stress fracture had an influence on outcomes, the cohort was divided into cases with and without fracture. Patients with a stress fracture had worse ASES ($p = 0.028$) and WOOS ($p = 0.048$) scores. Additionally, osteoporosis was present more commonly in the fracture group (80% vs 17%; $p = 0.01$). A statistically significant difference was identified when comparing the rates of scapular notching between standard RSA and BIO-RSA cohorts (68% vs 33%; $p = 0.028$). Furthermore, when notching was present, significantly worse outcome scores were present in all outcome measures ($p < 0.001$).

Conclusion: The BIO-RSA technique was associated with an increase in scapular stress fracture rate when compared to the standard RSA; however, this was not found to be significant. Furthermore, both techniques resulted in similar improvements in the measured functional outcomes. BIO-RSA, however, was associated with a lower scapular notching rate, justifying further evaluation of this technique.

Level of evidence: Retrospective cohort study, level III

Keywords: Reverse shoulder arthroplasty, BIO-RSA, Scapular insufficiency fractures, Scapular notching, Functional outcomes

* Correspondence: Nathan.kirzner@gmail.com; nathan.kirzner@gmail.com
[1]Orthopaedic Registrar, Alfred Hospital, 55 Commercial Rd, Prahran, Melbourne, VIC 3004, Australia
Full list of author information is available at the end of the article

Background

Reverse shoulder arthroplasty (RSA) has been shown to be a safe and effective procedure for the management of difficult shoulder problems. Indications include massive and irreparable rotator cuff tears with and without glenohumeral arthritis [1–3], proximal humeral fractures [4–6] and revision after failure of prior arthroplasty [7]. Postoperative complications however remain a concern. Inferior scapular notching, prosthetic instability, limited postoperative shoulder rotation and loss of shoulder contour have all been reported in the literature and largely attributed to the medialized design [2, 8, 9].

To address the problems of a medialized center of rotation reverse design, several design modifications have been introduced, including lateralized glenospheres, humeral lateralization and use of a bone graft under the baseplate, the so-called bony increased-offset reversed shoulder arthroplasty (BIO-RSA) [10]. Whilst this has shown good effect in decreasing the rates of scapular notching [11] and improving Constant scores, range of motion and pain scores [10, 12], the increased deltoid tension produced by excessive lateralization and humeral lengthening may also lead to complications. One possible complication may be of a scapular stress fracture, with rates between 0.9% and 10% reported in the literature [3, 13, 14].

Crosby et al. [15] suggested a classification and treatment strategy for scapular stress fractures on the basis of a retrospective review of 400 patients treated with RSA over 4.5 years. They identified three discrete patterns: avulsion fractures of the anterior acromion (type I); fractures of the acromion posterior to the acromioclavicular joint (type II); and fractures of the scapular spine (type III). Whilst the best treatment options remain uncertain, acromial fractures can be treated conservatively without major dysfunction of the shoulder, whereas scapular spine fractures lead to painful dysfunction and may require open reduction and internal fixation [16, 17].

To date, there have been no comparative studies to determine whether BIO-RSA is more likely to cause scapular stress fractures than a standard RSA. The aim of this study was to compare fracture rates, notching rates and functional outcomes between patients who have undergone BIO-RSA and those who have had a standard RSA at a minimum of 12 months follow-up. We hypothesised that the BIO-RSA cohort would have a higher rate of scapular stress fractures; however, lower notching rates and improved functional outcome scores would still be present.

Methods

Study design and outcome measures

A retrospective review of prospectively collected data was performed of patients that had undergone RSA by the senior author (A.M.) between January 2013 and October 2016. A retrospective comparative cohort study was designed to compared patients with a standard Grammont-style RSA to those with a BIO-RSA, using the same implant. The following inclusion criteria were used: (1) all skeletally mature adults; (2) either a standard RSA or BIO-RSA technique employed by a single-orthopaedic surgeon; (3) at least 12 months follow-up; (4) contactable and agreeable to inclusion in the study. Patient's with pre-operative acquired or congenital acromial abnormalities such as os acromiale or stress fractures were excluded from the study. The institution's human research ethics committee provided ethical approval for the study.

Patient characteristics including age, gender, arm dominance, osteoporosis, diagnosis of injury, operative characteristics, postoperative complications and follow-up data were retrieved. The senior surgeon (A.M.) maintains a prospectively collected database for all patients undergoing shoulder arthroplasty. Using this database, we identified all patients who had undergone a Grammont-style reverse shoulder arthroplasty. The decision to perform a standard versus BIO-RSA was predominantly made at the senior surgeon's discretion. Factors such as availability and quality of the proximal humerus bone, size of the patient, degree of pre-operative bone loss and the degree of soft tissue tension all influenced this decision-making. These factors are very difficult to quantify; however, we did ensure that the two cohorts were matched for patient demographics (including age, gender, hand dominance and osteoporosis) as well as the length of follow up. Functional outcomes were measured by the American Shoulder and Elbow Surgeons (ASES) Shoulder Score [18], the Subjective Shoulder Value (SSV) [19] and Western Ontario Osteoarthritis of the Shoulder (WOOS) index [20]. The ASES scores were expressed in a range from 0 (maximum disability) to 100 (no disability) and are comprised of pain and functional portions. The SSV is a validated method for shoulder assessment in arthroplasty and is expressed as a percentage of an entirely normal shoulder, which would score 100%. The WOOS index is a patient-reported, disease-specific questionnaire for the measurement of the quality-of-life in patients undergoing arthroplasty. It is scored as a percentage with 100 signifying an extreme decrease in the shoulder-related quality of life. Pain scores were also recorded with a range from 0 to 100.

Radiological evaluation including initial preoperative CT scans were reviewed to classify the glenoid morphology according to the Walch classification [21]. Shoulder radiographs were obtained for all patients at final follow-up and assessed for the presence of a scapular insufficiency fracture and graded according to the Crosby classification [15]. Scapular notching was rated on the anteroposterior scapular radiograph according to the system of Sirveaux et al. [8]. For the BIO-RSA cohort, graft incorporation assessed as either incorporated or resorbed. Radiographs were evaluated by two independent reviewers, and any differences were discussed until a consensus was reached.

Surgical technique

All operations were performed by a fellowship-trained shoulder surgeon (A.M.), using the Aequalis Reversed prosthesis (Wright-Tornier, Memphis, TN, USA). The procedure was performed through a standard deltopectroal approach, with detachment of any remaining subscapularis and tenodesis of the long head of biceps. In the BIO-RSA, a 10-mm-thick cylindrical autograft was harvested from the humeral head [2]. A glenoid baseplate with an extended 25-mm central post was used to ensure host bone contact. All baseplates were placed in the same position on the inferior margin of the glenoid rim. To ensure that the deltoid was appropriately tensioned and the implant was properly positioned, we (1) looked for absence of pistoning of the prosthesis during application of axial traction on the arm, (2) ensured stability throughout a full range of motion, (3) palpated for tension in the conjoint tendon after trial reduction [2]. The humeral stem was cementless, with a neck-shaft angle of 155 degrees.

The rehabilitation protocol was similar in both groups, with the use of a sling for 4 weeks, allowing both passive- and active-assisted range of motion. After 4 weeks, the sling was discontinued and active range of motion commenced. Strengthening was commenced after 10 weeks.

Statistical analysis

Descriptive statistics, including means and standard deviations, were reported for demographic data and outcome variables. Differences between groups were made using Student's t test for normally distributed continuous variables and Wilcoxon rank-sum test for continuous variables with skewed distributions. Comparisons of categorical data between groups were made using chi-square test for equal proportions or Fisher's exact test where numbers were small. The relationship between scapular notching and functional outcomes was determined using Spearman rank correlation. The level of statistical significance was set at $p < 0.05$. Statistical analysis was performed with SPSS 18.0 software (SPSS Inc., Chicago, IL, USA).

Results

A total of 40 patients who had undergone a reverse shoulder arthroplasty met our inclusion criteria and were enrolled in the study. Standard RSA was performed in 22 patients (55%) with the BIO-RSA technique employed in 18 patients (45%). There were 9 males and

31 females with a mean age of 74.7 years (range 59–91). The average postoperative follow-up was 20 months (12–48 months) with a minimum of 12 months follow-up. Patient demographics, pre-operative diagnosis and glenoid morphology (Walch classification) are presented in Table 1. Baseline characteristics including age, gender, length of follow-up, dominant side and osteoporosis were similar in both groups.

The overall scapular stress fracture rate was 12.5%, with 2 patients having Crosby type III scapular spine fractures, 2 patients with type II and 1 patient with a type 1 acromion avulsion fracture. Surgery was offered to the 2 patients with a type III scapular spine fracture but declined in both cases. The scapular notching rate was 52.5%, with 13 of 40 patients showing grade 1 notching, 7 patients with grade 2 notching and 1 patient with grade 3 notching. There was bone graft incorporation in all BIO-RSA patients at the final radiological follow-up, with no evidence of resorption.

Patient outcomes, scapular stress fracture and notching rates, stratified by standard RSA or BIO-RSA are presented in Table 2. No differences were identified at the latest follow-up between cohorts when comparing functional scores, including the ASES score ($p = 0.53$), SSV score ($p = 0.67$), WOOS index ($p = 0.59$) and overall pain scores ($p = 0.19$). The scapular stress fracture rates were also similar ($p = 0.64$). A significant difference was observed in the scapular notching rates, occurring in 68% of standard RSA patients compared with 33% in the BIO-RSA cohort ($p = 0.028$). In the standard RSA group, 9 patients (41%) had grade 1 notching, 5 patients (23%) had grade 2 notching and 1 patient (4%) had grade 3 notching. In the BIO-RSA group, 4 patients (22%) had grade 1 notching, 2 patients (11%) had grade 2 notching and no patients had grade 3 or 4 notching.

To determine whether the presence of a scapular stress fracture had an influence on outcomes, the entire cohort was divided into cases with and without fracture (Table 3). Comparing between the fracture cohort (5 patients) and the non-fracture cohort (35 patients), no significant difference was seen in terms of age, gender and length of follow-up. There was, however, a statistically significant difference in the rate of osteoporosis, present in 80% of patients with a fracture compared to just 17% without a fracture ($p = 0.01$). There were also statistically significant differences observed in both ASES ($p = 0.028$) and WOOS ($p = 0.048$) scores, with the fracture patients having worse outcomes.

Patients were also divided into two cohorts comprising those with scapular notching and those without to determine how notching impacted outcome (Table 4). This showed no significant difference in terms of patient characteristics. Statistically significant differences could be seen; however, when comparing ASES, SSV, WOOS and

Table 1 Pre-operative comparison of standard RSA and BIO-RSA

Variable*	RSA (n = 22)	BIO-RSA (n = 18)	p value
Age, years	74.50 (60–91)	75.06 (59–89)	0.65
Gender			
Male	3 (14)	6 (33)	0.25
Female	19 (86)	12 (66)	
Follow-up, months	20 ± 8.9 (12–37)	19 ± 8.4 (12–36)	0.71
Dominant side	11 (50)	8 (44)	0.85
Osteoporosis	7 (32)	3 (17)	0.46
Diagnosis			
Osteoarthritis	1 (4)	11 (61)	
Rotator cuff arthropathy	5 (23)	5 (28)	
Proximal humerus fracture	10 (45)	0	
AVN, malunion, dislocation	6 (27)	2 (11)	
Glenoid morphology (Walch classification)			
A1	20 (90)	8 (44)	
A2	0 (0)	5 (28)	
B1	0 (0)	0 (0)	
B2	1 (5)	4 (22)	
C	1 (5)	1 (6)	

BIO-RSA bony increased-offset reverse shoulder arthroplasty, *RSA* reverse shoulder arthroplasty
*Continuous data are presented as the mean ± standard deviation (range) or as indicated and categorical data as number (%) or number

pain scores between the two groups with the notching cohort showing worse outcomes. This was further confirmed by performing a Spearman correlation which demonstrated evidence of a moderate correlation between WOOS score and scapular notching (Spearman correlation coefficient 0.51; $p < 0.001$) and mild correlations between all other outcome measures and notching.

Discussion

In relation to our original hypothesis, our study found that the BIO-RSA technique almost doubled the rate of scapular stress fractures when compared to the standard RSA, but the difference did not reach statistical significance. Furthermore, both techniques resulted in similar improvements in the measured functional outcomes, including the ASES, SSV, WOOS and pain scores. We did, however, find a significant association between BIO-RSA and a lower scapular notching rate.

Postoperative scapular fracture is a common complication following RSA, affecting patient outcome [16] and at times, requiring secondary surgery [15, 22]. Our study showed a scapular stress fracture rate of 16.7% in the BIO-RSA cohort compared to 9.1% in the standard RSA cohort (p value = 0.64). This equated to an overall fracture rate of 12.5%, slightly higher than that reported in previous literature [1, 3, 13]. This may relate to under-reporting of this complication, due to the difficulty in diagnosis [14, 23] and failure of several key studies to report this complication [11, 24, 25].

Table 2 Comparison of standard RSA versus BIO-RSA at mean 20 months' follow-up

Variable*	Standard RSA (n = 22)	BIO-RSA (n = 18)	p value
ASES	67.5 ± 23.8 (23–100)	73 ± 18.7 (24–93)	0.53
SSV	60.2 ± 1.8 (20–95)	63.5 ± 25.7 (5–100)	0.67
WOOS	35.9 ± 30.3 (3–94)	31.4 ± 24.3 (0–84)	0.59
Pain scores	25.7 ± 27.2 (0–75)	15.3 ± 21.5 (0–70)	0.19
Scapular stress fracture	2 (9.1)	3 (16.7)	0.64
Scapular notching	15 (68.2)	6 (33.3)	0.028

BIO-RSA bony increased-offset reverse shoulder arthroplasty, *RSA* reverse shoulder arthroplasty;
ASES American Shoulder and Elbow Surgeons Shoulder Score, *SSV* Subjective Shoulder Value, *WOOS* Western Ontario Osteoarthritis of the Shoulder index
*Continuous data are presented as the mean ± standard deviation (range) or as indicated and categorical data as number (%) or number

Table 3 Comparison of scapular stress fracture versus non-fracture cohort at mean of 20 months' follow up

Variable*	Scapular stress fracture (n = 5)	Non-fracture (n = 35)	p value
Age, years	74.7 (59–91)	75 (60–84)	0.79
Male	1 (20)	8 (23)	1.0
Osteoporosis	4 (80)	6 (17)	0.01
ASES	51.4 ± 23.0 (23–75)	72.8 ± 20.2 (24–100)	0.028
SSV	52 ± 23.9 (30–80)	63.1 ± 17.9 (5–100)	0.22
WOOS	54.8 ± 20.5 (35–84)	30.9 ± 27.3 (0–94)	0.048
Pain scores	19.4 ± 23.4	32 ± 35.6	0.30

ASES American Shoulder and Elbow Surgeons Shoulder Score, SSV Subjective Shoulder Value, WOOS Western Ontario Osteoarthritis of the Shoulder index
*Continuous data are presented as the mean ± standard deviation (range) or as indicated and categorical data as number (%) or number

Furthermore, both patient and surgical factors have been shown to increase the risk of postoperative scapular fractures following RSA (Fig. 1). Otto et al. in a case-controlled study of 265 patients found osteoporosis to be a significant risk factor, present in 30.8% of fracture patients compared with 18.4% of control patients [23]. Osteoporosis was prevalent in our cohort (present in 25% of our patients), with 80.0% of the fracture patients having osteoporosis, compared to 17.1% of non-fracture patients ($p < 0.001$).

Surgical factors include a deltopectoral approach [26], suboptimal superior and posterior screw length and position [10, 15] and excessive deltoid tension produced either by excessive lateralization of the glenoid or humeral lengthening [14, 26, 27]. In our series, we tried to minimise the risk of a stress fracture by placing our superior screw into the base of the coracoid process [14, 15] and judiciously balanced the shoulder, ensuring to avoid over tensioning as previously described.

Our study showed similar improvements in pain and functional outcomes with both standard and BIO-RSA. This finding is comparable to studies by Athwal et al. [11] and Greiner et al. [25]. There is, however, conflicting information about the possible advantages of the BIO-RSA technique. Collin et al. [24] reported significantly higher Constant scores in the BIO-RSA group (69.0 ± 9.4) versus RSA (61.4 ± 12.7). Other studies have

shown an improved range of motion [10, 12], reduced prosthetic instability [11, 28] and better shoulder contour [10] with BIO-RSA technique.

A proposed disadvantage of glenoid lateralization is it places the deltoid lever arm at a mechanical disadvantage when compared with a more medialized implant [29]. This was hypothesised to result in reduced deltoid strength. To date, no significant difference has been found in deltoid strength when comparing the two designs [11]. The technique can also be used to address angled multiplanar glenoid deformity [30].

Scapular notching is the erosion of the scapula neck as well as polyethylene wear, secondary to inferomedial impingement of the humeral implant against the scapula [31] (Fig. 2). Sirveaux et al. [8] classified this into four grades: grade 1 describes a defect contained within the inferior pillar of the scapular neck, a grade 2 is considered when erosion of the scapular neck extends to the level of the inferior fixation screw, grade 3 when it was over the lower screw and grade 4 when it extended under the baseplate. A recent systematic review reported an overall notching rate of 35%, with an increased rate of 50% in the Grammont-style RSA [17]. Similar to findings by Athwal [11], we found an increase in the rate of notching (68% in the standard RSA group versus to 33% in the BIO-RSA group, $p = 0.028$). Whilst early studies reported no effect of scapular notching on pain and functional outcomes,

Table 4 Comparison of scapular notching cohort versus non-notching cohort at mean 20 months' follow-up

Variable*	Scapular notching (n = 21)	Non-notching (n = 19)	p value
Age, years	72.3 (59–88)	77.4 (60–91)	0.056
Male	6 (28.6)	3 (15.8)	0.46
Osteoporosis	6 (28.6)	4 (21.1)	0.72
ASES	58.7 ± 21.7 (23–97)	85.2 ± 13.3 (51–100)	< 0.001
SSV	49.9 ± 19.9 (5–80)	74.7 ± 20.1 (25–100)	< 0.001
WOOS	51.0 ± 25.7 (13–94)	14.8 ± 13.3 (0–44)	< 0.001
Pain scores	34.1 ± 28.1	6.6 ± 7.8	0.001

ASES American Shoulder and Elbow Surgeons Shoulder Score, SSV Subjective Shoulder Value, WOOS Western Ontario Osteoarthritis of the Shoulder index
*Continuous data are presented as the mean ± standard deviation (range) or as indicated and categorical data as number (%) or number

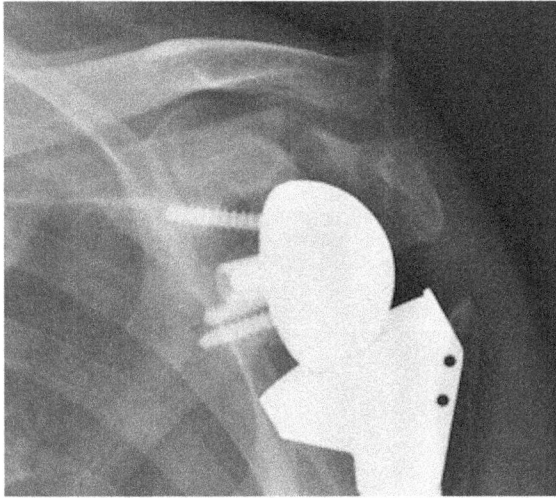

Fig. 1 Postoperative fracture of the scapular spine after BIO-RSA

recent studies with longer follow-up have demonstrated notching is associated with reduced shoulder ROM, strength, decreased SSV and Constant-Murley scores, and the potential for implant loosening [8, 32]. Our study similarly showed that patients with scapular notching had significantly worse functional outcome measures and pain scores.

The strength of our study is that all patients were operated on by a single surgeon, with regular follow-up using radiographs and validated outcome measures. The main limitations of the study are its relatively small sample size, retrospective nature, as well as lack of physical examination to document shoulder range of motion and strength.

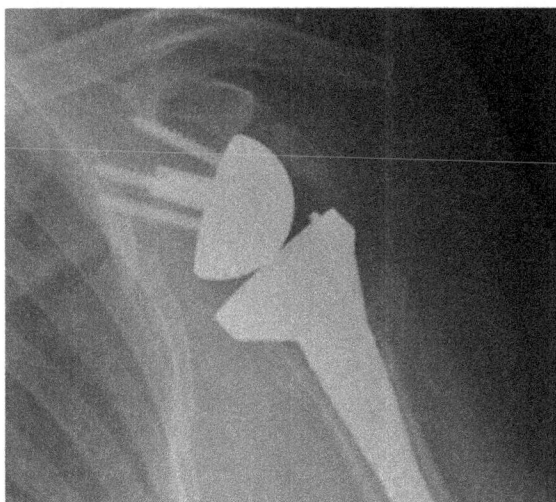

Fig. 2 Anteroposterior radiographs of BIO-RSA with Sirveaux grade 2 scapular notching

Conclusions

In conclusion, lateralization of a Grammont-style prosthesis with bony increased-offset techniques is associated with a reduction in scapular notching. Of concern is the possible increase in the rate of scapular insufficiency fractures. Both notching and scapular insufficiency fractures seem to compromise the outcome of reverse arthroplasty. Although with the numbers available, the difference in fracture rate did not reach statistical significance, further research into this area may be of benefit.

Abbreviations

ASES: American Shoulder and Elbow Surgeons Shoulder Score; BIO-RSA: Bony increased-offset reverse shoulder arthroplasty; RSA: Reverse shoulder arthroplasty; SSV: Subjective Shoulder Value (SSV); WOOS: Western Ontario Osteoarthritis of the Shoulder index

Acknowledgements

The authors thank Kelly Story and Madeleine Scicchitano for their assistance.

Authors' contributions

NK performed a literature search, participated in the design of the study, carried out the data collection, analysis and interpretation, helped to draft the manuscript and perform critical revisions. EP helped carry out data analysis and perform data interpretation. AM conceived of the study, participated in its design and coordination and helped to draft the manuscript. All authors read and approved the final manuscript.

Competing interests

The authors declare that they have no competing interests.

Author details

[1]Orthopaedic Registrar, Alfred Hospital, 55 Commercial Rd, Prahran, Melbourne, VIC 3004, Australia. [2]Department of Epidemiology and Preventive Medicine, Monash University, Victoria, Australia. [3]Orthopaedic Consultant, Alfred Hospital, 55 Commercial Rd, Prahran, Melbourne, Victoria 3004, Australia.

References

1. Boileau P, Watkinson D, Hatzidakis AM, Hovorka I. Neer Award 2005: The Grammont reverse shoulder prosthesis: results in cuff tear arthritis, fracture sequelae, and revision arthroplasty. J Shoulder Elb Surg. 2005;15(5):527–40.
2. Boileau P, Watkinson DJ, Hatzidakis AM, Balg F. Grammont reverse prosthesis: design, rationale, and biomechanics. J Shoulder Elb Surg. 2005; 14(1 Suppl S):147S–61S.
3. Frankle M, Siegal S, Pupello D, Saleem A, Mighell M, Vasey M. The reverse shoulder prosthesis for glenohumeral arthritis associated with severe rotator cuff deficiency. A minimum two-year follow-up study of sixty patients. J Bone Joint Surg Am. 2005;87(8):1697–705.

4. Boyle MJ, Youn SM, Frampton CM, Ball CM. Functional outcomes of reverse shoulder arthroplasty compared with hemiarthroplasty for acute proximal humeral fractures. J Shoulder Elb Surg. 2013;22(1):32–7.

5. Bufquin T, Hersan A, Hubert L, Massin P. Reverse shoulder arthroplasty for the treatment of three- and four-part fractures of the proximal humerus in the elderly: a prospective review of 43 cases with a short-term follow-up. J Bone Joint Surg Br. 2007;89(4):516–20.

6. Garofalo R, Brody F, Castagna A, Ceccarelli E, Krishnan SG. Reverse shoulder arthroplasty with glenoid bone grafting for anterior glenoid rim fracture associated with glenohumeral dislocation and proximal humerus fracture. Orthop Traumatol Surg Res. 2016;102(8):989–94.

7. Ortmaier R, Resch H, Matis N, Blocher M, Auffarth A, Mayer M, et al. Reverse shoulder arthroplasty in revision of failed shoulder arthroplasty-outcome and follow-up. Int Orthop. 2013;37(1):67–75.

8. Sirveaux F, Favard L, Oudet D, Huquet D, Walch G, Mole D. Grammont inverted total shoulder arthroplasty in the treatment of glenohumeral osteoarthritis with massive rupture of the cuff. Results of a multicentre study of 80 shoulders. J Bone Joint Surg Br. 2004;86(3):388–95.

9. Gerber C, Pennington SD, Nyffeler RW. Reverse total shoulder arthroplasty. J Am Acad Orthop Surg. 2009;17(5):284–95.

10. Boileau P, Moineau G, Roussanne Y, O'Shea K. Bony increased-offset reversed shoulder arthroplasty: minimizing scapular impingement while maximizing glenoid fixation. Clin Orthop Relat Res. 2011;469(9):2558–67.

11. Athwal GS, Faber KJ. Outcomes of reverse shoulder arthroplasty using a mini 25-mm glenoid baseplate. Int Orthop. 2016;40(1):109–13.

12. Neyton L, Boileau P, Nove-Josserand L, Edwards TB, Walch G. Glenoid bone grafting with a reverse design prosthesis. J Shoulder Elb Surg. 2007;16(3 Suppl):S71–8.

13. Matsen FA 3rd, Boileau P, Walch G, Gerber C, Bicknell RT. The reverse total shoulder arthroplasty. J Bone Joint Surg Am. 2007;89(3):660–7.

14. Mayne IP, Bell SN, Wright W, Coghlan JA. Acromial and scapular spine fractures after reverse total shoulder arthroplasty. Shoulder Elbow. 2016;8(2):90–100.

15. Crosby LA, Hamilton A, Twiss T. Scapula fractures after reverse total shoulder arthroplasty: classification and treatment. Clin Orthop Relat Res. 2011;469(9):2544–9.

16. Walch G, Mottier F, Wall B, Boileau P, Mole D, Favard L. Acromial insufficiency in reverse shoulder arthroplasties. J Shoulder Elb Surg. 2009;18(3):495–502.

17. Zumstein MA, Pinedo M, Old J, Boileau P. Problems, complications, reoperations, and revisions in reverse total shoulder arthroplasty: a systematic review. J Shoulder Elb Surg. 2011;20(1):146–57.

18. Michener LA, McClure PW, Sennett BJ. American Shoulder and Elbow Surgeons Standardized Shoulder Assessment Form, patient self-report section: reliability, validity, and responsiveness. J Shoulder Elb Surg. 2002;11(6):587–94.

19. Gilbart MK, Gerber C. Comparison of the subjective shoulder value and the Constant score. J Shoulder Elb Surg. 2007;16(6):717–21.

20. Lo IK, Griffin S, Kirkley A. The development of a disease-specific quality of life measurement tool for osteoarthritis of the shoulder: the Western Ontario Osteoarthritis of the Shoulder (WOOS) index. Osteoarthr Cartil. 2001;9(8):771–8.

21. Walch G, Badet R, Boulahia A, Khoury A. Morphologic study of the glenoid in primary glenohumeral osteoarthritis. J Arthroplast. 1999;14(6):756–60.

22. Werner CM, Steinmann PA, Gilbart M, Gerber C. Treatment of painful pseudoparesis due to irreparable rotator cuff dysfunction with the Delta III reverse-ball-and-socket total shoulder prosthesis. J Bone Joint Surg Am. 2005;87(7):1476–86.

23. Otto RJ, Virani NA, Levy JC, Nigro PT, Cuff DJ, Frankle MA. Scapular fractures after reverse shoulder arthroplasty: evaluation of risk factors and the reliability of a proposed classification. J Shoulder Elb Surg. 2013;22(11):1514–21.

24. Collin P, Liu X, Denard PJ, Gain S, Nowak A, Ladermann A. Standard versus bony increased-offset reverse shoulder arthroplasty: a retrospective comparative cohort study. J Shoulder Elb Surg. 2018;27(1):59–64.

25. Greiner S, Schmidt C, Herrmann S, Pauly S, Perka C. Clinical performance of lateralized versus non-lateralized reverse shoulder arthroplasty: a prospective randomized study. J Shoulder Elb Surg. 2015;24(9):1397–404.

26. Farshad M, Gerber C. Reverse total shoulder arthroplasty-from the most to the least common complication. Int Orthop. 2010;34(8):1075–82.

27. Scarlat MM. Complications with reverse total shoulder arthroplasty and recent evolutions. Int Orthop. 2013;37(5):843–51.

28. Jones RB, Wright TW, Zuckerman JD. Reverse total shoulder arthroplasty with structural bone grafting of large glenoid defects. J Shoulder Elb Surg. 2016;25(9):1425–32.

29. Henninger HB, Barg A, Anderson AE, Bachus KN, Burks RT, Tashjian RZ. Effect of lateral offset center of rotation in reverse total shoulder arthroplasty: a biomechanical study. J Shoulder Elb Surg. 2012;21(9):1128–35.

30. Boileau P, Morin-Salvo N, Gauci MO, Seeto BL, Chalmers PN, Holzer N, et al. Angled BIO-RSA (bony-increased offset-reverse shoulder arthroplasty): a solution for the management of glenoid bone loss and erosion. J Shoulder Elb Surg. 2017;26(12):2133–42.

31. Nicholson GP, Strauss EJ, Sherman SL. Scapular notching: recognition and strategies to minimize clinical impact. Clin Orthop Relat Res. 2011;469(9):2521–30.

32. Simovitch RW, Zumstein MA, Lohri E, Helmy N, Gerber C. Predictors of scapular notching in patients managed with the Delta III reverse total shoulder replacement. J Bone Joint Surg Am. 2007;89(3):588–600.

30

Adjacent segment degeneration or disease after cervical total disc replacement

Shuai Xu[†], Yan Liang[†], Zhenqi Zhu, Yalong Qian and Haiying Liu[*]

Abstract

Background: Anterior cervical discectomy and fusion (ACDF) has been widely used in cervical spondylosis, but adjacent segment degeneration/disease (ASD) was inevitable. Cervical total disc replacement (TDR) could reduce the stress of adjacent segments and retard ASD in theory, but the superiority has not been determined yet. This analysis aimed that whether TDR was superior to ACDF for decreasing adjacent segment degeneration (ASDeg) and adjacent segment disease (ASDis).

Methods: A meta-analysis was performed according to the guidelines of the Cochrane Collaboration with PubMed, EMBASE, Cochrane Library and CBM (China Biological Medicine) databases. It included randomized controlled trials (RCTs) that reported ASDeg, ASDis, and reoperation on adjacent segments after TDR and ACDF. Two investigators independently selected trials, assessed methodological quality, and evaluated the quality of this meta-analysis using the grades of recommendation, assessment, development, and evaluation (GRADE) approach.

Results: Eleven studies with 2632 patients were included in the meta-analysis. The overall rate of ASD in TDR group was lower than ACDF group (OR = 0.6; 95% CI [0.38, 0.73]; $P < 0.00001$). Both the incidence of ASDeg and the reoperation rate were statistically lower in the TDR group than in the ACDF group (OR = 0.58, $P < 0.00001$; OR = 0.52, $P = 0.01$, respectively). Subgroup analysis was performed according to the follow-up time and trial site; the rate of ASDeg was lower in patients underwent TDR no matter the follow-up time, and TDR tended to increase the superiority across time. The rate of ASDeg was also lower with TDR both in the USA and China ($P < 0.0001$, $P = 0.03$, respectively). But the cost-effectiveness result might be prone to neither of the two surgery approaches. According to GRADE, the overall quality of this meta-analysis was moderate.

Conclusions: TDR decreased the rates of ASDeg and reoperation compared with that of ACDF, and the superiority may become more apparent over time. We cautiously and slightly suggest adopting TDR according to the GRADE but may not believe it excessively.

Keywords: Adjacent segment degeneration, Adjacent segment disease, TDR, ACDF, Meta-analysis

* Correspondence: 393805151@qq.com
[†]Shuai Xu and Yan Liang contributed equally to this work.
Department of Spinal Surgery, Peking University People's Hospital, Peking University, No. 11 Xizhimen South Street, Xicheng District, Beijing, People's Republic of China

Introduction

Anterior cervical discectomy and fusion (ACDF) is widely performed for the treatment of cervical diseases, estimated to provide relief for more than 90% of radicular and myelopathic complaints [1]. However, ACDF has been associated with the development of new degeneration at levels adjacent to the fused segments [2, 3]. This operation affected normal cervical spine alignment, and loss of mobility at one functional spinal unit increased the load sustained by the remaining units [4]. Hilibrand et al. [5] classified degeneration of adjacent segments as "adjacent segment degeneration" (ASDeg) and "adjacent segment disease" (ASDis) to formulate unified standards and to avoid confusion when researching these problems. ASDeg was defined as radiographic changes at the adjacent segments, whereas ASDis was used to refer to the development of new clinical symptoms, such as mechanical neck pain or coronal-sagittal imbalance. However, the etiology and symptomatology of these adjacent segment changes have remained intensely controversial. Some experts believe it is the natural progress of cervical disc disease [6–8], while others insist fusion can change the biomechanics of adjacent segments, accelerating adjacent segment degeneration/disease (ASD) [2, 9].

Total disc replacement (TDR) on cervical vertebra has been greatly improved over the last decade. Based on a large amount of biomechanical testing, TDR can theoretically decrease the incidence of adjacent segment degeneration by maintaining normal disc kinematics [10–12]. But few clinical studies, especially controlled trials, have specifically investigated ASDeg, ASDis, or reoperation after TDR or ACDF together with less relevant evidence-based medicine, including several systematic reviews that could not determine whether TDR is superior in ASD due to the poor qualified studies [13–15].

To focus on this issue, many studies on ASD have been published in recent years, and performing meta-analysis is necessary to describe the results. The present study aimed to determine whether TDR is superior to ACDF in reducing the incidence of ASD.

Materials and methods

We performed this meta-analysis using the guidelines of the Cochrane Collaboration [16].

Criteria for selecting studies for the meta-analysis
Types of studies

In view of the currency of randomized controlled trials (RCTs), the highest-grade evidence, comparing TDR with fusion, only RCTs were evaluated.

Types of participants

The study population included patients (>18 years) with radiculopathy or myelopathy cervical spondylosis, or other degenerative diseases. The two treatment groups were similar demographically, with no statistically significant differences on the variables of age, sex, or work status. Patients had failed active conservative management for at least 6 months.

Types of interventions

Jawahar et al. [17] indicated the non-statistical significance of single or double segment degenerative disc diseases for the prevalence of ASDeg and ASDis. Therefore, we compared the results of surgical treatment of single or double disc diseases treated by TDR or ACDF.

Types of outcomes studied

According to Hilibrand's [5] definitions of ASDeg and ASDis, the incidence of ASDeg and ASDis can be described as direct results and primary outcomes. Reoperation on adjacent segments indirectly reflected the rate of ASD, and we adopted it as a secondary evaluation standard.

Search strategy and selection criteria

The databases used to search included PUBMED, EMBASE, Cochrane Library, CBM (China Biological Medicine Database), CNKI, and Wanfang Data.

Since the first study describing a commercially available TDR device was published in 2002 [18], the range was from January 2002 to December 2017. The following keywords were used: cervical vertebrae, total cervical disc replacement OR TDR OR arthroplasty OR prostheses OR dynamic stabilization device AND anterior cervical discectomy and fusion OR ACDF OR cervical

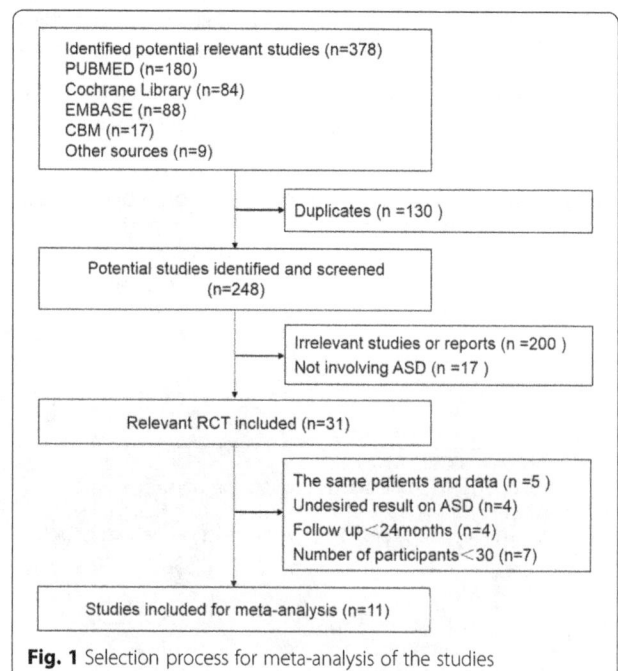

Identified potential relevant studies (n=378)
PUBMED (n=180)
Cochrane Library (n=84)
EMBASE (n=88)
CBM (n=17)
Other sources (n=9)

Duplicates (n =130)

Potential studies identified and screened (n=248)

Irrelevant studies or reports (n =200)
Not involving ASD (n =17)

Relevant RCT included (n=31)

The same patients and data (n =5)
Undesired result on ASD (n=4)
Follow up<24months (n=4)
Number of participants<30 (n=7)

Studies included for meta-analysis (n=11)

Fig. 1 Selection process for meta-analysis of the studies

arthrodesis AND "randomized controlled trials."The inclusion criteria were (1) RCTs of cervical degenerative diseases involving single or double segments underwent TDR and ACDF; (2) definite, diagnostic, and direct evidence for ASD; (3) a minimum of a two-year follow-up; (4) at least a minimum of 30 patients per population; (5) containing specific data information on ASD for meta-analysis. Incompatible studies that may have been excluded were (1) case reports; (2) reviews; (3) studies with follow-up time less than 2 years; and (4) just with undesirable result although referring to ASD such as only a mention on ASD with no specific data, secondary surgeries not totally resulting from ASD, and confounding subjects of ASDis and ASDeg for a hardly data extraction. (Additional file 1: Table S1).

Data extraction and management

Both reviewers (SX and ZQZ) assessed potentially eligible trials and extracted information independently from each potential study. Any discrepancies were resolved through a third reviewer (YLQ) to reach consensus. Extracted data included the general characteristics and outcome measures. General characteristics included study design, first author, sample size, intervention, and types of artificial total disc. Measures of outcomes included the number of ASDeg or ASDis and reoperation (Additional file 2: File S1).

Risk of bias assessment

Two investigators independently graded each eligible study. We used the Cochrane Handbook for Systematic Reviews of Interventions, version 5.0 [19] for RCTs. The following domains were assessed: randomization, blinding

Table 1 Characteristics of the included studies

References	Design	Intervention		Patients		Level		Age(years)		FU (months)	ASDeg		ASDis		Reoperation		Quality[a]
		F	NF	F	NF	F	NF	F	NF		F	NF	F	NF	F	NF	
Phillips, F M(US) [31]	RCT (R:1:1 C:unclear B:unclear L:114/403)	ACDF	TDR (PCM)	185	218	S	S	comparable		60	92	72			11	4	B
Davis, R J(US) [30]	RCT (R:ratio1:2 C:Yes B:patients L:18/330)	ACDF	TDR (Mobi-C)	105	225	D	D	46.2	45.3	48	48	92					B
Zhang, H X(CHA) [29]	RCT (R:ratio1:1 C:unclear B:unclear L:0/111)	ACDF	TDR (Mobi-C)	56	55	S	S	46.7	44.8	48					4	0	B
Burkus, J K(US) [28]	RCT (R:ratio1:1 C:Yes B:patients L:146/541)	ACDF	TDR (Prestige)	265	276	S	S	43.9	43.3	84					10	8	B
Li, Z H(CHA) [27]	RCT (R:ratio1:1 C:unclear B:unclear L:0/81)	ACDF	TDR (Scient'x)	42	39	S	S	49.5	45.3	27	6	5					C
Guan, T (CHA) [26]	RCT (R:ratio1:1 C:unclear B:unclear L:6/66)	ACDF	TDR (Active-c)	34	32	S	S	52.6	49.6	34	21	13					B
Tian, W(CHA) [25]	RCT (R:ratio1:1 C:unclear B:unclear L:30/93)	ACDF	TDR (Bryan)	48	45	S/D (23/12)	S/D (20/8)	48.7	45	80	21	12					B
Nunley, P D(US) [24]	RCT (R:ratio1:2 C:unclear B:Patients L:12/182)	ACDF	TDR (unclear)	62	120	S/D (43/19)	S/D (71/29)	43	45	42	18	31	9	19			C
Coric, D(US) [23]	RCT (R:ratio1:1 C:unclear B:unclear L:35/269)	ACDF	TDR (Kineflex-C)	133	136	S	S	43.9	43.7	24	68	42			5	1	B
Sasso, R C(US) [22]	RCT (R:ratio1:1 C:Yes B:Both L:154/463)	ACDF	TDR (Bryan)	221	242	S	S	46.1	42.5	48			9	9	9	9	A
Jawahar, A(US) [17]	RCT (R:randomization number C:unclear B:Patients L:29/93)	ACDF	TDR (Kineflex-C/ Mobi-C/ Advent)	34	59	S/D (28/6)	S/D (43/16)	comparable		37			6	9			B

Abbreviations: RCT randomized controlled trial, *R* randomization, *C* concealment of allocation, *B* blinding, *L* losses to follow-up, *ACDF* anterior cervical discectomy and fusion, *TDR* total disc replacement, *S* single level, *D* double levels, *FU* follow-up, *ASDeg* adjacent segment degeneration, *ASDis* adjacent segment disease
[a]*Quality* was classified as A level (A), B level (B), or C level (C) by Cochrane Handbook for Systematic Reviews of Interventions

(of patients, surgeons and assessors), allocation concealment, and follow-up coverage. Each domain of quality assessment was classified as adequate (A), unclear (B), or inadequate (C). If all domains were A, the study was A-level; if at least one domain was B, the study was B-level; if at least one domain was C, the study was C-level (Additional file 3: Table S2).

GRADE approach

The GRADE (the grades of recommendation, assessment, development, and evaluation) approach was used to evaluate the strength of evidence [20]. Based on parameters, the quality assessment was classified as very low, low, moderate, or high according to the GRADE handbook(version 3.2), with the GRADE profiler software (version 3.6). A Summary of Findings Table (SoF Table) was used to explain the final results.

Data analysis

Review Manager Software (RevMan Version 5.3) was used to conduct the statistical analysis.

Measures of treatment effect

Only dichotomous outcomes were presented in this study; the odds ratio (OR) and 95% confidence intervals (95% CI) were calculated for outcomes.

Assessment of heterogeneity

Results were regarded as statistically significant if $P < 0.05$. I^2 was used to estimate the size of the heterogeneity [21]. $I^2 < 50\%$ indicated low heterogeneity, and the results of comparable groups could be pooled using a fixed-effects model.

Subgroup analysis

Subgroup analysis that could reduce statistical heterogeneity to facilitate factor definition was worthwhile. If the overall heterogeneity was $I^2 < 50\%$, we could still divide studies into subgroups depending on professional principles and clinical meaning.

Bias of publication

We constructed a funnel plot for overall outcomes to assess publication bias and to examine the relationship between sample size and the effect.

There was no protocol.

Results

Description of the studies

The process of identifying relevant studies is summarized in Fig 1. Three hundred seventy-eight references were obtained from the databases mentioned and a total of 11 studies [17, 22–31] met inclusion criteria with a total of 2632 patients: 1185 underwent ACDF and 1447 underwent TDR. As some studies were continuations of previous articles, we used the latest publication to avoid duplication. Thus, the search range was from 2002 to 2016, but the 11 included studies were published between 2010 and 2016.We recorded the characteristics of the 11 included RCTs in Table 1.

Risk of bias in the studies

According to the quality assessment criteria recommended by the Cochrane Handbook for Systematic Reviews of Interventions [19], 9 out of 11 were of high quality. One study was A-level quality [22], 8 articles were B-level [17, 23, 25,

	Random sequence generation (selection bias)	Allocation concealment (selection bias)	Blinding of participants and personnel (performance bias)	Blinding of outcome assessment (detection bias)	Incomplete outcome data (attrition bias)	Selective reporting (reporting bias)	Other bias
Burkus, J K 2014	+	+	+	+	+	+	?
Coric, D 2011	+	?	?	?	+	+	?
Davis, R J 2015	+	+	+	+	+	+	?
Jawahar, A 2010	+	?	+	+	+	+	+
Li, Zhonghai 2014	+	–	?	?	+	?	?
Nunley, P D 2012	+	?	+	?	+	+	–
Phillips, F M 2015	+	?	?	?	+	+	?
Sasso, R C 2011	+	+	+	+	+	+	+
Tao,guan 2014	+	?	+	+	+	+	?
Wei, TIAN 2013	+	?	?	?	+	+	?
Zhang, H X 2014	+	?	?	?	+	?	?

Fig. 2 Risk of bias summary. The review authors' judgments about each risk of bias item for each included study: + is "yes", – is "no", ? is "unclear"

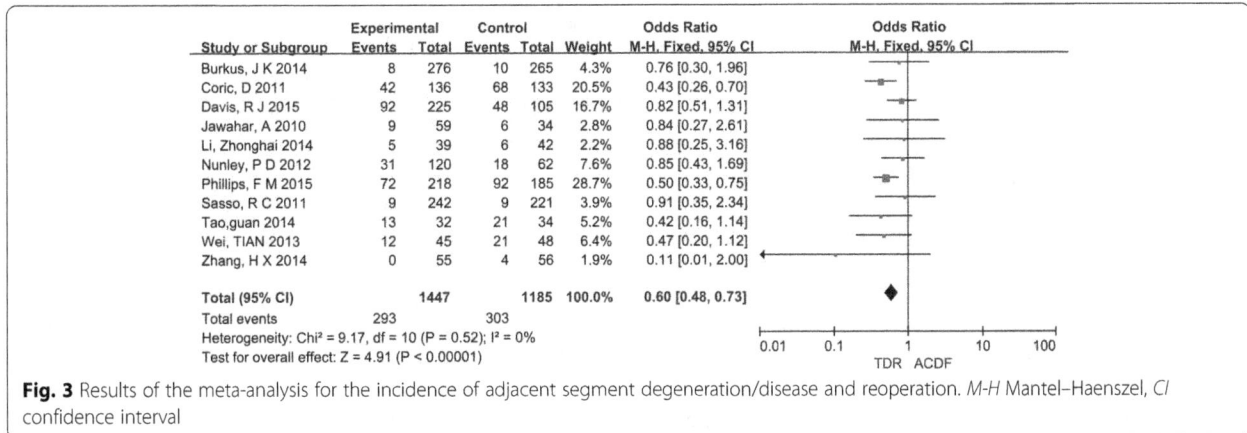

Fig. 3 Results of the meta-analysis for the incidence of adjacent segment degeneration/disease and reoperation. *M-H* Mantel–Haenszel, *CI* confidence interval

26, 28–31], and 2 articles were C-level [24, 27] Fig. 2. The review authors' judgments about each risk of bias item for each included study: + is "yes", – is "no", ? is "unclear".

Measures of overall outcomes

In this meta-analysis, the rates of ASDeg and ASDis were described as the direct outcomes, reoperation on adjacent segments was adopted as the indirect standard. All 11 RCTs used unified standards on ASD in line with Hilibrand's [5] definitions. None of the studies simultaneously involved the three results of the rates of ASDeg, ASDis, and reoperation; 7 RCTs [23–27, 30, 31] mentioned ASDeg, 3 RCTs [17, 22, 24] mentioned ASDis, and 5 RCTs [22, 23, 28, 29, 31] mentioned reoperation. If both direct outcomes and indirect outcomes were involved in a study, the former was preferentially adopted.

After a meta-analysis, there was no statistical heterogeneity among all 11 studies (I^2 = 0%). With the fixed-effects model, the overall rate of ASD was lower in the TDR group (20.2%) compared with ACDF group (25.6%), and the difference was statistically significant (OR = 0.6; 95% CI [0.38, 0.73]; $P < 0.00001$) with no heterogeneity (I^2 = 0%), which was showed in Fig. 3.

Adjacent segment degeneration (ASDeg)

Seven studies [23–27, 30, 31] reported ASDeg. The rate of ASDeg was lower in patients who underwent TDR, and the difference was statistically significant (OR = 0.58, 95% CI [0.46, 0.72]; $P < 0.00001$), which was showed in Fig. 4.

Adjacent segment disease (ASDis)

Three studies [17, 22, 24] reported ASDis. The rate of ASDis was similar in two groups (8.8%, 7.6% respectively) with no statistical significance (OR = 0.97, 95% CI [0.56, 1.69]; $P = 0.91$) and it is shown in Fig. 5.

Reoperation

Five studies [22, 23, 28, 29, 31] and reported reoperation on adjacent segments. The reoperation rate was lower in patients with TDR (2.4%) than in patients who underwent ACDF (4.5%) (OR = 0.52, 95% CI [0.30, 0.87]; $P = 0.01$), which is shown in Fig. 6.

Subgroup analysis

Subgroup analysis was performed according to follow-up time. Table 2 listed the average follow-up time spanned 24–84 months. We divided the follow-up time into two periods: < 5 years and ≥ 5 years.

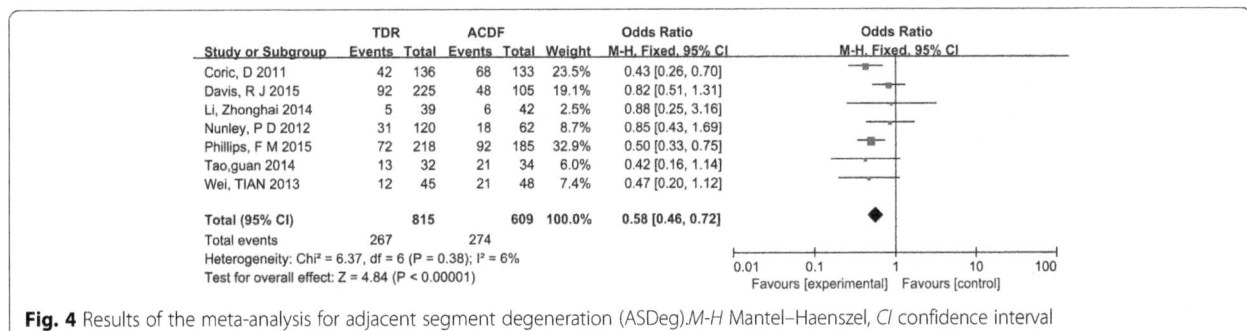

Fig. 4 Results of the meta-analysis for adjacent segment degeneration (ASDeg). *M-H* Mantel–Haenszel, *CI* confidence interval

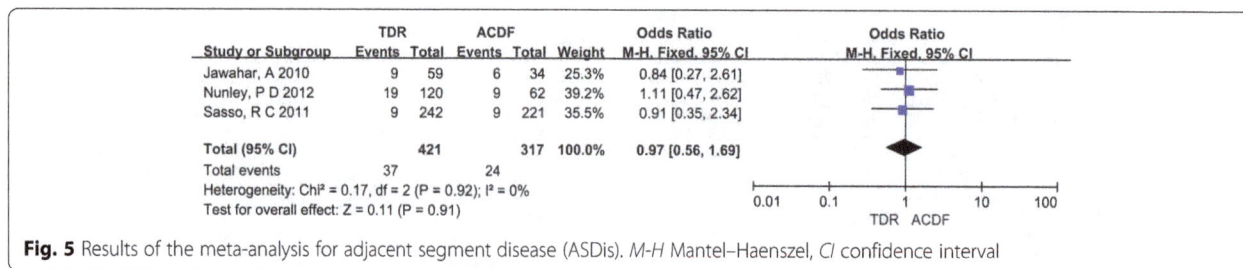

Fig. 5 Results of the meta-analysis for adjacent segment disease (ASDis). *M-H* Mantel–Haenszel, *CI* confidence interval

Eight studies involving < 5 years of follow-up [17, 22–24, 26, 27, 29, 30] showed that the rate of ASDeg was lower in TDR (*P* = 0.001), but the rates of ASDis and reoperation were not significantly different (*P* = 0.98 and *P* = 0.1, respectively). Three studies involving ≥ 5 years of follow-up [25, 28, 31] showed that the rate of ASDeg was much lower in TDR group (*P* = 0.0002).

Subgroup analysis was also performed according to the trial sites. The trial sites in the 11 RCTs were from two countries: the USA and China. We divided 11 studies into two subgroups in Table 3.

Seven studies performed in the USA [17, 22–24, 28, 30, 31] showed the rate of ASDeg and the reoperation rate for adjacent segments were lower on TDR (*P* < 0.0001 and *P* = 0.03, respectively) but not ASDis (*P* = 0.98). Four studies performed in China [25–27, 29] showed the rate of ASDeg was lower in patients who underwent TDR than ACDF (*P* = 0.03) but not the rate of reoperation (*P* = 0.13).

The meta-analysis of ASDin Fig. 7 showed no evidence of publication bias.

The GRADE of this meta-analysis

The SoF Table presents the grade of the ultimate outcome (ASD) under the intervention of TDR and ACDF according to academic and clinical experiences as well as the quality grade of this meta-analysis in Table 4. According to the GRADE [20], the grade of the ultimate outcome (ASD) was critical, and the overall grade quality of our meta-analysis was moderate.

Discussion

ACDF has been recognized as a classic surgical treatment of cervical disease [32, 33], but limitations in range of motion, increased stress on adjacent segments made it defective at simulating physiology. Many publications have reported their observations of this and summarized pathological causal factors of ASD [33–35]. Some experts believe it is a natural process; Hilibrand's results indicated that ASD was indeed a common problem but may reflect the natural history of the underlying cervical spondylosis [5]. Some have suggested that the alignment, curvature, and activity of the cervical spine are relevant factors that result in ASD [33, 35]. Takeshima [36] concluded cervical dynamic change may increase the adjacent intervertebral stress and accelerate degeneration of adjacent segments.

Since 2002, progressive superiority of TDR in biomechanics theory has been applied in clinical practice and the more technological mature is accepted. The mechanical difference between TDR and ACDF made us increasingly concerned about ASD and hereafter meaningful comparison. But poor qualified studies led to lots of bias and many patients unfit to experimental or control group caused unsatisfactory efficacy, in addition substantial costs made it difficult to perform a multi-center RCT.

There were several articles referred to ASD between TDR and ACDF, but few conclusions indicated ASD has radiological or clinical statistical difference [37–39]. Probable reasons were (1) ASD was a natural process unrelated to surgery, corresponding to the view of Hilibrand and

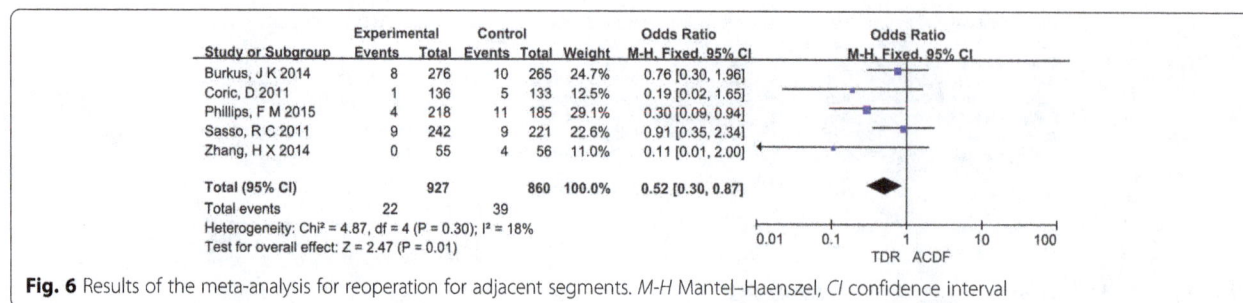

Fig. 6 Results of the meta-analysis for reoperation for adjacent segments. *M-H* Mantel–Haenszel, *CI* confidence interval

Table 2 Subgroup analysis according to follow-up time

FU	<5y						≥5y					
	OR [95%CI]	P value	I²(%)	NO. of P	NO. of ASD	NO. of S	OR [95%CI]	P value	I²(%)	NO. of P	NO. of ASD	NO. of S
ASDeg	0.63 [0.48, 0.84]	0.001	23	928	344	5	0.49 [0.34, 0.71]	0.0002	0	496	197	2
ASDis	0.99 [0.57, 1.73]	0.98	0	738	61	3	–	–	–	–	–	0
Reop	0.52 [0.24, 1.13]	0.1	40	843	28	3	0.51 [0.25, 1.04]	0.07	35	944	33	2

Abbreviations: FU follow-up, ASDeg adjacent segment degeneration, ASDis adjacent segment disease, Reop Reoperation, NO. of P the number of patients, NO. of ASD the number of ASD, NO. of S the number of studies

Herkowitz [7, 8]; (2) inconsistencies in surgical indications between TDR and ACDF, non-controlled trials, and demographical differences could bring about clear bias. Therefore, RCTs of high grade were optimal to perform a meta-analysis, then prospective cohort studies. Many meta-analysis publications comparing TDR to ASD have had ambiguous outcomes. Yang, B.et al. [14] mentioned the defect of including only five studies without stratification on factors and exclusion of publication bias.

This meta-analysis contained two poor quality studies [24, 27] of inadequate (C) grade, and most were high quality with low risk of bias. Overall, there was a statistically confirmed lower occurrence of ASD in TDR group and TDR could be considered as a treatment of deferring ASD in comparison with ACDF, so was ASDeg and reoperation in subgroup. The positive outcome of rate may be based on cost-effectiveness analysis, patients believed the efficacy of TDR should be better than ACDF with a higher cost, leaving them a bias of no-attribution to ASDis on TDR with relevant symptom and prefer not to selection a second surgery. With extended follow-up, it may be difficult to explain the difference in reoperation rate; Coric, D [23] mentioned it was ambiguous to draw conclusions with fewer patients added lower incidence on ASDis. The rate of ASDis of no significance likely resulted from the inadequate number of positive population, in addition, ASDis occurred postpone as a symptomatology compared with ASDeg, with no difference between the two groups till current endpoint.

In subgroup analysis, the difference in incidence of ASDeg was still statistically different whether it was shorter than 5 years or not. Furthermore, the results were better with 5 years of follow-up than follow-up

within 5 years, probably implying that the longer the follow-up, the more superiority in TDR. But Davis, R J [30] mentioned that the underlying mechanism defining the relationship between decreased radiographic degeneration in patients treated with TDR remains uncorrelated, and further long-term follow-up should continue to correlate these results. The incidence of ASDeg was statistically different between TDR and ACDF both in the USA and China, and TDR may have an advantage over ACDF. However, no matter in China or the USA, there are both tendency in clinical trials towards to the positive results with a larger selection bias, and overall, ensuing a certain lack of representation in incidence of ASD, which may be also related to the policy on cost reimbursement.

There were some limitations in this meta-analysis. Eleven studies may still limit our assessment of potential publication bias and more relevant studies should be included. Then, the various types of disc may affect the occurrence of ASD, so it should be stratified for further analysis. However, there were too many types of discs referred in the literatures, 8 kinds mentioned in 11 documents, and the kind of prosthesis mentioned by Nunley, P D is unclear [24] and even the document by Jawahar, A [17] includes three discs (Kineflex-C/ Mobi-C/Advent) at the same time. Therefore, it was difficult to process a stratified analysis with inconsistency and disorganization.

In addition, we did not but it was of vital importance to perform a cost-effectiveness analysis, and most countries was dealing with a nearly unaffordable costs of health care. Qureshi SA [40] suggested in single-segment operation between TDR and ACDF indicated TDR must remain functional for at least

Table 3 Subgroup analysis according to study sites

SITE	U.S.						CHINA					
	OR [95%CI]	P value	I²(%)	NO. of P	NO. of ASD	NO. of S	OR [95%CI]	P value	I²(%)	NO. of P	NO. of ASD	NO. of S
ASDeg	0.59 [0.46, 0.75]	0.0001	44	1184	463	4	0.52 [0.29, 0.92]	0.03	0	240	78	3
ASDis	0.99 [0.57, 1.73]	0.98	0	738	61	3	–	–	–	–	–	0
Reop	0.56 [0.32, 0.96]	0.03	11	1676	57	4	0.11 [0.01, 2.00]	0.13	–	111	4	1

Abbreviations: FU follow-up, ASDeg adjacent segment degeneration, ASDis adjacent segment disease, Reop Reoperation, NO. of P the number of patients, NO. of ASD the number of ASD, NO. of S the number of studies

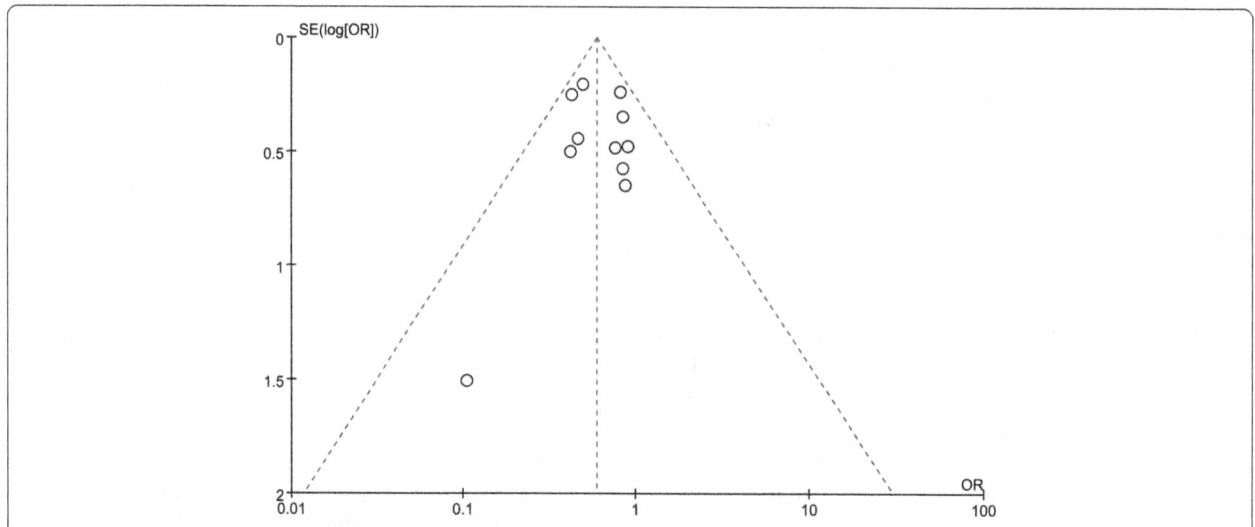

Fig. 7 Funnel plot for the occurrence of ASD

14 years to establish greater cost-effectiveness than ACDF. Ament, J D et al. [41, 42] in cost-effectiveness analysis with two-level segments reaffirmed TDR a stability of the model and the sustainability of this intervention. In this meta-analysis, the difference referred to the ASDis between TDR and ACDF is 2.1% and the NNT is 43.5 but 11 articles did not involve the detailed calculations on cost-effectiveness issues. It is of no meaning if we offered huge cost to make up a little disadvantage, and it could have resulted in an overestimation of the effectiveness of interventions.

The overall grade quality of our meta-analysis was moderate according to the GRADE, and we suggest adopting TDR for the reduction of incidence of ASD to a certain degree. TDR can reduce the rate of reoperation and ASDeg compared with ACDF with probable obvious advantages as the time prolonged basing the prerequisites of a larger sample, but the result should be accepted with caution.

Conclusion

TDR decreased the rates of ASDeg and reoperations compared with ACDF, and the superiority may be more

Table 4 Preview SoF table of the GRADE for this meta-analysis

TDR compared to ACDF for ASD

Patient or population: patients with ASD
Settings:
Intervention: TDR
Comparison: ACDF

Outcomes	Illustrative comparative risks[a] (95% CI)		Relative effect (95% CI)	No of participants (studies)	Quality of the evidence (GRADE)	Comments
	Assumed risk	Corresponding risk				
	ACDF	TDR				
ASD Follow-up: 24–84 months	Study population		OR 0.6 (0.49 to 0.73)	2632 (11 studies)	⊕⊕⊕⊖ moderate	
	256 per 1000	171 per 1000 (144 to 201)				
	Moderate					

GRADE Working group grades of evidence

   High quality: Further research is very unlikely to change our confidence in the estimate of effect.

   Moderate quality: Further research is likely to have an important impact on our confidence in the estimate of effect and may change the estimate.

   Low quality: Further research is very likely to have an important impact on our confidence in the estimate of effect and is likely to change the estimate.

   Very low quality: We are very uncertain about the estimate.

Abbreviations: CI Confidence interval, *OR* Odds ratio, *GRADE* grading of recommendations assessment, development and evaluation, *TDR* total disc replacement, *ACDF* anterior cervical discectomy and fusion, *ASD* adjacent segment degeneration/disease
[a]The basis for the assumed risk (e.g., the median control group risk across studies) is provided in footnotes. The corresponding risk (and its 95% confidence interval) is based on the assumed risk in the comparison group and the relative effect of the intervention (and its 95% CI)

apparent overtime. TDR can be selected purely in terms of mitigation on ASD, but the overall efficacy through cost-effectiveness analysis that values. The overall grade quality of our meta-analysis was moderate according to the GRADE, and we cautiously and slightly suggest adopting TDR.

Abbreviations

ACDF: Anterior cervical discectomy and fusion; ASD: Segment degeneration disease; GRADE: Grades of recommendation, assessment, development and evaluation; TDR: Total disc replacement

Acknowledgements

We acknowledge Houshan Lv who contributed towards the study by making substantial contributions to the design and the acquisition of data.

Device statement

Types of artificial discs	Manufacturer's name	Address
PCM	Waldemar Link GmbH & Co., KG	Barkhausenweg 10, 22339 Hamburg
Mobi-C	LDR Medical	BP2 10902 Troyes Cedex 9 France
Prestige	Medtronic	Memphis, TN 38132, USA
Scient'x	Scient'x	Guyancourt Cedex France
Active-c	Aesculap	Tuttlingen, Germany
Bryan	Medtronic	Memphis, TN 38132, USA
Kineflex-C	USA	USA
Advent	/	USA

Authors' contributions

SX carried out the molecular genetic studies, participated in the sequence alignment, and drafted the manuscript. YL participated in the design of the study and performed the statistical analysis. HYL conceived of the study and participated in its design and coordination, and helped to draft the manuscript. ZQZ and YLQ performed the experiments. All authors read and approved the final manuscript.

Competing interests

The authors declare that they have no competing interests.

References

1. Robinson RA, Smith GW. Anterolateral cervical disc removal and interbody fusion for cervical disc syndrome. SAS Journal. 2010;4(1):34–5.
2. Baba H, Furusawa N, Imura S, et al. Late radiographic findings after anterior cervical fusion for spondylotic myeloradiculopathy. Spine. 1993; 18(15):2167–73.
3. Wu W, Thuomas KA, Hedlund R, et al. Degenerative changes following anterior cervical discectomy and fusion evaluated by fast spin-echo MR imaging. ACTA RADIOL. 1996;37(5):614–7.
4. Matsunaga S, Kabayama S, Yamamoto T, et al. Strain on intervertebral discs after anterior cervical decompression and fusion. Spine (Phila Pa 1976). 1999;24(7):670–5.
5. Hilibrand AS, Robbins M. Adjacent segment degeneration and adjacent segment disease: the consequences of spinal fusion? SPINE J. 2004, 4;(6 Suppl):190S–4S.
6. Lund T, Oxland TR. Adjacent level disk disease--is it really a fusion disease? Orthop Clin North Am. 2011;42(4):529–41.
7. Herkowitz HN, Kurz LT, Overholt DP. Surgical management of cervical soft disc herniation. A comparison between the anterior and posterior approach. Spine (Phila Pa 1976). 1990;15(10):1026–30.
8. Song KJ, Choi BW, Jeon TS, et al. Adjacent segment degenerative disease: is it due to disease progression or a fusion-associated phenomenon? Comparison between segments adjacent to the fused and non-fused segments. Eur Spine J. 2011;20(11):1940–5.
9. Gore DR, Sepic SB. Anterior cervical fusion for degenerated or protruded discs. A review of one hundred forty-six patients. Spine (Phila Pa 1976). 1984;9(7):667–71.
10. Puttlitz CM, Rousseau MA, Xu Z, et al. Intervertebral disc replacement maintains cervical spine kinetics. Spine. 2004;29:2809–14.
11. Diangelo DJ, Foley KT, Morrow BR, et al. In vitro biomechanics of cervical disc arthroplasty with the ProDisc-C total disc implant. Neurosurg Focus. 2004;17(3):E7.
12. Wigfield C, Gill S, Nelson R, et al. Influence of an artificial cervical joint compared with fusion on adjacent-level motion in the treatment of degenerative cervical disc disease. J Neurosurg. 2002;96(1 Suppl):17–21.
13. Botelho RV, Moraes OJ, Fernandes GA, et al. A systematic review of randomized trials on the effect of cervical disc arthroplasty on reducing adjacent-level degeneration. Neurosurg Focus. 2010;28(6):E5.
14. Yang B, Li H, Zhang T, et al. The incidence of adjacent segment degeneration after cervical disc arthroplasty (CDA): a meta analysis of randomized controlled trials. PLoS One. 2012;7(4):e35032.
15. Luo J, Gong M, Huang S, et al. Incidence of adjacent segment degeneration in cervical disc arthroplasty versus anterior cervical decompression and fusion meta-analysis of prospective studies. Arch Orthop Trauma Surg. 2015; 135(2):155–60.
16. Moher D, Cook DJ. Eastwood S, et al. Improving the quality of reports of meta-analyses of randomized controlled trials: the QUOROM statement. Rev Esp Salud Publica. 2000;74(2):107–18.
17. Jawahar A, Cavanaugh DA, Kerr ER, et al. Total disc arthroplasty does not affect the incidence of adjacent segment degeneration in cervical spine: results of 93 patients in three prospective randomized clinical trials. Spine J. 2010;10(12):1043–8.
18. Goffin J, Casey A, Kehr P, et al. Preliminary clinical experience with the Bryan cervical disc prosthesis. Neurosurgery. 2002;51:840–7.
19. Higgins JP, Altman DG, Gotzsche PC, et al. The Cochrane Collaboration's tool for assessing risk of bias in randomised trials. BMJ. 2011;343:d5928.
20. Atkins D, De Briss PA, Eccles M, et al. Systems for grading the quality of evidence and the strength of recommendations II: pilot study of a new system. BMC Health Serv Res. 2005:5.
21. Deeks JJ, Higgins JPT, Altman DG. Analysing data and undertaking meta-analyses. In: Higgins JPT, Green S, editors. Cochrane handbook for systematic reviews of interventions version 5.1.0 (updated march 2011). London: The Cochrane Collaboration. Chapter 9; 2011.
22. Sasso RC, Anderson PA, Riew KD, et al. Results of cervical arthroplasty compared with anterior discectomy and fusion: four-year clinical outcomes in a prospective, randomized controlled trial. Orthopedics. 2011;34(11):889.
23. Coric D, Nunley PD, Guyer RD, et al. Prospective, randomized, multicenter study of cervical arthroplasty: 269 patients from the Kineflex|C artificial disc

investigational device exemption study with a minimum 2-year follow-up: clinical article. J Neurosurg Spine. 2011;15(4):348–58.

24. Nunley PD, Jawahar A, Kerr ER, et al. Factors affecting the incidence of symptomatic adjacent-level disease in cervical spine after total disc arthroplasty: 2- to 4-year follow-up of 3 prospective randomized trials. Spine (Phila Pa 1976). 2012;37(6):445–51.

25. Tian W, Yan K, Han X, et al. Comparison of the mid-term follow-up results between Bryan cervical artificial disc replacement and anterior cervical decompression and fusion for cervical degenerative disc disease. Chinese Journal of Orthopedics. 2013;33:97–104.

26. Guan T, Hu Z, Xiu L, et al. Effect of cervical disc arthroplasty and anterior cervical decompression and fusion on adjacent segment degeneration. Zhongguo Xiu Fu Chong Jian Wai Ke Za Zhi. 2014;28(9): 1100–5.

27. Li Z, Yu S, Zhao Y, et al. Clinical and radiologic comparison of dynamic cervical implant arthroplasty versus anterior cervical discectomy and fusion for the treatment of cervical degenerative disc disease. J Clin Neurosci. 2014;21(6):942–8.

28. Burkus JK, Traynelis VC, Haid RJ, et al. Clinical and radiographic analysis of an artificial cervical disc: 7-year follow-up from the prestige prospective randomized controlled clinical trial: clinical article. J Neurosurg Spine. 2014; 21(4):516–28.

29. Zhang HX, Shao YD, Chen Y, et al. A prospective, randomised, controlled multicentre study comparing cervical disc replacement with anterior cervical decompression and fusion. Int Orthop. 2014;38(12): 2533–41.

30. Davis RJ, Nunley PD, Kim KD, et al. Two-level total disc replacement with Mobi-C cervical artificial disc versus anterior discectomy and fusion: a prospective, randomized, controlled multicenter clinical trial with 4-year follow-up results. J Neurosurg Spine. 2015;22(1):15–25.

31. Phillips FM, Geisler FH, Gilder KM, et al. Long-term outcomes of the US FDA IDE prospective, randomized controlled clinical trial comparing PCM cervical disc arthroplasty with anterior cervical discectomy and fusion. Spine (Phila Pa 1976). 2015;40(10):674–83.

32. Zoega B, Karrholm J, Lind B. Plate fixation adds stability to two-level anterior fusion in the cervical spine: a randomized study using radiostereometry. Eur Spine J. 1998;7(4):302–7.

33. Katsuura A, Hukuda S, Saruhashi Y, et al. Kyphotic malalignment after anterior cervical fusion is one of the factors promoting the degenerative process in adjacent intervertebral levels. Eur Spine J. 2001;10(4):320–4.

34. Auerbach JD, Anakwenze OA, Milby AH, et al. Segmental contribution toward total cervical range of motion: a comparison of cervical disc arthroplasty and fusion. Spine (Phila Pa 1976). 2011;36(25):E1593–9.

35. Eck JC, Humphreys SC, Lim TH, et al. Biomechanical study on the effect of cervical spine fusion on adjacent-level intradiscal pressure and segmental motion. Spine (Phila Pa 1976). 2002;27(22):2431–4.

36. Takeshima T, Omokawa S, Takaoka T, et al. Sagittal alignment of cervical flexion and extension: lateral radiographic analysis. Spine Phila Pa 1976. 2002;27:E348–55.

37. Kelly MP, Mok JM, Frisch RF, et al. Adjacent segment motion after anterior cervical discectomy and fusion versus Prodisc-c cervical total disk arthroplasty: analysis from a randomized, controlled trial. Spine (Phila Pa 1976). 2011;36(15):1171–9.

38. Hauerberg J, Kosteljanetz M, Boge-Rasmussen T, et al. Anterior cervical discectomy with or without fusion with ray titanium cage: a prospective randomized clinical study. Spine (Phila Pa 1976). 2008;33(5):458–64.

39. Mummaneni PV, Burkus JK, Haid RW, et al. Clinical and radiographic analysis of cervical disc arthroplasty compared with allograft fusion: a randomized controlled clinical trial. J Neurosurg Spine. 2007;6(3):198–209.

40. Qureshi SA, Mcanany S, Goz V, et al. Cost-effectiveness analysis: comparing single-level cervical disc replacement and single-level anterior cervical discectomy and fusion: clinical article. J Neurosurg Spine. 2013;19(5):546–54.

41. Ament JD, Yang Z, Nunley P, et al. Cost-effectiveness of cervical total disc replacement vs fusion for the treatment of 2-level symptomatic degenerative disc disease. JAMA Surg. 2014;149(12):1231–9.

42. Warren D, Andres T, Hoelscher C, et al. Cost-utility analysis modeling at 2-year follow-up for cervical disc arthroplasty versus anterior cervical discectomy and fusion: a single-center contribution to the randomized controlled trial. Int J Spine Surg. 2013;7:e58–66.

Permissions

The contributors of this book come from diverse backgrounds, making this book a truly international effort. This book will bring forth new frontiers with its revolutionizing research information and detailed analysis of the nascent developments around the world.

We would like to thank all the contributing authors for lending their expertise to make the book truly unique. They have played a crucial role in the development of this book. Without their invaluable contributions this book wouldn't have been possible. They have made vital efforts to compile up to date information on the varied aspects of this subject to make this book a valuable addition to the collection of many professionals and students.

This book was conceptualized with the vision of imparting up-to-date information and advanced data in this field. To ensure the same, a matchless editorial board was set up. Every individual on the board went through rigorous rounds of assessment to prove their worth. After which they invested a large part of their time researching and compiling the most relevant data for our readers.

The editorial board has been involved in producing this book since its inception. They have spent rigorous hours researching and exploring the diverse topics which have resulted in the successful publishing of this book. They have passed on their knowledge of decades through this book. To expedite this challenging task, the publisher supported the team at every step. A small team of assistant editors was also appointed to further simplify the editing procedure and attain best results for the readers.

Apart from the editorial board, the designing team has also invested a significant amount of their time in understanding the subject and creating the most relevant covers. They scrutinized every image to scout for the most suitable representation of the subject and create an appropriate cover for the book.

The publishing team has been an ardent support to the editorial, designing and production team. Their endless efforts to recruit the best for this project, has resulted in the accomplishment of this book. They are a veteran in the field of academics and their pool of knowledge is as vast as their experience in printing. Their expertise and guidance has proved useful at every step. Their uncompromising quality standards have made this book an exceptional effort. Their encouragement from time to time has been an inspiration for everyone.

The publisher and the editorial board hope that this book will prove to be a valuable piece of knowledge for researchers, students, practitioners and scholars across the globe.

List of Contributors

Dejan Kernc and Vojko Strojnik
Faculty of Sport, University of Ljubljana, Gortanova 22, 1000 Ljubljana, Slovenia

Rok Vengust
Faculty of Medicine, University of Ljubljana, Vrazov trg 2, 1000 Ljubljana, Slovenia

Shenghan Lou
Department of Spine Surgery, The First Affiliated Hospital of Harbin Medical University, No. 23 Youzheng Road, Harbin 150001, Heilongjiang, People's Republic of China
Department of Orthopedics, Chinese PLA General Hospital, No. 28 Fuxing Road, Beijing 100853, People's Republic of China

Houchen Lv, Zhirui Li and Peifu Tang
Department of Orthopedics, Chinese PLA General Hospital, No. 28 Fuxing Road, Beijing 100853, People's Republic of China

Yansong Wang
Department of Spine Surgery, The First Affiliated Hospital of Harbin Medical University, No. 23 Youzheng Road, Harbin 150001, Heilongjiang, People's Republic of China

Guheng Wang, Tian Mao and Shuguo Xing
Department of Hand Surgery, Affiliated Hospital of Nantong University, 20 West Temple Road, Nantong 226001, People's Republic of China

Renguo Xie
Department of Hand Surgery, Affiliated Hospital of Nantong University, 20# West Temple Road, Nantong 226001, People's Republic of China
Department of Hand Surgery, Shanghai General Hospital, 650 Songjiang Road, Shanghai 201620, People's Republic of China

Zhifang Mou
Department of Critical Care Medicine, The Affiliated Lianyungang Hospital of Xuzhou Medical University/ the First People's Hospital of Lianyungang, Lianyungang, China

Wanpeng Dong, Zhen Zhang and Aohan Wang
School of Materials Engineering, Shanghai University of Engineering Science, Shanghai, China

Guanghong Hu
Institute of Plasticity Forming Technology and Equipment, Shanghai Jiao Tong University, Shanghai, China

Bing Wang and Yuefu Dong
Department of Orthopedics, The Affiliated Lianyungang Hospital of Xuzhou Medical University/ the First People's Hospital of Lianyungang, Lianyungang, China

Håkon With Solvang, Robin Andre Nordheggen and Per-Henrik Randsborg
The Department of Orthopedic Surgery, Akershus University Hospital, 1478 Lørenskog, Norway

Ståle Clementsen and Ola-Lars Hammer
The Department of Orthopedic Surgery, Akershus University Hospital, 1478 Lørenskog, Norway
The Faculty of Medicine, The University of Oslo, Oslo, Norway

Xuedong Sun
Department of Orthopaedics, Weifang People's Hospital, no. 151 Guangwen Road, Weifang 260041, China

Zheng Su
Department of Medical Oncology, Weifang People's Hospital, no. 151 Guangwen Road, Weifang 260041, China

Vito Pavone, Emanuele Chisari, Andrea Vescio, Ludovico Lucenti, Giuseppe Sessa and Gianluca Testa
Department of General Surgery and Medical Surgical Specialties, Section of Orthopaedics and Traumatology, University Hospital Policlinico-Vittorio Emanuele, University of Catania, Via Plebiscito, 628, 95124 Catania, Italy

Takeshi Kataoka, Takeshi Kokubu, Tomoyuki Muto, Yutaka Mifune, Atsuyuki Inui, Ryosuke Sakata, Hanako Nishimoto, Yoshifumi Harada, Fumiaki Takase, Yasuhiro Ueda, Takashi Kurosawa, Kohei Yamaura and Ryosuke Kuroda
Department of Orthopaedic Surgery, Kobe University Graduate School of Medicine, 7-5-1 Kusunoki-cho, Chuo-ku, Kobe, Hyogo 650-0017, Japan

Ann-Kathrin Schubert
Tissue Engineering Laboratory and Berlin-Brandenburg Center for Regenerative Therapies, Charité - Universitätsmedizin Berlin, corporate member of Freie Universität Berlin, Humboldt-Universität zu Berlin and Berlin Institute of Health, Augustenburger Platz 1, Südstråe 2, 13353 Berlin, Germany
CO.DON AG, Teltow, Germany

Jeske J. Smink
CO.DON AG, Teltow, Germany

Matthias Pumberger and Michael Putzier
Center for MusculoskeletalSurgery, Department of Orthopaedics, Charité - Universitätsmedizin Berlin, corporate member of Freie Universität Berlin, Humboldt-Universität zu Berlin and Berlin Institute of Health, Berlin, Germany

Michael Sittinger and Jochen Ringe
Tissue Engineering Laboratory and Berlin-Brandenburg Center for Regenerative Therapies, Charité - Universitätsmedizin Berlin, corporate member of Freie Universität Berlin, Humboldt-Universität zu Berlin and Berlin Institute of Health, Augustenburger Platz 1, Südstråe 2, 13353 Berlin, Germany

Dennis Silvester Maria Gerardus Kruijntjens, Jacobus Johannes Chris Arts and René Hendrikus Maria ten Broeke
Department of Orthopaedic Surgery, Research School Caphri, Maastricht University Medical Centre, P. Debyelaan 25, 6202 AZ Maastricht, the Netherlands

Per Kjaersgaard-Andersen, Peter Revald and Jane Schwartz Leonhardt
Department of Orthopaedic Surgery, Vejle Hospital, Beriderbakken 4, 7100 Vejle, Denmark

Guang-Ming Guo, Jun Li1, Qing-Xun Diao, Tai-Hang Zhu, Zhong-Xue Song and Yang-Yang Guo
Department of Orthopaedics, Henan Zhoukou Union Orthopaedic Hospital, East Section, Taihao Road, Zhoukou 466000, Henan, China

Yan-Zheng Gao
Department of Orthopaedics, Henan Province People's Hospital, Zhengzhou 450000, Henan, China

Yuta Tsubouchi
Oita University Hospital Rehabilitation Center, Oita University, 1-1 Idaigaoka, Hasama-machi, Yufu-city, Oita 879-5593, Japan

Shinichi Ikeda
Department of Rehabilitation Medicine, Faculty of Medicine, Oita University, 1-1 Idaigaoka, Hasama-machi, Yufu-city, Oita 879-5593, Japan

Masashi Kataoka
Physical Therapy Course of Study, Faculty of Welfare and Health Sciences, Oita University, 700 Dannoharu, Oita 870-1192, Japan

Hiroshi Tsumura
Department of Orthopaedic Surgery, Faculty of Medicine, Oita University, 1-1 Idaigaoka, Hasama-machi, Yufu-city, Oita 879-5593, Japan

Yung-Cheng Chiu and Horng-Chaung Hsu
School of Medicine, China Medical University, Taichung 404, Taiwan
Department of Orthopedic Surgery, China Medical University Hospital, Taichung 404, Taiwan, Republic of China

Ming-Tzu Tsai
Department of Biomedical Engineering, Hungkuang University, Taichung 433, Taiwan

Cheng-En Hsu
Department of Orthopaedics, Taichung Veterans General Hospital, Taichung 407, Taiwan
Sports Recreation and Health Management Continuing Studies-Bachelor's Degree Completion Program, Tunghai University, Taichung 407, Taiwan

Heng-Li Huang
School of Dentistry, College of Dentistry, China Medical University, 91 Hsueh-Shih Road, Taichung 40402, Taiwan
Department of Bioinformatics and Medical Engineering, Asia University, Taichung 413, Taiwan

Jui-Ting Hsu
Department of Bioinformatics and Medical Engineering, Asia University, Taichung 413, Taiwan

Bin Feng, Shiliang Cao, Jiliang Zhai, Yi Ren, Jianhua Hu, Ye Tian and Xisheng Weng
Department of Orthopedics Surgery, Peking Union Medical College Hospital, Chinese Academy of Medical Sciences and Peking Union Medical College, Beijing 100730, China

Sjur Oppebøen, Annette K. B. Wikerøy and Per-Henrik Randsborg
Department of Orthopaedic Surgery, Akershus University Hospital, Lørenskog, Norway

Hendrik F. S. Fuglesang and Filip C. Dolatowski
Department of Orthopaedic Surgery, Akershus University Hospital, Lørenskog, Norway
Faculty of Medicine, University of Oslo, Oslo, Norway

Kenichi Yoshikawa, Ayumu Sano and Kazunori Koseki
Department of Physical Therapy, Ibaraki Prefectural University of Health Sciences Hospital, 4773 Ami, Ami-machi, Inashiki-gun, Ibaraki 300-0331, Japan

Hirotaka Mutsuzaki
Department of Orthopaedic Surgery, Ibaraki Prefectural University of Health Sciences, 4669-2 Ami, Ami-machi, Inashiki-gun, Ibaraki 300-0394, Japan

Takashi Fukaya
Department of Physical Therapy, Faculty of Health Sciences, Tsukuba International University, 6-8-33 Manabe, Tsuchiura, Ibaraki 300-0051, Japan

Masafumi Mizukami
Department of Physical Therapy, Ibaraki Prefectural University of Health Sciences, 4669-2 Ami, Ami-machi, Inashiki-gun, Ibaraki 300-0394, Japan

Masashi Yamazaki
Department of Orthopaedic Surgery, Faculty of Medicine, University of Tsukuba, 1-1-1 Tennodai, Tsukuba, Ibaraki 305-8575, Japan

Jialing Shi and Rongzhi Huang
Guangxi Medical University, No. 22, Shuang Yong Road, Nanning 530021, Guangxi Zhuang Autonomous Region, China

Guang Liang and Liang Liao
The first affiliated Hospital of Guangxi Medical University, The First Clinical Medical College, No. 6, Shuang Yong Road, Nanning 530021, Guangxi Zhuang Autonomous Region, China

Danlu Qin
Department of the Second Endocrinology Ward, Jiangbin Hospital of Guangxi Zhuang Autonomous Region, Nanning 530021, Guangxi Zhuang Autonomous Region, China

Ismail Hadisoebroto Dilogo
Integrated Service Unit of Stem Cell Medical Technology, Dr. Cipto Mangunkusumo General Hospital (RSCM), Jl. Diponegoro No 71, Salemba, Cental Jakarta 10430, Indonesia
Stem Cell and Tissue Engineering Cluster, Indonesian Medical Education and Research Institute (IMERI), Faculty of Medicine, Universitas Indonesia, Jl. Salemba Raya No 6, Salemba, Cental Jakarta 10430, Indonesia
Department of Orthopaedic and Traumatology, Faculty of Medicine, Universitas Indonesia - Dr. Cipto Mangunkusumo General Hospital, Jl. Diponegoro No 71, Salemba, Cental Jakarta 10430, Indonesia

Fajar Mujadid
Integrated Service Unit of Stem Cell Medical Technology, Dr. Cipto Mangunkusumo General Hospital (RSCM), Jl. Diponegoro No 71, Salemba, Cental Jakarta 10430, Indonesia

Retno Wahyu Nurhayati
Stem Cell and Tissue Engineering Cluster, Indonesian Medical Education and Research Institute (IMERI), Faculty of Medicine, Universitas Indonesia, Jl. Salemba Raya No 6, Salemba, Cental Jakarta 10430, Indonesia
Department of Biochemistry and Molecular Biology, Faculty of Medicine, Universitas Indonesia, Jl. Salemba Raya No. 6, Central Jakarta 10430, Indonesia

Aryadi Kurniawan
Department of Orthopaedic and Traumatology, Faculty of Medicine, Universitas Indonesia - Dr. Cipto Mangunkusumo General Hospital, Jl. Diponegoro No 71, Salemba, Cental Jakarta 10430, Indonesia

Zhao Wang
Department of Orthopedics, Jingjiang People's Hospital, Jingjiang, China

Hao-jie Zhang
Department of Orthopaedics, The 82rn Hospital of People's Liberation Army of China, No. 100, Jiankangdong Road, Huai'an, Jiangsu, China.

Hiroshi Uei, Yasuaki Tokuhashi, Masafumi Maseda, Masahiro Nakahashi, Hirokatsu Sawada, Koji Matsumoto and Hiroyuki Miyakata
Department of Orthopaedic Surgery, Nihon University School of Medicine, 30-1 Oyaguchi Kami-cho, Itabashi-ku, Tokyo 173-8610, Japan

Jianzhong Bai, Pei Zhang and Meiying Liu
Dalian Medical University, Dalian 116044, Liaoning, China

Yongxiang Wang, Jingcheng Wang and Yuan Liang
Clinical Medical College, Yangzhou University, Yangzhou 225001, China

Peian Wang
Heze Mudan People's Hospital, Heze 274000, China

Xiang Salim and Richard Carey Smith
Department of Orthopaedics, Sir Charles Gairdner Hospital, 55 Viewway Nedlands, Perth, WA 6009, Australia

Peter D'Alessandro and Piers Yates
Department of Orthopaedics, Fiona Stanley Fremantle Hospital Groups, Perth, Australia

Orthopaedic Research Foundation of Western Australia (ORFWA), Perth, Australia

James Little
Department of Orthopaedics, Fiona Stanley Fremantle Hospital Groups, Perth, Australia

Kulvir Mudhar
Department of Orthopaedics, Royal Perth Hospital, Perth, Australia

Kevin Murray
Centre for Applied Statistics, University of Western Australia, Perth, Australia

Yimin Qi
Nanjing Medical University, Nanjing, China

Yiwen Zeng, Dalin Wang, Jisheng Sui and Qiang Wang
Department of Orthopaedic Surgery, Nanjing First Hospital, Nanjing Medical University, 68 Changle Rd, Qinhuai District, Nanjing 210000, Jiangsu, China

Aoyuan Fan, Tianyang Xu, Lin Fan, Dong Yang and Guodong Li
Department of Orthopedics, Shanghai Tenth People's Hospital of Tongji University, 301 Yanchang Rd, Shanghai 200072, China
Tongji University School of Medicine, Shanghai, China

Xifan Li
Tongji University School of Medicine, Shanghai, China
Department of Radiology, Shanghai Tenth People's Hospital of Tongji University, Shanghai, China

Lei Li
Department of Orthopedics, Shanghai Tenth People's Hospital of Tongji University, 301 Yanchang Rd, Shanghai 200072, China
Department of Neurosurgery, Shanghai Tenth People's Hospital of Tongji University, Shanghai, China

Yi-Ming Ren, Yuan-Hui Duan, Yun-Bo Sun, Tao Yang and Meng-Qiang Tian
Department of Joint and Sport Medicine, Tianjin Union Medical Center, Jieyuan Road 190, Hongqiao District, Tianjin 300121, People's Republic of China

Bo Wang, Chang-Ping Zhao, Lian-Xin Song and Lian Zhu
Department of Orthopedic Trauma Centre, 3rd Hospital of Hebei Medical University, No. 139 ZiQiang Road, Qiaoxi District, Shijiazhuang 050051, China

Jing Wang, Jin Zhang, Tie Ge Chen, Kai Sheng Zhou and Hai Hong Zhang
Department Of Orthopedics, Orthopedics Key Laboratory of Gansu Province, Lanzhou University Second Hospital, Cuiyingmen, Lanzhou 730030, Gansu province, China

Rui Xu
Radiology Department, Lanzhou University Second Hospital, Cuiyingmen, Lanzhou 730030, Gansu province, China

Tomoyuki Kuroiwa, Koji Fujita, Toru Sasaki and Atsushi Okawa
Department of Orthopaedic and Spinal Surgery, Graduate School of Medical and Dental Sciences, Tokyo Medical and Dental University, 1-4-5, Yushima, Bunkyo-ku, Tokyo 113-8519, Japan

Akimoto Nimura and Takashi Miyamoto
Department of Functional Joint Anatomy, Graduate School of Medical and Dental Sciences, Tokyo Medical and Dental University, 1-4-5, Yushima, Bunkyo-ku, Tokyo 113-8519, Japan

Nathan Kirzner
Orthopaedic Registrar, Alfred Hospital, 55 Commercial Rd, Prahran, Melbourne, VIC 3004, Australia

Eldho Paul
Department of Epidemiology and Preventive Medicine, Monash University, Victoria, Australia

Ash Moaveni
Orthopaedic Consultant, Alfred Hospital, 55 Commercial Rd, Prahran, Melbourne, Victoria 3004, Australia

Shuai Xu, Yan Liang, Zhenqi Zhu, Yalong Qian and Haiying Liu
Department of Spinal Surgery, Peking University People's Hospital, Peking University, No. 11 Xizhimen South Street, Xicheng District, Beijing, People's Republic of China

Index

www.ingramcontent.com/pod-product-compliance
Lightning Source LLC
Chambersburg PA
CBHW080456200326
41458CB00012B/3988